THE PSYCHOLOGY OF RELIGION

THE PSYCHOLOGY OF RELIGION

An Empirical Approach

Third Edition

BERNARD SPILKA

RALPH W. HOOD, JR.

BRUCE HUNSBERGER

RICHARD GORSUCH

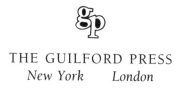

THE GUILFORD PRESS
New York   London

© 2003 The Guilford Press
A Division of Guilford Publications, Inc.
72 Spring Street, New York, NY 10012
www.guilford.com

Printed in the United States of America

This book is printed on acid-free paper.

Last digit is print number: 9   8   7   6   5   4   3   2   1

Library of Congress Cataloging-in-Publication Data

The psychology of religion : an empirical approach / Bernard Spilka . . .
 [et al.].—3rd ed.
     p.   cm.
Previous edition entered under: Spilka, Bernard.
Includes bibliographical references and indexes.
    ISBN 1-57230-901-6 (alk. paper)
    1. Psychology, Religious.   I. Spilka, Bernard, 1926–
BL53.P625   2003
200'.1'9—dc21   2003011806

We dedicate this edition to very significant people in our lives:

*To Ellen for 50 years of love, support, and guidance.
My love for her continually grows. —Bernie*

To Betsy, Laura, and Linda. —Ralph

To Emily, Paul, and Carol. —Bruce

To Sylvia for continuing love and support. —Richard

ABOUT THE AUTHORS

Bernard Spilka, PhD, is Professor Emeritus of Psychology at the University of Denver. He is a past president of the Psychology of Religion division of the American Psychological Association and a recipient of its William James Award. Dr. Spilka has also been vice president of the Society for the Scientific Study of Religion, and president of the Colorado Psychological Association and the Rocky Mountain Psychological Association. Now retired, he continues to write on the psychology of prayer and on religion, evolution, and genetics.

Ralph W. Hood, Jr., PhD, is Professor of Psychology at the University of Tennessee at Chattanooga. He is a past president of the Psychology of Religion division of the American Psychological Association and a recipient of both its William James Award and its Mentoring Award. He is a cofounder of the *International Journal for the Psychology of Religion,* for which he has served as coeditor and as a book review editor. Dr. Hood has also been editor of the *Journal for the Scientific Study of Religion,* and is currently a member of the executive committee of the Internationale Gesellschaft für Religionspsychologie.

Bruce Hunsberger, PhD, is Professor of Psychology and former department chair at Wilfrid Laurier University. A prolific researcher relating the psychology of religion to prejudice, socialization, attitudes, doubt, fundamentalism, and life transitions, Dr. Hunsberger is coauthor of the book *Amazing Conversions: Why Some Turn to Faith and Others Abandon Religion.*

Richard Gorsuch, PhD, is Professor of Psychology at Fuller Theological Seminary. He is a past president of the Psychology of Religion division of the American Psychological Association and a recipient of its William James Award. An extremely productive scholar in the psychology of religion, psychometrics, and statistics, Dr. Gorsuch has written more than 20 books, manuals, monographs, and book chapters, as well as more than 120 papers published in refereed journals. His most recent book is *Integrating Psychology with Spirituality.*

PREFACE

At the beginning of the 20th century, those who were to become highly esteemed figures in the history of psychology and its sister disciplines focused much of their interest and attention upon religion. In academic psychology, names such as William James and G. Stanley Hall not only helped to found psychology, but manifested great interest in the psychological study of religion. In psychoanalysis, a new field was created outside of academic psychology that nevertheless immensely influenced psychology. One cannot read Freud or Jung for long without encountering extensive discussions of religion.

The second quarter of the 20th century saw a rapid decline in the study of religion among psychologists. Behaviorism was indifferent to the topic, while psychoanalysts relegated it to the province of psychopathology. The net effect was that research in this area remained on the periphery of scientific respectability. The mid-1950s, however, saw a renaissance in the study of religion. Perhaps more secure as a science, psychology could once again look with some interest upon the serious investigation of religion. This time the study was less speculative, not as concerned with grand theory, and focused on issues other than the origin of religion. In a word, an *empirical* psychology of religion emerged. This was a more limited view, to be sure, but it demanded that statements about religion be formulated as hypotheses capable of empirical verification or falsification.

In rapid succession, journals devoted to the empirical study of religion emerged in the middle of the last century. Among these are the *Journal for the Scientific Study of Religion*, the *Journal of Religion and Health*, the *Review of Religious Research*, and the *Journal of Psychology and Theology*. More recently, additional journals and annuals have appeared, including the *International Journal for the Psychology of Religion*, the *Journal of the Psychology of Religion, Research in the Social Scientific Study of Religion*, and (most recently) *Mental Health, Religion and Culture*. Specific religious interests have also sponsored such publications as the *Journal of Psychology and Christianity* and *The Psychology of Judaism*. In 1988 the *Annual Review of Psychology* included, for the first time, a summary of the psychology of religion, affirming by its presence that a significant body of empirical research in the area is now available. As this text goes to press, a second *Annual Review of Psychology* summary has been completed. Likewise, the *Archiv für Religionspsychologie* (*Archives for the Psychology of Religion*), the yearbook of the Internationale Gesellschaft für Religionspsychologie (International Association for the Psychology of Religion), founded in 1914, has been revived; this indicates that the psychology of religion has proven to be a topic of truly international interest. The pertinent literature continues to grow at a rapid rate across the globe. The domination of interpretative and conceptual discussions of religion in psychology is gradually yielding to data-based research and writing that are pulling the psychology of religion into the mainstream of academic psychology. Studies in which religious variables are central are no longer as rare as they once were in such mainstream references as the *Journal of Personality and Social Psychology*. The appearance of the third edition of this text is itself an indication of the vigor of our field as we begin another century.

Our aim remains the same in this third edition as in the first two: to present a comprehensive evaluation of the psychology of religion from an empirical perspective. We are not concerned with purely conceptual or philosophical discussions of religion, or with theories that have little empirical support. Interesting as these approaches may be, they generate few if any hard data of relevance to their evaluation. We do not, however, ignore these theories when meaningful empirical predictions follow from their claims. When this occurs, they are considered, as are other hypotheses, tentative claims to be judged by the facts. We have not imposed a single theoretical perspective across all the chapters. Much of the text is organized in terms of attribution theory, at least as a way of providing some consistent theoretical summary of each of the chapters. However, we have also organized the findings within each chapter according to the theory or theories that best illuminate them. Although we are sensitive to the difficulties and limitations of a purely empirical approach, we have not abandoned the commitment to empiricism as the single most fruitful avenue to understanding the psychology of religion. However, as several of the chapters also reveal, the same empirical data can lend credence to radically different ontological claims. Since William James, texts on the psychology of religion have suggested various metaphysical options under which the same empirical data can be viewed with radically different consequences. All we ask is that one not lose sight of the empirical data, so that various theoretical interpretations can be recognized and evaluated in terms of their relationship to these data.

While the basic structure of the second edition remains, we have expanded our coverage of religion and biology in a chapter new to this edition. We have greatly broadened our discussions of religion and prejudice and helping behavior, as well as the roles and functions of religion in adult life. This expansion reflects increased empirical research in these areas and justifies their treatment in separate chapters. The rich variety of empirical research that continues to be published is itself a testimony to the vitality of the field. Our hope is not only that this new edition fairly represents the research and scholarly literature, but that it will encourage young psychologists to participate in the empirical study of religion, regardless of how they otherwise identify their own psychological expertise.

Bernard Spilka
Ralph W. Hood, Jr.
Bruce Hunsberger
Richard Gorsuch

ACKNOWLEDGMENTS

The third edition of a book represents a long history of searching for information, as well as support and direction, from others. We have relied strongly on guidance from scholars who convey to us points of view we might otherwise have overlooked. Despite our best efforts, we can never thank all who deserve recognition.

Bernard Spilka: Michael Donahue of the Graduate Psychology Department at Azusa Pacific University brought the viewpoints of teachers and students to us and pointed out how we might make some improvements in our presentation. We hope we have succeeded. Michael Nielsen of the Department of Psychology at Georgia Southern University is a fount of information. When I encountered what appeared to be the limits of research in an area or needed further entrée into a troublesome topic, I knew Mike would offer something I had overlooked—a necessary study or a new direction. Michael Kearl from the Department of Sociology at Trinity University has been thanked in previous editions of this work and is a scholar who works compulsively to keep his knowledge up to date. In his areas of expertise, he has few peers, if any. Daniel Helminiak of the Psychology Department at The State University of West Georgia is, to this author, the Dean of scholarship in spirituality, and his extensive writings provided much guidance. He is also a specialist in other topics, and offered significant help in these areas as well. In addition, there are those people in the background who simply see themselves as doing nothing more than their job. I must recognize Christopher Brown and Lois Jones of the University of Denver library. Their genius at finding the most obscure but essential sources continually amazes me. To all these helpers, I express my deepest appreciation. Finally, my fullest gratitude will always go to my wife, who secretly believes there is a virtual lover hidden in my computer.

Ralph Hood: I have benefited greatly from discussions with my colleagues and frequent coauthors Ron Morris and Paul Watson on issues related to the psychology of religion. I am also very grateful for friendly and pertinent discussions with Jacob Belzen and David Wulff on the range and scope of psychology in general and of the psychology of religion in particular. I am extremely thankful for a few days with Antoine Vergote that reminded me that scholarship and faith need not be antagonistic.

Bruce Hunsberger: I thanked various people for their kind assistance in the previous edition of this book, but most became far too busy to help this time. Even my wife, Emily, found quilting to be much more fun than giving me feedback on chapters. Bob Altemeyer, Mike Pratt, Lynn Jackson, Scott Veenleit, and others did give my plodding brain a much-needed kick here and there. The truth, however, is that I am entirely to blame for any mistakes in my chapters of this work. I do want to thank my ever optimistic oncologist, Dr. Bob

Stevens, who has kept me alive and kicking, and who is so interested in his patients that he even asked me about my research—but only once.

There is no doubt that as coauthors we feel a great debt to each other. In spite of diverse backgrounds and research interests, varying expertise, and geographical separations of over 1,000 miles, we were able to work together smoothly and without conflict. We remain good friends and greatly appreciate each other's scholarship and help.

Special thanks to the editorial team at The Guilford Press. Editor-in-Chief Seymour Weingarten has always been highly supportive of our efforts. Senior Editor Jim Nageotte provided much needed guidance and whipped some of us into line more than once. The relaxed efficiency of Chris Coughlin and Craig Thomas was always reassuring. Above all, we were blessed with a copyeditor, Marie Sprayberry, whose brilliance, dedication, and proficiency were truly exceptional—if not, at times, literally awe-inspiring. She could teach all of us much about writing.

CONTENTS

ॐ

Chapter 1

THE PSYCHOLOGICAL NATURE
AND FUNCTIONS OF RELIGION

There is only one religion, though there are a hundred versions of it.

I assert that the cosmic religious experience is the strongest and the noblest driving force behind scientific research.

I am an atheist still, thank God.

Things have come to a pretty pass when religion is allowed to invade the sphere of private life.

My religion is to do good.[1]

WHY SHOULD WE STUDY RELIGION PSYCHOLOGICALLY?

"Why should we study religion psychologically?" This significant question demands an answer before we can go any further, and the answer is surprisingly simple. Indeed, religion, including spirituality (which we discuss later), is a fascinating realm, and that may be enough reason to study it. Of much greater significance is the fact that religion is of the utmost importance to people all over the earth. Every day, the mass media report instances of religious conflict throughout the world among those who adhere to different faiths. How often have we heard about tragic cult practices that resulted in mass suicides and other inhuman actions? Allport (1954) has said, "The role of religion is paradoxical. It makes prejudice and it unmakes prejudice" (p. 444). Concurrently, religion is also inextricably tied to altruistic and helping behavior. Those in dire straits commonly call upon their gods when they desperately need aid, and most feel strengthened by their faith. In addition, church members often help each other, or organize to aid a community when disaster strikes.

Research tells us that about 97% of U.S. residents believe in God, and about 90% pray (Gallup & Lindsay, 1999; Poloma & Gallup, 1991). That religion is a truly important part of human life cannot be questioned. Simply put, most North Americans see their religious faith as part and parcel of the larger picture of living their lives. Our role is to keep this larger picture before us as we attempt to understand the psychological role of faith in the individual personality.

---

1. These quotations come, respectively, from the following sources: Shaw (1931, p. 378); Einstein (1931, p. 357); Luis Buñuel, quoted in Rogers (1983, p. 175); Lord Melbourne, quoted in Cecil (1966, p. 181); and Paine (1897, p. 497).

Clearly, few human concerns are taken more seriously than religion. We surround ourselves with spiritual references, creating a context in which the sacred is invoked to convey the significance of every major life event. Birth is sanctified by christening or circumcision. Marriages are solemnized by clergy who readily interpret the roles of husband and wife in religious terms. Weekly religious meetings guide the faithful throughout life. Religion also helps people deal with death by associating it with gratifying images of an afterlife where only good and justice prevail. And, finally, some religious traditions assure the faithful of an ultimate resurrection at the end of time.

Religion is also an integral part of many other aspects of our existence. It is intimately tied to a wide variety of nonreligious beliefs and behaviors. Though we explore these in depth in later chapters, we can mention here that religion may be the best predictor of abstinence from the use of drugs and alcohol, as well as of nonparticipation in pre- and extramarital sexual activity (Gorsuch, 1988). Later chapters describe many ways in which religion affects people.

The preceding information answers another fundamental question: "Why has religion attained such status?" This is a problem not only for both the social sciences and psychology; it is also one for religion, particularly for the theologians who justify and support each faith. Though we may not directly deal with theology, the topics and issues discussed in these pages are central to both psychology and religion, and therefore to people everywhere. Particularly in Western civilization, and especially in the North American milieu (which is our primary focus), religion is an ever-present and extremely important aspect of our collective heritage.

Given the foregoing, it is incumbent upon us to understand the role religion plays in our personal and social lives. This is the task of the psychology of religion.

WHAT IS THE PSYCHOLOGY OF RELIGION?

The basic goal of psychology is to understand people. Psychologists attempt to do this by studying human motivation, cognition, and behavior. Within this rather broad definition of "psychology," over 50 specialties have been designated divisions of the American Psychological Association. These divisions represent such well-known psychological topics as personality, coping/adjustment, clinical psychology, psychological development, and social psychology, among many others. For us, the most pertinent one is Division 36, Psychology of Religion, which has approximately 1,600 members. Although these psychologists represent all of the other divisions and disciplines, they concern themselves with integrating their other specialties with religion, or at least with the way people relate to their faith. The members of Division 36 both conduct research on the role of religion in life, and apply what they learn to the problems people confront in the course of living. This requires that psychologists of religion learn about religious motivation, religious cognition, and religious behavior—the topics that are discussed in these pages.

The chapter titles in this volume indicate that virtually every aspect of life has the potential for religious involvement and significance. Our job is to comprehend the many ways in which a person's faith operates in his or her particular world. Religion is thus functional. It expresses and serves many individual, social, and cultural needs. Even though the approach employed here examines the person in the sociocultural context, it focuses primarily on the individual; this distinguishes psychological analysis from sociology and anthropology, which examine religion in society and culture. (In many instances, the distinction is difficult to make.) Furthermore, since we four authors of this book are primarily researchers, our desire is to show how religion is scientifically studied and what we have learned from research. The resulting knowledge reveals the phenomenal richness of a person's religious world. We hope that these findings will be as exciting for you, our readers, as they are for us.

Our approach emphasizes the empirical and scientific; we go where theory and data take us. Since most psychological research has been conducted within the Judeo-Christian framework, this material provides us with the overwhelming majority of our citations. Where information is available outside of this realm, however, we pursue it. Our role is to search in mind, society, and culture for the nature of religious thinking and behavior. We primarily want to know what religion is *psychologically*. We must always keep in mind that there is a major difference between religion per se and religious behavior, motivation, perception, and cognition. We study these human considerations and not religion as such.

To follow this theme for a moment, our proper role as psychologists in this endeavor must be understood. A disclaimer is therefore in order. Let us recognize that psychologists have no calling to challenge religious institutions and their doctrines. God is not our domain; neither is the world vision of churches. We do not enter into debates of faith versus reason, of one theology versus another, or of religion with science. In addition, it is not our place to question revelation, tradition, or scripture. Psychology as a social and behavioral science is our resource, and we expend our energies on this level of understanding.

The Empirical Scientific Approach

Psychology strives to be scientific. From this perspective, a psychologist desires to gather objective data—that is, information that is both public and capable of being reproduced. Even though there is contention in scientific circles about how to go about collecting information, the problem of the empirical scientist is to carry out research without letting his or her biases affect the outcome. The sociologist C. Wright Mills is reported to have declared, "I will make every effort to be objective, but I do not claim to be detached." As we will see, it is often not easy to remain "detached" and objective.

In explaining the task of the scientist more fully, Reich (2000) thus tells us that

> the task of science is to come to some (tentative) conclusions concerning order or patterns with respect to the objects of study, to explain them by elucidating the variables involved and demonstrating relationships between them, and finally to understand the underlying mechanisms in depth, whenever possible, in terms of a coherent theory. (p. 193)

This is an impressive set of requirements; they are scientific goals toward which we aspire. We have proposed what must be taken as aims and purposes—hopeful intentions, which are idealistic to say the least. Although scientists have often fallen short of attaining these ambitious heights, it is important that we attempt to attain objectivity, despite the complexity and difficulty of doing this.

We may further ask, "What about the psychologist of religion who is also devoutly religious?" Pointing out that this issue has been discussed for almost a century, Reich (2000) has again addressed it by noting the problem of "extreme positions," which exacerbate conflicts. Extreme positions are "extreme" in the eye of the beholder; hence what is reasonable to either the committed believer or the committed scientist may seem unreasonable and extreme to the other. When the same person is both believer and scientist, there may be a continuing struggle for definitive answers. Reich does not provide us with a simple and final response to the dilemma of belief versus science, but he points out the pitfalls in our scientific endeavor. Examination of the "objective" realm may necessitate parallel examination of our "subjective" commitments. Self-examination is a prerequisite to self-understanding and the avoidance of short-sighted prejudices.

But note that theological conviction is a problem not just for the religious psychologist, but for any psychologist who also takes a stand regarding religion. The agnostic and atheist likewise are constantly seeking to avoid prejudices that may jeopardize their objectivity. Indeed, one cannot understand Freud's treatment of religion unless we recognize his *assumption* that all religion is irrational (see Chapter 2).

A scientific treatment of religion may be subject to the criticism that science is usurping religious prerogatives—something we have already stated we are trying to avoid. There are several ways to consider the relationship. First, in order to accomplish this goal, one might want to adopt an approach described by Gould (1999). That is, no inherent conflict between religion and science exists when one recognizes that they represent separate, nonoverlapping domains of teaching authority. This is a version of "giving to God that which is God's, and to Caesar that which is Caesar's." A second approach available to the religiously committed scholar is to consider science as an avenue to God. This implies that God primarily works through natural law and processes. Another religious judgment might claim that we gain insight into God's way in the world, and that humanity may possibly be endowed with a naturalistic awareness of God's existence. As interesting as these perspectives may be, if we are to be psychologists of religion, we must wear the scientific mantle when we conduct our research and formulate our theories about faith in the life of the individual.

Let's Be Realistic

We have stated our hopes and ideals. The problem is the way people, including psychologists, tend to think and behave in real life. Professional psychologists are quite as subject to prejudices against religion as their religious peers have been to prejudices against psychology. Some clinicians perceive religion as inducing mental pathology and countering constructive thinking and behavior (Cortes, 1999). The research of Pargament (1997) represents a much more balanced and positive position. We show in the chapter on religion and mental disorder (Chapter 16) that religion can indeed be a "hazard to one's health," but it seems to function in a much more constructive manner for the majority of people. We further show that the kind of religion being judged and the standards used to judge religion have an impact on any evaluation of the usefulness of personal faith. Indeed, anyone can selectively employ psychological research to make a case either for or against religion. The better quest is to understand religion in its manifold varieties.

Historically, the issue of "the rise and fall of the psychology of religion" as a function of a scientific bias in psychology has become contentious (Hood, 2000b), but behavioristic and psychoanalytic antipathy toward religion has been well documented (Cortes, 1999). Unhappily, personal theological and antitheological positions have been shown to affect research and interpretation within the psychology of religion (Kirkpatrick & Hood, 1990). Our goal in these pages is to note the potential of slanted views entering the picture, and to reduce such bias. Indeed, although all of us authors adhere to the Judeo-Christian tradition, we are deliberately a multifaith group, and we hold varying values. We indeed attempt to recognize and avoid the possibilities of distortions from our personal theological positions.

The Necessity of Theory

For over a century, thousands of studies have been carried out in the psychology of religion. Unless these are organized in some manner that tries to inform us why these findings exist, we have little more than a random and confusing collection of research results. In order to resolve this dilemma, theories must be developed. Our knowledge has to be meaningfully ordered, and theories do just that. They tell us what factors or variables may or may not be pertinent when certain problems and issues are examined. Theories should first be formulated in interaction with any available data, and then guide research.

Psychologist Kurt Lewin is reported to have said that "there is nothing as practical as a good theory." Theories are the ways we have of organizing our thoughts and ideas, so that the data we collect make sense because all of the relevant variables have been studied. Without theories, we could never fully comprehend data.

But where do these theories come from? The prime source for the psychology of religion has usually been mainstream psychology, primarily personality and social psychology. The psychology of religion has formally been regarded as a subfield of social psychology (Dittes, 1969). It therefore makes sense that psychologists of religion look first to social psychology for direction. Consider three examples. First, attribution theory has been instrumental in guiding our thinking, as we discuss both later in this chapter and in Chapter 2. Second, many issues in the study of personal faith involve personality, mental disorder, and adjustment; hence coping theory is of great importance. Third, there is much concern about how personal religion develops in early life and changes over the lifespan. To deal with these matters, many scholars have turned to child psychology, drawing upon the contributions of Piagetian theory (and, more recently, attachment theory). As these examples suggest, psychology is a complex field with a large number of subdisciplines. All have the potential to provide theories for the psychology of religion.

Even though we usually look to the main body of psychological knowledge to guide us theoretically, there is no reason why the psychology of religion itself may not eventually provide us with new and constructive directions. Indeed, some of its findings do not fit well with other parts of psychology; this implies that these other subareas may be able to benefit from the psychological study of religion. (We suggest that you look for examples as you read this book.)

Clearly, we are not confined to psychology and its subdisciplines for theoretical guidance. Sociology, anthropology, and biology cannot be ignored. Indeed, the significance of religion is of such breadth and magnitude that we cannot deny the possibility of fruitful ideas coming from other scientific and nonscientific sources. Even theologies themselves can serve as psychological theories (Spilka, 1970, 1976). But to say that we take ideas from such other areas does not mean that the ideas remain unchanged. They may be altered because the psychology of religion has somewhat different interests, or because modifications are necessary to enhance their fit with our data. The theories we hold are "open"; they are always amenable to new information. To close our minds is the most impractical thing we can do. Our approach is therefore both theoretical and empirical, because neither aspect by itself is meaningful.

WHAT IS RELIGION?

For thousands of years, scholars have been writing and talking about religion. Chances are that more books have been written on this topic than any other in the history of humanity.

With such impressive evidence of concern, who would have the temerity to ask, "Just what is it you are talking about?" Boldness notwithstanding, this is a very good question to pose to anyone.

Even though data and observations in the social sciences point to the universality of religion, any attempt at definition immediately runs into trouble. We feel quite confident that we can come to a meeting of the minds if we deal with the Judeo-Christian heritage and the Islamic tradition, but once we go beyond these to the religions of eastern Asia, Africa, Polynesia, and a host of other localities that are not well known in North America and Europe—or even to the Native religious traditions of the United States and Canada—we find ourselves in great difficulty. Religion may encompass the supernatural, the non-natural, theism, deism, atheism, monotheism, polytheism, and both finite and infinite deities; it may also include practices, beliefs, and rituals that almost totally defy circumscription and definition.

The best efforts of anthropologists to define "religion" are frustrated at every turn. Guthrie simply asserts that "a definition of the term [religion] still eludes consensus" (Guthrie, 1996a, p. 412). He further claims that "the term religion is a misleading reification, labeling a probabilistic aggregate of similar, but not identical ideas in individual heads" (Guthrie, 1996b, p. 162). In other words, we select a number of ideas and observations that we think belong together, and call it religion. The fact that we use one word to describe a complex of beliefs, behaviors, and experiences as "religious" is often enough for us to believe that religion is really one entity, and that we can expect to find the same or similar phenomena anywhere else in the world.

The assumption that the term "religion" really represents one entity leads to a second question: "On what basis do we group the components we now call 'religion'?" The evident answer is that we call upon our experiences, obviously in our own society and culture, and then uncritically generalize these to other peoples. For example, if idols are found, they are often considered representations of the Judeo-Christian God; rituals are frequently viewed as religious ceremonies; and trances are commonly termed "mystical religious states." We distinguish religion from other aspects of our culture, but such a distinction may be invalid elsewhere, and our interpretations can be very wrong. The noted anthropologist Murray Wax affirms "that in most non-Western societies the natives do not distinguish religion as we do" (Wax, 1984, p. 16).

Returning to the premise that religion is universal, we may now ask, "If religion can't be defined, how do we know it is universal?" Wax (1984) implies that whatever is said to be religious must be manifested in both the individual and the culture. A psychologist of religion would now propose that people are likely to express their faith through behavior (e.g., rituals), belief (e.g., belief in the supernatural), and experience (e.g., mystical states). Writing about religion, the biologist R. A. Hinde (1999) suggests that these characteristics are "pan-societal" or universal.

As psychologists, we also have statistical tools to help us. One such tool is "factor analysis," which groups related variables through more general underlying factors. One example of such a factor is the concept of a loving God. Many adjectives expressing this concept go together empirically as a set. Other sets of variables are those that distinguish liberal from conservative interpretations of the Bible. These form two separate but related factors. By such data, we organize the many possible facets of religion. (For additional information on factor analysis, see the Appendix to this chapter.)

Defining Religion: Is It Possible?

We have asked some very basic questions about the definition of religion and come away without the kind of answers that truly satisfy our scientific curiosity. Are we now to resort to that popular and vague saying, "I don't know how to define it, but I know it when I see it"? Unhappily, this is not scientifically gratifying, and we cannot agree with such a proposition. The famous theologian Paul Tillich (1957) strongly believed that we need to clarify our muddled thinking about religion. He observed:

> There is hardly a word in the religious language, both theological and popular, which is subject to more misunderstandings, distortions, and questionable definitions than the word "faith." . . . It confuses, misleads, creates alternatively skepticism and fanaticism, intellectual resistance and emotional surrender, rejection of genuine religion and subjection to substitutes. (p. ix)

Despite his unhappiness with the terminology, Tillich (1957) could not find a substitute for "the reality to which the term 'faith'" (p. ix) refers, and he devoted a volume to its exposition. We are confronted with a similar task, but our method and approach are different, and we hope that they will help to clarify Tillich's "reality."

Social scientists and religionists have teased out every abstraction, nuance, and implication in each word in any definition of religion that has ever been offered. We therefore agree with the sociologist J. Milton Yinger (1967) that "any definition of religion is likely to be satisfactory only to its author" (p. 18). Nevertheless, in a later book, Yinger (1970) struggled with the problem of definition in a very scholarly manner for some 23 pages. It may have been similar frustration that much earlier caused a noted psychologist of religion, George Coe (1916), to state:

> I purposely refrain from giving a formal definition of religion . . . partly because definitions carry so little information as to facts; partly because the history of definitions of religion makes it almost certain that any fresh attempts at definition would necessarily complicate these introductory chapters. (p. 13)

We do not feel that the situation has basically changed in the nearly 90 years since Coe took his stand. We can, however, take the advice of another early scholar (Dresser, 1916) who claimed that "religion, like poetry and most other living things, cannot be defined. But some characteristic marks may be given" (p. 441). Let us therefore avoid the pitfalls of unproductive, far-ranging, grandly theoretical definitions of religion. We are simply not ready for them. Many are available in the literature, but the highly general, vague, and abstract manner in which they are usually stated reduces their usefulness either for illuminating the concept of religion or for undertaking research. Our purpose is to enable our readers to understand the variety of ways in which psychologists have defined religion.

Indeed, we are in a quandary. We deal largely in this book with the Western religious tradition (because that is where most research has been conducted), but we are saying that religion performs many functions for many different people. Though these functions may vary greatly in terms of their surface appearance, at their core we feel they represent the same elemental human needs and roles, about which we will have more to say. In order to understand the research on these issues, we utilize a class of definitions that at least yield clear criteria: "operational definitions," which we discuss in detail later in this chapter. This is not to say that there may not be debate about what operational definitions really represent, since their selection should be based on theory.

Spirituality and/or Religion?

> "Spirit" and "spiritual" are words which are constantly used and easily taken for granted by all writers upon religion—more constantly and easily, perhaps, than any of the other terms in the mysterious currency of faith. (Underhill, 1933, p. 1)

This observation is as significant today as it was 70 years ago. After reviewing the available literature on spirituality in 1993, Spilka, in his frustration, claimed that spirituality is "a word that embraces obscurity with passion" (p. 1). He further labeled the concept "fuzzy." Though Daniel Helminiak (1987, 1996) has written a number of impressive scholarly psychological/ philosophical treatises on spirituality, psychologists of religion have not taken his theoretical guidance and provided the kind of objective assessment we are stressing here. On the other hand, Gorsuch and Miller (1999) have suggested that the term "spirituality" can have meaning in the psychology of religion if clear operational definitions are made.

In the past decade, "spirituality" has become a popular word. It is now common to refer to "spirituality" instead of referring to "religion," but without drawing any clear distinction between them. This has been sufficiently the case in treatment issues. Gorsuch and Miller (1999) employ "spirituality" predominantly in this practical sense. They review classical measures used within the psychology of religion as measures of spirituality. Little changes except that "spirituality" is substituted for "religion." This substitution has also occurred in many assessment scales, in which, again, the term "spirituality" is used as a synonym for "religion." There is some justification for the usage of these two terms as synonyms, since research has shown that most people see them as highly similar. When people report valuing religion, they also claim to value spirituality (Spilka & McIntosh, 1996; Zinnbauer, Pargament, Cowell, & Scott, 1996).

Psychometric Problems in Measuring Spirituality

This confusion further applies to the labels used to identify the various "spirituality" measures, as they are usually not distinguished from each other. Thus, for example, there are both objective and subjective measures of "spiritual well-being" (Bufford, Paloutzian, & Ellison, 1991; Ellison, 1983; Ellison & Smith, 1991; Moberg, 1984). There is also a multidimensional Spiritual Gifts Inventory, although it clearly needs more work (Ledbetter & Foster, 1989). Genia (1991, 1997) has offered a two-factor Spiritual Experience Index that looks promising. Unhappily, few of those who have constructed these scales provide data on relationships among their measures and others purporting to assess different or similar indices of spirituality. In addition, correlations with well-known scales of religiosity are lacking. With regard to the latter concern, Genia (1997), who provides much useful information, reports correlations as high as .84 between the Spiritual Support factor of her measure and a widely used measure of Intrinsic religion as defined by Allport. (See this chapter's Appendix for an explanation of correlation, and Chapter 2 for a discussion of Intrinsic religion as defined by Allport.) Given associations of this magnitude, one may properly ask what the difference is between Genia's measure of Spiritual Support and Allport's Intrinsic religion. Clearly, we need much more assessment of these instruments.

The Spirituality–Religion Debate

The last few years have witnessed a growing response to the question of spirituality that draws some distinctions between spirituality and religion. It is as if a "critical mass" of vague definitions has been reached. This has stimulated a new concern with the conceptualization of spirituality that directs our thinking toward its objective assessment and application through research (Hill et al., 2000; Hood, 2000b; Miller, 1999; Pargament, 1999; Pargament & Mahoney, 2002; Zinnbauer et al., 1997; Zinnebauer, Pargament, & Scott, 1999). Many current thinkers are therefore attempting to create theoretical and operational definitions of spirituality that either distinguish it from personal religiosity or show how the two concepts are related.

A traditional distinction exists between being spiritual and being religious that can be used to enhance our use of both terms (Gorsuch, 1993). The connotations of "spirituality" are more personal than institutional, whereas the connotations of "religion" are more institutional, so spirituality is more psychological (and religion more sociological). In this usage, the two terms are not synonymous but distinct: Spirituality is about a person's beliefs, values, and behavior, while religiousness is about the person's involvement with a religious tradition and institution.

One may ask why the change from the term "religion" to the term "spirituality" is occurring now, rather than, for example, with the major research done in the early days of psychology. Two facts suggest a possible lead. The first is that only a minority of psychologists are religious in the classical sense of being affiliated with religious organizations, but many more see themselves as spiritual (Shafranske & Malony, 1985). This indicates that most psychologists, to whom religion is unimportant, have little wish to be identified with it. But spirituality is another matter; it can be part of one's self-concept without a need to relate to any institution, or even to know anything about religion.

The second fact that may support the increasing use of the term "spirituality" is that, despite the negative reaction "religion" engenders in most psychologists, aspects of it have become recognized as important for major areas of life. These include the benefits of meditation (Benson, 1975; Benson & Stark, 1996), as well as the evidence that religious people are less likely to use illegal substances, abuse alcohol, or be sexually promiscuous (Gorsuch, 1988, 1995; Gorsuch & Butler, 1976). As a result, religious persons possess better physical health than those engaging in these undesirable actions (e.g., Larson et al., 1989).

Psychologists want what is good from spirituality, but, as noted above, they often do not want religion. A possible answer is that they can be spiritual without changing their views about religion. Some would say that this is "easy religion" or "cheap grace," whereas others might claim that it is "separating the valuable from the superstitious." Clearly, there is considerable debate regarding the potential separation of these concepts. Donahue (1998) forcefully claims that "there is no true spirituality apart from religion." Pargament (1999) views the separatist trend with ambivalence, and offers guidance to prevent a polarization of these realms. Regardless of how the professionals phrase this issue, on the popular level the distinction may be sharpening, with spirituality the favored notion (Roof, 1993).

It is still an open question whether the practice of spirituality outside of religion can be adequately defined. If it can, will it then be found to relate to the same variables as religion? The proponents of Transcendental Meditation provide support that some effects of meditation are separate from those of religion (see Chapter 12), but this is a difficult area to research, for training people in a meditation style independent of a religion does not mean that they practice meditation apart from their faith. No one knows at this point whether spirituality will be a more viable psychological construct than religion once it is operationally distinguished from religion.

Distinguishing Spirituality from Religion: Is It Possible?

Defining "spirituality" in a manner distinct from "religion" can start from the past meanings of "spirituality," which is an ancient and complex term. In Western thought, it has been a part of classical dualistic thinking that pits the material world against the spiritual world. The former consists of things we can see, hear, smell, or touch, whereas the latter consists of elements that exist in the mental world but can at best only be inferred from the material world. Non-Western thinkers have seen these two areas as more closely intertwined, but spirit still has the sense of being immaterial. For example, in Thailand a house must be provided for the spirits of a parcel of land before it can be used (many Thai restaurants in the United States have such houses); although the spirits themselves dwell outside of ordinary experience by the human senses, they must still be appeased by a physical dwelling.

A contemporary illustration of setting the spiritual apart comes from the way church governance is distinguished within the Disciples of Christ, the Christian Church movement, or the Churches of Christ (as this group of Protestant congregations is variously known). In these congregations, there are two governing bodies: the "deacons" and the "elders." The deacons are concerned with the material aspects of congregational life, including physical property and taking food to the needy. The elders are responsible for the spiritual welfare of the church. This includes taking the comforts of the faith to the sick and grieving, and encouraging activities that enhance the members' relationships to God. In other words, the elders are concerned with the inner being of the person, and the deacons with the more worldly aspects of existence. Members of these congregations never have a problem defining the "spiritual" matters of the congregations. But what these church members know, the psychology of religion (including the psychology of spirituality) needs to spell out—that is, to define operationally.

Another approach to defining spirituality from classical usage is to identify it with "spiritual disciplines." These include such acts as prayer and meditation, but have also included fasting and doing penance for sins. For example, monks retire to a monastery to practice such disciplines, in order to lead a more spiritual life than is commonly possible outside the monastery. With the traditional Disciples of Christ (etc.) usage noted above and the set of spiritual disciplines, we could just divide the psychology of religion into personal practices (the spiritual) and communal practices (the religious). That is, we could employ both terms but would not use them synonymously.

There are other ways of defining spirituality that shift the construct to new grounds, and so allow testing of whether religion and spirituality are just interchangeable terms. Here is one: "Spirituality is the quest for understanding ourselves in relationship to our view of ultimate reality, and to live in accordance with that understanding" (Gorsuch, 2002, p. 8). It resembles Tillich's (1957) notions as presented above, and many would say that Tillich was more concerned with spirituality than with faith or religion. Some differences between spirituality in this definition and a definition of religion include the following:

- Spirituality does not require an institutional framework.
- Spirituality is personal.

- A spiritual person is deeply concerned about value commitments.
- A person can be spiritual without a deity (although some would say that the "view of ultimate reality" always includes what Alcoholics Anonymous refers to as a "higher power").
- Religiousness is a subset of spirituality, which means that religiousness invariably involves spirituality, but that there may be nonreligious spirituality as well.

In the current psychology of religion, there is no common acceptance of any of these positions on the meaning of "spirituality" as compared to "religion." Furthermore, it is not our intention in this text to force any distinction on the profession. Instead, our point here is that the use of these two terms is highly ambiguous. Only by checking what an investigator actually measures can one be sure what, regardless of the investigator's usage of these terms, is being researched.

Defining Religion Operationally

It is not what psychologists claim to define as religious, but what they actually use to measure it in their research, that is crucial. "Operational definitions" literally focus on "operations"—the methods and procedures used to assess something. They are the experimental manipulations plus the measures and instruments employed. With respect to religion, what does it mean to be religious? How do we indicate religiousness? Operationally, we often identify people as religious if they are members of a church or other congregation, attend religious services, read the Bible or other sacred writings, peruse congregational bulletins, contribute money to religious causes, observe religious holidays and fast days, pray frequently, say grace before meals, and accept religiously based diet restrictions, among other possibilities. Many psychologists also look to the beliefs that the devout express, as well as the experiences they report. Frequently, respondents fill out questionnaires about these expressions, and the questions they answer are the operational definitions for that study. There are a great many such operations that illustrate commitment to one's faith.

Basically, operational definitions tell us what the researcher means when religious language is used. For example, suppose we desire to evaluate the degree to which individuals believe in "fundamentalist" doctrines. We might then administer a questionnaire specifically designed to obtain agreement or disagreement with such principles. The Hunsberger Fundamentalism Scale might be selected, and we could report its scores for the sample tested (Altemeyer & Hunsberger, 1992). Fundamentalism is thus operationally defined by this measuring instrument. Fulton, Gorsuch, and Maynard (1999) have used a somewhat different scale that they call Fundamentalism; using this scale provides a second operational definition of fundamentalism. When the same term is associated with two measures, it is important to examine both measures closely to determine how similar and how different their items are. Throughout this volume, we emphasize operational definitions of different aspects or forms of faith. This is the only way we can understand religion from a scientific standpoint.

The quality of an operational definition is evaluated by two criteria, both of which are discussed more fully in the Appendix to this chapter. The first is "reliability." Once reliability is established, we know that a scale is measuring something consistently—but does it measure what we want it to? If so, the scale has "validity." The validity of most psychology-of-religion scales is based on an expert's evaluation of the content of the items (so-called "content validity"). For example, if we had a set of items all referring to whether or not the

Bible was dictated by God, then the scale questions would be considered valid as a Biblical Inerrancy Scale. But those same items would be invalid if they were used to measure Christian commitment, since many Christians hold that the Bible was *inspired* rather than literally *dictated* by God.

Gorsuch (1984) suggests that we psychologists have been quite successful in evaluating personal religion. That is, the scales developed for this purpose generally show both good reliability and good validity. In his eyes, while this is a boon, it carries with it a number of banes. Success itself is a bane if it prevents us from developing techniques other than questionnaires. Concurrently, another bane is that we may spend too much time and effort dealing with measurement rather than with the phenomena that should be assessed. Too many psychologists who begin to study religion fail to learn what measures are already available, and too often call the same operations by several different labels.

Unfortunately, many modern-day writers are attempting to create not only theoretical but also operational definitions of spirituality that neither distinguish it from personal religiosity nor show how the two concepts are related. Many aspects of spirituality are well measured by traditional psychology-of-religion scales. Any new scales should show empirically how they are superior to current scales.

The fact that we have, so far, mentioned only questionnaires does not mean that there are no other ways of gathering information about the place of religion in the lives of those we study. For example, valuable data can be gained from interviews. These need to be carefully developed and skillfully administered in a standardized manner. They can be of special significance in the study of religious experience. Sometimes projective tests, such as drawing pictures of God, have been successfully employed.

Defining and observing religious behavior (e.g., how often people pray, the nature of their prayers, when they are said, etc.) can tell us much about one's personal faith. Methodologically, we want to gather data with procedures that (1) are consistent and (2) clearly assess what we want to measure. These two points capture the ideas of reliability and validity, respectively, which are the cornerstones of good psychological measurement.

Qualitative and Quantitative Research Methods

"Qualitative" data collection ranges from writing the biography of a religious person to chatting with several people about a religious topic, conducting interviews with open-ended questions, or having people tell a story about a picture they are given. For example, determining what people do in certain specific settings may call for a novel procedure. This could include observing missionary activity in a native village undergoing cultural change, or the behavior of congregants during a church service (Wolcott, 1994). In contrast, "quantitative" data collection techniques might ask people to rate how strongly they agree with a particular statement or to report how often they attend worship services. The major distinction is that quantitative measures give scores directly, but qualitative data must be processed by a rater (or, more often these days, by a computer program) for information.

A similar distinction can be made between qualitative and quantitative analyses of data. Qualitative treatment can involve a more or less subjective review that enables a scholar to make sense of the information and draw conclusions. A researcher employing quantitative analysis uses statistics such as means, standard deviations, significance levels, and correlations (defined in the Appendix to this chapter) in order to draw conclusions.

Although quantitative methods have been typical of data collection and analysis in the sciences as well as in the psychology of religion, there is no doubt that they miss something. A description of a sunset in terms of physics is quantitative, but none would argue that a painting of that sunset is replaced by the physical description. Physics has never claimed to contain the whole of human experience regarding physical phenomena; nor does the psychology of religion claim to contain the whole of human experience regarding religion. Just as a personal experience with a sunset is meaningful in addition to the physics of a sunset, so a personal religious experience cannot be replaced by the psychology of that experience. In like manner, psychology does not cover the history of religions, the biographies of religious leaders, nor the anthropology of religions. The psychology of religion is an application of scientific methods to enhance our psychological understanding of religion.

The acceptability of both quantitative and qualitative methods within the psychology of religion depends on whether they can be shown to meet the scientific criteria of reliability and validity. For example when Ponton and Gorsuch (1988) used an instrument called the Quest scale in Venezuela, its reliability was low, so the authors were hesitant to draw any conclusions from it.

Qualitative measures also need to demonstrate reliability. Do different persons or judges agree in their observations and/or interpretations? If they reach different conclusions as to whether a person feels God's presence during meditation, then they not only do not communicate well with each other; there is no reliability.

Once it has been shown that the qualitative or quantitative method is reliable, validity must then be established. Usually "content validity" is used, as noted earlier. This means that psychologists examining the method agree that the items or interview or rating criteria are appropriate for whatever descriptive term is employed.

Since both qualitative and quantitative methods are acceptable if they meet the standards of being reliable and valid, why are quantitative methods so popular? One important problem is that reliable qualitative methods are rather expensive to use. Consider the question of how a victim becomes a forgiving person after major harm has been done to that person. Using an interview-based qualitative approach, a researcher might ask each of 100 people to describe a time when a person harmed them, and then, in their own words, to explain how they forgave that person and how their religious faith was a part of that process. The interviewing would take about 300 hours (including setting up the interviews, doing the interviews, finding new people to reduce the "no-shows," transcribing the interviews, etc.). Then the interviews would need to be rated by two people trained to use the same language to describe the processes that were reported, and differences would need to be reconciled with the help of a third rater (all this would take another 300 hours). At this point, a total of 600 hours would be needed for collecting and scoring the data.

By contrast, in quantitative measurement utilizing a questionnaire, a group of 100 people might take 2 hours to fill out the questionnaire. Scoring these responses would take another 4 hours. The quantitative approach would thus take an estimated 6 hours, versus 600 hours for the qualitative approach. Which procedure would you rather use in a research project?

In some cases, qualitative methods are the only ones we currently have to tap into the psychological processes being studied. It is, for example, difficult to understand children's concepts of God without using their drawings of God, which are then rated. And in models where a person makes a choice, it is also a problem to find out what options *spontaneously* occur to that person without utilizing at least somewhat qualitative methods. When qualitative research that has demonstrated reliability and validity is available, we include it in this text, just as we do quantitative research that has demonstrated reliability and validity.

PERSPECTIVES ON THE PSYCHOLOGY OF RELIGION

Psychology in Context

The sociocultural context is the external foundation for religious beliefs, attitudes, values, behavior, and experience. The essential psychological point here is that psychologists of religion do not study religion per se; they study people in relation to their faith, and what this faith may mean to other facets of their lives. Whereas sociologists and anthropologists look to the external setting in which religion exists, we psychologists focus on the individual. Ours is an internal perspective. Even while we adopt the psychological stance, we must never lose sight of the fact that people cannot really be separated from their personal and social histories, and that these exist in relation to group and institutional life. Families, schools, and work are part of the "big picture," and we cannot abstract a person from these influences. They constitute a large part of what we discuss in the following chapters.

The Objective/Empirical Position

From what has been said above about the scientific and empirical viewpoint, it is obvious that this is the perspective we authors take in this volume. We desire to minimize subjectivity by stressing objective methods of investigation and research. As also noted above, psychologists must be flexible in creating appropriate instruments to measure the variables we select for research. Our primary concern is to obtain data that can be objectively treated, quantitatively analyzed, and confirmed when the studies are repeated.

Quantification within this framework invariably means that findings will be statistically analyzed. Ideally, we would like to phrase our results in terms of causes and effects. This would, however, entail the construction of experiments in which independent, dependent, and control variables are rigorously defined operationally. Unfortunately, the psychological aspects of religion have rarely been amenable to such treatment. Since we may not be able to construct experiments, we can sometimes conduct "quasi-experimental" research, in which we study naturally occurring groups (Batson, Schoenrade, & Ventis, 1993; Cook & Campbell, 1979). Though there are many different quasi-experimental research designs, an example for the psychology of religion might compare two seemingly equivalent groups of churchgoers; however, the members of only one of these groups might have had religious mystical experiences. Differences between the two groups might then be assessed. Work of this nature has been undertaken (Spilka, Ladd, McIntosh, & Milmoe, 1996).

The dominant methodology used by psychologists of religion is "associational." For instance, the fact that couples who take their children to church have more religious children does not necessarily mean that attending church produces religious children. It could be the modeling of religion by the parents in the home that is important, or the social networks created through church attendance. All we know is that the variables are associated.

With other variables, a correlation coefficient may be used to describe the association. This approach may tell us that our personal religious measures vary together, meaning that if one changes, so does the other. If engaging in prayer (Variable 1) makes people feel better

(Variable 2), it usually means that the more they pray, the better they feel. Technically, maybe the better they feel, the more they pray. Since we use theory and evidence to decide which choice is probably true, the data tell us that people pray much more when they are in distress. This could be a simplification, for there are likely to be people for whom an extremely high frequency of praying could reflect psychological problems. Under such circumstances, it might be wiser to say that "on the average," as the frequency of prayer increases, so does one's feeling of well-being.

The computation of correlations is probably the most widely employed statistical method used in the empirical psychology of religion. But some readers may be inexperienced with correlation coefficients and the factor analyses that are often used with them. These are explained in the Appendix to this chapter, along with other essential concepts for understanding the many research findings we present in this book.

A FRAMEWORK FOR STUDYING THE PSYCHOLOGY OF RELIGION

In each succeeding edition of this book, we have tried to make our framework for understanding the psychology of religion more inclusive. The attributional approach that we employed in earlier editions is now subsumed under a more general perspective that stresses a search for meaning. For all religious people, religion is indeed a struggle to comprehend their place in the scheme of things and what this entails for their relations with the world and others. Though this frame of reference is applicable to all of the chapters that follow, those dealing with religion and biology (Chapter 3) and with religion, coping, and adjustment (Chapter 15) are probably most explicit in its utilization.

Despite the serious problems of definition with which we wrestled earlier, our approach assumes that religion is truly a worldwide phenomenon. Invariably, behavior, experience, and belief express different aspects of this complex unity wherever it is found. As we indicate in Chapter 3, genetic and evolutionary arguments and data are part of this problem. On the level of psychology, we ask what human characteristics appear to be universally applicable, in one of the three general realms of cognition, motivation, and social life. Our framework suggests that these three realms offer us the directions necessary for a rather "grand" psychological theory for understanding the role of religion in human life. When we look to cognition, we are concerned with meaning. Motivation focuses us on the need of people to exercise control over themselves and their environment. Social life, which we encapsulate in the concept of "sociality," recognizes that people necessarily exist within relationships. They must relate to others to survive and prosper. In other words, people need people.

The Need for Meaning

Aristotle's dictum "All men by nature desire to know" (McKeon, 1941, p. 689) set the stage for a host of philosophers and psychologists to stress the importance of knowledge in coping with the world. In the psychological literature, the concept of meaning has been tied not only to knowledge, but also to a variety of other overlapping (if not identical) notions, such as "information processing" and "cognitive structure." Though there is a kind of scientific vagueness to the idea of "meaning," no other word seems to capture as well its inherent significance, and thus we employ the term without concern. In essence, people need to make sense out of the world in order to live; it must be made meaningful. When we turn to religion, we focus on higher-level cognitions and some understanding of ourselves and our relationship to others and the world. The result is meaning—the cognitive significance of sensory and perceptual stimulation and information to us.

The Attributional Aspect of Meaning

For over 40 years, attribution theory has been a staple of social psychology (Fiske & Taylor, 1991; Heider, 1958; Hewstone, 1983). In the mid-1980s, it became a significant basis for research in the psychology of religion (Spilka, Shaver, & Kirkpatrick, 1985). Attribution theory is concerned with explanations—primarily causal explanations about people, things, and events. These are expressed in statements and ideas that assign certain roles and influences to various situational and dispositional factors. For instance, we might attribute a person's getting lung cancer to being exposed to the smoking of coworkers, to his or her own smoking, or to the view that "God works in mysterious ways." All of these are attributions. Research examining such meanings and their ramifications became the cornerstone of cognitive social psychology, and attributional approaches were soon extended to explain how people understand emotional states and much of what happens to them and to others (Fiske & Taylor, 1991). As an effort to acquire new knowledge, the attributional process appears to be a first step in making things meaningful (Kruglanski, Hasmel, Maides, & Schwartz, 1978). Among the factors that may be involved in understanding the kinds of attributions people make are situational and personal-dispositional influences; the nature of the event to be explained (whether it is positive, negative, or neutral); and the event domain (e.g., medical, social, economic). We will also want to know what cues are present in the situation. For example, does the event take place in a church, on a mountaintop, or in a business office? In like manner, when we turn to personal-dispositional concerns, we may need to get information on the attributor's background, personality, attitudes, language strengths and weaknesses, cognitive inclinations, and other biases. Research Box 1.1 presents a representative attributional study in the psychology of religion.

Religion and the Search for Meaning

Argyle (1959) claims that "a major mechanism behind religious beliefs is a purely cognitive desire to understand" (p. 57). Similarly, Clark (1958) asserts that "religion more than any other human function satisfies the need for meaning in life" (p. 419). A number of sociologists have further conceptualized "religion as a form of knowledge . . . which answers preexistent and eternal problems of meaning" (Budd, 1973, p. 79). On one level, religion fills in the blanks in our knowledge of life and the world, and offers us a sense of security. This is especially true when we are confronted with crisis and death. Religion is therefore a normal, natural, functional development whereby "persons are prepared intellectually and emotionally to meet the non-manipulable aspects of existence positively by means of a reinterpretation of the total situation" (Bernhardt, 1958, p. 157).

The Need for Control

Like the idea of "meaning," the idea of "control" has a long history in both philosophy and psychology. Control in the sense of power is central in the philosophies of Hobbes and

---

Research Box 1.1. General Attribution Theory for the Psychology of Religion: The Influence of Event Character on Attributions to God (Spilka & Schmidt, 1983a)

This research focused on the components of events that occur to people. When seeking explanations, is a person influenced by (1) whether the event happens to oneself or others; (2) how important it is; (3) whether it is positive or negative; and (4) what its domain is—economic, social, or medical? Given these possible influences, the emphasis of this study was on the degree to which attributions are made to God.

A total of 135 youths from introductory psychology classes and from a church participated in the study. Twelve short stories were written to depict various social, economic, and medical occurrences. Of the four stories in each of these domains, two described minor to moderate incidents, and two described important happenings. One of each pair was positive, and one was negative. In half of the stories, the referent person was the responder; the other half of the stories referred to someone else. The participants were thus dealing with variations in incident domain, plus the dimensions of importance, whether the occurrence was positive or negative, and whether it was personal or impersonal. In addition, each participant was able to make attributions to (1) the characteristics of the person in the story; (2) possible others, even if not present in the story; (3) the role of chance; (4) God; or (5) the personal faith of the individual in the story. Lastly, two experiments were constructed. In the first, all of the participants filled out the forms in a school setting; in the second study, half the participants were in a church and half in school. This was an attempt to determine situational influences.

No situational differences were found, but all of the other conditions yielded significance. Attributions to God were mostly made for occurrences that were medical, positive, and important. Many significant interactions among these factors occurred, and though the personal–impersonal factor per se was not statistically significant, it was in its relationships to the other effects. Other research on attributions to God has revealed similar influences (Gorsuch & Smith, 1983).

Nietzsche. Reid (1969) spoke of power as one of the basic human desires. Adler termed it "an intrinsic 'necessity of life'" (quoted in Vyse, 1997, p. 131). Though the ideal in life is *actual* control, the need to perceive personal mastery is often so great that the *illusion* of control will suffice. Lefcourt (1973) even suggests that this illusion "may be the bedrock on which life flourishes" (p. 425). Baumeister (1991) believes the subjective sense of personal efficacy to be the essence of control.

The Attributional Aspect of Control

We have noted above that the process of attribution reflects a search for meaning, a need to know. It also represents a need for mastery and control. One of the central figures in attribution theory and research, Harold Kelley, stated: "The theory describes processes that operate as if the individual were motivated to attain a cognitive mastery of the causal structure of his environment" (Kelley, 1967, p. 193). Especially when threatened with harm or pain, all higher organisms seek to predict and/or control the outcomes of the events that affect them

(Seligman, 1975). This fact has been linked by attribution theorists and researchers with novelty, frustration or failure, lack of control, and restriction of personal freedom (Berlyne, 1960; Wong, 1979; Wong & Weiner, 1981; Wortman, 1976). It may be that people gain a sense of control by making sense out of what is happening and being able to predict what will occur, even if the result is undesirable.

Religion and the Need for Control

We have seen that religion helps people make sense out of their personal worlds by offering them meaning for virtually every life situation, particularly those that are most distressing, such as death and dying. Often when people obtain such "information," they feel that they have a measure of control over their lives. Various techniques strengthen a person's feeling of mastery—for example, prayer and participation in religious rituals and ceremonies. An argument can be made that religious ritual and prayer are mechanisms for enhancing the sense of self-control and control of one's world. Gibbs (1994) claims that supernaturalism arises when secular control efforts fail. Vyse (1997) further shows how lack of control relates to the development of and belief in superstition and magic. Indeed, the historic interplay of magic and religion has often been viewed as a response to uncertainty and helplessness.

Earlier we have noted the remarks of Lefcourt (1973) and Baumeister (1991) with regard to the importance of the illusion of control. We have further noted that the conception of control that is personally significant is subjective. Many times in life, people must recognize that their secular attempts at control are limited (e.g., when a death is impending). When such events occur, people need that illusory, subjective sense of control—and they frequently turn to their faith, possibly by prayer, to regain the feeling that they are doing something that may work. The subjective feeling of control is thus enhanced. They hope that turning to the source of ultimate power, in whatever way they define that source, will work. The notion of mastery is often powerful, however, and though it may not be objectively efficient, there is no doubt that it can offer people the strength they need to succeed.

Sociality: The Need for Relationships

Defining Sociality

A truly fundamental principle is that we humans cannot live without others. We are conceived and born in relationship and interdependence, and, throughout our entire lives, connections and interactions with others are indispensable to life. "Sociality" refers to behaviors that relate organisms to one another, and that keep an individual identified with a group (Brewer, 1997). Included here are expressions of social support, cooperation, adherence to group standards, attachment to others, altruism, and many other actions that maintain effectively functioning groups. Faith systems accomplish these goals for many people, and in return the cultural order embraces religion.

Religion and Sociality

Religion connects individuals to each other and their groups; it socializes members into a community, and concurrently suppresses deviant behavior. As Lumsden and Wilson (1983) put it, religion is a "powerful device by which people are absorbed into a tribe and psychically strengthened" (p. 7). In this way, both religious bodies and the societies of which they are a part strengthen themselves in numbers and importance.

There is a circular pattern in this linking of social life to faith. Religion fosters social group unity, which further strengthens religious sentiments. Current data show that church members possess larger social support networks than nonmembers do; in addition, there is more positive involvement in intrafamily relationships among the religiously committed than among their less religious peers (Pargament, 1997). Many of these observations have been attributed to enhanced feelings of social belonging and integration into a community of like-minded thinkers. This may mean that church members and those reared in churchgoing families also join more social groups than nonmembers in later life. Data support this inference (Graves, Wang, Mead, Johnson, & Klag, 1998).

Moreover, the importance of marriage and reproduction is invariably stressed by religious traditions (Hoult, 1958). Expectations to marry and have children probably influence reproductive success in couples where both spouses attend the same church, as such couples generally show high birth rates (Moberg, 1962). There is a strong need for new research in this area, as there may be much variation across different religious bodies. It does seem to be true of some growing conservative groups, such as the Church of Jesus Christ of Latter-Day Saints (also known as the Mormons). This mutually reinforcing pattern is also likely to limit access to those whose religious beliefs differ, and could contribute to relatively high divorce rates plus low marital satisfaction when people of diverse religious affiliations marry (Lehrer & Chiswick, 1993; Levinger, 1979; Shortz & Worthington, 1994).

One may thus view religious faith as strengthening ingroup bonds, welfare, and positive social evaluation. In addition, religion appears to eventuate in heightened reproductive and genetic potential. Obviously, religious affiliation opens important social channels for interpersonal approval and integration into society on many levels.

Framework: Directions and Implications

Our framework has been presented in this chapter in an introductory and rather condensed manner. In the following chapters (particularly Chapters 3 and 15, as noted earlier), these ideas are expanded. Relative to biology, reference is made to the evolutionary and genetic possibilities underlying our scheme. When all of these framework views are put together, the result is a general psychological theory of religion that is quite useful in understanding how people relate to their faith.

OVERVIEW

This chapter's brief introduction to the psychology of religion has attempted to distinguish the major dimensions of the discipline. Just as a standard introductory textbook in psychology overviews the major facets of the field, each of the areas cited in this chapter has resulted in volumes that analyze and treat the specifics of the issue in question.

We have also presented an orientation that stresses theory and objective measurement. We seek knowledge that is both public and reproducible. Our aim is to achieve a scientific circumscription of the psychology of religion, and to convey the importance of such a framework. The next chapter describes this approach in further detail. When this effort has been completed, we show how religion relates to biology, as well as to individual development throughout the lifespan; describe the experiential expressions of religion; and finally discuss the significance of faith in social life, coping, adjustment, and mental disorder. Simply put, religion is a central feature of human existence, the psychological appreciation of which we try to communicate in these pages.

From a scientific point of view, the most important feature of our integrating framework is that it is testable. In brief, measures tapping the need for meaning, control, and sociality should relate positively to religious commitment, and we hypothesize that they will evidence stronger genetic involvement than religious devotion currently demonstrates. Statistically removing these needs from data supporting the genetic component in religion should significantly reduce indications of direct genetic influence on religion, or even cause them to disappear. Such findings cannot prove that religion totally originates from the needs specified here. However, they will speak strongly to the idea that religion is a powerful factor in meeting human needs for meaning, control, and sociality. Needless to say, the expression of these needs will be shaped by culture.

APPENDIX: STATISTICAL PROCEDURES AND CONSIDERATIONS

As we have stated in the chapter text, this book emphasizes the empirical psychological study of religion. Frequent references are made throughout the book to various statistical procedures, the chief ones of which are correlation, factor analysis, and reliability and validity. To aid readers, we offer a brief explanation of these techniques.

Correlation

"Correlation" is a procedure that determines the strength of a relationship between two variables. The statistical calculations result in a number called a "correlation coefficient." This number can range from −1.00 through 0 to +1.00. A correlation of 0 means that there is no relationship. The higher the correlation coefficient, meaning the closer it is to either −1.00 or +1.00, the stronger is the relationship between the two variables being studied. Correlations are important, for they imply prediction. Using the appropriate formulas, the researcher can use the correlation coefficient to predict how a person might respond in one area from how that individual reacts in another area. Of course, the closer the correlation coefficient is to either −1.00 or +1.00, the stronger the predictions that can be made.

If the computed correlation coefficient is in the 0 to +1.00 range, the association between the variables is said to be "positive." As the values of one of the variables increases, so do the values of the other variable. Stated differently, the scores of the two measures increase and decrease together. To illustrate, we know that perceptions of a loving God correlate positively with church attendance. The more one believes that God is loving, the greater is the likelihood that one attends church. If everyone who believed in a loving God always attended church, while none of those who did not believe in a loving God ever attended church, the correlation would be 1.00. Of course, "always" and "never" leave out such possibilities as these: Illness might prevent some from attending church, despite believing in a loving God; a male atheist might go to church to "get in good with a very attractive girl"; and some people might always interpret the question differently than the rest of us do. So correlations never reach 1.00, and in fact seldom reach .50.

Is a correlation of .50 worthwhile? Speaking in a probabilistic way, yes, it is. If we square the .50, we get .25, which might be interpreted roughly as a percentage that tells us we can predict something at 25% above chance level. If the correlation between church attendance and belief in a loving God computes at .50, we can predict at 25% above chance level the degree of such belief from knowing how often a person attends church.

Note that the relationship is not perfect. Part of the imperfection would result from inaccuracies in our measures. Our sample might contain people who attend church from once a year to once a week or even more frequently. We may fail to account for every response possibility in our question. Respondents may include under "church attendance" being at church suppers, attending board meetings, taking courses, and so on. Also, there are numerous other variables affecting church attendance, in addition to belief in a loving God. Still, the .50 correlation shows a meaningful relationship between the two indices.

If the coefficients are in the −.01 to −1.00 range, the relationship between the variables is said to be "negative." This means that as the value of one of the variables increases, the other decreases. In other words, the scores of the two variables are related in opposite directions. For example, the variable of extrinsic religion may correlate negatively with self-esteem, so a person who rejects extrinsic religion is more likely to have higher self-esteem.

The psychology of religion has commonly found correlations of .20 between various aspects of religious belief or motivation. A .20 correlation is relatively low, but it may nevertheless be meaningful and useful.

The interpretation of a correlation coefficient is also a function of the size of the sample in which the relationship between the variables was calculated. The larger the sample, the smaller the coefficient that can be said to be "statistically significant." When a correlation is statistically significant, even though numerically low, it indicates an association that has a very low probability of arising on the basis of chance alone. When this probability is less than, say, 5% (or $p < .05$, as it is usually expressed), we are inclined to infer that the association (relationship) between the variables exists in the population; the variables are then assumed to be related. In other words, suppose we observe that intrinsic faith and the likelihood of having a religious mystical experience are positively correlated (e.g., .40). If the sample is large enough to show that this is a statistically significant correlation coefficient, we are likely to infer that the more one is intrinsically religious, the greater the chance that a person will have had or will have a religious mystical experience.

Finally, we must state that if a correlation is not statistically significant, the two variables are considered to be "independent" of each other; that is, they evidence a correlation that for all practical purposes is equal to 0. No meaningful relationship is said to exist.

Factor Analysis

"Factor analysis" is a useful tool in deciding whether several variables measure a single construct or different things. Let us assume that we have administered six religious motivation items to 100 people. Should we keep the items separate, or should we add them together to give a single score for each person? Adding them together would give us a more simple description, but would we lose valuable information? Factor analysis might give us the answer.

Let us also assume that we have a large set of items. A subset of the items might intercorrelate well among themselves, but these questions might correlate little with those constituting another set that shows high correlations among its variables. For illustrative purposes, let us assume that the items in the first set are variations on the theme "I pray to commune with God." For that reason, factor analysis might group them together, and we could label the set Intrinsic Religious Motivation. We would conclude that being intrinsically motivated leads to the responses on these items.

As for the second group of intercorrelated variables, which correlates poorly with the first set, we could group them together as well. A typical item is "I am religious so I can meet nice people." We might call these items Extrinsic Social Religious Motivation, for the motivation producing these responses is extrinsic to religion and revolves around a social benefit that can be gained from acting as if one were religious.

In this example, we have identified two factors of religious motivation, Intrinsic and Extrinsic Social, and we can measure each by scoring its items.

Factor analysis is a statistical procedure that does mathematically what we have just done logically. It groups together those variables that correlate most highly and calls their common element a factor. If there are several sets of items that can be represented by several factors, then factor analysis does so.

Factor analysis is used primarily in scale development to identify which items are sufficiently alike so that they might be scored together as an inventory and other items that might be tallied similarly for another scale. Obviously, if we have two variables, we have one correlation; if we have three variables, we have three intercorrelations. Given n variables, the formula $n(n-1)/2$ tells us how many correlation coefficients there will be. Fifty items produces a table with 1,225 correlations. Examining 1,225 correlations to subjectively identify which go together and should be considered a factor would produce more eyestrain and headaches than factors.

Fortunately, today we have computers to do the complex calculations that explain the large numbers of correlations through a much smaller number of underlying factors. It is possible that five or six factors might result from the analysis of the 1,225 correlations among the 50 variables noted above. This approach was used by many of the researchers whose various dimensions of religion are discussed throughout the text.

A major danger in factor analysis lies in grouping together variables from different domains. A "domain" consists of an area within which the psychological principles are expected to be the same. For example, "belief" (defined as the probability that a statement is true) differs from "affect" (defined as emotions). The phrase "The saints believe in God and rejoice; the Devil believes in God and shudders" shows how a conclusion in one domain (belief in God) does not always generalize to another (affect). Factoring different domains together mixes "apples and oranges." One historical example is Allport's Religious Orientation scale (Allport & Ross, 1967). It mixed items from several domains—for example, religious motivation as to why one prays, and behaviors such as participating in worship services. It could not, therefore, aid in understanding the relationship between domains of religious motivation and religious behavior. When correlations were found between this scale and another variable, no one could tell whether it was associated with religious motivation for prayer, or worshipping, or both. (If both correlations and factor analysis are new topics for you, mark these sections and refer to them later when the discussion uses one of these constructs.)

Reliability and Validity

As noted in the chapter text, there must be some assurance that psychology-of-religion measures really accomplish what they are intended to. We have briefly alluded to the two criteria of "validity" and "reliability."

Unfortunately, there are some very basic arguments about the possible discrepancy between "real life" and what the inventories tell us. Though we are unable to respond to this issue in detail, we do have reason to believe that questionnaires usually get at the information researchers seek. This last inference deals with the concept of validity: Does the test measure what it is supposed to measure?

Probably the best way of determining this is by employing the test to confirm what theory says it should confirm.

Validity presupposes reliability—namely, consistency in the measure's assessment. This consistency may occur over time, or over the test items when the scale has been administered only once. Do they all measure the same thing? If a test is reliable, it may still not be valid, but not vice versa. Reliability has been termed "poor person's validity." If one cannot demonstrate reliability, the questionnaire must be invalid, so this is a good place to start. (Though we refer primarily to questionnaires in this discussion, the other procedures mentioned in the chapter text may also yield reliability coefficients.)

Reliability and validity can be evaluated by a variety of statistical procedures akin to correlation, so we may speak of reliability and validity coefficients. For the former, we would like these to be above .75, but for research purposes sometimes we go as low as .60, and then try to find out how to improve scale reliability. For example, we may write more items, or edit and improve those in use. There are no guidelines for the size of validity coefficients. We simply start by hoping to have these attain statistical significance, and the higher they are, the better.

When we have a questionnaire that demonstrates good reliability, we term it a "scale." This generally refers to a set of items that are summed to give a score for that scale. But this label has other meanings in mathematics and the social sciences, so the interested reader should look to other sources and references for further information. Here we are concerned with the realm of "psychometrics," which treats issues of psychological measurement such as those just mentioned.

We have just touched on a few statistical and psychometric concepts among many that are pertinent to work in our area. To be a psychologist, especially an empirical researcher, means that one must become familiar with a wide variety of other statistical concepts and procedures. It is our hope that our presentations in this volume will not be too abstruse and difficult. You may want to make a list of psychometric and statistical terms that appear in these pages, and check them out in greater depth than we can do here.

Chapter 2

FOUNDATIONS FOR AN EMPIRICAL PSYCHOLOGY OF RELIGION

> Without knowledge of self there is no knowledge of God.
>
> That's God's signature. God's signature is never a forgery.
>
> . . . like most Americans, my faith consists in believing in every religion, including my own, but without ill-will toward anybody, no matter what he believes or disbelieves.
>
> Religion is different from everything else; because in religion seeking is finding.
>
> Man without religion is the creature of circumstances.[1]

EXAMINING RELIGION EMPIRICALLY

Since its earliest days, psychology has examined religion. In 1902, William James—a U.S. philosopher and one of the founders of our field—gave his famous Gifford Lectures at the University of Edinburgh. These were soon published in book form as *The Varieties of Religious Experience* (James, 1902/1985; see also Gorsuch & Spilka, 1987). This work is a candidate for the most successful book in the history of psychology, since it has been continuously in print for over 100 years!

The success of James's *Varieties* lies in several features that guide our discussions in this book. First is the question of the nature of religion, compared to such concepts as psychic phenomena and superstition. For instance, James wrote books and papers on both religion and psychic phenomena; what distinguishes them? Second is the question of whether religion is a help or a hindrance; that is, does the good it brings outweigh the harm that can be associated with it? These questions are as much a part of the scientific study of religion today as they were in 1902.

Each of these issues is discussed throughout this text. For example, the nature of religion has been touched on already in Chapter 1, especially in regard to the recent emergence of a preference for the term "spirituality." The second question—that of whether religion improves human relationships or creates prejudices and other problems that harm rela-

---

1. These quotations come, respectively, from the following sources: John Calvin, quoted in Kunkel, Cook, Meshel, Daughtry, and Hauenstein (1999, p. 193); Eddie Joe Lloyd, quoted in the online version of *The New York Times* (August 26, 2002); Saroyan (1937, p. 130); Cather (1926/1990, p. 94); and Julian Charles Hare and Augustus William Hare, quoted in *The Oxford Dictionary of Quotations* (1959, p. 237, No. 19).

tionships—is considered in a number of the chapters that follow. In the present chapter, however, we focus first on separating religion from other concepts that are often considered similar. We then examine dimensional and social-psychological approaches to the study of religion, and consider some other issues that are basic to establishing the foundations for an empirical psychology of religion.

DISTINGUISHING RELIGION FROM OTHER CONCEPTS

In Chapter 1, we have avoided defining religion. Still, it needs to be distinguished from other, possibly overlapping concepts. Such distinctions allow us to deal in a more focused fashion with theory and empirical research in the psychology of religion. James's *The Varieties of Religious Experience* provides us with an entrée into this realm. He viewed religion as most laypeople might, without possessing any special information about it. As James saw it, religion mainly involves beliefs about "ultimate reality" and our relationship to it. "Ultimate" has been popularly and commonly defined in terms of a final referent—a God or gods—or the realm of religious institutions and their representatives.

Although James's *Varieties* works from traditional descriptions of religion, James did not confine himself to studying religion as thus defined. He also investigated, and published work on, psychic phenomena. In this portion of the chapter, both psychic phenomena and superstition are considered in relation to religion.

Psychic Phenomena

James's researches in psychic phenomena (e.g., foretelling the future, reading cards, numerology, astrology, psychokinesis, etc.) culminated in a collection of letters, essays, and book reviews on reports of such non-natural behaviors and occurrences (Schmeidler, 1992). He also discussed extrasensory perception, dissociation (e.g., automatic writing, in which one hand writes while the person apparently does not know what is being written), and communication with spirits (see Murphy & Ballou, 1960). In these essays, James's strong commitments to data are evident. He sought facts instead of speculation, and was highly critical of scientists who simply assume that psychic phenomena do not occur. He was equally skeptical of those who believe that they do occur because someone claims they do. Based on his lifelong search for evidence of psychic phenomena, he concluded that almost all such events have naturalistic explanations. Nevertheless, he continued to feel that, given the number of people who claim to have had psychic experiences, there must be some degree of truth in these reports. In other words, consensual agreement—an unscientific and nonempirical criterion—was accepted by James.

One of the areas for which James felt some explanations could be proposed was dissociation. As noted above, dissociation includes automatic writing; it also includes posthypnotic suggestion and other acts and words that a person performs or says without conscious awareness. Central to his thinking about these phenomena was the importance of the subconscious (which he suggested causes them), along with a cosmic consciousness, a reflection of a universal mind over all people (which may also be involved).

James did consistently note the problem of duplicity. That is, he found that psychic mediums and similar individuals distorted their experiences and cheated extensively. What James eventually accepted, however, was thin evidence based upon equally thin assertions that there may have been an occasional valid event in so much material.

In this framework, religion appears distinct from psychic phenomena. Extrasensory perception, dissociative events, and communication with spirits via mediums are rare in religion. Despite an undeniably overlapping border between psychic claims and religious experiences, a number of differences are evident. The psychic realm is totally individualistic, highly transitory, magically loose in its structure, antithetical to reason, and lacking in historical-cultural foundation. In addition, psychic claims are usually considered morally irrelevant and unalterably opposed to scientific investigation. Their nature makes them unreliable and hence invalid in the sense discussed in Chapter 1. James's own belief was that religion is valid because it changes people's lives, whereas psychic phenomena, if they exist at all, have dubious effects and therefore remain of questionable validity.

Superstition

A "superstition" has been defined as "any belief or attitude, based on fear or ignorance, that is inconsistent with the known laws of science or with what is generally considered in the particular society as true and rational; esp., such a belief in charms, omens, the supernatural, etc." (Guralnik, 1986, p. 1430). A superstitious person is one who acts on such beliefs. Examples of superstitious actions include walking under a ladder, avoiding the number 13, and tugging on one's cap before throwing a pitch in a ball game.

These examples of superstition contain nothing that is called religious or spiritual. But does the "superstition" label properly extend to religion as studied by psychology? *The Oxford Universal Dictionary on Historical Principles* (Onions, 1955) includes in its definition: "esp. in connection with religion" (p. 2084). This definition explicitly links the two concepts, but it also distinguishes between superstition and religion, since the two realms are not equated with each other.

One basis of superstition can be found in learning research. Though this type of research was originally conducted on animals by the noted psychologist B. F. Skinner (1948, 1969), superstition is obviously present in humans and may occur in one-trial learning, particularly with strong negative reinforcement (Morris & Maisto, 1998). Primarily when threat, pain, or much emotion is present, and is then resolved, irrelevant stimuli present in the situation become meaningful. For example, let us suppose that an athlete was wearing a specific pair of socks when a problem was alleviated; hence they become his "lucky socks," which he wears just in case they might make a difference in future similar circumstances. The athlete knows full well that there is no rational basis for the lucky socks to affect the game, but he just feels better when wearing them. Of course, if success occurs, the incident will be cited as proof of the superstition's truth.

It is not surprising that some religious behaviors are also superstitious for a particular person. They meet the twin conditions of being nonrational and of avoiding a major negative outcome (i.e., being based in fear). We must, however, ask whether religion is superstition.

Most religion does not meet the conditions of superstition. Whether right or wrong, religions usually have well-developed theologies that make religious behaviors rational, at least to those who hold them. The threat of avoiding a major negative outcome also seldom enters into daily religious behavior. Furthermore, the promise of hell is unlikely to take hold after one-trial learning. The idea of hell requires much complex social learning, plus both cognitive and motivational inputs. Later it will be shown that the subculture in which one is raised is a major determinant of religious behavior in general. Although religion includes conditioned responses, it is far more than just these responses, in that much social learning may be involved and may even be influenced indirectly by genetic and evolutionary factors. These factors are detailed in Chapter 3.

Research Comparing Psychic Phenomena and Superstition to Religion

As a science, the psychology of religion is quite interested in data comparing psychic phenomena and superstition to religion itself. If religion involves the same psychological processes as the other two concepts, then either of two conditions must be met. First, those who believe most strongly in psychic manifestations or who are most superstitious should also be the most religious. In other words, positive correlations would be predicted between measures of religion on the one hand, and measures of superstition and psychic beliefs on the other. The second condition under which psychic phenomena, superstition, and religion can be psychologically theorized to be identical is if they answer the same needs. Perhaps fears of the future can be lessened through consulting a psychic, through superstition, or through religion. Theoretically, then, if one had superstitions, one would not need religion. This view predicts a negative correlation between religion and these other phenomena. Of course, if different needs are met by these phenomena or if different psychological processes are involved, then negative correlations should also be observed among them.

Research has included questions and statements about beliefs in all three areas. An entire pool of items reflecting belief in psychic phenomena, superstitions, and religion is factored (see Chapter 1). There are three possible outcomes. If items from two or more areas load on the same factor, then the data support the contention that these two areas are "functionally the same." If the items from two of the areas load in the opposite direction on the same factor or form two separate factors that are negatively correlated, then the "substitution" theory cannot be rejected. (It is not, however, directly supported, because religion may prevent the development of psychic or superstitious beliefs, just as we hope a good college education will decrease irrational beliefs.) If the religious items load on a separate, uncorrelated factor, the "functionally the same" and "substitution" theories would both be unsupported.

Studies are few in this area, and further work is necessary. Johnston, de Groot, and Spanos (1995) have factored a set of items representing the constructs discussed above. They found separate factors for the paranormal, superstition, extraordinary life forms, and religion; these results counter the "functionally the same" hypothesis. Sparks's (2001) review of work in this area confirms the distinctiveness noted by Johnston et al. (1995). Goode (2000), however, claims that there may be paranormal elements in certain religious concepts (e.g., creationism, angels, the Devil), and provides data to this effect.

Contrary to the "substitution" hypothesis is Hynam's (1970) finding that superstition correlated positively with a lack of clear social norms or rules, while both religiousness and scientific training were negatively related.

These data suggest three conclusions. First, a definition of superstition that does not mention religion is more accurate than a definition that does. Second, James was correct in writing separately on religious and psychic phenomena. Third, psychologists of religion in general, and we authors of this book in particular, are investigating neither psychic phenomena nor superstition per se. Of course, superstition and psychic reports occur in almost all areas of life, and occur among religious people as well. They are, however, peripheral to the psychology of religion.

HOW IS RELIGIOUSNESS DEFINED IN
THE PSYCHOLOGY OF RELIGION?

If superstition and psychic phenomena are not part of the psychology of religion, then what is included in this discipline? To answer this question, we first discuss several dimensional approaches that have been used in past research to provide both broad and narrow definitions of various areas of religion. Logical, logical–empirical, and factor-analytic approaches are all discussed. Another method of defining the psychology of religion is to consider it in relation to the major areas of psychology. How do social psychology, abnormal psychology, or developmental psychology treat religion? In this chapter, we concentrate on the social-psychological approach.

DIMENSIONAL APPROACHES TO RELIGIOUSNESS

The human passion to be efficient, to summarize the complex, to wrap it all up in "25 words or less," is often an enemy to real understanding. Words are symbols that place many things under one heading, and the term "religion" is an excellent example of this tendency. When psychologists first began research in this area, they simply constructed measures of religiousness or religiosity. Sophisticated thinkers, however, soon put aside notions that people simply vary along a single dimension with antireligious sentiments at one end and orthodox views at the other end. These proved unsatisfactory, and many new sets of dimensions—some covering a broad range, some narrower in their focus—began to appear in the research literature.

When we examine the many dimensional schemes that have been proposed, we see that some stress the purpose of faith, whereas others look to the possible personal and social origins of religion. Although some appear to mix psychology and religion, there are also those that take their cues exclusively from psychology and focus on motivation or cognition. However, the real problem is twofold: the presence of a "hidden" value agenda that implies "good" and "bad" religion, and a lack of conceptual and theoretical clarity. There is also great overlap among the various proposals, with essentially the same idea being phrased in different words—testimony to the excellent vocabularies of some social scientists. There is, however, one point on which all agree: namely, that even though there is only one word for "religion," there may be a hundred possible ways of being "religious."

Logical Approaches

Some dimensional approaches to religiousness are logically derived; that is, they are based on concepts and ideas derived from induction. In other words, some theorists have observed and thought logically about religion, and from their many observations, they suggest what its multifaceted essence is. One particularly wide-ranging, comprehensive logical system of understanding religion is that proposed by Glock (1962), a well-known sociologist of religion. This system identifies and measures the following areas of religion (all quotes are from Glock, 1962, p. S99):

• *Experiential dimension*: "Religious people will . . . achieve direct knowledge of ultimate reality or will experience religious emotion."

- *Ideological dimension*: "The religious person will hold to certain beliefs."
- *Ritualistic dimension*: "Specifically religious practices [are] expected of religious adherents."
- *Intellectual dimension*: "The religious person will be informed and knowledgeable about the basic tenets of his faith and its sacred scriptures."
- *Consequential dimension*: This covers "what people ought to do and the attitudes they ought to hold as a consequence of their religion."

The inclusion of ritual ties Glock's system to anthropology and psychology, as well as sociology. Also, the Ideological dimension is separated from the Intellectual, since religious adherents always hold a set of beliefs but may or may not be knowledgeable about the details of the faith.

In addition to Glock's dimensions, it is possible to develop sets of logically derived psychological categories for understanding religion. One system for doing so would separate the personal from the interpersonal. This system is narrower in its focus than that of Glock, but it can be highly useful when detail on religious practices is desired. Because religion is at the same time unique to each person and yet part of a community, religion can be subdivided within each of these two areas. Here is one possible breakdown of religious practices:

- Personal
  - Prayer
  - Reading of scriptures
  - Meditation
- Interpersonal
  - Worshiping with others
  - Committee participation
  - Receiving and providing social support

Examining Logical Systems Empirically

Logical systems such as Glock's (1962) and our categories of religious practices (see above) help to organize our thinking and research. Although they are obviously useful, how they relate to each other is an empirical question. Proponents of a more empirical approach note that logical approaches to understanding religion may have poor psychometric properties. Glock's dimensions as described above are a good example. Although the *logic* distinguishing Experiential from Consequential is clear, *empirically* the two are strongly related (Faulkner & DeJong, 1966; Weigert & Thomas, 1969). This is true of all the categories—they correlate highly with each other. Statistically, then, one only needs to measure one or two, because the same conclusions will be reached regardless of which dimension is used. For instance, a person who has a religious experience is therefore likely to be concerned with the consequences of adhering to the faith.

Similar objections can be raised to the logically derived system of religious practices we have described. If a person engages in one personal category of religious behavior, it is quite likely that this person utilizes the other personal practices. And if the person engages in an interpersonal category of religious behavior, he or she probably also employs other interpersonal practices.

Logical–Empirical Approaches

Logical approaches can evolve into systems that blend the logical and the empirical. This is what happened to a system proposed by Gordon Allport (1959, 1966). In attempting to understand prejudice, he noted that some Christians, in keeping with the Christian tenets of love toward all, are less prejudiced than non-Christians. He also noted, however, that some Christians are more prejudiced than other Christians, even though this is in violation of Christian doctrines of love. To explain this difference, Allport suggested that some are Christian for the sake of the faith itself, and thus are "intrinsically" committed. They try to live in accordance with Christian doctrines. Others are Christian for what they can personally get out of it; these "extrinsically" committed Christians pick what they need and ignore the rest, such as the teachings on loving others. Allport called these "religious orientations" and saw them as opposite ends of an Intrinsic–Extrinsic (abbreviated here as I-E) continuum. Others developed similar constructs, including Allen and Spilka's (1967) Committed versus Consensual scales, and Batson's Internal versus External scales (Batson & Ventis, 1982).

Christians and others do have an immediate question about Allport's placing I and E as opposites. For example, one item on a scale of religiousness may state that God answers prayers; another item may state that prayer is for communion with God. The former item is E, in the sense that an extrinsic benefit is gained from being Christian (e.g., the answered prayer might provide a higher income, a desire extrinsic to the prayer itself). The wish for communion is I, since there is no benefit extrinsic to the prayer experience itself. Christians have always held that both E and I experiences are benefits—a point also made by Pargament (1992). Allport recognized this, but he was not interested in multiple benefits. He was concerned with what people saw as the main goal. So each item of Allport's I-E scales contains a phrase such as "the only reason" or "the main reason." This permits investigation of what is most central to a person's religiousness. Without such qualifiers, we would not be able to identify those who report receiving intrinsic benefits, and who also feel they are privy to extrinsic benefits as well (Gorsuch, Mylvaganan, Gorsuch, & Johnson, 1997). With verbal qualifiers such as Allport's, people choose what they consider to be the central reason for being religious.

Empirical research develops constructs in ways that are not always predictable. In research on I versus E as opposite ends of a continuum, a problem soon arose: E items did not correlate strongly negatively with I items, which they should do if I and E are opposites. Even the wording "the only reason" was not sufficient for people to treat I and E as mutually exclusive (people are not bound by logic). The wording did keep the scales from correlating positively. Allport and Ross (1967) then modified their stance from I versus E as the ends of a single dimension, to I and E as two distinct dimensions, each with its own separate set of items. Although I and E were clearly distinct, there was, and generally continues to be, a low negative correlation between the I and E scales.

Batson and Ventis (1982) still felt that the I-E distinction was insufficient, as it did not fulfill the requirements for which it was originally proposed. Allport suggested that even intrinsically religious people would be prejudiced if they felt that religion was closed and exclusionary, but that they would be less judgmental if they saw religion as an open quest. So he added a Quest dimension, which is empirically distinct from both I and E (Batson & Ventis, 1982). People who are intrinsically committed to their faith should be as likely as not to view it as an ongoing quest. To date, this has been shown to be true.

In 1989, Kirkpatrick discovered one reason why the original E scale had low internal-consistency reliability: It was composed of two different ways of being religious for extrinsic reasons. One is that of receiving a *personal* benefit, such as comfort in times of stress for an answered prayer. This has been labeled Extrinsic Personal (Ep). The other form is *social* and focuses on the people with whom one associates when participating in the religion. This might further mean making them friends, and has been termed Extrinsic Social (Es).

By the 1980s and 1990s, it was evident that the widely used 1967 versions of the Allport–Ross I-E scales needed revisions. The E dimension was shown to be complex, and the reliability of the original scale was low. The thoroughness of the E scale was also questioned. Gorsuch et al. (1997) asked students in Hawaii, a multicultural and multireligious setting, to suggest reasons for being religious. The items were then statistically analyzed in several cultures, and the I, Ep, and Es factors were replicated. They also found suggestions of other extrinsic factors, primarily one for Extrinsic Morality (Em), in which one is moral because it is utilitarian to be moral. Em describes a facet of one's religious motivations as stemming from religion's decision-making moral basis. A common moral base for a culture is also a part of this construct, and supports a religious–moral stance.

Obviously the concepts of I and E have developed considerably since Allport's original formulation, which is now primarily of historical interest. Not only have the concepts changed; we also know more about what other variables I and E relate to and what they do not relate to (see later chapters). This is typical of the cumulative nature of science.

Many researchers besides Allport and his colleagues have taken combined logical–empirical approaches to defining dimensions of religion. A sampling of the results is given in Table 2.1.

Factor-Analytic Approaches

One method of identifying the dimensions that are needed is to employ factor analysis. As noted in Chapter 1, factor analysis distinguishes the basic dimensions within a set of variables, with "basic" being defined by high correlations among the variables within dimensions, and low correlations between dimensions.

Factor analysis has several critical points that we need to note. First, the variables must be assessed systematically with a clearly defined sample. They must also be pertinent and relevant to the issue studied; sampling of a hodge-podge of variables results in a hodge-podge of factors. Moreover, factor analysis provides a view of the variables that is solely determined by the correlations among them. In particular, the factors themselves may or may not be correlated. This is important for religion, because so many of the constructs within religion are related to each other. Clearly, one must determine whether the factors are correlated.

Even though some of the dimensions listed in Table 2.1 were finally established via factor analysis, factor-analytic approaches were more fully undertaken in three attempts to understand the way people conceptualize God. Table 2.2 illustrates these attempts.

The three patterns of concepts/images of God shown in Table 2.2 suggest the variation that can result when different methods of analysis and different content are used to describe God. The statistical complexity of these advanced procedures might convince unsophisticated people of their total objectivity; however, subjectivity is always present and can affect such methods (Horn, 1967). For example, one has to decide on criteria for stopping the extraction of factors or select a minimum size for a factor loading to be meaningful. In sum, there are few simple answers to the problem of describing God or any other religious concept to which these analyses are applied.

TABLE 2.1. Some Logically and Empirically Derived Dimensional Approaches to the Study of Individual Religion

Allen and Spilka (1967)	
Committed religion	"Utilizes an abstract philosophical perspective: multiplex religious ideas are relatively clear in meaning and an open and flexible framework of commitment relates religion to daily activities" (p. 205).
Consensual religion	"Vague, nondifferentiated, bifurcated, neutralized" (p. 205). A cognitively simplified and personally convenient faith.
Batson and Ventis (1982)	
Means religion	"Religion is a means to other self-serving ends than religion itself" (p. 151).
End religion	"Religion is an ultimate end in itself" (p. 151).
Clark (1958)	
Primary religious behavior	"An authentic inner experience of the divine combined with whatever efforts the individual may make to harmonize his life with the divine" (p. 23).
Secondary religious behavior	"A very routine and uninspired carrying out . . . of an obligation" (p. 24).
Tertiary religious behavior	"A matter of religious routine or convention accepted on the authority of someone else" (p. 25).
Fromm (1950)	
Authoritarian religion	"The main virtue of this type of religion is obedience, its cardinal sin is disobedience" (p. 35).
Humanistic religion	"This type of religion is centered around man and his strength . . . virtue is self-realization, not obedience" (p. 37).
Hunt (1972)	
Literal religion	Taking "at face value any religious statement without in any way questioning it" (p. 43).
Antiliteral religion	A simple rejection of literalist religious statements.
Mythological religion	A reinterpretation of religious statements to seek their deeper symbolic meanings.
James (1902/1985)	
Healthy-mindedness	An optimistic, happy, extroverted, social faith: "the tendency that looks on all things and sees that they are good" (p. 78).
Sick souls	"The way that takes all this experience of evil as something essential" (p. 36). A faith of pessimism, sorrow, suffering, and introverted reflection.
Lenski (1961)	
Doctrinal orthodoxy	"Stresses intellectual assent [to] prescribed doctrines" (p. 23).
Devotionalism	"Emphasizes the importance of private, or personal communion with God" (p. 23).
McConahay & Hough (1973)	
Guilt-oriented, extrapunitive	"Religious belief . . . centered on the wrath of God as it is related to other people . . . emphasizes punishment for wrong-doers" (p. 55).
Guilt-oriented, intropunitive	"A sense of one's own unworthiness and badness . . . a manifest need for punishment and a conviction that it will inevitably come" (p. 56).
Love-oriented, self-centered	"Oriented toward the forgiveness of one's own sins" (p. 56).
Love-oriented, other-centered	"Emphasizes the common humanity of all persons as creatures of God, and God's love . . . related to the redemption of the whole world" (p. 56).
Culture-oriented, conventional	"Values . . . are more culturally than theologically oriented" (p. 56).

TABLE 2.2. Factorial Conceptualizations of God from Adjective Ratings

Spilka, Armatas, and Nussbaum (1964): Factor analysis

Positive God[a]	*Harsh God*	*Omni-God*
Considerate	Damning	Omnipotent
Comforting	Punishing	Omnipresent
Helpful	Avenging	Omniscient
Warm	Jealous	All-wise
Benevolent Ruler	*Impersonal God*	*Formal Ruler*
Just	Impersonal	Formal
Blessed	Distant	Democratic
Kind	Inaccessible	Firm
Sovereign	Mythical	Unchanging
Timeless Father	*Supreme Ruler*	*Psalmist's God*
Eternal	Kingly	Gentle
Everlasting	Majestic	Guiding
Holy	Glorious	Forgiving
Redeeming	Divine	Loving

Gorsuch (1968): Hierarchical factor analysis

Third-order factor:

Traditional Christian
(a very large factor)
Glorious, Strong, Matchless, Majestic, etc.

Second-order factors:

Benevolent Deity	*Companionable*
All-wise	Warm
Forgiving	Fair
Loving	Faithful
Redeeming	Considerate

Primary factors:[b]

Kindliness	*Wrathfulness*	*Deisticness*
Kind	Severe	Inaccessible
Merciful	Wrathful	Impersonal
Gentle	Hard	Distant
Forgiving	Avenging	Mythical
Omni-ness	*Evaluation*	*Eternality*
Omnipresent	Valuable	Everlasting
Omniscient	Timely	Eternal
Omnipotent	Vigorous	Divine
Infinite	Important	Holy

Kunkel et al. (1999): Concept analysis, multidimensional scaling, and cluster analysis[c]

Dimensions:

Nurturant vs. *Punitive*
Mystical vs. *Anthropomorphic*

Concept clusters:[d]

Vengeful	*Human Roles*	*Regulating*
Life-taking	Family members	Ruler
Unfair	Judge	Lawmaker
Punishing	Teacher	Guide
Hates evil	Man/Woman	Messiah

continued

TABLE 2.2. *continued*

Mysterious	*Powerful*	*Inspirational*
Mysterious	Superior	Inspirational
Logical	Powerful	Exciting
Simple	Strong	Amazing
Spiritual	Everlasting	Charming
Benevolent		
Forgiving		
Wonderful		
Unselfish		
Welcoming		

[a]The top four loaded adjectives are presented for all factors in all studies. This selection was used in later test construction.

[b]Eleven factors are given, but only the six most pertinent and comparable are given here.

[c]Cluster analysis may use any of a wide number of measures of similarity among variables. These measures are "clustered" or grouped by the researcher, and criteria are selected that maximize the relationships among the variables within a cluster and minimize those between the clusters. Factor analysis, as described in Chapter 1, starts with correlations, measures of relationships among the variables. It has been called "a refined cluster analysis" (Guertin & Bailey, 1970, p. 14).

[d]These descriptive terms are simply selected from a number within each cluster to illustrate the concept as well as possible.

A PERSPECTIVE FROM PSYCHOLOGY: SOCIAL PSYCHOLOGY

The structure of psychology is not as logically organized as introductory psychology texts often imply. Although there are specific subfields within psychology, psychologists from different subfields are often concerned with what turn out to be the same processes. Though we look at areas such as developmental psychology and abnormal psychology (among others) later in this volume, here we concentrate on social psychology.

The psychology of religion falls primarily within social psychology in general, and within the domain of individual differences in particular (Dittes, 1969). Social psychology studies the person in the social context. Because religiousness varies from one person to another, the psychology of religion stresses the individual-variability aspect of social psychology. The person's own attitudes and behavior are studied as dependent and independent variables. Social psychology further examines how independent variables, such as religiousness, affect people and their relationships with others. Much of this research is devoted to social-cognitive processes, particularly attributions. In Chapter 1, we have discussed the making of attributions as an important part of the search for meaning—a core theme in our framework for the psychology of religion. The attribution process is described in further detail, following the discussion of individual differences.

Individual Differences

Traditionally, social psychology sees the domain of individual differences as having three subdomains within it; these are the realms of "cognition," "affect," and "behavior." To these three, we add "habit." Cognition is primarily concerned with beliefs and how they are learned—in other words, how the ideological aspect of religion is conceptualized. The affective realm emphasizes feelings and attitudes—the emotional, "like–dislike" facet of belief or behavior. Behavior, of course, consists of what people do, how they act. Finally, habit stresses what one does regularly and consistently. These brief descriptions are expanded upon below. The psychology of religion looks at individual religious differences within each of these areas. Items representing these subdomains are exemplified in Table 2.3. The first illustration in the cognitive area uses a response format that emphasizes the definition of the subdomain, mostly here belief. The second illustration uses a common response format that emphasizes belief but includes an element of affect—namely, value, which we discuss below. This distinction is not made for the other subdomains.

The concept of "attitude" is ambiguous. Standard social psychology texts use "attitudes" to refer to a domain that unites cognition and affect with the potential of producing behav-

---

TABLE 2.3. Illustrations of Items Assessing Aspects of Cognition, Affect, Habit, and Behavior

Cognition

Belief
1. Rate what you feel are the "odds" (%) that God exists.
   There is no God 0 25 50 75 100 God definitely exists

Value
2. God exists.
   Strongly disagree 1 2 3 4 5 Strongly agree

Belief
3. Rate how important attending church weekly is.
   Unimportant 1 2 3 4 5 Important

Value
4. Everyone should attend church each week.
   Strongly disagree 1 2 3 4 5 Strongly agree

Affect (attitudes)

Belief
5. Rate how much you enjoy worship services.
   Not at all 1 2 3 4 5 Very much

Value
6. I enjoy worship services.
   Strongly disagree 1 2 3 4 5 Strongly agree

Habit

7. How long have you had your current pattern of church attendance?
   a. 1 year or less
   b. 1–2 years
   c. 3–4 years
   d. 5 years or more

Behavior

8. How often do you attend church?
   a. Never
   b. A couple of times a year
   c. Once a month
   d. Several times a month
   e. Once a week
   f. More than once a week

ior. Research often uses the term in reference to affect or emotion toward an object, as in "positive attitude" to mean that a person likes something and "negative attitude" to mean that a person doesn't like it. "Value" is a more involved and somewhat conflicted concept, as it deals with the importance or worth to a person of an object, situation, or event. Rokeach (1968) called values "abstract ideals, positive or negative . . . representing a person's beliefs about ideal modes of conduct and ideal terminal goals" (p. 124). When we measure a person's orientation toward religion, beliefs, values, attitudes, behavior, and habits are all part of the total picture.

Because each subdomain has a different purpose, it is important to keep them distinct. Research can then identify the conditions under which they relate to each other. For example, Allport (1959) was interested in total religiousness based on both the I and E scores (Allport & Ross, 1967). He stressed affect or motivation in these orientations, and ignored cognition. Later versions of the I and E scales also dropped the behavioral items.

Cognition

The cognitive realm consists of the two subareas mentioned above, beliefs and values. Since these are a function of experience, usually with others (e.g., parents, friends, etc.), they imply that learning theory is the basis for psychological models of how one acquires religious beliefs. A major emphasis is on social learning theory—that is, how a person learns from others. This can range from watching someone model a particular belief to accepting a belief on the basis of another person's authority.

Cognitions are organized into "schemas," which are sets of interrelated beliefs and values. Because schemas are interrelated, people want the constructs to be consistent with one another. If they are not consistent, a person may compartmentalize them so that the inconsistency is no longer apparent. The person may, however, change one or more constructs to make them consistent.

Beliefs. To make sense of people's personal experiences, we need to know what they consider true—that is, their beliefs. Examples of beliefs include accepting the ideas that God did (or did not) create the world, that the Bible was dictated by God, or that one's fellow believers would be proud if they knew what one did.

Beliefs provide information about the physical and psychological surroundings to which people must adapt. They are "cognitive maps" of the reality through which individuals navigate to reach a goal. As cognitive maps, they do not in themselves provide motivation. Rather, beliefs are used as people become motivated to achieve some goal.

The concepts of God listed in Table 2.2 are beliefs. For example, people who agree with Gorsuch's (1968) Traditional Christian concept hold that God is primarily glorious, strong, matchless, majestic, and so on.

Beliefs are defined here solely as cognitive constructs. They do not contain emotions such as liking or disliking. The saying "the Devil believes in God [i.e., the Traditional Christian God] and shudders" shows the distinction between a belief and understanding the implication of that belief. It also suggests possible approval of that belief.

This is, of course, a narrow definition of "belief." Elsewhere in this text, the term is used more broadly. The phrase "believe in" includes thoughts as to what is true and implies a commitment as well. In the United States, to "believe in God" suggests to many people that one both believes God exists and is a follower—probably a joyful follower—of God.

This extends the idea of belief to the notion of assent. Belief as cognition is supplemented by motivation, implying commitment to the system of which individual beliefs are one aspect. Believers now become followers of a faith.

One can also believe in a variety of spirits, and do what is necessary to placate the spirits. We must keep in mind that beliefs plus assents are key components of attitudes. In other words, attitudes are composites of beliefs plus motivations to act in a certain way.

Values. Values are cognitive constructs of the good, and consist of the ideals, principles, and moral obligations held by an individual or group. Though values are not a central focus in social psychology, most social psychologists assume that they reflect beliefs with an element of affect, as noted earlier. To consider values broadens the definition of beliefs beyond the criterion of apparent truth. In this model, values are not a part of affect per se; however, they add to prediction over and above classical attitude scales in a wide range of situations (Gorsuch & Ortberg, 1983).

Values differ from beliefs in that they are motivational, which beliefs, in and of themselves, are not. Values acquire motivation when the observed belief describing "what is" differs from the valued situation of "what should be." In Table 2.3, the belief that God exists is treated as a probability, a likelihood. When value alone is considered, there is no doubt: "God exists." This follows from God's existence being regarded as the ideal state of affairs. Again, note that values are also part of attitude scales (see Table 2.2).

Affect

Affect is the emotional response to an object or situation. "Object or situation" is defined broadly here; it may be a particular place of worship or a contemplated action. We are concerned with how the person feels about the independent and objective "object or situation." We are also concerned with operationalizing that element of emotion by checking how a person responds to it (see Table 2.2). The presence of feeling implies that values are involved. This kind of affect is what most attitude scales measure. Affect is developed by classical conditioning. If a neutral object is associated with something that is very pleasant, then the neutral object is also judged to be pleasant. For example, a person may associate a particular religious setting with a reassuring feeling of being close to God; the setting then comes to provide a reassuring feeling by itself.

Technically, affect includes the whole range of emotions (fear, delight, awe, disgust, etc.). So far, research on human emotions has had little impact on the psychology of religion, and vice versa. A disproportionate emphasis has been placed on cognition, but slowly social psychology is increasingly stressing the association of belief with affect. Although future research will round out the area, affect is currently just measured as positive and negative.

Habit

Beliefs, values, and affect all have an impact on a decision. When the same choice/question arises several times, a person remembers the decision that was previously made. Unless the person perceives that something has changed, he or she can just use the prior decision and do the same thing again. Instead of "reinventing the wheel" every time people encounter familiar situations, they develop habits. This is very effective, for if they did not develop habits, every act would need to be consciously evaluated.

Habits extend over a long time. They can be developed in childhood and carried into adulthood. They can lie dormant because the situation calling them forth does not occur, only to be activated once again when the same situation recurs. Much religious behavior is habitual.

One important and unique aspect of a habit is its relationship to beliefs, values, and affects. Whereas the original behavior leading to a habit may be based on an explicit decision based on a person's beliefs, values, and affects, the habit itself replaces thinking. In the early stages of a habit, reasoning remains accessible. As time passes, the rationale for the habit tends to be forgotten, and the reasoning becomes increasingly inaccessible. This means that the behavior may be carried on even if the situation changes in ways the person does not perceive. The original reasoning may not apply in new circumstances.

People are born into social orders in which religion already exists and is both formally and informally learned. Religious behavior can be reinforced by parents, friends, and society, so many people express their faith habitually and mechanically. Parents teach it to their children, and these lessons are further reinforced by society through the fact that births, marriages, deaths, and most other noteworthy personal and cultural/societal/communal events are solemnized by religious institutions, rituals, language, and concepts.

Behavior

Behavior results from multiple variables. These include cognitive (belief and value) and affective components. In utility and reasoned-action models, behavior is a function of both. In reasoned-action models (e.g., Fishbein & Ajzen, 1975), belief pertains to the consequences that follow actions. As we have mentioned in Chapter 1, the local religion in Thailand teaches that there is a spirit associated with a piece of land. If the spirit is somehow offended, the building on that land or the people in it will have bad luck. To prevent this, a Thai person builds a spirit house on the property. This behavior depends on a belief that such action will appease the spirit, and that it is valuable to do so. Positive affect will also result from erecting a spirit house, ranging from relief of fear to pride from building an attractive spirit house. The following equation is a typical way of including the elements just noted:

$$\text{Behavior} = (\text{Belief} \times \text{Value}) + (\text{Belief} \times \text{Affect}) + \text{Habit}$$

This assumes that belief, value, and affect are all measured with a true zero. When any one of the elements in the equation is zero, then that part of the equation drops out, regardless of the other values. If a person does not believe that a spirit house will appease the spirits of the land, then it makes no difference to build one, regardless of whether appeasing the spirits is seen as valuable or generates positive affect. In like manner, if value, affect, or habit is zero, this will eliminate it from the equation.

In addition to beliefs, values, and affect, behaviors are influenced by a host of other variables, including situational constraints. For example, an adolescent's church attendance may be more a function of that adolescent's parents' beliefs, values, and affect toward the church than of the adolescent's. If the whole family attends church, then the adolescent goes. The teenager's presence at services is an example of situational constraints that affect religious behavior.

Advantages of the Multivariate Individual-Differences Model

The overall individual-differences model just proposed is helpful because each of the areas (e.g., beliefs, affects, etc.) functions by different psychological means. Beliefs are developed by the principles of cognition and learning theory; different places of worship provide information for a variety of beliefs. These include a whole host of data, including the congregants' degree of liberalism or conservatism, their style of worship, and a variety of demographic characteristics. We would be able to build a cognitive map of these places of worship.

Religious affects either result from direct emotion that is immediately elicited, or are learned through classical conditioning. Direct emotions often occur in worship services and become components of religious experience. These can include awe, forgiveness, a feeling of belonging, and the warmth of being accepted by those with the same beliefs and values. Other emotions become associated with specific situations and behaviors through classical conditioning. For instance, particular songs may later bring back pleasant memories, as the desirable emotions associated with those songs in past situations are attached to the songs themselves.

Value and affect should be positively related. One normally enjoys maximizing a value, and this distinction permits exploration of intrapsychic conflicts about religion. Those who place a high value on religious behavior but do not personally enjoy it could be under special stress.

The Intrinsic (I)–Extrinsic (E)–Quest line of research has yet to be broken down into constituent components. I and E are considered motivations and appear to comprise affect and value items (Gorsuch, 1994). Quest is more difficult to understand; it may be a personality- and conflict-based orientation toward religion (Gorsuch, 1994; Kojetin, McIntosh, Bridges, & Spilka, 1987).

Habits, as already noted, may be founded on beliefs, values, and affects that are accessible or inaccessible. If they are accessible, it is easy to evaluate whether the habit is still reasonable. When beliefs, values, or affects are inaccessible, assessing habit applicability may be quite difficult.

Because each of the areas functions differently, it is often important to distinguish among them. Still, at other times we may wish to investigate some overriding concern, and measure across several of these areas. As noted earlier, Allport (1959) introduced I and E as "orientations" that assessed both attitudes and behaviors. Further development of the topic has shown that the primary element in these concepts is religious motivation. Newer versions of the I-E scales have eliminated religious behavior in order to make the constructs more exacting and useful.

Attribution in the Psychology of Religion

A major theoretical position in social psychology has been termed "attribution theory." As indicated in Chapter 1, it is a core element in our framework, particularly in understanding how religion helps people make sense out of the world.

Over 40 years ago, the noted psychologist Fritz Heider (1958) theorized that people often explain social situations in terms of both the characteristics of those who interact within these settings and the nature of the environment itself. The relationship of someone with his or her God might also be conceptualized in interpersonal terms. A process of organization, interpretation, and explanation takes place. Heider stated that "this ordering and classifying can be considered a process of attribution" (p. 296). In other words, as we have noted in Chapter 1, attribution is primarily concerned with causal explanations about people, things, and events. Such explanations are couched in ideas and statements that assign certain powers and positions to various situational and dispositional factors. By examining such meanings and their ramifications, attributional research became a major cornerstone of cognitive social psychology, and it was soon extended to explain how people understand their emotional states and many of the things that happen to them and to others (Fiske & Taylor, 1991; Hewstone, 1983a).

Motivational Bases of Attributions: Needs for Meaning, Control, and Esteem

The question of why people make attributions returns us to some basic motivational themes that underlie much religious thinking and behavior—namely, to needs for meaning, control, and esteem. Here we define "esteem" as a personal sense of capability and adequacy, which is a central part of sociality (as defined in Chapter 1) and is reflected in our relationships with others. Though other activating elements will be important, depending on the topic and situation, we see meaning, control, and esteem as central concerns for the psychology of religion.

Forms of personal faith—for example, Allport's I, E, and Quest orientations—can be viewed as motivationally concerned with meaning, control, and esteem. Allport's (1966) idea of I faith as a sentiment flooding "the whole life with motivation and meaning" (p. 455), and as a search for truth, is explicitly directed toward the attainment of ultimate meaning. Quest is a similar effort to attain answers to basic questions. Further analyses of these religious orientations easily yield connections with these motivations

In addition to being activated by a "need to know," a "need for mastery and control" enters the picture, as Kelley (1967) and other central figures in attribution theory and research have noted. Bulman and Wortman (1977) suggested yet another motivational source of attributions, which has been buttressed by much research—namely, that "people assign causality in order to maintain or enhance their self-esteem" (p. 351). Self-esteem is also likely to be a consequence of the presence of meaning and a sense of control.

Our theoretical position asserts that attributions are triggered when meanings are unclear, control is in doubt, and self-esteem is challenged. There is, as suggested, much evidence that these three factors are interrelated.

Naturalistic and Religious Attributions

Given these three sources of motivations for attributions, the individual may attribute the causes of events to a wide variety of possible referents (oneself, others, chance, God, etc.). These referents may be classified into two broad categories: "naturalistic" and "religious." The evidence is that most people in most circumstances initially employ naturalistic explanations and attributions (e.g., references to people, natural events, accidents, chance, etc.) (Lupfer, Brock, & DePaola, 1992). Depending on a wide variety of situational and personal characteristics, there is a good likelihood of shifting to religious attributions when naturalistic ones do not satisfactorily meet the needs for meaning, control, and esteem (Hewstone, 1983b; Spilka, Shaver, & Kirkpatrick, 1985). The task is to identify and comprehend those influences that contribute to the making of religious attributions. For example, we already know that the attributions of intrinsically religious individuals differ from those who are extrinsically oriented (Watson, Morris, & Hood, 1990a). In addition, Gorsuch and Smith (1983) have examined the bases of attributions to God. Spilka and Schmidt (1983a) and Lupfer et al. (1992) have also looked at a number of personal and situational possibilities that affect religious and secular attributions. Hunsberger (1983c) has focused on biases that enter this process. Even though there is much potential in this theoretical framework, it has only been applied in a few areas.

Extending Attribution Theory

Theories usually become more useful when they are combined with other theoretical speculations, and Wikstrom (1987) has joined our attributional framework with Sundén's role theory of religion. Sundén's theory proposes that religion "psychologically speaking, seem[s] to provide models and roles for a certain kind of perceptual 'set'" (Wikstrom, 1987, p. 391). A frame of reference is established in which the person's actions and cognitions are now structured by a religious role. Wikstrom further tells us that "when the frame of reference is activated, stimuli which would otherwise be left unnoticed are not only observed but also combined and attributed to a living and acting 'other,' to God" (1987, p. 393). Moreover, "as a condition and as a result of the feedback from the role-taking experience . . . [the self-perception] . . . can be seen as something that provides meaning and a feeling of identity, and strengthens self-esteem" (1987, p. 396). Control is also brought into the picture, showing how role and attribution approaches seem to parallel each other. There is unexplored potential here: van der Lans (1987) shows how this kind of role theory predicts various aspects of religious experience. Unfortunately, this approach has not stimulated much research.

Our contention is that these two cornerstones of social psychology—the attributional process and role taking—are products of interactions between external situational factors and internal dispositional factors (Magnusson, 1981). In other words, all thinking and behavior takes place in an interpersonal and sociocultural context in which situations are elements. We now identify some of these influences that contribute to the making of religious attributions.

Situational Influences

For many years, social psychology in general and attribution research in particular have emphasized the role of immediate environmental factors in the determination of thinking and behavior (Ross & Nisbett, 1991). This implies that much religious experience, belief, and behavior are subject to the vagaries of current circumstances. In other words, the information we researchers obtain may largely be a function of the settings in which people are studied and data collected. There is evidence to support this approach. Schachter (1964) claims that an individual "will label his feelings in terms of his knowledge of the immediate situation" (p. 54). Dienstbier (1979) has referred to this labeling as "emotion attribution theory," in order to explain how people define the causes of emotional states when ambiguity exists. Proudfoot and Shaver (1975) use the same basic idea to denote the bases of religious experience. Research suggests that up to three-quarters of intense religious experiences occur when individuals are engaged in religious activities or are in religious settings (Spilka & Schmidt, 1983a). Still, one must be cautious, for some studies have not shown the influence of religious situations on religious attributions (Lupfer et al., 1992). There is also reason to believe that personal factors need to be considered (Epstein & O'Brien, 1985). Since we want to understand attributions in general, rather than those that involve only emotion or ambiguity, we have called our approach "general attribution theory" (Spilka et al., 1985).

We perceive situational influences as falling into two broad categories: "contextual factors" and "event character factors." The first category is concerned with the degree to which situations are religiously structured, while the latter stresses the nature of the event being explained.

Contextual Factors.   Situations may be religiously structured by the locale in which activities or their evaluation take place (e.g., church or nonchurch surroundings; the presence of others who are known to be religious, such as clergy; or participation in religious activities, such as prayer or worship). The presence of such circumstances should elicit religious attributions, and, as noted above, this is obviously true when religious mystical or intense religious experiences occur. Certainly if other people are present and are religiously involved, their actions should aid in the selection of a religious interpretation. We might say that the likelihood of religious explanations is heightened by such factors. Work by Hood (1977) has further demonstrated the importance of situational influences in the creation of nature and spiritual experiences. Contextual elements apparently increase the chances that those affected will attribute what occurs to the intervention of God. The *salience* of religion seems to be the key influence here. That is, the more important, noticeable, or conspicuous religion is in a situation, the more probable it is that religious attributions will be offered. This suggests what has been called the "availability hypothesis" or "availability heuristic." Religious influences in situations increase the probability of making religious associations or arousing religious ideas (Fiske & Taylor, 1991). One may argue that church settings in which religious attributions are not made may not be salient for religion. For example, research has shown that simply being present in a religious institution may not be enough (Spilka & Schmidt, 1983a).

Event Character Factors.   Religious attributions may also be affected by the nature or character of the event being explained. A number of such influences are possible: (1) the importance of what takes place; (2) whether the event is positive or negative; (3) the domain of the event (social, political, economic, medical, etc.); and (4) whether the event occurs to the attributing person or to someone else. These factors have been shown to affect the intensity and frequency of religious attributions, and we feel that they are influential to the extent that they enhance meaning, control, and esteem.

Lupfer et al. (1992) speak of "meaning belief systems" (p. 491). This concept emphasizes the adequacy of naturalistic versus religious explanations. As one set proves to be satisfactory, the alternative set may be ignored, at least in terms of what the relative availability of explanations suggests. Another possibility that reintroduces questions of meaning and control concerns the degree of ambiguity and threat that events convey. For example, medical problems may be least understood and have the greatest potential for threatening life. In contrast, as serious as economic disasters are, they seem to be understood more easily; they also leave the individual the possibility of starting over again. In other words, we hypothesize that situations involving high ambiguity and high threat may have the greatest likelihood of calling forth religious explanations. One problem is to determine the relative degrees of threat for the different domains.

Event Importance.   Considering the awe with which the power of God is regarded, one might perceive a role for the deity only when events of the greatest significance are involved. A disaster takes place, and the insurance company defines it as an "act of God." A young person unexpectedly dies, and it is said to be an expression of "God's will." People who win millions of dollars in lotteries commonly see the "hand of God" in their success. The unanticipated is often explained by such phrases as "God works in mysterious ways." Despite the fact that science has provided detailed naturalistic interpretations of birth and death, as well as reasons for good fortune and victory or failure and defeat, for most people there still remains a sense of the miraculous about the rare and unique events that can greatly change their lives. From a personal perspective, science and common sense often do not satisfactorily answer such questions as "Why now?", "Why me?", or "Why here?" If someone is suffering from a severe illness or a terminal condition, attributions and pleas to God seem quite appropriate. Instances of remission when all appeared hopeless are frequently regarded as signs of God's mercy, compassion, favor, or forgiveness. Research confirms this view that God becomes part of the "big picture" for the significant things that happen (Spilka & Schmidt, 1983a). Defining what is important has a very individual quality: Sports teams may pray for extra achievement in the "big" game, or gamblers may plead for divine intervention on a roll of the dice (Hoffman, 1992). Attributions therefore are a function of event importance—a subjectively determined concept.

The Valence (Positivity–Negativity) of an Event.   If there is one tendency in making attributions to God, it is that people rarely blame God for the bad things that happen to them. Attributions to God are overwhelmingly positive (Bulman & Wortman, 1977; Johnson & Spilka, 1991; Lupfer et al., 1992). Bulman and Wortman (1977) studied the reasons given by young people who became paraplegic because of serious accidents. They saw a benevolent divine purpose in what happened to them. As one such youth put it, "God's trying to put me in situations, help me learn about Him and myself and also how I can help other people" (quoted in Bulman & Wortman, 1977, p. 358). In another study, a patient with cancer told one of the authors, "God does not cause cancer . . . illness and grief do not come from God. God does give me the strength to cope with any and all problems" (quoted in Johnson & Spilka, 1991, p. 30). Rabbi Harold Kushner's (1981) well-known book *When Bad Things Happen to Good People* supports this idea that bad things should not be attributed to God.

Even though positive attributions to God prevail, some people feel that they are being punished for their sins and may make negative attributions, but this is relatively rare. Clearly, the valence of events influences religious attributions, but we need to know more about why and under what circumstances positive or negative attributions are made to the deity.

Event Domain.   Certain domains appear "ready-made" for the application of secular understandings, while others seem more appropriate for invoking religious possibilities. We know that medical situations elicit more religious attributions than either social or economic circumstances, and it may be that, historically and culturally, the latter realms have largely been associated with naturalistic explanations (Spilka & Schmidt, 1983a). In addition, religious institutions have been quite averse to glorifying money and wealth. References in the Bible to "filthy lucre" and the difficulty the rich will encounter in attempting to enter heaven leave little doubt that economic and spiritual matters are not regarded as harmonious.

Without question, when people are in dire straits in any domain, it is not uncommon to seek divine help. The issue may, however, revolve around the clarity of meanings and the sense of control a person has in various situations. Religion may best fill the void when the person cannot understand why things are as they are, and control is lacking. In other words, when ambiguity is great and threat is high.

The Personal Relevance of Events.   Personal relevance is one of those variables that overlaps the broad categories of situational and dispositional (see "Dispositional Influences," below). It shares both realms. There is little doubt that when events occur to us, they are much more personally important than when they happen to others. We can be deeply moved when we hear about a friend or relative's serious illness, but when we suffer from such a condition ourselves, the question "Why me?" is suddenly of the greatest significance, and attributions to God are commonly made. If something particularly good happens to someone else, such as the winning of a great deal of money, we might say "That's luck for you," and feel happy for that person. The one benefited is more likely to claim that "God was looking out for me." The idea that personal relevance may elicit more religious attributions has gained support, but not consistently. It does seem to be involved in interactions with other variables, so additional research is called for to resolve these ambiguities (Lupfer et al., 1992; Spilka & Schmidt, 1983a).

Situational Complexity and Event Significance.   Reality tells us not only that any particular event includes all of the dimensions described above—importance, valence, domain, and personal relevance—but also that event contexts vary greatly. It is also quite probable that event characteristics interact differently in different settings. It may be contended that each situation is a unique, one-time occurrence, and without question this is true. Still, there are commonalities across events and situations that need to be abstracted and categorized. Even within-situation dimensions remain to be discovered. An empirical scientific approach must keep these considerations in mind when theories such as the one proposed here are employed to direct research.

Though we somewhat arbitrarily distinguish situations and people, in life this really makes little sense. There are no situations or events that are meaningful without people to create such meanings. In the last analysis, person and situation are in "transaction." It is a conceptual convenience to separate the two with the word "interaction" when in actuality they are inseparable. To many psychologists, the ultimate purpose of our discipline is to develop a psychology that treats the situation and the individual as a unit (Magnusson, 1981; Rowe, 1987). Though this is a goal to which we may aspire, we are forced to consider the individual in the same way that we look at the situation.

Dispositional Influences

The Individual in Context.   The strong emphasis on individualism in North American society causes us to look at people as if they act independently of their surroundings. Just as events take place in contexts, persons always exist in their individual life spaces, which vary with time and place. It may make a big difference if someone reacts in the morning before breakfast, or in the evening after supper. A religious experience that takes place in a church may have different repercussions than one that occurs when the individual is alone on a mountain top. Personal response is surprisingly situationally dependent.

Personal Factors.   Individual characteristics may be termed "dispositional," and these fall into three overlapping categories: "background," "cognitive/linguistic," and for lack of a better word, "personality." Since we are not in a position to denote constitutional and genetic influences or their effects, these three realms imply that people pattern their attributions regarding the causes and nature of events so that some explanations are much more congenial (meaning more "available" and/or "better-fitting") than other possibilities. This would hold true for the selection of naturalistic as opposed to religious referents. Specifically, it would be true for their decisions as to whether positive or negative event outcomes are a result of their own actions or those of others; are due to fate, luck, or chance; or are attributable to the involvement of God. Research in this area is still needed, and slowly the challenge is being taken up (Bains, 1983; Lupfer et al., 1992; Schaefer & Gorsuch, 1991).

Background Factors.   It is a psychological truism to state that people are largely products of their environment as far as most behavior is concerned. The overwhelming majority of us are exposed early in life to religious teachings at home and by our peers and adults in schools, churches, and communities. These childhood lessons often follow us throughout life, and are expressed by the use of religious concepts in a wide variety of circumstances. A common observation suggests that the stronger a person's spiritual background, the greater the chance that the person will report intense religious experiences and undergo conversion (Clark, 1929; Coe, 1900). Frequency of church attendance, knowledge of one's faith, importance of religious beliefs, and the persistence of religious ideas over many decades are correlates of early religious socialization (McGuire, 1992; Shand, 1990). In other words, the more conservatively religious or orthodox the home and family in which a person was reared, the greater the person's likelihood of using religious attributions later in life.

Cognitive/Linguistic Factors.   Attributions depend on having available a language that both permits and supports thinking along certain lines. Bernstein (1964) tells us that "Language marks out what is relevant, affectively, cognitively, and socially, and experience is transformed by what is made relevant" (quoted in Bourque & Back, 1971, p. 3).

Such relevance is well demonstrated by studies showing that religious persons possess a religious language and use it to describe their experience. There is reason to believe that the presence of such a language designates an experience as religious instead of aesthetic or some other possibility (Bourque, 1969; Bourque & Back, 1971). Meaning to the experiencing individual appears in part to be a function of the language and vocabulary available to the person, and this clearly relates to the individual's background and interests. There is much in the idea that thought is a slave of language, and the thoughts that breed attributions are clearly influenced by the language the attributor is set to use (Carroll, 1956).

Personality/Attitudinal Factors.   The broad heading of "personality/attitudinal factors" includes a wide variety of dispositional factors that almost seem to defy classification. The language of personality is both difficult and complex, and different thinkers often employ different concepts to cover the same psychological territory. Schaefer and Gorsuch (1991) propose a "multivariate belief–motivation theory of religiousness" in an effort to integrate the often scattered ideas and research notions that associate traits and attitudes with religion. These scholars first recognize what they term a "superordinate domain" of religiousness, which comprises a number of subdomains. Their intention is to define the components of these latter spheres. The three they select for study are religious motivation, religious beliefs, and religious problem-solving style. Depending on the variables chosen to represent these subdomains, there may be room for argument as to whether one is looking at a cognitive or a motivational factor. Unhappily, most workers in the field have not been as rigorous as Gorsuch and his students where definition of variables is concerned. For example, many "personality" factors have been examined in relation to religiousness. Among these are self-esteem, locus of control, the concept of a just world, and form of personal faith. All four seem to possess a motivational quality, yet the last two strongly involve belief systems. The Schaefer–Gorsuch theory implies a need to distinguish motivational from belief components, or to identify a third, overlapping domain (Schaefer & Gorsuch, 1991). This has been discussed earlier in this chapter. Obviously, this work is in its infancy, but it suggests a potentially fruitful way of organizing a mass of piecemeal findings into a coherent framework.

To illustrate the meanings of personality/attitudinal dispositions relative to the making of religious attributions, let us look briefly at what we know about two well-researched factors: self-esteem and locus of control.

Self-esteem. Research on self-conceptions has been conducted for almost 60 years. For more than 30 years, many psychologists have focused on self-esteem—the regard people have for themselves (Wylie, 1979). The evidence suggests that this variable is quite basic to personality. One view is that attributions are often made to validate and enhance self-esteem; they perform a self-protective function (Hewstone, 1983b).

Needless to say, a fair number of researchers have examined self-esteem relative to religiosity. In general, high self-esteem relates to positive and loving images of God, and similarly to Allport's I religious orientation (Benson & Spilka, 1972; Hood, 1992; Masters & Bergin, 1992). There may be a need here for consistency; this suggests that those who have negative self-views perceive God as unloving and punitive (Benson & Spilka, 1972). In other words, the person with a negative opinion of the self may think "I am unlovable; hence God can't love me." Consistency further implies that favorable attributions to God ought to be associated with positive event outcomes as opposed to negative occurrences. This hypothesis has been supported (Lupfer et al., 1992; Spilka & Schmidt, 1983a).

Self-esteem does not stand by itself. It is enmeshed in a complex of overlapping personality traits and religious concepts and measures, such as sin and guilt, as well as the nature of the religious tradition with which one is identified (Hood, 1992). This work indicates that different patterns of self-esteem and God attributions may be a function of one's religious heritage and its doctrines. If a prime role of attributions is to buttress self-esteem, we need to ask how religion performs such a function—especially in traditions such as fundamentalism, which may seem quite harsh on an individual's effort to express positive self-regard.

Locus of control. Locus of control was initially conceptualized as a tendency to see events as either internally determined by the person or externally produced by factors beyond the control of the individual. This formulation has been extended and refined a number of times. External control was originally viewed as fate, luck, and chance until Levenson (1973) added control by powerful others, and Kopplin (1976) brought in control by God. Pargament et al. (1988) recognized the complexity of control relationships relative to the deity, and developed measures to assess what they termed a "deferring" mode (an active God and a passive person), a "collaborative" mode (both an active God and an active person), and a "self-directive" mode (an active person and a passive God). These notions illustrate different patterns of attribution for control to the self and God. In the deferring mode, individuals may pray and, having done that, attribute all the power to God: "It's in the hands of God." Those with a collaborative style are basically saying that both they and God have control: "God helps those who help themselves." Utilizing these coping styles relates to further attributions to the nature of God. Though the associations are stronger with the collaborative than with the deferring mode, the tendency for persons who adopt such control perspectives is to attribute generally positive qualities to the deity, along with their recognition of God's power (Schaefer & Gorsuch, 1991).

Although belief in supernaturalism affiliates with external control, Shrauger and Silverman (1971) found that "people who are more involved in religious activities perceive themselves as having more control over what happens to them" (p. 15; see also Randall & Desrosiers, 1980). This sounds like intrinsic religion, or at least orthodoxy, for this relationship is strongest among fundamentalists (Furnham, 1982; Silvestri, 1979; Tipton, Harrison, & Mahoney, 1980). Studying highly religious people, Hunsberger and Watson (1986) found that attributions of control and responsibility are made to God when outcomes are positive—a well-confirmed finding—but that when the result is negative, the tendency is to attribute the blame to Satan ("The Devil made me do it"). Issues of control, and questions of to whom or what control is attributed, have been extensively studied both within and outside the psychology of religion. These are concerns that should be kept in mind throughout this book.

The Social-Psychological Perspective: A Brief Summary

In this portion of the chapter, we have looked at a few major aspects of the psychology of religion that derive from mainstream social psychology. Our intent is to keep the psychological study of religion within the overall field of psychology per se; still, as already noted, the psychology of religion is primarily regarded as a subfield of social psychology. Here we have looked at some central aspects of the latter—namely, beliefs, values, attitudes, religious habits, and behavior—as well as the broad realm of attribution theory. Keeping these considerations in mind, we now turn to some very basic issues for psychology, social psychology, and the psychology of religion.

REDUCTIONISM IN CONCEPTUALIZING RELIGIOUS ISSUES

In addition to distinguishing between cognitive and affective aspects of religiousness, the present social-psychological model allows for nonreductionistic understandings of religiousness. Conceptually, "reductionism" occurs when a topic is explained by variables independent of the topic itself. Sometimes this is appropriate, such as reducing a preschool child's church attendance to parental religiousness.

Three traditions in the psychology of religion illustrate reductionism: those of Sigmund Freud, R. B. Cattell, and William James. In each of these traditions, many of the reasons people give for being religious—primarily, beliefs—are ignored.

In the introduction to *The Future of an Illusion*, Freud (1927/1961) makes an important point:

> . . . in past ages in spite of their incontrovertible lack of authenticity, religious ideas have exercised the strongest possible influence on mankind. This is a fresh psychological problem. We must

ask where the inner force of those doctrines lies and to what they owe their efficacy, independent as it is, of the acknowledgement of reason. (p. 51)

Clearly, Freud assumed that religion is false. He therefore asked why people are religious when it is irrational to be so; since they believe in nothing that is real, there must be other foundations for these beliefs. In his theory, religion is reduced to infantile projection of the parental figure, a form of neuroticism. Other psychologists endorsed variants of this theme (e.g., Faber, 1972; Suttie, 1952; Symonds, 1946). If this is so, there can be nothing of importance to religious beliefs—so why measure them?

R. B. Cattell represents another tradition of reductionistic research. It starts with the fact that Cattell himself was a behaviorist who literally could not think in terms of beliefs. His stance ends with his personal view of religion as just "silly superstition" (Gorsuch, 2002). Like Freud, Cattell (1938, 1950) did give credit to religion for being a powerful force in people's lives. Given this beginning, Cattell posited motivational bases for being religious. Cattell and Child (1975) reported that religion is a function of strong needs to avoid fear, to be nurtured, and to nurture others. Others working in this tradition explained religion as a result of being deprived and therefore turning to a belief in life after death to meet currently unmet needs (Dewey, 1929). Beliefs are thus created by the person to resolve various problems. Again, since there can be nothing of importance to religious beliefs per se, why measure them?

William James, a founder of the psychology of religion, treated religion with great respect (James, 1902/1985). Why people hold religious beliefs to be true was not an issue for James, since he approached religion pragmatically: Does it help people live? To this he resoundingly answered, "Yes." Others have continued in this mode, and a major part of the increased attention given to spirituality (see below) stems from religion's having been shown to be beneficial (e.g., Gorsuch, 1976, 1988; Larson et al., 1989; Pargament, 1997).

James's form of reductionism is more subtle than that of Freud or Cattell, since James did not clearly take an atheistic position. In his view, nothing religionists claim as a basis for their religious faith needs to be examined; all such beliefs can be reduced to other variables. Religious beliefs become irrelevant.

The social-psychological model we have presented in this chapter has an explicit place in its category of beliefs for the claims of truth made by religion. To include beliefs in the model does not require that investigators hold such views themselves—only that they respect the fact that beliefs are a factor in religiousness. An example is Shermer's (2000) book *How We Believe*. Shermer is an explicit agnostic and an active leader of the Skeptics Society, a group in which 67% of the members are skeptical about the existence of God. The questions asked by Shermer for his book included why people do or do not believe in God. The most important reasons his respondents offered were arguments for the existence of God; another popular category was having had a personal experience with God (e.g., "I believe he exists because I met Him"). Both types of reasons clearly involve beliefs by our social-psychological definition.

Another example of measuring beliefs is the study of Christian attitudes toward homosexuals, which are described at length in Chapter 7. In sum, conservative Christians claim that God has stated in several places in the Bible that homosexuality is a sin. Hence they feel that the question of whether homosexuality is an acceptable behavior has been answered: God has said "No." It turns out that a belief in the Bible as the explicit word of God is a major predictor of rejecting homosexual behavior (Fulton, Gorsuch, & Maynard, 1999). This analysis suggests that Christians with this outlook can only be understood if their view of the Bible is known. Change in their values about homosexuality could occur only if their beliefs about the Bible were modified. This is a nonreductionistic analysis, because it takes seriously what religious people themselves say is important—namely, their beliefs.

In addition to beliefs, motivations found in affect and values may be important bases of religiosity. Proponents of faiths such as Christianity have always held that these faiths are helpful because they encourage people to come to them for extrinsic gratifications, such as solving personal problems or developing a clear set of moral values. These are very important reasons why people turn to religion and are included in our model. The point here is that any model can only be reductionistic unless beliefs are added to that model.

Note that the nonreductionistic approach based in social psychology does not suggest that all beliefs are based on rational arguments. Instead, by separating beliefs, values, and attitudes, it makes the question of the source and role of beliefs an empirical question. Advocates of reductionistic approaches eliminate beliefs by making assumptions, not by presenting data.

Reductionism as an Aspect of the Idiographic–Nomothetic Controversy

Reductionism is an attempt at explanation; however, the phenomenon to be clarified is usually considered a unit—a totality in itself, whether it be a belief, a value, or a behavior. Reductionism may or may not preserve that complex unity. This brings us to an awareness of one of the great classical problems in psychology, which is of considerable importance in the psychology of religion (Allport, 1937, 1942). It was originally termed the "idiographic–nomothetic" distinction, but Brand (1954), in relation to the broad realm of personality, utilized the more easily understood terms "individual-behavioral" and "general-behavioral." The major characteristics of these concepts are briefly presented in Table 2.4.

In essence, the idiographic (individual-behavioral) approach relies largely on the judgment of an expert, invariably one steeped in clinical or pastoral methods—possibly a cleric, pastoral counselor, or therapist. The bases for expert judgment are covert and not readily available for analysis or understanding. In contrast, the nomothetic (general-behavioral) orientation seeks to obtain information that is empirical, public, reproducible, and reliable. It is the main traditional scientific avenue to demonstrating valid knowledge. Gordon Allport, who was a great advocate of the idiographic method in both personality and religion, recog-

TABLE 2.4. Two Major Approaches to the
Psychological Study of Religion

Idiographic	Nomothetic
Individual-behavioral	General-behavioral
Qualitative	Quantitative
Concern with depth	Attention to the surface
European origin	American origin
Clinical	Experimental
Intuitive (subjective)	Objective
Holistic	Atomistic
Phenomenological	Positivistic
Source: Medicine	Source: Physical science

nized that much of his own work utilized nomothetic procedures (Marceil, 1977). It should be evident that the approach espoused in this text is essentially nomothetic. Harsh as it may sound to advocates of an idiographic approach, for those seeking scientific answers there is validity in the judgment of Paul Meehl (1954): "Always . . . the shadow of the statistician hovers in the background. Always the actuary will have the final word" (p. 138). We do believe that those who utilize holistic, idiographic techniques should be taken seriously; their applied contributions cannot be overestimated. However, they may often be best conceived and utilized as a source of hypotheses for assessment by nomothetic methods.

The holistic–atomistic distinction is not a sharp dichotomy; many levels exist between these endpoints. The human being, conceptualized as a holistic entity, is commonly fractionated into traits, attitudes, beliefs, values, habits, responses, and underlying physiology. Regardless of the level of analysis, it is highly likely that the human entity is amenable to some form of quantitative treatment. When behaviorism ruled psychology, there were psychologists who felt that human actions should eventually be reduced to the level of physics and chemistry (Weiss, 1929). Though that time has largely passed, some observers now argue that each of these concepts, when abstracted by an "objective" analysis, can only give a false and incomplete picture of the person—a partial interpretation with a grain of truth to it. Instead, a holistic, phenomenological, clinical approach is considered best. We are saying that this approach has serious shortcomings. Let us now examine these issues in action with a major concern in the psychology of religion–spirituality.

Spirituality: From a Holistic/Idiographic Concept to an Atomistic/Nomothetic One

In Chapter 1, we have attempted to circumscribe the concept of "spirituality"; now we confront it as an issue in the idiographic–nomothetic controversy. As noted in the preceding chapter, we have to be careful in dealing with spirituality. It is not a word to be easily substituted for "religiosity"; nor is it really meaningful when those who have left an organized, formal religious body define themselves as "spiritual." This essentially tells us nothing, as we don't know specifically what they are talking about.

Preparing to Assess Spirituality

Holistic versus Atomistic Considerations.   Even though there are problems with understanding what spirituality is, most commonly it is viewed holistically/idiographically— that is, as a characteristic of a person *in toto*. As soon as we question its nature within the individual, we start to move away from that idiographic ideal. Initially, many efforts have been made to distinguish between religiosity and spirituality (Hood, 2000b; Pargament, 1999; Zinnbauer, Pargament, & Scott, 1999). Next, a variety of spiritualities are described, such as "world-oriented," "people-oriented," "God-oriented," and "nature-oriented" spiritualities, among other possibilities (Spilka, 1993). One controversial issue is whether spirituality can be separated from religion. Each side of this debate has presented its views without resolving the matter (Emmons & Crumpler, 1999; Hill et al., 2000; Pargament, 1999; Zinnbauer et al., 1997). Hood (2000b) further points out that there is evident overlap between religion and spirituality. This problem holds for the various other forms of spirituality noted above: They may overlap with each other or with religion per se.

A holistic, personal approach is still possible; however, once the foregoing distinctions are made, attention becomes directed toward the criteria that identify spirituality per se. This again raises the question of whether we are dealing with a feature of the entire person or with some cognitive or motivational aspect of the individual, such as experience.

Spirituality as a General Characteristic.   With regard to spirituality as a general characteristic of a person, a number of overlapping systems have been proposed (Elkins, Hedstrom, Hughes, Leaf, & Saunders, 1988; LaPierre, 1994). Table 2.5 illustrates these two schemes. First, these systems are related; LaPierre used the Elkins et al. framework when he developed his own. Second, Elkins et al. attempted a broad stance not exclusively wedded to religion, while LaPierre remained solidly within the religious tradition.

The Elkins et al. (1988) and LaPierre (1994) criteria suggest directions for operationalizing spirituality, but still possess an idyllic quality that remains unclear and ethereal. They also strongly suggest that it will be difficult if not impossible to assess spirituality in a holistic manner. The equation of spirituality with "authenticity" by Helminiak (1996a, 1996b) could holistically subsume these criteria, but authenticity itself needs to be anchored in a defining and assessing methodology—something Helminiak, in a most scholarly manner, has been working on for some time.

Spirituality as Experience.   Implying that spiritual experience is at the heart of spirituality, if not almost the whole of spirituality, Hardy (1979) continued the movement from

TABLE 2.5. Some Suggested Dimensions of Spirituality

	Elkins et al. (1988)
Transcendental dimension	"Experientially based belief [in] a transcendent dimension to life" (p. 10).
Meaning and purpose to life	Authentic sense that life has purpose and meaning.
Mission in life	Sense that one has a calling, a mission.
Sacredness of life	Belief that "all of life is holy" (p. 11)
Material values	Sense that material things do not satisfy spiritual needs.
Altruism	Belief that we are all part of humanity.
Idealism	Being committed to ideals and life's potential.
Awareness of the tragic	Awareness of and sensitivity to pain and tragedy in life.
Spiritual fruits	Sense that life is infused with spiritual benefits and experience.
	LaPierre (1994)
Journey	Belief that life has meaning and purpose.
Transcendent encounters	As above, belief in a higher level of reality.
Community	Belief that personal growth should occur within a loving community.
Religion	Beliefs and practices relating one to a supreme being.
Mystery of creation	Sense of connection to an environment, its creation and creator.
Transformation	Sense of personal change in relation to social involvement—of becoming.

a holistic, phenomenological perspective to an objective, nomothetic analysis (see also Chapter 9 on religious experience). Offering "a provisional classification" (p. 25) of reported experiential elements, Hardy grouped the elements into 12 major categories, each with further subdivisions until a total of 90 components were given. An exhaustive questionnaire treatment could undoubtedly result in many more items than this last number suggests.

Following an in-depth review of the religion–spirituality issue, Hood (2000b) focused on a core component in spirituality—namely, mystical experience. Researching the matter, he found that mystical experience often ties religion and spirituality together. This is detailed in the later chapters on religious experience and mysticism (Chapters 9 and 10).

Sometimes things aren't what they seem to be. After presenting an impressive list of 12 criteria for a spiritually mature faith, Genia (1997) developed what she termed a Spiritual Experience Index, as noted in Chapter 1. Even though the instrument yielded good reliability, "support[ing] its use as a unitary measure" (p. 345), she factor-analyzed the items and obtained two factors, which she labeled Spiritual Support and Spiritual Openness. In terms of our earlier discussion, these scales overwhelmingly assess beliefs and explicitly have little to do with experience. They appear to be useful as preliminary instruments for the assessment of spirituality per se, but not for spiritual experience. Correlations above .80 were obtained between Spiritual Support and Allport's I religious orientation, implying the identity of these two concepts. Much more work is necessary relative to the initial criteria proposed in order to understand what Genia seems to have accomplished with regard to spirituality.

The Current State of Spirituality Assessment

The last decade has witnessed a flurry of efforts to evaluate spirituality. The term seems to have become more popular than "religion," as we have noted in Chapter 1. Despite extensive lists of characteristics associated with spirituality, the holistic–atomistic problem remains unresolved. Gorsuch and Miller (1999) indicate the many qualifications researchers should consider in their assessment attempts, but few have been taken seriously. Still, there has been no dearth of efforts to measure spirituality. One survey located 16 scales (Spilka & McIntosh, 1996).

To illustrate the kind of work undertaken by researchers concerned with the measurement of spirituality, a few examples in addition to Genia's work should be noted. Hall and Edwards (1996) have published a Spiritual Assessment Inventory that focuses on one's relationship with God. Despite the singular implication of its name, this instrument has been shown to be multidimensional. The Armstrong (1995) Measure of Spirituality has four subscales, reduced from an original nine. The latter constitute the criteria for spirituality that Armstrong utilized. Considering the nature of the items in the scales, we suspect that their correlations with standard indices of religiosity might show this approach to be strongly associated with widely used religiosity scales. Such tendencies have been shown above between the Genia instrument and Allport's I religiousness, and have also been reported with the Elkins et al. (1988) Spiritual Orientation Inventory (Scioli et al., 1997). The same appears to be true of the most recently developed measure in this area, the Spiritual Transcendence Index (Seidlitz et al., 2002). Tightly developed and comprising only eight items, this index seems to overlap with religion, but when a measure is constructed with such care, there is need for further study in order to understand what it is actually assessing.

Emphasizing research on African Americans, Taylor and his coworkers have developed a multidimensional framework with supporting scales to assess spirituality. Their higher-order dimensions are termed Integrative and Disintegrative, each of which possesses three meaningful factorially developed subscales (Taylor, Rogers, Jackson-Lowman, Zhang, & Zhao, 1995). Conceptually, this work is in line with the multiform criteria offered by Genia (1997), Elkins et al. (1988), and LaPierre (1994). Face indications are that the items may be quite useful in a broad range of populations.

Probably the most well-known concept in this area is that of "spiritual well-being." Originally advanced by Moberg (1971, 1979), and further developed in questionnaire form by Ellison (1983), it is closely affiliated with religion and primarily stresses personal well-being in relationship to one's deity. This is also termed "transcendence" and includes a search for purpose and meaning in life. A fair amount of research with Ellison's instrument suggests its utility, though it seems to overlap considerably with indices of religious involvement and commitment (Ellison, 1983; Bufford, Paloutzian, & Ellison, 1991).

The foregoing review of the literature on both the concept of spirituality and its operationalization demonstrates very clearly how a notion that was originally conceived idiographically necessarily found expression nomothetically. As it was analyzed and measured, various beliefs and values of people entered the realm of scientific knowledge, and became useful both for research and for application to real-life problems.

OVERVIEW

In this chapter, we have first attempted to distinguish what psychologists of religion study from possible overlaps with superstition and psychic phenomena. We have then directed our attention toward the operationalization of religious concepts. To this end we have examined various dimensions of religiousness, both logical and logical–empirical, in order to make our thinking clear about how we construct the instruments we employ. In addition, the notion of factor-analytic models is carried over and expanded from Chapter 1.

Our long-term goal is to keep the psychology of religion integrated with the mainstream of psychology itself. Since the study of personal faith is largely regarded as part of social psychology, we have shown how various basic ideas in social psychology are realized in our work. We must clearly know the details and parameters of what we are talking about; hence our emphasis on attitudes, beliefs, values, habit, and behavior, as well as on attribution theory.

Recognizing that the psychology of religion shares in (and is often plagued by) the same issues that the overall field of psychology continually confronts, we have then looked at questions concerning reductionism and the idiographic–nomothetic controversy, which overlaps with the issue of holistic versus atomistic analysis. Maintaining our inclination toward the scientific, with its concern for making information public, reproducible, reliable, and valid, we have illustrated the idiographic–nomothetic and holistic–atomistic issues by returning to the problem of spirituality, first discussed in Chapter 1. In the last decade, this has become a "hot" topic. Psychologists have heretofore avoided spirituality, because it was (and still is) so much easier to assess religiosity in its various forms. We have shown how spirituality, which has usually been conceptualized as holistic, rapidly becomes multiform in both conceptual and psychometric analyses. We are thus forced to return to Meehl's (1954) conclusion that "the actuary will have the final word" (p. 138). We see no scientific alternative at the present time.

Chapter 3

RELIGION AND BIOLOGY

Man is by constitution a religious animal.

Biology has nothing directly to do with religion, and by no possibility can religion, such as we know, be based on biology.

Darwin was a most careful observer . . . there was great truth in the theory and there was nothing atheistic in it if properly understood.

If you are a Darwinist, I pity you, for it is impossible to be a Darwinist and a Christian at the same time.

Truly, he who unfolds to us the way in which God works through the world of phenomena may well be called the best of religious teachers.[1]

RELIGION AND BIOLOGY: A TROUBLED RELATIONSHIP

The foregoing quotations linking biology to religion cover the spectrum of possibilities. The common point among them is, however, well stated by Hearn (1968): "Probably in no other area has the encounter between Christianity and science generated so much misunderstanding or left such deep scars as in that of biological science" (p. 199).

The Trials of Evolution

If there were ever a point of contention between biology and religion, the theory of evolution is that point. In 1859, when Darwin (1859/1972) published his *The Origin of Species,* it immediately became a target for conservative religionists. The famous debate between Thomas Huxley and Bishop Samuel Wilberforce (also known as "Soapy Sam") acquired the status of legend, and few could question that the winner in this clash of verbal arms was Huxley, also known as "Darwin's bulldog" (Irvine, 1955). Science and the theory of evolution won the war, and rather rapidly many Christians placed evolution within a Christian framework (Fiske, 1883; Himmelfarb, 1962; Kennedy, 1957; McCosh, 1890). Still, the conflict continues to reappear—as in the John Scopes trial of the 1920s, the more recent controversy over "creationism" and "creation science," and now the debate over "intelligent design."

---

1. These quotations come, respectively, from the following sources: Burke (1790/1909, p. 239); Haldane (1931, p. 43); McCosh (1890, p. vii); Russell (1935, p. 76), quoting his boyhood tutor; and Fiske (1883, p. 369), speaking about Darwin.

"Creationism" is a fundamentalist religious doctrine that avers the literal truth of the creation of the world and life as pictured in Genesis; any notion of evolution is therefore denied (Carter, 2000). "Creation science" is a more recent development, whose proponents seek to attach the idea of science to creationism. Their motivations to do so are perhaps twofold: (1) to endow creationism with the intellectual, worldly stature of science per se, and (2) to permit the incorporation of scientific ideas into the conservative faith of creationists (Gilbert, 1997; Wilcox, 1996). Science is thus seen as in harmony with the account of creation in Genesis. However, the premises, interpretations, and conclusions of creation science are at considerable variance with traditional scientific theories, methods, and findings (Gould, 1997, 1999). In recent years, another attempt to unite science and the religious concept of creation has emerged in the idea of "intelligent design." Advanced by sophisticated, religiously orthodox scientists, this theory accepts evolution in a modified form, and basically claims that many observed facts of nature cannot be explained by evolution and require the action of a creator. Just as a watch is made by a watchmaker, it is claimed that many complex biological and biochemical phenomena can only be accounted for through the intervention of God, the creator (Behe, 1996). This analogical argument at the root of "intelligent design" probably constitutes the most elemental critique of the doctrine as well (Shreve, 1996).

These developments illustrate the complicated, and sometimes uneasy, interplay at work between traditional religious beliefs and the theories propounded by biological science. Whether an attempt is made to expunge evolution from religion (creationism) or to incorporate it (intelligent design), the need clearly exists in religious believers to come to terms with modern biology. This chapter outlines several ways in which this interplay between religion and biological science has been conceptualized, and examines a range of scientific theories designed to help account for the various roles and functions of religion.

The Search for a Religious Instinct

In the late 19th and early 20th centuries, any discussion of evolution entailed a search for internal, biological sources of complex behavior. The classic concept of "instinct" came to the fore. Though full agreement has never been achieved regarding the nature of instinct, it generally refers to complex, unlearned behavior with a physiological basis and evidence of evolutionary involvement (Bateson, 2000). These are rather exacting criteria, and until the early 1920s they were loosely applied to humans (Bernard, 1924). With the rise of behaviorism, learning and the influence of environment became the preferred explanations.

A common idea among religionists was that God had implanted religion in humans; hence there existed a religious instinct. This instinct has been claimed to encompass a wide range of phenomena: animism, myth, ritual, beliefs in God, Christianity, the necessity of Sunday observance, the seeking of ideals and perfection, self-abasement, and the potential for other religious beliefs, behaviors, and experiences. One review of this literature found that some 83 types of religious instinct had been theorized (Bernard, 1924). Their vagueness, cultural relevance, and hypothetical character also suggested that learning, not instinct, was probably the real element being observed.

The Influence of Environment versus Heredity in Religion

For over a century, psychology has been plagued with the basic question of whether some psychological phenomena are the result of genetics or environment. This issue has been raised with respect to virtually every facet of psychology—intelligence, abilities, perceptual phenomena, personality, and mental disorder, among others. For us, the issue is religion.

How do we separate environmental influence from genetics? There is a potential exit from this dilemma, and it involves twins. One can study identical twins (who share 100% of their genes) as opposed to fraternal twins (who only share 50% of their genes). Some studies have focused on identical and fraternal twins who have been separated from each other at birth or very soon after. A little mathematics from quantitative genetics tells us that we can make reasonable assumptions and state the proportions of some psychological concern (e.g., religion) that seem to be a function of environment and heredity (Falconer, 1981; Wright, 1999).[2] Research Box 3.1 offers some insight into this work.

As interesting as the study described in Research Box 3.1 is, a few words are in order concerning the issues of twins raised apart. In any country (here, the United States), separated twins are never raised in a random set of environments (Cattell, 1950). In much of the work on twins, the biological distinction between identical and fraternal twins may be more significant than issues of environmental difference.

If we assume that a culture maximizes the spiritual or religious potential of its people, and if we assume at most a minor direct impact of heredity, the only differences left would be indirect heredity. Finding a high correlation with heredity does not mean that religious development cannot be affected by environment. It may mean that in the culture studied, the environment is relatively consistent.

Religion and Genetics: A Direct or Indirect Connection?

Using mostly very large samples of twins (e.g., from 3,000 to over 14,000 pairs of twins), behavior geneticists have shown that religious affiliation is (as might be expected) a cultural phenomenon, but that genetic factors manifest a moderate degree of influence on religious devotion and conservatism (D'Onofrio, Eaves, Murrelle, Maes, & Spilka, 1999).

On the face of it, this could imply that a *direct* connection exists between religiosity and heredity—in other words, that religion is in the genes. However, because the statistics involved in separating environmental and genetic possibilities are fundamentally correlational, it behooves us to distinguish sharply between correlation and causation. Causation builds in correlation, but not vice versa. If *A* causes *B*, they will yield a significant correlation coefficient, but if the two variables are only correlated, they simply vary together without either causing the change in the other.

These sobering second thoughts, coupled with observations that intimate a connection (or at least a correlation) between genetics and religion, suggest that this relationship might not be simple. One possibility is an *indirect* connection between religion and genetics, in which a number of factors "intervene" between genetics and faith. More specifically, genetic factors are most likely to be expressed through cognitive, motivational, and social avenues, which are involved in personal religious expressions (Spilka, 1999).

---

2. To be more precise, heritability is the proportion of the total variance of some characteristic that can be assigned to genetics or heredity (Falconer, 1981). The remainder of the variance is associated with environmental influences.

∂▲

Research Box 3.1. Genetic and Environmental Influences on Religious Attitudes, Interests, and Values: A Study of Twins Reared Apart and Together (Waller, Kojetin, Bouchard, Lykken, & Tellegen, 1990)

Utilizing respondents from the famous Minnesota Twin Study, Waller and colleagues were able to obtain data on five measures of religious attitudes, interests, and values. These were well-known scales: Religious Fundamentalism (Wiggins, 1966), Religious Occupational Interests (Waller, Lykken, & Tellegen, 1995), the Religious Interest subscale of the Strong–Campbell Vocational Interest Inventory (Hansen & Campbell, 1985), Religious Leisure Time Interests (Waller et al., 1995), and the Allport–Vernon–Lindzey Religious Values Scale (Allport, Vernon, & Lindzey, 1960).

The participants were 53 pairs of monozygotic (identical) twins and 31 pairs of dizygotic (fraternal) twins who had been reared apart. The measures were also given to 458 pairs of identical and 363 pairs of fraternal twins who were raised together. Data analyses suggested that about 50% of the variation in the scores on the religious measures was a function of genetic influences. In other words, in this study, genetic and environmental factors were equal in their effects regarding the origins of religious inclinations.

RELIGION, GENETICS, AND EVOLUTION: A THEORY

We have already claimed that religion appears to be a universal human phenomenon. This suggests a need to look for universal psychological mechanisms; if such exist, their presence hints at a role for evolution in this process. Evolution's role may, however, be indirectly expressed through what religion does for people. For whatever reasons, evolution has endowed us humans with large brains in order to adapt to the exigencies of living (Barash, 1977; Pinker, 1997; Stanford, 2001). Regardless of why our big brains evolved, there is good reason to believe that they can be employed for many things for which they were not designed. Gould (1991) terms this "exaptation," in which an organ or physiological process that developed for one purpose can also be used to attain other goals.

According to the Darwinian perspective, the goal of adaptation is basically twofold—to enable organisms to survive and to reproduce (Dawkins, 1976). This is the essence of natural selection, and we may theorize that religion meets at least three basic needs, which we have posited in our integrating framework in Chapter 1. Broadly speaking, these are cognitive, motivational, and social. For our purposes, we label these as needs for meaning, for control, and for relationships with others (i.e., sociality). The position taken here is that the religion–genetics connection may be diagrammed thus:

(Evolution and Genetics) → (Meaning, Control, and Sociality) → Religion

Before we discuss these factors, we might offer a few directions intimating a relationship between evolution and genetics on the one hand, and religion on the other, that could be either direct or indirect. As noted above, we favor the latter possibility. Data pointing toward such a possibility may be inferred first from evidence of religion during Paleolithic times (Mithen, 1996; Thompson, 1981). In addition, even though most anthropologists conceptualize religion as a specifically human phenomenon (Guthrie, 1993; Spiro, 1966), we should expect some signs of prereligious activity among animals. Goodall's (1971) observations of animism and ritual behavior among chimpanzees suggest precursors to religion. Specifically, Goodall describes collective gesturing toward the sky during storms and associated marching behavior, both of which are patterned. These primate behaviors appear to meet some of the needs that religion gratifies among people.

The Naturalistic Basis of the Need for Meaning

Broadly speaking, meaning is inherent in responses to stimuli and implies personally relevant knowledge. We are interested in the psychological reactivity of people, and overwhelmingly invoke consciousness and awareness on some level. Even though this might to some degree involve conditioned responses and habit, when we turn to religion, we focus on higher-level cognitions and some understanding of ourselves and our relationship to others and the world. The result is meaning, the cognitive significance of sensory and perceptual stimulation and information to us.

Maslow (1963) believed that the need to understand is part of human biological nature. In parallel, anthropologist Margaret Mead (1966/1972) universalized the search for meaning, labeling it the "cosmic sense . . . a basic human characteristic . . . a need found in every child and expressed in every culture" (pp. 155–156). The evolutionary psychologists Cosmides and Tooby (1987) take the final step by asserting that "information systems . . . actually link the evolutionary process to manifest behavior" (p. 277).

Many similar observations by other scholars lead to the inference that the search for knowledge, information, and meaning is a fundamental evolutionary drive that is basic to survival and to furthering one's genetic lineage.

We aver that seeking meaning is fundamental to evolutionary success and therefore plays a central role in religion, as well as aiding people to adapt to the exigencies of life.

The Naturalistic Basis of the Need for Control

Gibbs (1994) places the need for control in an evolutionary framework, suggesting its necessity on both human and nonhuman levels. Wilson (1993) offers the hypothesis that evolution might select humans with a long-range view of their interests, as impulsive action is likely to place an individual in jeopardy.

Twin studies have found that from one-third to one-half of the variance in measures of control and locus of control can be attributed to genetics (Finkel & McGue, 1997; Hur & Bouchard, 1997; Pedersen, Gatz, Plomin, Nesselroade, & McClearn, 1989). Finally, control and mastery confer survival and reproductive advantages upon those who possess power.

In summary, control motivation—regardless of its expression, whether social, magical, or religious—appears to rest on firm ground in evolutionary theory and genetics. Among humans, learning and culture dominate; however, the underlying biological substrate is far too extensive to be overlooked.

The Naturalistic Basis of Sociality (The Need for Relationships)

The evolutionary origins of social behavior were first suggested by Darwin, who viewed the association of pleasure with social relationships as contributing to success in natural selection (see Gardner, 1999). Brewer (1997) feels that "coordinated group living is the primary survival strategy of the species" (p. 55). To develop this idea fully would take volumes. Suffice it to say that sociality would include social responsiveness, cooperation, altruism, and attachment/bonding. The significance of language and communication in the expression of sociality cannot be minimized. In fact, the centrality of communication among humans and animals indicates its evolutionary significance.

Social behaviors such as affiliation and attachment can be shown to have biological foundations. Many studies among mammals reveal neuroendocrine influences empowering attachment behavior—in particular, the hormones oxytocin and vasopressin (Carter, 1998; Insel, 1993; Porges, 1998). These influences involve genetic and evolutionary factors. They constitute the biological substrate of much social behavior.

A similar potential exists with respect to social cooperation. Over a half-century ago, Ashley Montagu (1950) articulated the radical assertion that cooperation "is the most important factor in the survival of animal groups" (p. 41). Cooperation is allied with evolution in general and natural selection in particular. This recommends that natural selection "informs" the organism that its own interests are best met by supporting the social body. This is certainly true for humans.

Conceptually, altruism and social cooperation are closely affiliated. Summarizing a large and impressive amount of informed writing from the first half of the 20th century, Herrick (1956) stated that altruism is "deeply rooted in the prehuman ancestry of mankind" (p. 215). It is clearly present among a broad spectrum of animals, ranging from social insects through birds to primates (Breed & Page, 1989; De Waal, 1996). Selective pressures for genes that promote neural complexity may be a result of the need to cope with intricate relationships (Sigmund & Nowak, 2000). Like cooperation, altruism brings people together, and cultures reinforce such connections. Still, evolution and genetics lurk in the background.

Batson (1983) has nicely summarized the relative universalization of what were originally thought to be "kin-specific altruistic impulses" (p. 1385). He notes that "religious kinship images may promote prosocial behavior by increasing the range of application of a highly limited natural impulse toward altruism" (p. 1385). Similar thoughts hold for cooperation and any other form of positive social responsiveness.

SOME ALTERNATIVE PERSPECTIVES

Religion and Natural Selection

The door to modern biological speculation about evolution and religion was opened by Alister Hardy (1976) in his noted book *The Biology of God*, which is basically an appeal for reconciliation of Darwinian natural selection and genetics with religion. Hardy turned Darwinian theory upside down. Whereas the traditional perspective views behavior change as following physical change, Hardy saw "a powerful behavioral selection to bring about a relatively rapid bodily change" (p. 62). He considered this pattern an appropriate "behavioral selection" (p. 62) for human evolution. How this selection works was not specified, and this constitutes a weakness in Hardy's theory. This view, however, was pioneering, and is currently quite popular in evolutionary psychology (Bonner, 1980; Durham, 1982). The problem can be resolved if the concept of exaptation is introduced, as the behavior in question could easily be the result of existing anatomy and physiology. The underlying physical body may not have been designed for what occurred in behavior; rather, it may have been co-opted for what took place. Once again, the big human brain was used for something other than that for which it evolved.

Hardy, then, saw religious experience as a core element aiding adaptation, and hence as involved in natural selection. To buttress his biological substrate, he quoted another scholar to the effect that "there is a profound human instinct to seek something personal behind the processes of nature" (p. 96). Next, Hardy analogized from a dog's allegiance to his human master to humanity's dependence on God. Religion is thus a natural creation.

Hardy broadened his scholarly effort to include a theology with biological underpinnings. He explicitly offered what he hoped was a scientific and biological justification for religion, rather than simply a biological integration that would meet the criteria of contemporary science.

Rayburn and Richmond (1998, 2000) have also linked biology to religion in what they term "theobiology." Since this emanates more from a religious than from an empirical-psychological framework, we simply mention it here. It merits consideration as a theory for further exploration of possible links between biology and religion.

Religion and the Naturalistic Basis of Cognition

Several other scholars have advanced theories of religion that, on one level or another, involve biology and evolution. One impressive thinker is Pascal Boyer (1994), a noted anthropologist, who wrote a volume entitled *The Naturalness of Religious Ideas*. This is a cognitive theory of religion premised upon "universal cognitive processes." Natural selection is mentioned, but somehow the biological basis of these notions is never developed. Still, we are led to the classic evolutionary notion that religious ideas aid survival; however, even this notion remains obscure. Basically, we read that our thinking (cognition) is constrained in a variety of ways that support religious ideas. A constraint might be how past experience directs and focuses our present thinking. Biology remains in the shadows, and is never made explicit.

Sociobiology and Religion

The distinguished biologist E. O. Wilson of Harvard University has been termed the father of "sociobiology," a controversial field. He has defined sociobiology as "the systematic study of the biological basis of all forms of social behavior, in all kinds of organisms, including man" (Wilson, 1978, p. 16). Turning to religion, he calls it "one of the universals of social behavior" (p. 169). Wilson, then, perceives religion as involved in creating both evolutionary change and conferring genetic advantage. It may accomplish this through the exercise of power by religious leaders, who would choose and reward those who show conformity and loyalty to ecclesiastical authority, and who further display religious zeal and charisma. Insofar as faith might select for learning and motivation to acquire religious behaviors, the frequencies of genes that support such tendencies should increase in the population. Conversely, the frequencies of genes that support opposing propensities should be reduced. Implied here is the idea that religious leaders and religious practices weed out nonconformity, and enhance both the survival and reproduction of those who display valued religious responses. These inclinations would certainly be true for religious groups that separate themselves from the larger social matrix and sponsor ingroup marriages. Such groups include the Amish, Hutterites, Chasidic Jews, Mormons, Shakers, Doukhobors, and a host of other religious bodies (Stark, 1985b; Wilson, 1970).

Wilson has broadened his perspective to include a variety of religious expressions—myth, ritual, and magic. He has searched for the biological advantage religion and its components confers on believers, implying that religious indoctrination relates to learning rules that have evolved and are therefore genetically based.

In this section and the preceding one, we have presented a very brief summary of some contemporary thinking about possible roles for evolution and genetics in the development and expression of religion. Needless to say, the current popularity of evolutionary theorizing has spawned a variety of such notions. We can expect further refinement of these ideas from future studies of twins, plus the efforts of both evolutionary psychologists and anthropologists.

RELIGION AND THE BRAIN

Any approach to religion via biology raises questions about possible underlying anatomical and physiological correlates of religion. On a theoretical level, d'Aquili and his associates (d'Aquili, 1978; d'Aquili, Laughlin, & McManus, 1979; d'Aquili & Newberg, 1999) offer a complex neurobiological framework for understanding religion. Though it goes far beyond what we can deal with here, the theory is described as "a holistic neurophysiological model for the generation of mystical states, religious rituals, near-death experiences, culture, and consciousness itself" (d'Aquili & Newberg, 1999, p. 47). This approach clearly has no limits when it comes to explaining religious behavior, belief, and experience—or, for that matter, any form of human action. So far, this theoretical scheme has not resulted in much confirmatory research. Still, we describe some of its potentialities here.

Epilepsy: The Sacred Disease

Even though the ancient Greek physician Hippocrates wrote that epilepsy appeared to him "to be nowise more divine nor more sacred than other diseases" (Hippocrates, 1952, p. 154), the association of this condition with religion existed in his era and still persists. Today, of course, no one speaks of epilepsy as emanating from religious origins; however, it is still widely associated with expectations of religious expression. Formal medical recognition of such a likelihood first occurred in the 19th century (Dewhurst & Beard, 1970). A respected psychiatric text of the early 20th century referred to "a pathologic religiosity" as a major characteristic of epilepsy (Kraft-Ebing, 1904, p. 474). With greater qualification, the connection continued to be made in later psychiatric works (Strauss, 1959). Recognizing that the affiliation of religion and epilepsy in general is quite weak, White and Watt (1981) suggested a more specific link to temporal lobe epilepsy (TLE)—a view that is currently widespread. Additional caution in making this association is called for, though. Ogata and Miyakawa (1998) focused on the temporal lobe and limbic system in a sample of 234 patients with epilepsy; only three cases, or 1.3%, reported religious content during epileptic episodes. Thus, although the linkage of epilepsy and religion may be quite striking when it occurs, in actuality it seems rather uncommon. Expectations of such a connection have nevertheless stimulated some very significant research. The foregoing statistics explain, in part, why this work has employed very small samples.

Religion and Brain Stimulation

Persinger and his associates (Makarec & Persinger, 1985; Persinger, 1987, 1993; Persinger & Makarec, 1987; Persinger, Bureau, Peredery, & Richards, 1994) have studied the religious ideation accompanying the neuroelectric activity in TLE that Persinger terms "temporal lobe transients." More recently, Ramachandran and Blakeslee (1999) have reported God-associated mental content with TLE and limbic system involvement during epileptic episodes. Virtually every religious possibility has been reported (mystical experiences, conversions, strengthened religious beliefs, etc.). Ramachandran and Blakeslee feel that the content of these episodes is learned, and that such learning depends to a large extent on an individual's cultural context. As in near-death experiences, one can expect cultural shaping of religious content (Zaleski, 1987).

Even though Ramachandran and Blakeslee (1999) feel that the association of brain function with religious experience, belief, and behavior may be universal, they note that "it doesn't follow that the trait [here, religious experience] is genetically specified" (p. 184). They appropriately conclude that "there are circuits in the human brain that are involved in religious experience . . . and we still don't know whether these circuits evolved specifically for religion" (p. 188). Since the limbic system is central in such emotion-associated processes, these researchers stress the role of the limbic system in the production and regulation of emotional expressions in general. MacLean (1989) captures this notion well when he asserts that "under the abnormal conditions of a limbic discharge, the feelings that light up in the patient's mind are free-floating and out of context—being attached to no particular person, situation, or thing" (p. 449).

Ogata and Miyakawa (1998) stress "an underlying mechanism, enhanced affective association to previously neutral stimuli, events, or concepts. Experiencing objects and events shot through with affective coloration engenders a mystically religious world view" (p. 465). In other words, MacLean's (1989) "free-floating and out of context" unattached feelings do not last long.

Why "a mystically religious world view" would result when the appropriate limbic area is stimulated remains an open question. The position adopted here is that the brain structures are available for emotional and experiential usage, and that, through learning and culture, they are employed for religion.

Much research indicates that the process does not simply go from arousal to "religious" response. An intermediate cognitive step, variously termed "appraisal," "labeling" or "attribution," must be interposed here (Hewstone, 1983a; Shaver, 1975). For example, from a physiological perspective, religious, nature, and aesthetic emotional experiences appear to be equivalent; however, the individual selectively makes attributive interpretations on the basis of the language available to him or her, the context in which events take place, the person's past experience, and his or her attitudinal and personality propensities (Bourque, 1969; Back & Bourque, 1970; Proudfoot, 1985; Spilka, Shaver, & Kirkpatrick, 1985). Considering the prevalence, availability, and importance of religion in Western culture, it is appropriate to hypothesize that profound but ambiguous emotional experiences have a high probability of eliciting religious identifications, particularly in health-related situations (Spilka & Schmidt, 1983a).

Are We Hardwired for Religion?

When combined with research on brain stimulation, the recent emphasis on evolution and genetics has resulted in a movement claiming that much of our human behavior is predetermined by our genes. The Darwinian emphasis on adaptation and natural selection has convinced a number of biologists and evolutionary psychologists to focus on the genetic determination of complex human behavior (Buss, Haselton, Shackleford, Bleske, & Wakefield, 1998; Dawkins, 1976). The current mood proposes the question "Are we hardwired?" (Clark & Grunstein, 2000). It is then a short step to ask, "Are we hardwired for religion?" (Begley, 2001). In a logical extension of d'Aquili and Newberg's (1999) work *The Mystical Mind*, Newberg is quoted as asserting that "The human mind has been genetically wired to encourage religious beliefs" (Begley, 2001, p. 59). Newberg further states: "As long as our brain is wired the way it is, God will not go away" (Begley, 2001, p. 59). d'Aquili and Newberg (1999) label their view "neurotheology." In keeping with their previous work, this effort remains largely theoretical. They basically posit a direct connection between religion and specific aspects of biology—a position we challenge.

A fair amount of recent research indicates that activity occurs in various brain structures when one prays or has religious experiences. These studies simply show brain involvement in cognitive, emotional, or motor areas, as should occur for all behavior. They do not suggest that this neural activity either developed exclusively for religion or is solely dedicated to religious functions. This is a research realm that calls for considerable caution, qualification, and controlled enthusiasm. We are far from ready to embrace biology as a final answer to understanding religion. We need theory that eventuates in testable hypotheses. Nothing else will be satisfactory. We must also ask questions that may disprove some of the assertions being made about this topic. For instance, if we are "hardwired for religion," and "God will not go away," why is it that belief in God is often quite low in a number of European countries (see Greeley, 2002)?

We have tried to show that religion has become involved with evolutionary and genetic theorizing—in particular, through research on the action of the nervous system, as well as the results of twin studies. These ideas and research findings reveal new pathways to understanding the role of religion in how people function on the level of biology.

THE BIOLOGY OF RELIGIOUS BEHAVIOR

Let us continue our search for physiological correlates of religious behavior. We know how profoundly important religion is to many people; does this mean that religious activity may have biological repercussions? We do not have to look far to find a number of possible answers to this question. Ritual, rite, and ceremony are central to religion. Furthermore, ritual has a considerable evolutionary history, and is still significant in the functioning of the human nervous system. We humans can thus be rightfully called ritualizing animals. Clearly, we follow a long line of animal predecessors that have also engaged in ritualistic activities.

Before we go further, let us define "ritual," in order to clarify that religious ritual is only one realm in which such behavior is manifested. Among humans, ritual is individually and/ or socially organized and patterned behavior that is often repetitive in nature. Its roots lie deep in the genetic prehistory and neurophysiology of our species.

The Prevalence and Significance of Ritual

Human life is pervaded by ritual. It can, depending on the situation, be called "social," "political," "spiritual," "religious," or whatever adjective is elicited by immediate circumstances. When we meet someone we know, the ritual is "How are you?" The expected response is "Fine, how are you?" A pattern of small talk follows unless a ritual reaction to events dictates otherwise. The words we use and the gestures we make are all in the service of ritualistic design—at least in form, if not in content. As a rule, we are not usually aware of such actions in our everyday behavior. Even though similar tendencies hold for religious systems, there is much conscious learning of approved verbal and nonverbal communication modes, such as when to genuflect, kneel, adopt other postures or movements, say certain prayers, engage in dance, drink liquids or eat foods with religious significance (e.g., wine, wafers, matzoh), and so forth. Over the centuries, institutional religion has refined and redefined its rituals. Private and public forms of worship are specified for certain times of day (on arising, prior to sleep, at calls to prayer, etc.). Particular days of the week plus certain times of the month and year are set aside for special recognition and action by the faithful; all have their formally structured ceremonial expressions. Ritual circumscribes the entire process.

The Biology and Utility of Ritual

The prevalence and importance of ritual in animals and humans have led some biogenetic thinkers to theorize an underlying neurophysiology with specific brain sites (Bell, 1997; d'Aquili et al., 1979; d'Aquili & Newberg, 1999). d'Aquili and his associates have specifically applied their neurological analyses and interpretations to religious ritual and experience (d'Aquili et al., 1979; d'Aquili & Newberg, 1999).

There is general agreement that the basic purpose of ritual is communication, whether the ritual is the waggle dance of a bee to its fellow bees or the fervent prayer of a petitioner to a God. Messages are sent through whatever means an organism or a person apparently feels is most effective. These messages counter the stress of ambiguity and uncertainty. They contain information that endows the vague and indefinite with meaning. The discomfort, distress, and threat of uncertainty are lessened when one possesses ritualistic means of coping with troublesome situations. As Leach (1966) has pointed out, ritual summarizes a great deal of information that in many settings "is essential for the survival of the performers" (p. 405).

Communication, verbal or nonverbal, is a social control mechanism. Communication and language organize interpersonal and group situations to elicit behaviors that primarily maintain peace and harmony on all societal levels (Scheflen, 1972). Ritual thus coordinates religion, both in the public domain and within individuals (Ostow & Scharfstein, 1954). This relationship has led Rappaport (1999) to theorize that religion originated in ritual. There is a regularizing order to the way things are ritualistically done. This provides the kind of organization that supports consistency and comfort for individuals, and, in most instances, amity and understanding in community life. With this in mind, many scholars see ritual as reducing aggression and managing sexual impulses (Wulff, 1997). More broadly, rituals are viewed as means of encouraging and controlling emotion. Rituals in general and religious rituals in particular usually survive not because of the power of authorities, but because people want them, volunteer to participate in them, and probably gain pleasure from having roles to play in them.

To most people, religion represents an ideal state, with institutional faith emphasizing the discrepancy between reality and the ideal over which one frequently lacks control. Smith (1982/1996) perceives ritual as indicating the way things ought to be. Religious ceremonial participation confirms identification with the ideal, reestablishing a sense of mastery.

People frequently make religious attributions when serious medical problems arise (Spilka & Schmidt, 1983a). Ritual also becomes significant at such times (Helman, 1990). Healing rituals are efforts to transform illness into health. Psychologically, for both patients and their supporters, they reduce anxiety and uncertainty. These actions are in effect religious appeals and behaviors designed to bring supernatural forces to the aid of the afflicted. Prayer and participation in religious healing ceremonies often alleviate suffering and increase social integration.

Prayer: A Special Kind of Ritual

The Nature and Scope of Prayer

A ritual that lies at the core of religion is prayer. Since approximately 90% of U.S. residents pray, it is evident that prayer should have some positive effects—or theoretically, as behavior, it should simply be extinguished (Poloma & Gallup, 1991).

Prayer has often been compared and contrasted with meditation and the specific technique known as Transcendental Meditation (TM). Though "meditational prayer" has been identified and discussed (Paloma & Gallup, 1991), meditation does not always imply religion. Studies of meditation and prayer may be treating two phenomena that either are definitely religious or are actually opposed to each other, with only one having religious or spiritual significance. In Eastern religions such as Buddhism and Hinduism, meditation may be comparable to what we term "prayer"—specifically, to forms of prayer that attempt to foster identification with God or gods, a lessened sense of self-involvement while seeking salvation, enlightenment, and basically religious mystical experience (Hong, 1995; Puhakka, 1995). We must also keep in mind that both prayer and meditation are distinguished from mystical experience.

The overlap of prayer with meditation implies another problem—namely, the tendency of many people to think that "prayer is prayer is prayer." Prayer is not simple and unitary. There are many different kinds of prayer (Lucknow, McIntosh, Spilka, & Ladd, 2000; Paloma & Gallup, 1991). From one perspective, Foster (1992) suggests 21 different forms of prayer. Any study of the biological aspects of prayer should deal with this complexity. No such investigation has yet been made. Since prayer is important in religious coping, we return to it in Chapter 15.

The Biology of Prayer

Since prayer involves ritual, the neurobiological correlates of ritual may also hold for prayer. The results of research studies are not consistent in supporting the selective neural suppression postulated by d'Aquili and Newberg (1999). Noting that TM seems to slow down brain waves (as recorded by electroencephalograms or EEGs), Surwillo and Hobson (1978) claimed that TM was similar to prayer. They then expected to observe the same neural slowing effects in prayer as in TM. Using EEGs from a rather small sample, they were unable to confirm their hypothesis. Yoga and Zen meditation have, however, been associated with the production of alpha brain waves, which occur with feelings of well-being (Benson, 1975).

Utilizing the same theoretical approach, but with a much larger sample, Elkins, Anchor, and Sandler (1979) focused on tension reduction in subjects' muscles. They compared relaxation techniques with intercessory and reflective prayer. No information was provided as to how they defined these forms of prayer. Subjective claims of relaxation by the prayers were not objectively confirmed by the measurement of muscle potentials. The relaxation condition seemed to be more effective than prayer, but the latter demonstrated minor but non-significant tendencies toward tension reduction.

Though prayer may be aimed at reducing tension, its goal may not be relaxation per se, but rather an altered state of consciousness, either contemplative or mystical (Benson, 1975). Insofar as prayer may induce relaxation, Benson (1975) suggests that it should also result in a slowing of breathing, and thus a lowered exchange of oxygen and carbon dioxide. This relaxation response pattern has been observed in TM. Regardless of how it is elicited, such relaxation is considered a healthy body reaction (Benson & Stark, 1996). Benson and Stark further report that 80% of their patients selected prayer as an avenue to the relaxation response, and that 25% felt it enhanced their spirituality. Interestingly, this latter group manifested less medical symptomatology than those who did not experience any spiritual enlightenment.

Benson impressively conveys his belief that the use of religion as in prayer is physiologically and psychologically beneficial. This is buttressed by research showing that faith lowers anxiety, blood pressure, and depression, and that it counters the use of drugs, alcohol, and tobacco (see Chapters 13 and 15). These and other similar observations suggest to Benson that evolution has "hardwired" the brain for religion. In other words, beliefs in God and religion have aided humans to survive and perpetuate themselves through offspring—possibly, in part, because these beliefs have encouraged beneficial physiological reactions such as tension reduction and relaxation.

Prayer and Physical Health

The above-described biological correlates of prayer suggest that it may actually affect the health of those who pray. One way of looking at this potential is to conceive of prayer as an "emotion-regulating strategy" (Koenig, George, & Siegler, 1988). In one study of older adults, prayer appeared to reduce negative emotional expressions under stress (Koenig et al., 1988). Using a broad-based national sample, Ferraro and Albrecht-Jensen (1991) concluded that "people who pray and participate more actively in their religions have better health" (p. 199). A similar conclusion came from a study of patients undergoing coronary artery bypass, whose authors claimed that those who prayed evidenced better postoperative emotional health (Ai, Bolling, & Peterson, 2000). Though noting the positive effects and correlates of prayer relative to bodily health, those who have conducted extensive surveys of this literature are more cautious in their conclusions. They point out a variety of design, analytic, and interpretive problems in the research (McCullough, 1995). Prayer appears to be helpful, but the reasons are not so clear. Once again, controlled enthusiasm is merited.

THE BIOLOGY OF RELIGIOUS EXPERIENCE

Religious and mystical experiences are dealt with at length later in this volume (see Chapters 9 and 10), so we treat the biology of such experiences rather briefly at this point. We have referred earlier to the neurological investigations of Persinger and colleagues, and of Ramachandran and Blakeslee (1999); both groups of researchers associated religious experiential content with the limbic system. As already noted, this system is intimately involved with emotional expression.

d'Aquili and Newberg (1999) offer a rather involved theory of how the brain functions during altered states of consciousness. The main burden of the brain and consciousness with regard to religion falls on what they term "the emotional operator" (i.e., brain structures that mediate the control and expression of emotion). The complexity of emotion and evaluation is stressed. Cognition is afforded recognition, but the essence of the religious encounter is said to rely primarily on the emotional operator. The limbic system takes center stage in this view.

An example of research representing an alternate view is presented in Research Box 3.2. This work as a whole has attempted to locate empirically those brain regions that are active during religious experience. Despite the fact that the immense literature describing religious experiential states has emphasized emotion, cognitive elements—both psychological and neurological—have recently entered the picture. One indication that cognition might play an experiential role came in a study of meditation in Tibetan Buddhist meditators (Institute for the Scientific Study of Meditation, 2001). Single-photon emission computed tomography (SPECT) revealed frontal and parietal lobe activity in areas usually involved in cognition. A more direct experimental approach to this issue is described in Research Box 3.2. In the future, similar studies will undoubtedly be used to define further the relative roles of cognition and emotion in religious experiences. The seeds for such research have been sown, and much supportive theory is currently being created (Bower, 2001). To date, however, there is no definitive evidence that these patterns of brain response are unique to religion.

BIOLOGICAL INFLUENCE OF RELIGIOUS TEACHINGS AND PRACTICES

The Biological Effects of Forgiveness

The doctrine of forgiveness is often a primary ideal of religion. Studying a national sample, Gorsuch and Hao (1993) have shown that personal religiousness and a sense of forgiveness go together. Lack of a willingness to forgive correlates positively with hostility. In turn, the

---

Research Box 3.2. Neural Correlates of Religious Experience (Azari et al., 2001)

In pioneering research, Azari and her coworkers attempted to locate those areas in the brain that are active during religious experience. Utilizing positron emission tomography (PET) to image the brain during religious and other activities, six religious and six nonreligious participants took part in a total of six religious and control conditions. In all conditions, the state achieved was subjectively defined. While reading the 23rd Psalm, the religious respondents apparently attained a religious experiential state. Of most importance, the PET scans showed activation of cognitive areas in the frontal and parietal lobes of the religious subjects. Limbic emotional regions did not reveal involvement, unless specific feeling states were aroused. This cognitive emphasis is consonant with findings of roles for expectancy and desirability in religious experience (Spilka, Ladd, McIntosh, & Milmoe, 1996). Azari and her coworkers feel that religious experience is likely to be a cognitive process utilizing established neural connections between the frontal and parietal lobes.

finding that hostility is associated with unhealthy cardiovascular reactions has been well documented (Baum & Singer, 1987; Sarafino, 1990). In many people, hostility, stress, hypertension, and coronary heart disease constitute the main features of a syndrome known as the "Type A personality" (Friedman & Rosenman, 1974). The main destructive feature of Type A is its hostility component (Rhodewalt & Smith, 1991). As we have seen, research shows that forgiveness, not only counters hostility, but also lowers blood pressure and subjective and objective signs of stress (Witvliet & Ludwig, 1999). The positivity of the religion–health connection is more extensive than this work on forgiveness indicates. More such possibilities are presented in Chapter 15.

Neurological Correlates of Religious Practices

A worldwide perspective on the religious practices of individuals reveals virtually every human action that can be conceived. Altered states of consciousness are associated with such phenomena as meditation, dancing, and ritualistic frenzy, as well as the ingestion of stimulants, depressants, and "magic potions" of indefinite composition. Though we emphasize these practices in their religious forms, there is no reason to believe that their bodily effects are exclusively associated with religion.

d'Aquili and Newberg (1999) claim that these activities parallel the arousal of a variety of brain structures and functions. Much work on how neurons communicate with each other emphasizes, among other things, the role of the brain chemicals known as "neurotransmitters." A potent natural set of neurotransmitters produced in the brain is collectively termed "endorphins." Chemically related to drugs such as morphine, they are considered even more powerful than the usual opiates; they are said to heighten pleasure and reduce discomfort. One may hypothesize that endorphins are stimulated by religious practices that are designed to create a sense of exhilaration and ecstasy.

RELIGION AND BIOLOGY IN HEALTH AND ILLNESS

Health and disease raise crucial questions about biology and religion. First, do the practices of religious groups affect the bodily health and survival of their members? The answer is "Yes," and the Church of Jesus Christ of Latter-Day Saints (whose members are known as the Mormons) is an excellent example of how a church can favorably influence the health of its adherents. Second, can religious groups react in such a way that reproductive isolation (i.e., the confinement of sexual activity within the group) takes place, and genetic factors come to distinguish different religious populations? The answer again is "Yes," and the presence of various genetically based diseases among Jews testifies to the power of the historically conditioned aversion of Jews and non-Jews to intermarriage. The health situations of Mormons and Jews clearly illustrate how the biology of health and illness may be a function of the social expressions of a religious body's theology and practices.

The Effects of Health Behaviors: The Mormons

The virtues of a healthy lifestyle are central to Mormon theology and culture. From early childhood, Mormons are taught to avoid smoking, drinking, using stimulants (e.g., caffeine), and engaging in activities that might damage their bodies. In like manner, a nutritious diet and the elements of a positive and wholesome life are enthusiastically taught in Mormon communities. When one examines the health statistics for Utah, the so-called "Mormon state," the benefits of living such a carefully prescribed existence are well evidenced. With respect to the primary death-causing diseases, Utah has far lower death rates than the 48 contiguous United States as a whole (U.S. Bureau of the Census, 2000; see Table 3.1).

These data can, in part, be further specified by findings showing that Mormons have heart disease rates one-third to one-half those of their non-Mormon peers (Koenig, McCullough, & Larson, 2001). One should not lose sight of the fact that Utah has the highest birth rate in the United States, and therefore probably the youngest population. Still, there is much reason to believe that Mormon health practices do bear fruit.

The Mormons constitute an excellent example of the effects of engaging in healthful behaviors premised on religious doctrines. Similar results have been observed for the Seventh-Day Adventists, a group whose views are similar in many respects to those of the Mormons. Since many Adventists are vegetarians, they also evidence very low colon cancer rates (Koenig et al., 2001).

Problems of Inbreeding: The Jews

To a considerable degree, Jewish history in the past 2,000 years has been a tale of anti-Semitic discrimination and self-imposed separation from Christian neighbors. Long before Jesus, the early Hebrews sharply distinguished themselves from the other peoples who resided near them in the Near and Middle East. This pattern continued into the Christian era, when the separation of Jews into their own communities was finally formalized in the Middle Ages by the creation of the ghetto. Contrary to general belief, the ghetto was instituted by the Jews themselves, not by the Christian authorities (Wirth, 1928). "To the Jews the geographically separated and socially isolated community seemed to offer the best opportunity for following their religious precepts" (Wirth, 1928, p. 19). Administratively, the ghetto was an agency of social, political, and economic control that enforced the segregation of Jews from non-Jews. Considering the prevailing anti-Semitism of Christians, this separation also served their desires well. Simply put, the physical isolation of the Jews for millennia offered a lengthy opportunity for genetic mutations to develop.

Many religious groups have a long history of relatively high rates of inbreeding, with the associated possibility of developing and perpetuating genetic defects. Among such bodies are the Amish, the Hutterites, and other relatively isolated conservative religious com-

TABLE 3.1. Death Rates for the Main Death-Causing Diseases for Utah and the 48 Contiguous United States

Diseases	Utah	48 contiguous United States
Heart disease	146.0	271.6
Cancer	103.6	201.6
Cerebrovascular disease	42.5	59.7
Chronic pulmonary disease	21.5	40.7
Diabetes	21.0	23.4
Total (all causes)	562.3	864.7

Note. Data from U. S. Bureau of the Census, 2000, Tables 126 and 130, pp. 90 and 94. Rates are expressed as number of deaths per 100,000 population as of April 1, 1997.

munities. Since these groups are often distant from the social mainstream, reliable medical data on the health of their members are usually difficult to obtain. The situation of the Jews is quite different. Historically, as already noted, they were often separated from their Christian neighbors in Europe and America. This situation began changing rapidly in the 20th century. Prior to World War II, Jewish intermarriage rates were below 5%. By 1970, about 32% of Jews were intermarrying. In more recent years, incidences of 40–60% have been reported (Silberman, 1985). This is likely to change the genetic situation in the not too distant future.

Interesting recent genetic marker analyses reveal that Jews from Eastern and Western Europe, North Africa, and the Near and Middle East are related despite over 2,000 years of the Diaspora (i.e., the dispersion from their roots in Palestine during Biblical times) (Ostrer, 2000). These genetic indicators were probably preserved by centuries of Jewish segregation and inbreeding.

Medical information about a number of genetic mutations among Jews is not hard to find. Though Jews are prone to a wide variety of genetically based illnesses, in many instances one can argue that lifestyle and other factors contribute to the expression of certain diseases (Koenig et al., 2001). We must also keep in mind that in most cases genetics is more probabilistic than deterministic (Barkow, 1982; Gould, 1978). Still, a number of genetically based conditions evidence great discrepancies between Jews and non-Jews (Griffiths, Miller, Suzuki, Lewontin, & Gelbart, 2000; Post, 1973). For example, Gaucher syndrome—a metabolic disease that affects the liver, spleen, bones, blood, and possibly the nervous system—has an incidence of 1 per 2,500 among Ashkenazi Jews, but 1 per 75,000 among non-Jews. Another condition occurring disproportionately among Jews is Tay–Sachs disease, a degenerative disorder of the brain that results in blindness, deafness, paralysis, and death, usually by the age of 3 or 4. It is found in 1 per 3,500 Jews, but 1 per 35,000 non-Jews. Those who would like to peruse the medical literature might research other genetically based states, such as essential pentosuria, familial dysautonomia, Niemann–Pick disease, and torsion dystonia, plus other possibilities.

Concern among Jews about these conditions has resulted in a National Foundation for Jewish Genetic Diseases.[3] It is a voluntary, nonprofit health and research organization that gathers and provides information on research, care, and resources for those interested in and/or affected by any of the genetic diseases to which Jews are susceptible.

Inbreeding: Other Possibilities

So that the problems of relative reproductive isolation and genetic drift may be further appreciated, we briefly note such problems among the Amish, a strongly Bible-based Christian sect. They are reported to manifest disproportionate rates of hemophilia, phenylketonuria, two forms of dwarfism, and a rare type of anemia (Hostetler, 1968).

Since cancer also involves chromosomal and gene defects in cells, efforts have been made to see whether religious groups differ in the forms of cancer to which everyone is subject. Differences between Jews and non-Jews are evident for a variety of cancers. Sometimes Jewish rates are high, sometimes low (Shiloh & Selavan, 1973). The general picture, however, is that lifestyle characteristics such as diet, smoking, and environmental factors (e.g., occupational

---

3. The foundation can be contacted at 250 Park Avenue, Suite 1000, New York, NY 10177.

exposure to carcinogens) are the main factors inducing cancer (Post, 1973; Shiloh & Selavan, 1973).

Though the history of group separation has contributed to the development and spread of genetic diseases, the continuing breakdown of barriers between groups may well disseminate the undesirable mutations to a larger population. We live in an age where, we hope, progress in genetics should eventually counter and correct these conditions.

OVERVIEW

In this chapter, we have rather briefly examined the main questions surrounding the relationship of religion to biology. This is a realm about which volumes can be written. It is also one that rapidly becomes highly specialized and technical, invoking the esoterica of biochemistry and the neurosciences.

The relationship between religion and biology has been historically conditioned by the theory of evolution. Soon after Darwin presented his views, the religious community split—interestingly, with conservatives on both sides of the conflict. One group saw evolution as posing a dire threat to faith by doing away with the distinction between humans and other animals. The religious proponents of Darwinism saw evolutionary theory as testimony to the wondrous way God works through natural law. This battle is continuing into the 21st century. The basic issues remain the same, but in the contemporary world, the scientific mainstream occupies center stage.

Many thinkers have attempted to present scientific theories for the various roles and functions of religion. One such framework has been detailed here. Although we acknowledge the data from twin studies that speak to a genetic component in religious devotion, we suggest that there is no direct connection between religion and genetics. An indirect connection may be found because of the various functions religion performs in life. Our suggestion is that religious faith satisfies people's needs for meaning, control, and social relationships. Even though this approach is testable, it need not challenge the basic ideas of religion in general, or of any specific theology.

In current biological and social-scientific thinking, religion has become a popular topic. Anthropology, and the newly developed but very controversial field of sociobiology, have offered perspectives on possible origins and roles for religion. Grand, all-encompassing theories may be intellectually exciting, but unless they eventuate in fruitful evaluative research, they will essentially remain sterile.

Research on religion and the brain appears to be a "hot" research area today, but it is basically in its infancy. Work in this domain has, however, opened new avenues to understanding the biological correlates of religious experience and practice. Related research has further demonstrated that these facets of faith do have bodily effects that are primarily positive. In broader perspective, we must recognize that the use of certain substances (e.g., drugs), and ritualistic actions (e.g., starvation, mutilation, etc.) can be physically damaging. On a more general plane, much still needs to be done to unravel the issues of cause, correlation, and effects between religious expression and these physical processes.

Finally, religion and theological doctrines may act as independent variables to foster healthy or unhealthy body states. With our national emphasis on health directing our attention to such concerns as diet and the deleterious effects of smoking, alcohol, and drug abuse, there are obvious lessons that can be learned from the lifestyles practiced by such groups as the Mormons.

It is abundantly evident that religion, which seems so distant from biology, is actually intimately involved with it on many levels. The tip of this iceberg is now displayed, but more and more of its body is coming into view as science studies the various links between religion and biology.

Chapter 4

RELIGION IN CHILDHOOD

> He that spareth his rod hateth his son: but he that loveth him chasteneth him betimes.

> Seven children aged 6 to 14 have been removed from their homes in Aylmer, Ontario, because their parents, who accept the literal truth of the Bible, refuse to promise they will never again hit them with switches if they disobey.

> Around our house we try to keep our kids from having imaginary companions. I think they are associated with the devil and it would be very bad if they had imaginary companions.

> True love and religious experience are almost impossible before adolescence.

> King Solomon must have been fond of animals, because he had many wives and one thousand porcupines.[1]

BORN TO BE RELIGIOUS?

Does our human DNA carry some genetic code that predisposes us to be religious? Are we "naturally" religious, as Elkind (1970) has suggested? In Chapter 3, we have reviewed different theories and some empirical evidence suggesting that evolutionary processes might have "hardwired" humans to be predisposed to become religious beings. These ideas seem to be taken more seriously now than they were a few years ago, possibly because of the huge advances occurring in biology, medicine, and neuroscience with respect to our understanding of the genetic code and physiological functioning. Genetics and the nervous system clearly play important roles in human behavior, and this could include religious behavior. As we have seen in Chapter 3, there is no shortage of "instincts" that have been theorized to underlie religion.

However, many behavioral scientists remain skeptical that religious and other attitudes somehow result from genetic influence, just as they would be suspicious of a claim that we humans are "naturally" inclined to like (or dislike) heavy metal music, or that we have a genetic destiny to be "political" or to be "sports fans." Rather, many social scientists would argue that our love (or hate) of heavy metal music, and our inclinations towards politics and sports, come more from our socialization experiences and environmental factors than from the DNA

---

1. These quotations come, respectively, from the following sources: Proverbs 14:24; Saunders (2001, p. A1); a mother quoted by Taylor and Carlson (2000, p. 247); Kupky (1928, p. 70); and a child quoted by Goldman (1964, p. 1).

we inherited from our parents (see, e.g., Kagan, 1998). For example, Olson, Vernon, Harris, and Jang (2001) have concluded that "A truism in the social psychological literature on attitudes is that attitudes are learned" (p. 845). Albert Bandura's social learning theory (Bandura, 1977), which emphasizes the role of modelling and imitation of behavior, has been especially influential in promoting the view that many of people's attitudes and behaviors are learned.

However, authors and theorists from analyst Carl Jung (1933, 1938) to developmental psychologist David Elkind (1970) have concluded that at least some aspects of, or capacities for, religiousness may be inherited. Jung believed that we humans have an unconscious need to hunt for and to find a deity. Elkind suggested that cognitive-stage development is partially inherited. Therefore, at least some aspects of religion "can be traced to certain cognitive need capacities that emerge in the course of mental growth" (Elkind, 1970, p. 36). These "nativist" speculations were given an injection of new life when research on twins seemed to lend empirical support to the notion that religion is somehow innate. As noted in Chapter 3 (see Research Box 3.1), researchers at the University of Minnesota (Bouchard, Lykken, McGue, Segal, & Tellegen, 1990; Waller, Kojetin, Bouchard, Lykken, & Tellegen, 1990) followed monozygotic and dizygotic sets of twins who were separated in infancy and reared apart, as well as many more identical and fraternal twins who were raised together. They concluded that religiousness, like many other psychological characteristics, has fairly strong heritability components. More recent research on twins has generally confirmed this conclusion, but acknowledges that environmental factors seem to play an even stronger role in attitudes toward religion (Olson et al., 2001). Another study found that, at least during adolescence, there was no evidence of genetic influence on religious attitudes (Abrahamson, Baker, & Caspi, 2002).

Of course, the heritability research does not claim that one person is "born to be a Baptist" and another "born to be a Muslim." Rather, it is suggested that there may be some genetically inherited predisposition in all of us—for example, to find meaning in our existence—and that these might be satisfied by belief in a supreme power. Or an inborn need to affiliate with others might be easily satisfied by involvement in a religious group. In this chapter, however, we address the substantial evidence suggesting that religion affects and is affected by our experiences as we grow up.

"Religious development" has been an area of interest and study since the formative days of the psychology of religion (see, e.g., Hickman, 1926), and a number of major books and articles summarizing theory and research in this area have been published in the past half century (e.g., Allport, 1950; Hyde, 1990; Oser & Scarlett, 1991; Strommen, 1971; Tamminen, 1991; Tamminen & Nurmi, 1995). Also, Rosengren, Johnson, and Harris (2000) have produced a book titled *Imagining the Impossible: Magical, Scientific, and Religious Thinking in Children*, which offers a stimulating collection of articles with novel approaches to understanding religious thinking in childhood. The reader is referred to these scholars for more extensive treatment of the relevant research.

In this chapter we outline several major theoretical positions on religious development, consider relevant empirical work that has tested these theories, and we also review research in several related areas. First, Gordon Allport's insightful reflections on child religious growth are examined. We then turn to a consideration of Jean Piaget's stages of cognitive development, since they have served as the basis for much subsequent theory and research on cognitive religious development. This is followed by an exploration of the work of Elkind and Goldman, both of whom attempted to apply Piaget's concepts directly to religious growth.

Subsequent developments in stage theories are then considered, including Kohlberg's theory of moral development, Fowler's conceptualization of faith development, and Oser's thinking on the development of religious judgment. Then attention is directed to specific related topics, including the development of God concepts, prayer, and religious experience; links between religion and attachment theory; and work in other areas. Finally, in our chapter overview, we offer a critical assessment of previous efforts—especially with respect to "what's missing."

In general, in this chapter we restrict our consideration of "religious development" to theory and investigations involving *children*—here taken to include persons up to their midteen years. This purposely avoids many studies of college students and adults, unless such research has implications for child religious development, or unless it extends child-related findings to adolescent or adult samples. Most of the adolescent and adult material related to religious socialization is discussed in Chapter 5.

THEORIES OF RELIGIOUS DEVELOPMENT

Allport's Analysis

Gordon Allport (1950), in *The Individual and His Religion*, described his ideas about how the child moves from essentially no religion to the point where faith becomes an integrated part of the personality. Allport believed that religion is acquired, not inherited biologically, though he allowed that it does to some extent grow out of basic human needs. He suggested that, at least initially, babies are (psychologically) a bit like a ball of modeling clay—they can be shaped and molded into all sorts of interesting forms. Consequently, culture and environment shape religious orientation, just as they contribute to other aspects of the developing child. Thus babies move from a state of no religion through the acquisition of social responses and habits (e.g., bowing their heads, clasping their hands—things as routine as brushing their teeth). Children do not understand why they are doing these things, but are taught to "go through the motions" of some religious rituals.

According to Allport, young children are very egocentric, perceiving that the world revolves around them; thus prayer may be seen as a means of getting material things. Similarly, young children weave adult explanations and words into meanings that the *children* understand. For example, Allport told the story of a youngster who thought God must be the weathervane on top of the barn, because the child had heard that He is very high and bright, and the weathercock was the highest, brightest thing in the child's world. Furthermore, young children's religious concepts tend to be anthropomorphic (ascribing human characteristics to God); they may visualize God as a king, an old man, or a "superman."

Allport believed that children's egotism inevitably leads to disappointment and deprivations in the years preceding puberty; this process is initiated by such things as the death of pets or denial of material goods, and and in turn leads to revisions of their views of Providence. Essentially, Allport argued that children then pass from a "self-interested" type of religion to a "self-disinterested" religion. As time passes, older children begin to comprehend the abstract aspects of religiousness and no longer need to put everything in concrete terms. Also, they begin to identify with an "ingroup" (i.e., their religious group). All of this leads, usually in adolescence, to the development of religion as an integral part of the personality. This has been described as moving from a faith that is really "second-hand fittings" (i.e., understanding and "believing" parental religious teachings) to a religion of "first-hand fittings" during adolescence (i.e., religion becomes part of an adolescent's own personality) (Allport, 1950, p. 36).

This is an interesting and insightful analysis of children's religious development, but it is rather unsystematic compared to other theories of development that posit specific stages. Moreover, there has been little research to assess Allport's suggestions. Allport did acknowledge that Piaget's conceptualization of cognitive development influenced his own description of religious growth, but Piaget's impact was much stronger on some other theories of religious development, which in turn have stimulated many studies.

Stage Theories of Religious Development

Experiences relevant to faith development begin very early in our lives, and it has been suggested that there are common "stages" in religious growth. Allport did this in a general way, but we need to examine several important and more systematic theoretical positions in this regard. First, as Hyde (1990) pointed out over a decade ago, "The study of religion in childhood and adolescence has been dominated for thirty years by investigations of the process by which religious thinking develops" (p. 15), and this has been largely attributable to the influence of Piaget.

Piaget's Cognitive Stages

Jean Piaget, a dominant figure in developmental psychology, believed that the ways children think about their world change systematically as they grow up (Piaget, 1932/1948, 1936/1952, 1937/1954). That is, Piaget argued that "cognitive development" involves a series of stages. Beginning in the 1920s, he studied these stages in part by sitting on street corners and playing marbles and other games with his own and other children, asking about the "rules" of each game, posing problems for the children to solve, and so on. He was just as interested in the "errors" the children made as he was in "correct" answers to his questions, and noted that there were striking similarities among the ways in which children of the same age reasoned about things. Piaget concluded that there are four major identifiable stages of cognitive development, which reflect the general reasoning abilities of children of different ages:

1. *Sensorimotor stage* (birth to about 2 years). During this stage, children seem to understand things through their sensory and motor ("sensorimotor") interactions with the world around them (e.g., by touching and looking at things, and by putting them in their mouths). It is during this period that infants come to realize that objects continue to exist even though they are no longer immediately perceived ("object permanence"), and also that infants develop a fear of strangers ("stranger anxiety"). Both of these cognitive changes appear at about 8 months or soon thereafter.

2. *Preoperational stage* (about 2 to 7 years). During this second stage, children live in a very egocentric world, being unable to see things from others' perspectives. Preoperational children become quite at home in representing things with language and numbers, but lack sophisticated logical reasoning capability, and are unable to grasp more than one relationship at a time. Also, children at this stage are prone to errors, especially for concepts of conservation. That is, they have difficulty grasping the idea that such characteristics as volume, mass, or length of objects remain the same, in spite of changes in their outward appearance. For example, even when a child has seen the same amount of liquid poured back and forth

between a short, fat beaker and a tall, thin beaker, the youngster may fail to understand that the amount of liquid in the two containers is the same. Rather, he or she may think that the tall, thin beaker holds more water because it "looks bigger."

3. *Concrete operational stage* (about 7 to 12 years). During this stage, children become capable of understanding the concepts of conservation that gave them so much trouble at the previous level. They are also able to reason quite logically about concrete events, to understand analogies, and to perform mathematical transformations such as those involving reversibility (i.e., $4 + 3 = 7$; therefore $7 - 3 = 4$).

4. *Formal operational stage* (12 years and up). The last stage of cognitive development allows a move away from the concrete in thought processes. These older children are capable of complex abstract thinking involving the hypothetical—for example, by generating potential solutions to a problem, and then creating a plan to systematically test different possibilities in order to arrive at a "correct" solution.

Although Piaget's proposals have not escaped criticism, one of the most important contributions of his cognitive development stages seems to have been his recognition that children are not simply miniature adults and cannot think as adults do. Rather, cognitive growth proceeds sequentially in order to allow growing children to assimilate and deal with their environment, and also to make alterations in thinking in order to accommodate new information. Each stage builds on the previous stages in order to further cognitive development. This has important implications for religious development. For example, it suggests that children are not cognitively capable of understanding the complex and abstract concepts involved in most religions of the adult world. Piaget did not write directly about the religious growth of children (Hyde, 1990), even though he wrote a book on moral development (Piaget, 1932/1948). It was left to others to relate Piaget's theories of cognitive stages to religion.

Applications of Piaget's Stages to Religious Development

Elkind's Approach.   David Elkind proposed that religion is a natural result of mental development, such that biological roots of intellectual growth interact with individuals' experiences. Specifically, Elkind suggested that four basic sequential components of intelligence (conservation, search for representation, search for relations, and search for comprehension) are critical in religious development, and that this sequence parallels the cognitive stages described by Piaget (Elkind, 1961, 1962, 1963, 1964, 1970, 1971). Three studies investigating Elkind's ideas about cognitive religious development are described in Research Box 4.1. Essentially, his research supported a Piagetian kind of progression as religious understanding emerges in children. A subsequent study (Long, Elkind, & Spilka, 1967) revealed a similar cognitive sequence for children's ideas about prayer.

Some authors apparently saw in these findings implications for religious education. For example, it has been recommended that children not be taught basic concepts about God until they are capable of understanding them, at about age 6 (Williams, 1971). Abraham (1981) also found that it may be possible to hasten the transition from concrete to abstract religious thinking by deliberately stimulating cognitive conflict in religious education instructional materials at the sixth-grade level. As discussed below, Ronald Goldman in particular has extended Piaget's stages to the realm of religious education.

Research Box 4.1. The Child's Concept of Religion (Elkind, 1961, 1962, 1963)

In three separate studies, Elkind posed a series of questions to Jewish, Catholic, and Protestant children, respectively, concerning their understanding of their religious identity and ideas. For example, in his 1961 study, Jewish children were asked questions such as these: "Are you Jewish?", "What makes you Jewish?", "Can a cat or a dog be Jewish? Why?", and "How do you become a Jew?" Elkind found considerable age-related cognitive similarity in children's responses to such questions across his three major religious groups. The development of religious ideas seemed to parallel Piaget's cognitive stages to some extent.

In the 5- to 7-year range (comparable to Piaget's late preoperational stage), children seemed to think that their denominational affiliation was absolute, having been ordained by God, and therefore it could not be changed. A few years later (ages 7–9, comparable to Piaget's early concrete operational stage), religious ideas were indeed very "concrete." Religious affiliation was seen to be determined by the family into which one was born, and if a Catholic family had a pet cat, it was thought to be a Catholic cat. At the next stage of religious development (ages 10–14, corresponding to Piaget's late concrete and early formal operational stages), children apparently began to understand some of the complexities of religious practices and rituals, and they could conceive of a person's changing his or her religion because they understood religion to come from within the person rather than being determined externally. Abstract and differentiated religious thinking was beginning to appear. In the end, Elkind concluded that children were not capable of an abstract "adult" understanding of religion before the age of 11 or 12 (i.e., the beginning of Piaget's formal operational period).

The Work of Goldman.   Goldman applied Piaget's theory of cognitive development to religious thinking, claiming that "religious thinking is no different in mode and method from non-religious thinking" (Goldman, 1964, p. 5). Working in England, he asked 5- to 15-year-old children questions about drawings with religious connotations (e.g., a child kneeling at a bed, apparently praying), as well as questions about Bible stories (e.g., Moses at the burning bush). He then analyzed responses to the questions by looking for evidence of Piagetian stages of development. He concluded, as did Elkind, that religious thinking does indeed proceed in a fashion similar to more general cognitive development.

A number of studies have confirmed these general conclusions about "cognitive stages," especially the implication that children are capable of more abstract religious thinking as they grow older (see, e.g., Degelman, Mullen, & Mullen, 1984; Peatling, 1974, 1977; Peatling & Laabs, 1975; Tamminen, 1976; Tamminen & Nurmi, 1995). There has also been some confirmatory cross-cultural work (see Hyde, 1990). Some studies have examined specific predictions of the Piagetian approach for religious development. For example, Zachry (1990) concluded that his data, obtained from high school and college students, were "consistent with the prediction of Piagetian theory that abstract thought in a specific content area such as religion depends on an underlying formal logic" (p. 405).

Evaluating Goldman's Findings.   Some empirical work has not been entirely supportive of Goldman's conclusions about the development of religious thought. For example, Hoge and Petrillo (1978b) studied 451 high school sophomores in different Protestant and Catholic churches, and concluded that Goldman had overestimated the importance of cognitive capacity and underestimated the role of religious training in the development of religious thought. This conclusion, however, was apparently based primarily on differences between public and private school Catholics. Hoge and Petrillo attributed such differences to religious education at the private school, but there might well have been selection factors at work, such as socioeconomic status or parental religiosity. Hoge and Petrillo themselves acknowledged the bias in their sample, such that "the youth most alienated from the church refused [to participate] disproportionately often" (pp. 142–143).

Batson, Schoenrade, and Ventis (1993) reconsidered Hoge and Petrillo's (1978b) results and concluded that their conclusions were inappropriate. In fact, they suggested that Hoge and Petrillo's findings were "precisely what Goldman would have predicted" (1993, p. 62). The disagreement between these two groups of authors apparently hinges partly on a specific Goldman prediction concerning the level of religious *teachings* (e.g., "concrete thinking" about religious content) and adolescents' overall *capacity* for higher, more abstract ("formal operational") religious thinking. Hoge and Petrillo did not measure this "gap" directly, but assumed that higher absolute scores on a measure of abstract religious thinking meant that a smaller gap existed. Furthermore, their findings were not consistent across different measures of religious rejection or across different participant groupings, and the majority of reported correlations did not achieve statistical significance. It is not surprising that there was some disagreement as to the interpretation of these findings.

Some authors (e.g., Godin, 1968; Howkins, 1966; Kay, 1996; McCallister, 1995) have been quite critical of Goldman's general conclusions, especially the implications he drew for religious education. Apparently Elkind's research has escaped the severe criticism applied to Goldman's work, in part because Elkind avoided theological biases or assumptions (see Hyde, 1990), whereas Goldman "assumed a particular theological point of view" (Hyde, 1990, p. 35). For example, Greer (1983) has suggested that the cognitive tests of Goldman and those of Peatling, who developed a measure of religious cognitive development (Peatling, Laabs, & Newton, 1975), were biased in such a way that theologically conservative respondents would tend to endorse responses indicating concrete (rather than abstract) religious thinking.

In the end, although it has been argued that the religiosity of children is *not* dependent on cognitive development (Pierce & Cox, 1995), the works of Elkind, Goldman, and others have demonstrated the utility of a Piagetian framework for understanding the development of religious thinking. These researchers also set the stage for much subsequent work in related areas, such as moral development, faith development, and the emergence of the God concept and prayer.

Kohlberg's Stages of Moral Development

Lawrence Kohlberg's (1964, 1969, 1981, 1984) theory of moral development has served as a basis for the investigation of many issues related to morality. Building on Piaget's belief that the moral judgments of children derive from their cognitive development, Kohlberg attempted to identify cognitive stages that underlie the development of moral thinking. In a series of studies, he asked people what they thought about different "moral dilemmas."

His most famous dilemma involved a woman near death from cancer who could potentially be saved by a new drug developed by a nearby druggist. The druggist, however, wanted 10 times what the drug cost him to make—more than the sick woman's husband,

Heinz, could afford—and refused to sell it for less. So Heinz considered breaking into the druggist's store to steal the drug for his wife. Respondents were asked to comment on the morality of Heinz's potential decision to steal the drug, and to indicate the reasoning behind their response. Based on such responses to such dilemmas, Kohlberg proposed that individuals pass through three broad levels of moral development, each with substages. As Sapp (1986) stated, "each stage is distinguished by moral reasoning that is more complex, more comprehensive, more integrated, and more differentiated than the reasoning of the earlier stages" (p. 273). Table 4.1 outlines the levels and stages of moral development proposed by Kohlberg.

Kohlberg's theory has been criticized (Darley & Shultz, 1990), and Bergling's (1981) extensive assessment of its validity suggests that the theory may have limited utility outside of Western industrialized countries. But there is some support for Kohlberg's conclusions that children do progress through moral stages, especially from the preconventional level to the conventional level of morality. Also, Snarey's (1985) review of the literature suggests that this progression *is* reasonably similar in different cultures.

TABLE 4.1. Kohlberg's Stages of Moral Development

Preconventional level (develops during early childhood)

Stage 1. Punishment and obedience orientation
The first stage is characterized by avoidance of punishment and unquestioning deference to power as values in themselves. Morality is seen as based on self-interest, and the goodness or badness of actions is determined by their physical consequences, regardless of any human meaning attached to these consequences.

Stage 2. Instrumental relativist orientation
This stage is defined by a focus on instrumental satisfaction of one's own needs as the determiner of "right." Reciprocity may be present, but is of the "you scratch my back and I'll scratch yours" variety.

Conventional level (develops during late childhood and early adolescence)

Generally, this level involves a move towards gaining approval or avoiding disapproval as the basis for morality; law and social rules are seen as valuable in their own right.

Stage 3. Interpersonal concordance or "good boy/nice girl" orientation
Early in the conventional level, the individual is driven by behavior that pleases or helps others and that receives their approval.

Stage 4. "Law and order" orientation
Subsequently, in the conventional level, the person focuses on the maintenance of the social order and the importance of authority and strict rules.

Postconventional level (may develop from late adolescence on)

People at this level tend to be concerned with morality as abstract principles. They are able to separate their own identification with groups from the principles and moral values associated with those groups.

Stage 5. Social-contract/legalistic orientation
The fifth stage involves recognition of the relative nature of personal values, and the importance of having procedural rules to reach consensus. The individual can separate the legal world from individual differences of opinion.

Stage 6. Universal ethical principle orientation
The last and highest stage of moral development, according to Kohlberg, involves defining "right" in one's own conscience, consistent with one's own abstract ethical principles, but with a sense of responsibility to others. There is a clear emphasis on universality, consistency, logic, and rationality.

One might expect that Kohlberg's conceptualization of moral development would be closely linked to religious growth, or that religious development would directly affect (and possibly determine) the emergence of morality. However, Kohlberg was very clear that moral and religious development are quite separate, and the two should not be confused. For example, he suggested that it is a fallacy to think that

> basic moral principles are dependent upon a particular religion, or any religion at all. We have found no important differences in development of moral thinking between Catholics, Protestants, Jews, Buddhists, Moslems, and atheists. . . . Both cultural values and religion are important factors in selectively elaborating certain themes in the moral life but they are not unique causes of the development of basic moral values. (Kohlberg, 1980, pp. 33–34)

Research has confirmed Kohlberg's conclusion in this regard (Bruggeman & Hart, 1996; Cobb, Ong, & Tate, 2001; Gorsuch & McFarland, 1972; Selig & Teller, 1975), and other experts on moral development have taken a similar stance (e.g., Turiel & Neff, 2000). Moreover, Nucci and Turiel (1993) found that older children and adolescents were able to distinguish between moral and religious issues, and that they viewed moral rules as unalterable by religious authorities. However, this has not stopped many, many researchers from speculating about and investigating possible relationships between moral development and religiosity (e.g., Clouse, 1986; Fernhout & Boyd, 1985; Glover, 1997; Hanson, 1991; Kedem & Cohen, 1987; Mitchell, 1988). Such research has been facilitated by the development of a less subjective scoring system to evaluate stages of moral development.

Rest's (1979, 1983; Rest, Cooper, Coder, Masanz, & Anderson, 1974) Defining Issues Test (DIT) asks people to respond to a series of 12 statements concerning each of six moral dilemmas. The DIT was intended to be both simpler and more objective than Kohlberg's initial scoring of moral stages, and it has stimulated numerous studies on moral development and religion, though apparently few with children. These investigations have reported some relationships between level of moral judgment and religious orientation, though typically not strong ones (Clouse, 1991; Ernsberger & Manaster, 1981; Holley, 1991; Sapp, 1986). There have also been claims that people from fundamentalist denominations have lower DIT scores (Richards, 1991; Sapp, 1986). The validity of the DIT for conservative religious groups has been called into question, however, by Richards (1991; Richards & Davison, 1992). Recently an improved measure of moral judgment, the DIT2, was published (Rest, Narvaez, Thoma, & Bebeau, 1999). It remains to be seen whether this new measure will help to clarify the literature on moral development and religion.

Gilligan (1977) has criticized Kohlberg's theory and research for their failure to deal with unique aspects of women's moral development, especially the care and responsibility orientation of many women, as contrasted with the male justice orientation emphasized by Kohlberg. This could have implications for religious development—for example, in terms of gender differences in images of God, if God is seen as a person's anchor for morality. There is evidence that images of God diverge along gender lines, with women more likely to see God as supportive and men more likely to see God as instrumental (Nelsen, Cheek, & Au, 1985). Reich (1997) has pondered more generally whether such considerations might suggest the need for a theory specifically for women's religious development. However, he has concluded that there is no need to modify current theories of religious development, or to generate new ones in this regard. Others (DeNicola, 1997; Schweitzer, 1997) have been critical of Reich's stance; they have argued that, at the least, revisions to current theories are needed.

In general, Kohlberg's stages of moral development can at least stimulate our thinking about religious growth. For example, Scarlett and Periello (1991) have suggested that Kohlberg's ideas could help in understanding aspects of the development of prayer. Furthermore, religion has much to say about morality, and understanding how moral development occurs is certainly relevant to the communication and understanding of moral issues at different ages. At the same time, we must take Kohlberg's warning to heart and not assume—as some researchers have—that moral and religious development are necessarily directly and causally related.

Fowler's Stages of Faith Development

James Fowler (1981, 1991a, 1991b, 1994, 1996) has suggested that individual religious faith unfolds in a stage sequence similar to that described by Piaget for cognitive development and Kohlberg for moral growth. (For an analysis of similarities between Fowler's and Kohlberg's theories, see Hanford, 1991.) Faith is defined as "a dynamic and generic human experience . . . [that] includes, but is not limited to or identical with, religion" (Fowler, 1991a, p. 31). That is, although Fowler's use of the term "faith" does overlap with institutionalized religion, the two are also independent to some extent. Faith is seen as a deep core of the individual, the "center of values," "images and realities of power," and "master stories" (myths) involving both conscious and unconscious motivations. In other words, faith involves centers of values that vary from one individual to the next, but that are foci of primary life importance (such as religion, family, nation, power, money, and sexuality).

Furthermore, people tend to align themselves with power in this dangerous world—possibly religious power, but also sources of secular power, such as nations and economic systems. "Faith is trust in and loyalty to images and realities of power" (Fowler, 1991a, p. 32). Also, Fowler argues that faith involves stories or scripts that give meaning and direction to people's lives (e.g., what it means to be a good person or a part of a religious community).

Fowler and his colleagues have carried out extensive interviews with hundreds of people about these aspects of their faith. They have concluded that there are essentially seven stages in faith development, although some people never progress very far through these stages. Fowler's stages "aim to describe patterned operations of knowing and valuing that underlie our consciousness" (Fowler, 1996, p. 56), and are described in Table 4.2, with the approximate time of emergence of each stage shown in parentheses.

Fowler concluded that it is extremely rare for people to reach the seventh and final stage in his sequence, but people who have attained universalizing faith might include Mahatma Gandhi, Martin Luther King, Jr., and Mother Teresa. It is no coincidence that both Gandhi and King were assassinated. Fowler claims that people who achieve universalizing faith are in danger of premature death because of their confrontational involvement in solving serious problems in the world.

Fowler's analysis of stages of faith is rich in ideas, provides a framework for empirical work, and can potentially contribute to our understanding of what it means to be "religious." However, it has been pointed out that Fowler's conceptualization is complex and difficult to comprehend, and it has failed to generate relatively rigorous empirical research. Also, Fowler has generally declined to analyze his own results statistically and ignored related work in the psychology of religion (Hyde, 1990).

Recently the *International Journal for the Psychology of Religion* has devoted a special issue to critical discussion of what it calls Fowler's "faith development theory" (FDT) . Streib

TABLE 4.2. Fowler's Stages of Faith Development

1. *Primal faith* (infancy). This first stage involves the beginnings of emotional trust based on body contact, care, early play and the like. Subsequent faith development is based on this foundation.

2. *Intuitive/projective faith* (early childhood). In the second stage, imagination combines with perception and feelings to create long-lasting faith images. The child becomes aware of the sacred, of prohibitions, of death, and of the existence of morality.

3. *Mythical/literal faith* (elementary school years). Next, the developing ability to think logically helps to order the world, corresponding to the Piagetian stage of concrete operations. The child can now discriminate between fantasy and the real world, and can appreciate others' perspectives. Religious beliefs and symbols are accepted quite literally.

4. *Synthetic/conventional faith* (early adolescence). During the fourth stage, there is a reliance on abstract ideas of formal operational thinking, which engenders a hunger for a more personal relationship with God. Reflections on past experiences, and concerns about the future and personal relationships, contribute to the development of mutual perspective taking and the shaping of a world view and its values.

5. *Individuative/reflective faith* (late adolescence or young adulthood). The fifth stage involves a critical examination and reconstitution of values and beliefs, including a change from reliance on external authorities to authority within the self. The capacity for "third-person perspective taking" contributes to the development of consciously chosen commitments and to the emergence of an "executive ego."

6. *Conjunctive faith* (midlife or beyond). In the sixth stage, there is integration of opposites (e.g., the realization that each individual is both young and old, masculine and feminine, constructive and destructive), generating a "hunger for a deeper relationship to the reality that symbols mediate" (Fowler, 1991a, p. 41) "Dialogical knowing" emerges, such that the individual is open to the multiple perspectives of a complex world. This enables the person to go beyond the faith boundaries developed in the previous individuative/reflective stage, and to appreciate that "truth" is both multidimensional and organically interdependent.

7. *Universalizing faith* (unspecified age). The relatively rare final stage involves a oneness with the power of being or God, as well as commitment to love, justice, and overcoming oppression and violence. People who have attained this stage of faith development "live as though a commonwealth of love and justice were already reality among us. They create zones of liberation for the rest of us, and we experience them as both liberating and as threatening. These people tend to confront others concerning their involvement in, and attachments to, dehumanizing structures which oppose 'the commonwealth of love and justice'" (Fowler, 1991a, p. 41).

(2001) proposes that revisions to FDT are needed—for example, to free the theory from "its almost unquestioned adoption of the structural-developmental 'logic of development' . . . in order to account for the rich and deep life-world- and life-history-related dimensions of religion" (pp. 144–45). Similarly, Day (2001) claims that "contemporary research challenges the fundamental assumptions of the cognitive developmental paradigm" (p. 173); therefore, we need to look elsewhere if we are to understand religious development. He has suggested that greater attention should be addressed to (religious) speech and narrative. McDargh (2001) focuses his critique of EDT more on its theological foundations, and claims that a more individually focused approach would be useful. McDargh (2001) and Rizzuto (2001) have both argued for more incorporation of psychoanalytic concepts and processes in analyzing faith development. However, Fowler (2001) has defended FDT, arguing that it continues to serve as a useful framework for studying faith development at different levels (individual, family, and social group).

One problem with FDT has been the difficulty in operationalizing the stages, and consequently there have been attempts to simplify the measurement of Fowler's proposed stages.

Barnes and Doyles (1989) constructed a "faith development" version of Rest's Defining Issues Test (which itself was intended to simplify measurement of Kohlberg's moral stages). More recently, Leak, Loucks, and Bowlin (1999) have developed an 8-item Faith Development Scale intended to measure Fowler's proposed stages. However, attempts to validate this scale have generated mixed results. Leak et al. (1999) have suggested that this either might be due to limitations of the scale, or might suggest that we should have "reservations on the beneficence of mature faith within a Fowlerian framework" (p. 122). In light of these problems, Fowler's conceptualization of faith stages has yet to live up to its promise as a useful and important explanatory construct in the psychology of religion.

Oser's Stages of Development of Religious Judgment

Fritz Oser, with Gmunder and other colleagues (Oser, 1991, 1994; Oser & Gmunder, 1991; Oser & Reich, 1990, 1996; Oser, Reich, & Bucher, 1994), has focused on a related aspect of religious development called "religious judgment." Apart from the work of Elkind, Fowler and others, Oser (1991) concluded that

> there have been few investigations directed at building up a theory about the development of an individual's constructions and reconstructions of the religious experiences and beliefs. [Therefore we] are attempting to formulate a new paradigm of religious development, using a structural concept of discontinuous, stagelike development and the classical semiclinical interview method as our primary research strategy. (p. 6)

Oser's research has revealed five stages in the emergence of religious judgment, as qualitative changes occur in people's relationship to an "Ultimate Being" or God. Individuals move from a stage of believing that God intervenes unexpectedly in the world and that God's power guides human beings (Stage 1), through belief in a still external and all-powerful God who punishes or rewards depending on good or bad deeds ("Give so that you may receive") (Stage 2). Individuals in Stage 3 begin to think of God as somewhat detached from their world and as wielding less influence, with people generally responsible for their own lives, since they can now distinguish between transcendence (God's existence outside the created world) and immanence (God's presence and action from within). In Stage 4 people come to realize both the necessity and the limits of autonomy, recognizing that freedom and life stem from an Ultimate Being, who is often perceived to have a "divine plan" that gives meaning to life. Finally, in Stage 5 the Ultimate Being is realized through human action via care and love. There is "universal and unconditional religiosity" (Oser, 1991, p. 10).

Overall, there is a growing need for autonomy as people advance through the five stages, as well as a "deepening appreciation for the unity or 'partnership' of opposites" (Oser, 1991, p. 13). Elements of this stage analysis of religious judgment parallel aspects of the other stage theories considered above. For example, Oser's claim that people move from seeing God as all-powerful and as guiding human behavior to a much more autonomous, self-defined view of the deity and world is similar to Kohlberg's observation that people move from unquestioning deference to power (at the preconventional level) to the recognition of the relative nature of personal values and an emphasis on universality (at the postconventional level). This in turn is similar to Fowler's conceptualization of the early stages of faith development as a process of teasing apart the real from fantasy; of the middle stages as involving an increasing appreciation of other's perspectives, not just one's own; and of the later stages as characterized by the integration of opposites and the emergence of a universalizing faith.

Oser and Reich (1996) have pointed to limited empirical support for this stage conceptualization of the development of religious judgment; some recent research (e.g., Bucher, 1991; Di Loreto & Oser, 1996, as cited in Oser & Reich, 1996; Roco & Ticu, 1996; Zondag & Belzen, 1999) has provided further support for Oser's proposals. Huber, Reich, and Schenker (2000) have argued that it is important to match the technique of measurement to the goals of an investigation in this area; their findings suggest that combinations of methods may be appropriate.

Stage Theories: Enough Is Enough?

How many different stage conceptualizations of religious development are needed, especially with respect to the cognitive aspects of religion? Given the overlap among current stage conceptualizations, it might be productive to attempt an integration and synthesis of Piaget's, Kohlberg's, Fowler's, Oser's, and others' stage theories of development, in order to delineate the common elements of these theories as they apply to the development of religious thought processes. Such an integration has been attempted by Helmut Reich; his work is discussed later (see "Is a Unified Approach to Religious Development Possible?", below). However, it is clear that there has been a strong emphasis in existing theories of religious development on *cognitive* components of such growth, and a tendency to ignore or underemphasize other aspects of religious socialization (see Chapter 5).

More generally, is the "stage" approach the best way to conceptualize religious growth and change? Certainly this approach has increased our understanding of the general processes involved in the emergence of adult religiousness. However, it is possible that an obsession with stages may detract from our ability to understand the complexity and uniqueness of individual religious development. That is, the tendency to assume that such growth involves cognitive commonalities across all members of specific age groups can to some extent blind us to the idiosyncratic nature of religion in childhood and adolescence (see, e.g., Day, 1994, 2001; Streib, 2001). Furthermore, the stage approach implies a certain amount of discontinuity in religious development, whereas it may actually be a reasonably continuous process.

It has been argued that solid empirical investigations of the development of religious concepts are rare (Boyer & Walker, 2000), and the topic of religious development has been generally neglected (Harris, 2000). The studies that do exist are often "misguided" (Boyer & Walker, 2000, p. 140), because they compare how children think with "how adults ought to think, according to theological doctrine" (p. 141). Boyer and Walker have pointed out that we do not know whether adults' religious representations are indeed consistent with church doctrine; nor should we assume that children's religious development can be assessed by comparing it to adult religious thought. Possibly investigations of children's religion simply elicit "theologically correct" information. That is, children may say what their church, parents, or culture expect them to say, and this tells us little about, for example, religious concept development. In a similar vein, Harris (2000) has concluded that in spite of appearances to the contrary, the Piagetian legacy has actually led us to neglect the development of religious thinking. Maybe we need to rethink our thinking about children's religious thinking!

Is a Unified Approach to Religious Development Possible?

Helmut Reich (1993a, 1993b) has attempted to summarize the "smorgasbord" of differing theoretical and empirical approaches to the study of religious development. In addition, he has attempted to distinguish between the degree of "hardness" and "softness" of stage theories. "Hard" stages

> describe organized systems of action (first-order problem solving), are qualitatively different from each other and follow an unchanging sequence with a clear developmental logic: A later stage denotes greater complexity and improved problem solving capacity. Each hard stage integrates the preceding stage and logically requires the elements of the prior stage. (Reich, 1993a, p. 151)

The stage models of Piaget, Kohlberg, Elkind and Goldman would be considered "hard." "Soft" stages, on the other hand, "explicitly include elements of affective or reflective characteristics (metatheoretical reflection) that . . . do not follow a unique developmental logic" (Reich, 1993a, p. 151). Oser's and Fowler's theories above would fall into this "soft" category. The "hard–soft" distinction could be helpful in understanding and categorizing theories of religious development, and also the circumstances under which one theory might be more appropriate than another. However, Fowler (1993) has criticized this approach, suggesting that the use of "hard" and "soft" categories is obsolete; that Reich's formulation does not incorporate the important work by Gilligan (1977) on the ethics of responsibility and care; and that Reich fails to acknowledge important differences between Oser's and Fowler's stage theories.

Reich's work does a considerable service by mapping common elements in different theories and empirical investigations, critically evaluating and integrating theories, and suggesting the need for clarification and some standardization in terminology and approaches. In reaction to Reich's proposed integration, Wulff (1993) has suggested that "in the long run . . . the psychology of religion and its practitioners will be best served if we not only recognize the limitations of these theories and their associated research techniques, but also strive to develop new ones more faithful to the traditions and life experience of the persons we seek to understand" (p. 185). Reich's beginning could stimulate further integrative conceptualizations. However, a single major integrative theory of religious development remains an elusive goal (see also Tamminen & Nurmi, 1995).

Aside from the theoretical work described to this point, many studies have attempted to evaluate different aspects of "childhood" religion and its development. This research sometimes incorporates elements of the stage theories of religious growth described above, but specific issues are often studied empirically without direct reliance on the stage approach. We now turn to an examination of some additional theoretical work, as well as several empirical areas.

CONCEPTS OF GOD

When children think of God, what sort of an image forms in their minds? Many studies of religion in childhood have focused specifically on this issue. Some of this research was based on psychodynamic theories about the development of an image of God. For example, Freud (1913/1919, 1927/1961) interpreted the God image as a father figure, a kind of projection of one's real father in the context of the resolution of the Oedipus complex. Jung (1948/1969) apparently agreed that there is some projection of one's earthly father into one's God image, but he felt that "archetypes" (images/symbols with biological roots, found in many cultures) also play a role in concepts of God. Although such analytic theories of the origins and development of a God image are difficult to test directly, they suggest that there should be a firm link between how children see their real fathers and their images of God. What does the research show?

Parent and Gender Issues

Psychodynamic approaches tend to focus on the underlying psychoanalytic explanation of the origin of God concepts, and the relevant psychodynamic research has been criticized for serious methodological and conceptual problems, as well as an inadequate theoretical basis (Gorsuch, 1988; Kirkpatrick, 1986).

Some research has confirmed that God images are typically male-dominated in Western culture (Foster & Keating, 1992), possibly more so for girls than boys (Ladd, McIntosh, & Spilka, 1998). But empirical support for the prediction that God images should be related to children's views of their own fathers has been mixed (Spilka, Addison, & Rosensohn, 1975). Vergote and Tamayo (1981) suggested that the God image may actually bear more similarity to the mother than to the father, and Roberts (1989) found a correspondence between images of God and images of self. There is also evidence that general qualitative aspects of relationships with parents may be related to positive (e.g., warm, loving) images of God (Godin & Hallez, 1964; Potvin, 1977).

Krejci's (1998) investigation of college students, led him to concluded that God images were organized around three dimensions: "nurturing–judging," "controlling–saving," and "concrete–abstract." He found few gender differences, with the exception that control was more salient in men's God images. More gender differences appeared in another study (Dickie et al., 1997), which emphasized the importance of parents in affecting children's God images, both directly and indirectly. Dickie et al.'s results suggested that girls' God concepts were more closely related to attributes and discipline styles of parents than were boys' God concepts.

Hertel and Donahue (1995) examined more than 3,400 mother–father–youth triads from data obtained through the Search Institute in the United States in 1982–1983. The young people in this study were in fifth through ninth grades. Results showed that although relationships were not large, there were significant tendencies for parents' images of God to be reflected in young people's impressions of parenting styles. In particular, fathers' and mothers' loving God images both apparently affected children's images of their fathers and mothers as loving, respectively. In turn, parenting styles and parents' God images predicted youths' God images. These relationships remained even after social class, religious denomination, church attendance, and youths' ages were controlled for. Hertel and Donahue also concluded that there was a strong tendency for their participants to perceive God as love ("maternal") rather than as authority ("paternal"), and that mothers played a more important role in socializing their children's God images, especially for daughters.

At least one study has found evidence that teachers may be more important than parents in God concept development. De Roos, Miedema, and Iedema (2001) found that kindergarten children who evidenced a close relationship with their teachers also tended to display a loving God concept, whereas the mother–child relationship did not make a significant prediction in this regard.

In general, the literature on children's God images seems reasonably consistent in confirming the importance of parents in the development of these concepts. There is less agreement about gender differences in God images, the actual nature of those images (e.g., loving vs. authoritarian), and the relative impact of mothers and fathers in contributing to the development of God concepts.

Does a God Concept Develop in Stages?

Attempts to understand the developmental aspects of God concepts have typically focused on cognitive development. Some of these approaches are clearly Piagetian in orientation, whereas others have a more general cognitive focus. This area has benefited from research carried out in several different Western countries.

Harms (1944) suggested that previous investigations of children's images of God had erred by asking children to respond to fixed questions. Instead, he asked more than 4,800 U.S. children (aged 3–18) both to talk about and to draw their representations of religion, especially God. Their responses led Harms to conclude that there are three stages in the development of God concepts:

1. *Fairy-tale stage* (3–6 years). Children see little difference between God and fairy-tale characters.

2. *Realistic stage* (6–11 years). As children's cognitive capacities begin to expand, they see God as more concrete and more human. They are more comfortable using religious symbols.

3. *Individualistic stage* (adolescence). Adolescents no longer rely exclusively on religious symbols. They take a more individualized approach to God, resulting in very different conceptualizations from person to person.

Another major study of the development of God concepts was undertaken by Deconchy (1965) in France, though he did not include children under 7 years of age. He concluded that the development of God concepts occurs in three stages, revolving around themes of attribution, personalization and interiorization, respectively; these are described in Research Box 4.2.

There have been variations on these themes, but different authors describe similar stages in the development of God concepts (Ballard & Fleck, 1975; Fowler, 1981; Nye & Carlson, 1984; Williams, 1971), including some based on a Piagetian framework (Elkind, 1970; Goldman, 1964; Nye & Carlson, 1984). Others have simply noted the general change from fragmented, undifferentiated thinking through very simple, concrete God concepts to more abstract and complex images as children grow older (see, e.g., the review of European research on this topic by Tamminen, Vianello, Jaspard, & Ratcliff, 1988). However, attempts to further specify the parameters of such development, and the processes through which this unfolding occurs, have not been particularly successful (Ladd, McIntosh, & Spilka, 1998). For example, Janssen, de Hart, and Gerardts (1994) used open-ended questions about God in a study of Dutch secondary school students. They concluded that perceptions of God among their participants were complex and "can hardly be summarized" (p. 116). Furthermore, although there was evidence of abstract thinking among their Dutch adolescents, the authors pointed out that there was no proof that it resulted from a developmental process. However, it was questionable whether a developmental process *could* have been demonstrated in a study of teenagers only.

ʂ●

Research Box 4.2. The Idea of God: Its Emergence between 7 and 16 Years (Deconchy, 1965)

In this investigation, Catholic children and adolescents were asked to free-associate when they heard words such as "God." An analysis of their responses led Deconchy to conclude that these children exhibited three major stages in the development of God concepts. Those from about 7 or 8 to 11 years of age used predominantly "attributive" themes; that is, God was seen as a set of attributes, many anthropomorphic with overtones of animism. God concepts were relatively independent of other religious constructs, such as the historical events in the life of Jesus. The associations of children between 11 and 14 years of age emphasized "personalization" themes, such that God took on parental characteristics and was seen in more sophisticated anthropomorphic terms (e.g., "just," "strong," "good"). Finally, by approximately the age of 14 a further shift began to take place, focusing on "interiorization" themes. That is, in middle adolescence anthropomorphic characteristics of God disappeared, and God concepts became more abstract and tended to reflect relationships with God (e.g., involving love, trust) emanating from within the individual, rather than simply involving descriptive characteristics.

Does the development of God concepts vary across cultures or different religious groups? Vergote and Tamayo (1981) found that although there are commonalities in God images across cultures, at least some cultural differences do emerge with respect to maternal and paternal symbolism. Ladd et al. (1998) found that God concepts developed similarly across Christian denominations, in a manner generally consistent with Piagetian theory, in their study of almost 1,000 children from eight Christian groups in the United States. These authors have suggested that more research is necessary to understand how and why very different religious education experiences do not lead to divergent concepts of God by adolescence.

Diversity of Method and Direction

Harms's (1944) call for less constraining measures of ideas about God has not been ignored. In addition to his own attempt to allow subjects greater freedom in description of their God concepts, other researchers have used diverse techniques: pictures or drawings (Bassett et al., 1990; Graebner, 1964; Ladd et al., 1998); word associations (Deconchy, 1965); adjective ratings (Roberts, 1989; Schaefer & Gorsuch, 1992); open-ended questions (Janssen et al., 1994); letters written to God (Ludwig, Weber, & Iben, 1974); semantic differentials[2] (Benson & Spilka, 1973); Q-sorts[3] (Benson & Spilka, 1973; Nelson, 1971; Spilka, Armatas, & Nussbaum, 1964); other card-sorting tasks (Krejci, 1998); standardized scales (Gorsuch, 1968); combination techniques such as "concept mapping" (Kunkel, Cook, Meshel, Daughtry, & Hauenstein, 1999);

---

2. The semantic differential technique involves rating concepts on a series of bipolar adjective descriptors, such as "good___ : ___ : ___ : ___ : ___ : ___ : ___bad."

3. The Q-sort technique involves having a person sort cards with words (e.g., "loving") on them into various piles according to how well they describe, for example, one's concept of God.

and sentence completions, essays, and "projective photographs" (Tamminen, 1991). There has been some interest in comparing the utility of the different approaches. One study (Hutsebaut & Verhoeven, 1995) concluded that closed-ended questions concerning God offered slight advantages over open-ended questions, but the participants in that research were university students. Comparative studies involving children are needed.

Measures used can apparently influence research findings. Tamminen's (1991) extensive research with Finnish children and adolescents involved both structured questions about God and unstructured methods, such as sentence completion and "projective photographs." His results were generally consistent with the stage approach outlined above. However, Tamminen noted that the images of God that emerged varied somewhat, depending on the measures used: "For example, God's effect on people, making them be good to each other, which was considered very important in the alternative answers chosen in the questionnaires, was not often mentioned in the fill-in sentences or essays" (Tamminen, 1991, p. 192).

The first edition of this book (Spilka, Hood, & Gorsuch, 1985) pointed out that despite the value of studies in this area, research has tended to be descriptive rather than carefully designed to test theories of cognitive development. This is still generally true today. Also, relevant research sometimes involves only older adolescents or adults. Furthermore, Hyde (1990) has suggested that research on children's ideas of God has been "occasional and sporadic, with no continuous theme and [it] has tended to remain so, following the varied interests of those undertaking it" (p. 64). Additional research is needed, but it must address these problems.

PRAYER

Children's concepts of prayer seem to develop in a manner consistent with Piaget's cognitive-developmental stages. For example, Long et al. (1967) interviewed 5- to 12-year-olds about prayer (see Research Box 4.3). The authors concluded that there was a clear tendency for these children's concepts of prayer to evolve in three stages: They moved from habits and memorized passages, through concrete personal requests, to more abstract petitions.

Other studies seem generally to be consistent with this Piagetian view of prayer development (see, e.g., the review by Finney & Malony, 1985)—from relatively direct replication research by Worten and Dellinger (1986) to, for example, Brown's (1966) investigation of adolescents, which suggested less emphasis on the material consequences of prayer among older children. Scarlett and Perriello (1991) asked seventh- and ninth-grade Catholic school students, as well as college undergraduates, to write prayers for six hypothetical vignettes (e.g., a woman's best friend is dying of cancer). They found a shift from "using prayer to request changes in objective reality" (p. 72) among the younger students, toward prayer as a way to deal with feelings and become closer to God among the older participants. This shift is apparently consistent with the second and third stages of prayer outlined by Long et al. (1967), though at slightly older ages for the Scarlett and Perriello (1991) sample.

Tamminen (1991) also found some divergence from Long et al.'s (1967) stages in his Finnish young people. Personal conversation with God was important at younger ages (7–8 years) than Long et al. (1967) had found (9–12 years); moreover, petitionary prayer remained important up to age 20, whereas Long et al. reported decreasing importance of petitionary prayer as children grew older. Woolley (2000; Woolley & Phelps, 2001) also found that prayer and its connection to God developed years earlier (age 5) than Long et al. reported (9–10

~~~~~~

Research Box 4.3. The Child's Conception of Prayer
(Long, Elkind, & Spilka, 1967)

In a Piagetian context, these researchers interviewed 80 girls and 80 boys aged 5–12 about prayer. They asked them open-ended questions, such as "What is a prayer?" and "Where do prayers go?", as well as giving them sentence completion tasks (e.g., "I usually pray when . . ."). Three judges independently analyzed the children's responses according to a scoring manual that outlined levels of differentiation and degree of concretization–abstraction. The results suggested three stages of prayer concept development:

1. At the younger ages (5–7), children responded to the questions with learned formulas based on memorized prayers.

2. Children aged 7–9 identified prayer as a set of concrete activities, with time and place defined; the purpose was also concrete, typically centered on personal requests.

3. For children between the ages of 9 and 12, prayer was more abstract, and tended toward shared conversation rather than specific requests. Prayer was more focused on abstract goals than on material objects.

Thus, across the 5- to 12-year age range, prayer seemed to evolve from habits and memorized passages, through concrete personal requests, to more abstract petitions with humanitarian and altruistic sentiments. There was also an emotional shift noted: Praying was emotionally neutral for the younger children, but by the older ages prayer had important emotional implications (e.g., expression of empathy, as well as identification with others and the deity). All of this is quite consistent with the Piagetian conceptualization of cognitive development. The first two stages of prayer development parallel the preoperational (preconceptual substage) and concrete operational stages. Long et al.'s third stage is best characterized as transitional, giving evidence of the abstract thought characteristic of Piaget's stage of formal operations, which he felt did not begin until approximately 12 years of age.

---

years). Finally, Woolley and Phelps (2001) and Barrett, Richert, and Driesenga (2001) observed less tendency for children to anthropomorphize their concept of God than did Long et al. (1967). More research is necessary to determine the reasons for the differences across these studies. They could be attributable to culture, unique samples, method, time period of the research, and so on. For example, Woolley and Phelps (2001) pointed out that her sample came from religiously affiliated schools, compared to Long et al.'s private school sample. Also, her procedures involved new forced-choice questions and a variety of tasks, in addition to open-ended questions similar to those of Long et al.

Francis and Brown (1990, 1991) carried out investigations of influences on prayer, rather than cognitive stages in development of prayer. They found some denominational differences; for example, Church of England schools exerted a small "negative" influence on attitudes toward prayer, compared to the lack of influence in Roman Catholic schools. They also reported a shift in influence from parents (stronger among their 11-year-olds) to church (stronger among the 16-year-olds). They have interpreted their results as supporting a social learning or modeling interpretation of prayer, since prayer among children and adolescents seemed to result more from "explicit teaching or implicit example from their family and church community than as a spontaneous consequence of developmental dynamics or needs" (Francis & Brown, 1991, p. 120). This research is highlighted in Research Box 5.2 (see Chapter 5), in the context of our discussion of religious socialization.

Some research has also attempted to relate prayer to (nonreligious) aspects of adjustment in children. For example, Francis and Gibbs (1996), in an investigation of 8- to 11-year-olds, found no evidence to suggest that prayer contributed to the children's self-esteem, or that low self-esteem led to prayer. Other studies have reported negative links between prayer and psychoticism scores on a personality test (Francis, 1997b; Francis & Wilcox, 1996; Smith, 1996).

Prayer has also been associated with identity status, such that private prayer was less frequent for college students with higher "moratorium" scores (an indication of searching for answers to religious and other questions, but without ideological commitment; McKinney & McKinney, 1999; see Chapter 5 for a discussion of identity status). McKinney and McKinney also found that the social identity reflected in the prayers of adolescents tended to be limited. Prayers involved family and friends, but usually did not involve the broader community.

In an older sample (college students) that is potentially relevant here, Byrd and Boe (2001) studied three different types of prayer and found that colloquial (conversational) and meditative (contemplative) types of prayer were negatively related to high avoidance scores (indicating discomfort with interpersonal closeness) on a measure of attachment. Petitionary (material help-seeking) prayer was more common among individuals with higher anxiety scores on this measure.

These relationships suggest that prayer is linked to personality and adjustment characteristics, and this area deserves further investigation. However, some of these investigations involved older adolescents; the implications of the findings for prayer in children, or for early prayer development, are not clear.

It is surprising that more research attention has not focused on prayer as it relates to religious development. Although there are problems in operationalizing and studying prayer (especially spontaneous personal prayer), prayer is an important religious ritual that could potentially serve as a "window" into more general religious development, as well as the meaning of faith to religious persons. Furthermore, there remain many questions about the nature and function of prayer in individual lives, as well as the nature of social and contextual factors in shaping prayer (Francis & Brown, 1991). Brown's (1994) book *The Human Side of Prayer* has initiated an exploration of some of these issues and provided an integrative review of the diverse research in this area, especially in his chapter devoted to the development and meaning of prayer.

Finally, Woolley (2000) has pointed out that there are "clear connections between magic and religion" (p. 118); in particular, prayer is conceptually similar to wishing, which in turn is related to magical thinking. Goldman (1964) also referred to magical thinking in the early stages of children's thought processes related to religious development. However, Woolley (2000) has also concluded that prayer is a more complicated process than wishing, since, for example, it involves an intermediary (God) between thinking and physical events. Research is needed to further explore connections between magical thinking in childhood and the emergence of religious faith and prayer.

RELIGIOUS EXPERIENCE IN CHILDHOOD

Kalevi Tamminen's (1976, 1994; Tamminen & Nurmi, 1995; Tamminen et al., 1988) studies of the religious experiences of Finnish children and adolescents, highlighted in Research Box 4.4, deserve attention in this chapter for several reasons. First, almost 3,000 young people have been studied. Second, this research program has produced limited but important longitudinal data. Third, and possibly most important, these studies have moved a step beyond the more traditional cognitive-stage approach by investigating the meaning and implications of religious *experiences* for children's lives, in addition to aspects of religious cognitive development.

Tamminen's research program is not without problems. It is difficult to know what to make of written questionnaire responses from relatively young children; probably the younger children were not able to express themselves well in writing, and it is not clear that their self-reported "religious experiences" are consonant with what adults would call "religious experiences." Also, questionnaires were administered in school classrooms, suggesting that peer pressure, contextual influences, and other such factors may have influenced responses. For example, children may have been reluctant to reveal personal religious experiences to an unknown adult, especially while sitting among their classmates. As Scarlett (1994) has pointed out, "These are surveys carried out in impersonal settings not conducive to tapping into what God and religious experience *mean* to adolescents" (p. 88). Furthermore, the children and adolescents were fairly homogeneous in terms of their religious background (Lutheran), and it is not clear to what extent Tamminen's findings generalize to children from other religious backgrounds or no religious background at all. For a better appreciation of differences in religious experience across religious traditions (though not specifically in childhood), the reader might consult the first six chapters of Hood's (1995b) *Handbook of Religious Experience.*

In spite of these problems, this research program has made important contributions to our understanding of children's religious experiences. Tamminen's research has confirmed that there is a developmental sequence with respect to religious *experiences*, though his results are quite cognitive in nature. Although these investigations were not intended to test a Piagetian-based cognitive-developmental theory of religious development, the results are consistent with that approach (especially with respect to the shift from concrete to abstract thinking about religion as children move into adolescence). Also, the longitudinal trends in the data are consistent with cross-sectional findings.

Furthermore, it has been pointed out that these studies "enlighten by countering the old view that God becomes important only after childhood" (Scarlett, 1994, p. 88). Certainly there is a rich description of the nature and content of children's and adolescents' self-reported "close to God" experiences. Finally, this research should serve as a stimulus to other investigators to approach the topic of religious development from different perspectives, and not to be constrained by previous research carried out from within a Piagetian-based framework.

ATTACHMENT THEORY AND RELATED RESEARCH

Kirkpatrick (1992, 1994, 1995, 1997, 1998, 1999; Kirkpatrick & Shaver, 1990, 1992) has extended Bowlby's (1969, 1973, 1980) theory of parent–infant attachment to the realm of religion. In so doing, he has provided a unique approach for the study of links between early ze

Research Box 4.4. Religious Experience in Childhood and Adolescence: Finnish Research (Tamminen, 1994)

Tamminen began his series of investigations with a 1974 study that tested 1,588 children and adolescents (aged 7–20), who were mostly Lutheran and fairly evenly divided between boys and girls. Longitudinal data were collected 2 years later on 277 of the original participants, and a final longitudinal wave of data was collected in 1980 on 60 of those who had participated in the first and second stages. Also, 242 classmates of the "third-wave 60" were studied for comparison purposes. Finally, in 1986, a study was carried out to replicate and extend the 1974 investigation, involving 1,176 students. Most of the data were gathered by means of group questionnaires administered in classrooms, although the youngest students (first grade) were also interviewed. Tamminen acknowledges that many students up to fifth grade had difficulty expressing themselves in writing, and that this could have compromised his findings for the younger children.

Religious experience was operationally defined by the question "Have you at times felt that God is particularly close to you?" and its follow-up, "Would you like to tell me about it, when and in what situations?" Interestingly, 10–16% of the two youngest groups of students reported that they had *not* felt particularly close to God, and this figure grew steadily to 53% of the 17- to 20-year-olds. That is, older children and adolescents were significantly less likely to report any religious experiences involving closeness to God.

Closeness to God among the 7- to 11-year-old children was most likely to be linked with "situations of loneliness, fear, and emergencies—such as escaping or avoiding danger—or when they were ill" (p. 81). Tamminen notes that these reports correspond to a more general concreteness of thinking at these ages. Similar experiences were reported by the 11- to 13-year-olds, though they also linked closeness to God with encounters with death, loneliness, prayer, and contemplation. There was not much evidence of more abstract thinking until later ages.

The 13- to 15-year-olds evidenced a variety of religious doubts (e.g., concerning God's existence and trustworthiness, as well as the efficacy of prayer). Reports of decreased closeness to God were more common, and those reports of closeness that did appear were more often linked with death and external dangers. Finally, the religious experiences of older students (15- to 20-year-olds) tended to involve personal identity issues and existential questions (e.g., the meaning of life and death), and this material was more obviously abstract in nature.

Overall, Tamminen has concluded that the results of these far-reaching studies showed "a developmental line from concrete, separate, and external to more abstract, general, and internalized. In addition, experiences in childhood were related almost exclusively to everyday situations—as was the case also with evening prayer—whereas at the age of puberty and in adolescence, such experiences were more frequently related to congregational situations [i.e., church-related contexts]" (p. 82). In general, parallel findings appeared for other questions dealing with God's guidance and direction in life.

Note. A more extensive treatment of Tamminen's research on religion in Finnish young people can be found in his 1991 book *Religious Development in Childhood and Youth: An Empirical Study.*

development and religion, and their implications for children's and adult's lives. As Kirk-patrick (1992) describes Bowlby's work, attachment theory "postulates a primary, biosocial behavioral system in the infant that was designed by evolution to maintain proximity of the infant to its primary caregiver, thereby protecting the infant from predation and other natural dangers" (p. 4). Attachment theory is not without its critics (e.g., Kagan, 1998), but Kirk-patrick has pointed out that this theoretical basis may help to explain individual differences in religiousness. For example, he has noted the extent to which the God of Christian tradi-tions corresponds to the idea of a secure attachment figure. Similarly, religion more gener-ally may serve as a comfort and a sense of security, especially during times of stress or other difficulties.

These observations led Kirkpatrick and Shaver (1990) to suggest that attachment and religion may be linked in important ways. They posited a "compensation hypothesis," which predicts that people who have not had secure relationships with their parents (or other pri-mary caregivers) may be inclined to compensate for this absence by believing in a "loving, personal, available God." This was contrasted with a "mental model hypothesis," predicting that people's religiousness may be at least partially determined by early attachment relation-ships; that is, they may model their religious beliefs on the attachment relationships they experienced early in their lives.

In a study designed to test these ideas, Kirkpatrick and Shaver (1990; see Research Box 4.5) found some support for the compensation hypothesis, but only for people from rela-tively nonreligious homes. Findings generally contradicted the mental model hypothesis. Subsequent studies of adolescents (Granqvist, 2002b; Granqvist & Hagekull, 2001) and uni-versity students (Granqvist, 1998; Granqvist & Hagekull, 1999) in Sweden, and of adult women in the United States (Kirkpatrick, 1997), also lend some support to the compensa-tion hypothesis.

Kirkpatrick's writings on attachment and religion have provided a rich source of ideas for empirical investigation. For example, it has been suggested that attachment theory has relevance for understanding conceptualizations of God, religious behaviors such as prayer and glossolalia (speaking in tongues), and links between religious experience and romantic love (Kirkpatrick, 1992, 1994, 1997; Kirkpatrick & Shaver, 1992).

Subsequent research has confirmed the utility of attachment theory for understanding religion. Eshleman, Dickie, Merasco, Shepard, and Johnson (1999) interviewed 4- to 10-year-old children, and also surveyed their parents. Eshleman et al. concluded that their findings supported Kirkpatrick and Shaver's (1990) attachment theory model. For example, as chil-dren moved from early to middle childhood, their distance from parents increased as per-ceived closeness to God increased, just as attachment theory would predict. As a sidelight, these researchers also found that "perceiving God as male may distance God for girls and women" (p. 146). Dickie et al. (1997) also found evidence that seems to support attachment theory predictions; they concluded that "God becomes the 'perfect attachment substitute'" (p. 42) as children become more independent of parents.

Granqvist and Hagekull (1999) found that retrospective accounts of attachment to par-ents suggested a positive association between security of attachment and socialization-based religiosity. Avoidance in attachment to parents was associated with emotionally based reli-giousness. Insecure attachment was linked to sudden religious conversion. A subsequent study of Swedish teenagers found that attachment insecurity was linked to emotionally based religiosity, experience of religious changes, and a "new age orientation" (belief in alterna-tive medical treatment, belief in parapsychological phenomena, interest in alternative reli-

⟨⟨⟨ ❧ ⟩⟩⟩

Research Box 4.5. Attachment Theory and Religion
(Kirkpatrick & Shaver, 1990)

In this investigation, Kirkpatrick and Shaver tested the compensation and the mental model hypotheses (see text) with respect to links between childhood attachment to parents and adult religiousness. Data were collected from two surveys—one involving 670 respondents to a questionnaire in a Sunday newspaper, and the other including a subsample of 213 of these same people who agreed to participate in a further study. Various measures were used to tap aspects of religiousness, including the Allport and Ross (1967) scales for assessing Intrinsic and Extrinsic religious orientation (see Chapter 2). Child–parent attachment was measured in a standard way, which placed respondents into one of three categories (percentages in parentheses are from Kirkpatrick and Shaver's study): secure (51%), avoidant (8%), and anxious/ambivalent (41%).

Attachment did indeed serve as a predictor of religiousness, but in a somewhat complicated way. There was a tendency for those from avoidant parent–child attachment relationships to report higher levels of adult religiousness, and also for persons with secure attachments to report lower levels of religiousness, but only for respondents whose mothers were relatively nonreligious. The attachment classification apparently had a more direct relationship with reported sudden conversion experiences, with anxious/ambivalent respondents much more likely to report such conversions at some time in their lives (44%) than respondents from the other attachment groups (fewer than 10%). Home religiosity did not affect this relationship.

This study relied on adults' retrospective reports of earlier attachment and family religiousness, so memory and other biases may have affected responses. The authors pointed out that their investigation was very much an exploratory study of attachment–religion relationships. However, their initial findings are provocative and tend to support the compensation hypothesis (though only for people from relatively nonreligious homes in this study); they generally contradict the mental model hypothesis (i.e., that religiousness may be modeled after early attachment relationships). The reasons for this are not clear and call for further investigation.

gious ideas, etc.) (Granqvist & Hagekull, 2001). These findings seem consistent with attachment theory predictions.

Finally, it is important to note that the research discussed above attempted to relate *childhood* attachment experiences with adolescent and adult religion. Other research has explored relationships between *adult* attachment and adult religiosity. For example, Kirkpatrick (1998) concluded that university students who viewed themselves and others positively tended also to have positive images of God, as well as perceived positive relationships with God. Furthermore, longitudinal data from a subsample of these students revealed that a tendency to become more religious less than a year later was linked to negative views of self and positive models of others at the time of the original survey. These findings are consistent with other research on relationships between attachment and religion in adult lives (e.g., Kirkpatrick, 1995; Kirkpatrick & Shaver, 1992). Also, TenElshof and Furrow (2000) found that among conservative seminary students, secure adult attachment styles were positively related to a measure of spiritual maturity. Apparently attachment theory has implications for religion beyond child–parent attachment relationships.

OTHER WORK ON RELIGION IN CHILDHOOD

It is difficult to summarize the considerable literature on childhood religious development in a chapter such as this one. To this point, we have attempted to outline several major theoretical and empirical directions, and the resulting knowledge accumulated from many studies. We have given little attention to other theories (e.g., psychodynamic) and to the many articles that do not offer theoretical advances or that lack an empirical base (e.g., some in the religious education and pastoral counseling literature). Furthermore, many empirical studies have not fallen neatly into the subcategories used in this chapter. Other authors (e.g., Benson, Masters, & Larson, 1997; Hyde, 1990) have summarized much of this other work. Here we offer a sampling of recent research directions not discussed above.

Personality and Attitudes

Leslie Francis (1994) has summarized a considerable body of research on personality and mental aspects of religious development, relying heavily on the work and orientation of Hans Eysenck (e.g., Eysenck, 1981). Francis's own studies (e.g., Francis, Pearson, & Kay, 1982; Francis, Pearson, & Kay, 1983b) suggest that among children, religiousness and introversion are positively related, and that these in turn may be related to rejection of substance use (Francis, 1997a). An extensive literature on religion and substance use/abuse exists, but it tends to focus on postchildhood samples and is discussed in the chapter on morality (see Chapter 13). Bible reading has also been linked to increased purpose in life among 13- to 15-year-olds (Francis, 2000).

Another line of research has focused on influences on religiousness and attitudes toward religion among young people (especially the influence of parents, but also peers, schools, church, etc.). Some of this work has included samples of children or early adolescents (e.g., Francis & Gibson, 1993; Francis & Greer, 2001); however, most of these studies have involved older adolescents and young adults, so a review of these efforts is left to Chapter 5. Likewise, there has been some emphasis on the influence of religiously affiliated schools versus public institutions on values and other aspects of children's lives, but these have not shown much difference between the two types of schooling (see, e.g., McCartin & Freehill, 1986). However, Francis (1986) has found variations between the influences of Catholic and Protestant schools in England. The effects of schooling on religiousness are also considered in more detail in Chapter 5.

Much other work has included religion as simply one of many variables of interest. For example, Archer's (1989) investigation of gender differences suggests that among early to late adolescents, males and females use the identity process similarly with respect to religious development. de Vaus and McAllister (1987) concluded that gender variations in religiosity are not attributable to child-rearing roles of females, and Albert and Porter (1986) found that liberal Christian and Jewish backgrounds were related to less rigid conceptions of gender roles in 4- to 6-year-old children. An Israeli study (Florian & Kravetz, 1985) found that Jewish and Christian 10-year-olds had internalised a Western scientific conception of death to a greater extent than Muslim and Druze children. Other work (Saigh, 1979; Saigh, O'Keefe,

& Antoun, 1984) has pointed to a link between religious symbols worn by examiners and performance on intelligence tests, such that performance may be better when young people are tested by same-religion examiners.

There has been interest in the difficulty of getting children, especially at young ages, to understand and respond appropriately to questions about religion (e.g., Tamminen, 1994). Similarly, tendencies have been noted by Francis for children's scores on attitudes toward religion to be positively related to lie scores on other scales (Francis, Pearson, & Kay, 1988), and also for children to bias their responses in a proreligious direction when a priest, as opposed to a layperson, is the test administrator (Francis, 1979). Similar effects were not found by Hunsberger and Ennis (1982) in several studies of university students, however. The best conclusion seems to be that caution must be exercised in studies of children involving measurement of religion, and that appropriate checks should be included to assess possible biases or distortion of responses whenever possible.

Meaning and Implications of Religion in Childhood

We know relatively little about the meaning and implications of religion for children as they grow older, beyond the cognitive and experiential components discussed earlier in this chapter. We need to find novel ways of studying children's religious development without assuming that adult thought is the gold standard for comparison in this regard (see, e.g., Boyer & Walker, 2000). What impact, if any, does religion have on the day-to-day lives of children—including their physical and mental health, personal identity, and social relationships? How does childhood religion affect later religiosity, as well as nonreligious social attitudes? Does religious training affect a child's concept of death (see Florian & Kravetz, 1985; Stambrook & Parker, 1987)? What role, if any, does religion play in childhood psychopathology, and what role does (and should) religion play in the clinical treatment of children (see Wells, 1999)?

Findings suggest that a conservative or fundamentalist religious upbringing has implications for educational attainment and gender roles (see Sherkat, 2000; Sherkat & Darnell, 1999). A broad survey of children and young adolescents (fifth through ninth graders) led Forliti and Benson (1986) to conclude that religiosity was related to increased prosocial action, as well as to decreased incidence of sexual intercourse, drug use, and antisocial behavior. They also concluded that a restrictive religious orientation was linked to antisocial behavior, alcohol use, racism, and sexism. These latter conclusions are not always consistent with those reached for older adolescents and adults (see Chapters 5 on socialization and 13 on morality). Also, given the moderately strong associations among right-wing authoritarianism, religious fundamentalism, and prejudice observed by Altemeyer (1988, 1996; Altemeyer & Hunsberger, 1992), it would seem appropriate to investigate childhood antecedents of such relationships, as well as the developmental dynamics fostering such connections.

Child Rearing

Parenting Style

There is general agreement among developmental psychologists that parenting practices have important implications for child development (Darling & Steinberg, 1993). In spite of the likelihood that parental religious orientation influences parenting style (see Luft & Sorell,

1987), there has been little research relating parenting approaches, religion, and child development. A few early studies (e.g., Bateman & Jensen, 1958; Nunn, 1964) suggested the potential of such links. Subsequent theoretical and empirical work on "parenting styles" has provided new avenues for exploring the relationship between parenting and child religious development.

Baumrind (1967, 1991) has suggested that there exist four very different styles of parenting, based on parental responsiveness and demandingness: "authoritarian," "authoritative," "permissive," and "rejecting/neglecting." Authoritarian parents are high on demandingness but low on responsiveness, preferring to impose rules on their children and emphasize obedience. Authoritative parents tend to be both demanding and responsive, explaining why rules are necessary, and being open to their children's perspectives. Permissive parents make few demands, use little punishment, and are responsive to the point of submitting to their children's wishes. Rejecting/neglecting parents are neither demanding nor responsive, being generally disengaged from their children.

Correlational and longitudinal research has suggested that the authoritative style of parenting may have benefits for children's development, whereas the authoritarian and rejecting/neglecting styles may involve some negative implications (Buri, Louiselle, Misukanis, & Mueller, 1988; Rohner, 1994). Other research suggests that parental emphasis on obedience is related to "cognitive accomplishment" (Holden & Edwards, 1989) and to personality development (e.g., right-wing authoritarianism; Altemeyer, 1988). There is also tentative evidence that permissive parenting is associated with an extrinsic religious orientation, and that authoritative parenting may be related to an intrinsic religious orientation among adolescent offspring (Giesbrecht, 1995), and to greater religiosity among parents (Linder Gunnoe, Hetherington, & Reiss, 1999).

The authoritarian parenting style bears some similarity to Biblical injunctions to emphasize obedience among children, and not to "spare the rod." Zern (1987) has argued that from a religious perspective, obedience is a preferred trait. In fact, research by Ellison and Sherkat (1993) has revealed that conservative Protestants (and, to a lesser extent, Catholics) tend to endorse an authoritarian parenting orientation, valuing obedience in children. Religion has also been linked with parental disciplinary practices (Kelley, Power, & Wimbush, 1992)—including a preference, among more conservative groups and those who subscribe to a literal belief in the Bible, for the use of corporal punishment (Ellison, Bartkowski, & Segal, 1996; Gershoff, Miller, & Holden, 1999; Grasmick, Morgan, & Kennedy, 1992; Mahoney, Pargament, Tarakeshwar, & Swank, 2001; Wiehe, 1990). Similarly, religiousness has been linked with emphasis on obedience to cultural norms generally (Zern, 1984).

As described in Research Box 4.6, Danso, Hunsberger, and Pratt (1997) found evidence that more fundamentalist university students (Study 1) and parents (Study 2) were more likely to condone the use of corporal punishment and to value obedience (rather than autonomy) in child rearing. However, mediation analyses suggested that the greater desire of fundamentalists to socialize their children to accept the (parental) religious faith was linked more closely to right-wing authoritarianism than to religious fundamentalism per se. One wonders, then, whether conservative religious groups (or religious fundamentalists more generally) might be inclined to use an authoritarian parenting style, with consequent implications for their children. Also, what role does right-wing authoritarianism as a parental personality trait play in such a relationship?

Darling and Steinberg (1993) have suggested that parenting goals and values should be distinguished from parenting styles and parenting practices. In light of the discussion above,

ಶಿ.

Research Box 4.6. The Role of Parental Religious Fundamentalism and Right-Wing Authoritarianism in Child-Rearing Goals and Practices (Danso, Hunsberger, & Pratt, 1997)

These authors concluded that previous research had established links between stronger parental religiosity and a greater parental emphasis on obedience for their children, and also more positive attitudes toward corporal punishment (e.g., spanking) in child rearing. It was further hypothesized that parents' desire to raise their children to accept the family religion ("faith keeping") would have an influence on the goals that they set for their children. More fundamentalist parents were expected to place greater value on faith keeping, to emphasize obedience for children more strongly, and also to be more likely to condone the use of corporal punishment in child rearing. But beyond this, the authors explored how these factors were linked—suspecting, for example, that right-wing authoritarianism would mediate the relationship between religious orientation and child-rearing attitudes.

Two studies were carried out; the first involved 204 university students, and the second 154 mothers and fathers of university students. Measures included Faith Keeping, Attitudes toward Corporal Punishment, Autonomy, and Obedience scales developed for the research, as well as Religious Fundamentalism and Right-Wing Authoritarianism scales (the last scale administered in Study 2 only). The university students were asked to respond to parenting items by imagining that they had children of their own. The parents were asked about their actual child-rearing attitudes when their (university student) children were between 7 and 12 years old.

The results of both studies indicated that religious fundamentalism was positively correlated with greater valuation of obedience, stronger endorsement of corporal punishment in child rearing, and the importance of socializing children to accept their parents' faith. Fundamentalism was also linked with weaker valuation of autonomy in one's children. In both studies, it appeared that faith keeping seemed to play a mediating role between fundamentalism and obedience attitudes. That is, more fundamentalist parents' child-rearing attitudes (e.g., increased emphasis on obedience, endorsement of corporal punishment) seemed to be a result of their stronger desire to have their children uphold the family's religious faith.

However, the addition of the Right-Wing Authoritarianism scale in Study 2 indicated that it was actually a more powerful mediating variable in these relationships than was faith keeping. That is, the fact that religious fundamentalism was strongly positively correlated with right-wing authoritarian attitudes "explained" the links between fundamentalism and child-rearing attitudes (e.g., the tendency to emphasize obedience, and condone the use of corporal punishment). The authors suggested that future researchers should consider the role of parental personality variables such as authoritarianism in studies of religion and child rearing.

This study's limitations include the facts that university students were simply speculating about what their child-rearing attitudes would be *if* they had children (Study 1), and that parents had to reflect back 5–10 years to recall what their child-rearing attitudes had been at that time. We do not know the extent to which such speculations and memories are accurate. Also, the authors do not discuss the "chicken and egg" problem of whether fundamentalism or authoritarianism comes first, or whether they might be causally related. This issue reappears in Chapter 14.

it seems apparent that religious orientation is likely to have some impact on parenting goals and values. Certainly, some conservative Christian books on child rearing emphasize the importance of authoritarian-like goals for parents—for example, by explicitly advising parents that raising obedient children is an important goal (Fugate, 1980; Meier, 1977). Such goals in turn are likely to influence both general parenting style as delineated by Baumrind, and specific parenting practices such as the use of corporal punishment to teach obedience (e.g., Danso et al., 1997). The role of religion in this process might even help to explain variations in the prevalence of different parenting styles in North American ethnic groups (Steinberg, Lamborn, Dornbusch, & Darling, 1992).

Parenting goals and practices can have important real-world implications beyond their direct effects for the children themselves, as illustrated by the second quotation presented at the beginning of this chapter. To recapitulate, in Aylmer, Ontario, Canada, seven children whose family belonged to a conservative religious group were taken from their parents by child welfare authorities (Saunders, 2001). The parents reportedly sometimes disciplined their children by hitting them with a rod or strap. When the authorities met with the parents, the parents justified their disciplinary methods by reference to their literal belief in the Bible, and they refused to assure the authorities that this practice would stop. The children were eventually returned to the family when the parents reportedly provided some assurance that they would not use certain types of physical punishment to discipline the children. However, the broader issues of the legality of such religiously based justification for corporal punishment, and of whether or not authorities should remove such children from their homes, have yet to be resolved.

It is important to note that the research and ideas discussed above involve conservative or fundamentalist religion groups and measures, and that the hypothesized relationships between conservative/fundamentalist religion and authoritarian parenting style may not hold for more general measures of religiousness. For example, Linder Gunnoe et al. (1999) did *not* find a positive link between authoritarian parenting style and a measure of the extent to which parents' religious beliefs played a role in their daily lives. Furthermore, Wilcox (1998) found that the strict discipline characteristic of conservative Protestant religious parents is tempered by the finding that conservative parents are also *more* likely to praise and hug their children. Wilcox has therefore argued that parents who hold theologically conservative beliefs may show aspects of *both* authoritarian and authoritative parenting styles. This possibility, as well as its implications for child and adolescent development, needs further investigation.

Other Aspects of Parenting

Religion may play more subtle roles in child rearing as well. Carlson, Taylor, and Levin (1998) found that the ways in which children use pretend play can differ across religious groups, even for different varieties of Mennonites. Ojha and Pramanick (1992) studied mothers in India and found that Hindu mothers began weaning and toilet-training their children earlier than did Christian mothers, on average, who in turn were earlier than Muslim mothers. Of the three religious groups, Christian mothers were the most restrictive toward their children. The role of religion in these aspects of parenting and child rearing (and consequences for child development) has received little empirical attention to date.

Parenting techniques have been linked with religion in a somewhat different context. Nunn (1964) suggested that some parents invoke the image of a punishing God in an attempt to control their children's behavior. He hypothesized that relatively ineffective, powerless parents would be inclined to use God in an attempt to gain some semblance of power, telling their children such things as "God will punish you if you misbehave." Nunn's data supported this view of parents who formed a "coalition with God," and also suggested that this "God will punish you" approach had negative consequences for the children, who were reportedly more inclined to blame themselves for problems and to feel that they should be obedient.

Nelsen and Kroliczak (1984) have pointed out that there has been a general decline in people's belief in a punishing God, and that this decline is at least partly attributable "to parents being less likely to use coalitions with God. Hence, fewer children form this image" (p. 269). Nelsen and Kroliczak examined data from over 3,000 children in Minnesota elementary schools in an attempt to replicate Nunn's findings. They found a decreased tendency of parents to resort to the "God will punish you" approach (73% of respondents said that neither parent in a family employed this approach, compared to Nunn's 33%). But the children whose parents tended to use the "coalition" also tended to view God as malevolent, to have higher self-blame scores, and to feel a greater need to be obedient. Essentially, Nelsen and Kroliczak replicated Nunn's finding some 20 years later.

These studies have implications for the development of God images, but they also suggest that parents' approach to discipline may be important for children's religiosity, as well as for more general child development (e.g., tendencies toward self-blame and obedience). There may also be noteworthy ramifications for how parents deal with other child-rearing issues, such as illness. For example, research has indicated that parents who believe more strongly in divine influence are more likely to seek spiritual guidance in coping with (hypothetical) child illnesses (De Vellis, De Vellis, & Spilsbury, 1988). All of these findings are consistent with the suggestion that parenting goals, styles, and practices may have significant links with religious orientation.

Much of the research above has assessed the extent to which parenting affects religion in one's children. We should not forget that religion can also affect parenting and parent–child relationships (e.g., Pearce & Axinn, 1998). There is also evidence that parenting can itself contribute to religious change in fathers (Palkovitz & Palm, 1998).

Child Abuse and Religion

In the past decade, there has been increasing interest in possible links between religion and child abuse (e.g., Bottoms, Shaver, Goodman, & Qin, 1995; Capps, 1992; Greven, 1991). As we have noted earlier, evidence suggests that conservative and fundamentalist religious orientation is linked with a tendency to condone the use of physical punishment in child rearing (e.g., Ellison et al., 1996). Greven (1991) has argued that the inclination of some religious groups and individuals to legitimize and promote the use of corporal punishment in child rearing can effectively condone child abuse. Whether or not this is true, abuse can apparently have implications for religiosity. Rossetti (1995) found, not surprisingly, that people who were sexually abused as children by priests expressed less trust in the priesthood, the Catholic church, and relationship to God (see Chapter 13 regarding sexual abuse perpetrated by clergy). Similarly, others concluded that childhood sexual abuse more generally was associated with lower levels of religiosity (Doxey, Jensen, & Jensen, 1997; Hall, 1995; Stout-Miller, Miller, & Langenbrunner, 1997) or a more negative view of God (Kane, Cheston, & Greer, 1993).

However, some researchers have concluded that those who were sexually abused as children may turn to religion for support (Reinert & Smith, 1997), or at least may show some evidence of increased religious behavior, such as prayer (Lawson, Drebing, Berg, Vincellette, & Penk, 1998). Possibly such increased religiousness acts as a form of compensation, as discussed earlier in the context of attachment theory. Others (Gange-Fling, Veach, Kuang, & Hong, 2000) found that a group of individuals in psychotherapy for childhood sexual abuse did not differ in spiritual functioning from a group of people in psychotherapy for other reasons. However, both of these groups scored lower in spiritual well-being than people not in psychotherapy did.

In view of the apparently conflicting results of recent studies, more research is needed. Possibly there are gender differences in response to abuse, and factors such as the religious environment before and after the abuse need to be taken into account, as well as the type, perpetrator, and context of the abuse.

A Note on Psychoanalytic Work

A considerable body of relevant theoretical work from a psychoanalytic perspective exists, but it has received little attention in this chapter. The theories of Freud and Jung have been mentioned in the context of the development of concepts of God. However, usually we have not discussed more general implications of psychoanalytic theory for religious development (see, e.g., Coles, 1990; Fitzgibbons, 1987; Rizzuto, 1991, 2001). Nor have we mentioned the psychoanalyst Erik Erikson (1958, 1963, 1969), whose theory of psychosocial development could be interpreted as a model of religious development (Wright, 1982), although Erikson's influence is sometimes apparent in the work of others. Fowler, for example, made use of Erikson's theory in his conceptualization of faith development.

Although these psychoanalytic theories can offer rich sources of ideas and insights into religious development, in general we have not given them more attention because (1) they have not generated much empirical research; (2) the relevant research that has been carried out has been compromised by the difficulties inherent in operationalizing and testing some psychoanalytic concepts; and (3) the conclusions of related studies are somewhat ambiguous and contradictory.

OVERVIEW

Fresh conceptual approaches are needed to revitalize the study of children's religious development. The area of religious development is top-heavy in theory, especially stage theories of religious cognitive development. There has been a considerable amount of overlap in research that "tests" these theories, but not much integrative work has been done to make sense of it all. Furthermore, there has been little or no empirical research on many issues related to childhood religious development, and some studies of religious development have little to say about *children*, having focused on older adolescents or young adults.

Clearly, Piaget's original description of stages of cognitive development has been important in guiding theories and studies of religious growth. Probably because of the mostly *cognitive* theme of the theoretical approaches, there has been a relatively narrow focus on cognition in empirical investigations of religious development. The resulting accumulation of knowledge typically confirms the development of patterns of religious thinking that parallel stages of more general cognitive development. However, this emphasis on cognitive development may have diverted attention from many other issues in child religious development.

There is evidence to suggest that children's religious identity, morality, faith, images of God, and prayer all emerge in stages that parallel the Piagetian stages to some extent. In general, the progression involves a move from an inability to understand religious concepts at all early in life, through a very egocentric religion, to an understanding of religion limited to the concrete, and finally to a more abstract and complex religiousness.

Theoretical conceptualizations of religious growth generally (Elkind, Goldman), as well as of moral (Kohlberg) and faith (Fowler) development, have apparently been stimulated by Piaget's formulations. And much other work on religious development (e.g., images of God, concepts of prayer) has also used the Piagetian framework as the basis for empirical studies. The results of numerous investigations have confirmed the utility of Piaget's cognitive stages for understanding various aspects of religious growth. However, promising non-Piagetian theoretical conceptualizations and empirical work have also appeared in the psychology of religion. For example, Tamminen has directed attention to the religious experience of children, and Kirkpatrick has shown the potential of attachment theory for understanding aspects of religious growth.

In spite of attempts at integration of work on religious development, we are left with a kind of "smorgasbord" of differing directions (Reich, 1993b, p. 39). This is not necessarily a bad thing, since this diversity has stimulated many different creative and useful empirical studies of religious development. Further integration of this work could eventually lead to a more comprehensive theory of religion in childhood. Future research on religious growth could take many potentially fruitful directions. The role of religion in parenting goals, styles, and practices, and the consequences for child development, are especially promising in this regard.

We would encourage researchers to diversify their efforts in the area of child religious development. In particular, they might consider the implications of more traditional developmental and social-psychological theories in the context of child religious development—for example, attribution theory (Spilka et al., 1985), attitude theories (Gorsuch & Wakeman, 1991; Hill, 1994; Hill & Bassett, 1992), personality constructs (Altemeyer, 1996; Francis, 1994), attachment theory (Kirkpatrick, 1992, 1998), self-discrepancy theory (Higgins, 1989), schema theory (McIntosh, 1995), and so on. We need to escape from the confines of the Piagetian approach to religious development. It is possible that the Extrinsic, Intrinsic, and Quest religious orientations (Allport & Ross, 1967; Batson et al., 1993; see Chapter 2) may appear in developmental sequence (Batson et al., 1993). Furthermore, the implications of childhood religious development for the children themselves, as well as for other individuals and groups (e.g., peers, parents, social and athletic groups, schools), need to be investigated.

These issues have generated considerable research with adolescent and adult populations, but not with children. As one example, recent work suggests that religion may affect childhood fantasy behavior and parental interpretation of such behavior (Taylor & Carlson, 2000). There continues to be a distinct paucity of *longitudinal* research on child religious development issues. Such research is critical if we are to escape the serious limitations of cross-sectional studies (Gorsuch, 1988). Historically, there is also a lack of strong experimental research in this area (Gorsuch, 1988). Additional consideration needs to be given to the studies that have investigated isolated topics in childhood religious development (e.g., personality, gender differences, methodological issues, child abuse), with an eye to integrating and making sense out of the diverse findings.

Compared to other areas in the psychology of religion, relatively little new empirical work is being published on religion in childhood. There is a rich theoretical framework dealing with developmental aspects of religion, as discussed earlier in this chapter. But with a few exceptions (e.g., God concepts, parenting issues), there is a dearth of solid empirical work. Why? For one thing, research with children is often more challenging than comparable studies with adults. For example, ethical and related permission issues may be time-consuming and frustrating for researchers. New measuring instruments may have to be developed for child populations. Additional research staff may have to be hired, and extra training may be needed to insure that research assistants are qualified to work with children. Interpretation of research findings can be problematic, since it is often difficult to establish validity of measuring instruments, and the meaning of children's responses is not always clear. Simply put, research with children can be time-consuming, expensive, and difficult to carry out. And much-needed longitudinal research is even more time-consuming, expensive, and problematic.

Finally, we would suggest that the main theoretical focus over the years, based on a Piagetian framework, has become stale. We need new theoretical directions. Yet, there are indications of vitality in some areas of research on religion in childhood, and there is considerable potential for investigators to pursue a variety of important questions in this area.

Chapter 5

RELIGIOUS SOCIALIZATION AND THOUGHT IN ADOLESCENCE AND YOUNG ADULTHOOD

Adolescence is a crisis of faith.

Adults appear to seriously underestimate the interest teens have in religion.

[Doubt] is altogether a pernicious companion which has its origins not in the good creation of God but in the *Nihil*—the power of destruction . . .

. . . doubt is not the opposite of faith; it is an element of faith.

[The churches] are engaged in perpetuating attitudes and beliefs which are going to cause suffering, conflict, and disillusionment to all those young people intelligent enough to respond to modern culture. It is not that the moral principles are wrong, but that the developing adolescent will consider them wrong when he finds they are tied to positively childish dogma.[1]

RELIGIOUS SOCIALIZATION

Why do people believe what they do? Some people think that their religious beliefs arose from a careful consideration of different perspectives and their own thinking about religious issues. And they may feel that they would hold those beliefs regardless of their family upbringing, education, friends, cultural context, and so on. They feel that because they have reasoned things through, they have reached the best possible conclusions about religion, and because of the kind of people they are, they would have arrived at these same beliefs had they been raised in any family or culture. Others may feel that through divine revelation or historical precedent, they have special access to the "truth"—that God has singled them out to believe in the "one true religion."

The empirical evidence, of course, argues against such views. Study after study has shown the importance of the socialization process in determining people's present religious beliefs. In other words, your environment has played a major role in shaping your religious and other attitudes. If you had been born into a devout Muslim family, today you would probably be

---

1. These quotations come, respectively, from the following sources: Campbell (1969, p. 852); Bergman (2001, p. 46); Barth (1963, p. 131); Tillich (1957, p. 116); and Cattell (1938, p. 189).

bowing toward Mecca. If you had been raised as a Pentecostal, you would probably sometimes speak in tongues. If your parents had been confirmed atheists, you would probably *not* believe in God today. If you had grown up in a particular native culture, you would probably believe in many gods.

In earlier chapters, we have discussed various potential explanations for why people are religious. Similarly, a number of reasons have been proposed for people's underlying level of religious commitment, since the environment can influence individuals in many different ways. For example, deprivation theory, often associated with the work of Glock and Stark (1966; Stark, 1972), suggests that religious commitment may compensate for other deprivations in life. Status theory proposes that religious commitment may be socially useful by increasing one's social status (see, e.g., Goode, 1968). Localism theory suggests that local communities may have well-defined standards that encourage religious commitment; people living in more cosmopolitan contexts tend to be relatively free of such "local" expectations and may therefore be less involved in religion. It has also been argued that beliefs at least partly determine religious involvement and commitment. Finally, the socialization approach emphasizes the role of the culture in teaching children and adolescents religious beliefs and behaviors.

Other specific factors have been suggested as determinants of religious commitment. For example, Ryan, Rigby, and King (1993) have argued that guilt and fear determine religiousness; Burris, Batson, Altstaedten, and Stephens (1994) have found that loneliness predicts religiousness; and Erikson (1958) has linked religion to the "identity crisis" that supposedly occurs during adolescence. These various approaches have been useful in helping to explain religious commitment. However, in this chapter we focus on the socialization explanation of religiousness—an approach that has marshaled a considerable body of empirical support, and one that offers specific plausible explanations of religious influence, which have been studied in some detail.

"Socialization," as the term is used here, refers to the process by which a culture (usually through its primary agents, such as parents) encourages individuals to accept beliefs and behaviors that are normative and expected within that culture. Such socialization often involves a process of internalization, as noted by Ryan et al. (1993), "through which an individual transforms a formerly externally prescribed regulation or value into an internal one" (p. 586). Johnstone (1988) has argued that people internalize the religion of their family or culture in essentially the same way that they learn their sex role, their language, or the lifestyle appropriate to their socioeconomic status. This is not to deny that people can become religious in other ways (e.g., see Chapter 11 on conversion); rather, it is suggested that socialization serves as the usual basis for religiosity in adolescence and adulthood.

There is no single "socialization theory." Different theoretical traditions in the social sciences have influenced the study of socialization processes, including psychoanalytic, social learning, cognitive-developmental, and symbolic-interactionist/role-learning perspectives (see Slaughter-Defoe, 1995). All of these have made contributions to our understanding of socialization, though we would argue that social learning theory has particular relevance for our consideration of the religious socialization process. As proposed by Bandura (1977), social learning theory emphasizes the importance of observing and imitating others, as well as the role of reinforcement. An important implication of this approach is that religiousness is typically strongly influenced by one's immediate environment (especially parents), through both modeling and reinforcement processes.

Some people find it difficult to accept the fact that, had they been born into a different cultural context, their religious beliefs would almost certainly be very different. And yet that is what the evidence regarding socialization suggests. There are exceptions to the rule, and these require our attention. However, we first need to examine the childhood and adolescent religious socialization process; this then leads us to a discussion of adolescent and young adult thinking about religion, especially religious questions and doubts, and their resolution. Then we consider the processes involved in leaving the family religion (apostasy), which at first blush might seem to contradict socialization theory. Finally, we explore ways in which adolescent religiousness may be related to ego identity development. But first, how and why does socialization exert such a strong influence on religiousness?

INFLUENCES ON RELIGIOUSNESS
IN CHILDHOOD AND ADOLESCENCE

Many external influences have the potential to affect people's religiousness: parents, peers, schools, religious institutions, books, the mass media, and so on. They can affect individuals directly through, for example, explicit religious teachings or family practices. They can also affect people indirectly in many ways—for example, by influencing school, marital, and career choices, or through cultural assumptions, subtle modeling, or lack of exposure to alternative positions. People may be conscious of some religious socialization influences, but quite unaware of others. Cornwall (1988) has noted that the religious socialization literature has traditionally focused on three "agents" of socialization: parents, peers, and church. We examine each of these in turn, but consider church (or any other religious institution) simply as one of a number of "other factors" that have been suggested to affect the religious socialization process. We also examine an additional factor that has been studied, education.

Our coverage of these potential influencing factors is largely restricted to the empirical work on religious socialization. There exists a rich body of literature in the psychodynamic and object relations traditions, especially with respect to the role of parents in the socialization process. The reader may wish to consult other sources for differing perspectives on these issues (see, e.g., Coles, 1990; Rizzuto, 1979, 2001).

The Influence of Parents

Parents have both direct and indirect effects on the socialization of their children, who in turn may or may not be aware of their parents' influence. Of the many different possible socialization influences, parents have typically been found to be the most important. There is copious evidence that parents have considerable impact on the religiosity of their children, both when their offspring are younger and also when they are adolescents and young adults.

Some social scientists (e.g., Cornwall & Thomas, 1990) believe that parental influence occurs within the family as a "personal religious community" that may exist quite independently of institutionalized religion. This small community, of which the parents are an integral part, influences religiousness indirectly by affecting the "personal community relationship" (Cornwall, 1987, p. 44). It is possible that this focus on personal religious communities may be most applicable in such groups as the Mormons, which served as the empirical basis for Cornwall's (e.g., 1987) conclusions about the religious socialization process. Of course,

one's family of origin is potentially very important in affecting one's socialization and functioning in a number of systems, not just religion (Friedman, 1985; Slaughter-Defoe, 1995).
Also, in this chapter we consider various avenues of parental socialization influence, not just
that within "personal religious communities."

To some extent, children lead sheltered lives in terms of religion; they may not be aware
that there *are* other religions, or even that there are people whose beliefs differ from their
own. Parents often have a "captive audience" for their religious and other teachings, at least
when their children are younger. Social learning theory would predict that children will be
strongly influenced by these powerful and important parental models, as well as by the reinforcement contingencies controlled by the parents (Bandura, 1977). Much evidence is
consistent with this prediction, and social learning theory may be viewed as the theoretical
underpinning of the socialization process.

It is not a straightforward matter to tap parental influence in studies of religious socialization. Some investigators simply focus on "keeping the faith"—the extent to which children identify with the family religion as they grow older. These investigations typically assume that keeping the family faith must result in large part from parental influence. Other
researchers focus on parent–child attitudinal agreement regarding religious and other matters, assuming that greater agreement indicates more effective parental influence. Still others rely on direct self-reports of influence, asking children or adolescents about the extent
to which parents influence their religiousness. Similarly, some investigators have asked older
adolescents and adults to reflect back on their lives and consider to what extent parents (and
other factors) influenced their religion.

All of these approaches have their problems. For example, identification with a religious
group may mean different things for different denominations, and it may not always be a
good indicator of parental influence. Parent–child attitudinal agreement does not necessarily mean that parental influence was strong, and people's self-reports and memories may be
faulty. But, collectively, these different approaches offer insight into parental religious socialization influence.

Studies of "Keeping the Faith"

Hunsberger (1976) studied several hundred university students from Catholic, United Church
("liberal Protestant"), and Mennonite ("conservative Protestant") families in Canada. These
students were asked about the extent to which they accepted earlier religious teachings, as
well as the strength of the emphasis placed on religion in their homes. The correlation between these measures was +.44, indicating that a self-reported tendency for greater emphasis on religion in one's childhood home was linked with acceptance of religious teachings
during the university years. However, a significant tendency remained for Mennonite students to be more accepting of religious teachings than United Church students (with Catholics being intermediate), even after differential emphasis on religious teachings in these groups
was controlled for. This suggests that other factors unique to specific religious groups may
also be important.

A social-cognitive model of religious change in adolescence (Ozorak, 1989; see Research
Box 5.1) predicts that both social factors (such as parental or peer influence) and cognitive
variables (such as intellectual aptitude and existential questioning) influence adolescent religiousness. Ozorak's (1989) data supported the social-cognitive model, especially with respect to the positive link between parental and adolescent religiousness, and she concluded

ह⃝

Research Box 5.1. Influences on Religious Beliefs and Commitment in Adolescence (Ozorak, 1989)

Elizabeth Ozorak noted that various explanations exist for adolescent change in religious beliefs and practices. For example, it has been proposed that influence from parents, peers, or others may be powerful factors; that "existential anxiety" may be an initiating factor; or (as we have seen in Chapter 4) that cognitive development can serve as the stimulus for such change. Ozorak sought to test a variety of possible effects within a social-cognitive model of religious change. She proposed that social influences, especially parents, are the most powerful factors affecting adolescent religiousness; that there is a gradual polarization of religious beliefs in the direction established relatively early in people's lives; and that such cognitive factors as "existential questioning" are associated with decreased religious commitment.

After pilot-testing her materials on 9th and 11th graders, Ozorak studied 390 high school students and high school alumni from the Boston area. The subjects included 106 students in 9th grade, 150 students in 11th or 12th grade, and 134 alumni who had graduated 3 years earlier from two of the three high schools involved. Each participant completed a questionnaire including a wide variety of items and scales tapping religious affiliation, participation, beliefs, experiences, existential questioning, social "connectedness," family and peer influences, and religious change.

The data indicated that "middle adolescence is a period of [religious] readjustment for many individuals" (p. 455), with the average age of change being about 14.5 years. Social factors, especially parents, were powerful predictors of religiousness. For example, parents' religious affiliation and participation were positively related to children's religiousness. The influence of peers (discussed later in this chapter) was not so straightforward, though the data suggested that it too was related to adolescent religiosity. Cognitive factors also played a role; more existential questioning and higher intellectual aptitude were associated with religious change, but only for the oldest age group (high school alumni). In addition, there was support for a "polarization" interpretation of the data, such that the most religious participants tended to report greater change in a proreligious direction and the least religious participants reported decreasing religiosity over time.

Ozorak concluded that "parents' affiliation and their faith in that affiliation act as cognitive anchors from which the child's beliefs evolve over time. Family cohesion seems to limit modification of religious practices but exerts less pressure on beliefs, which become increasingly individual with maturation" (p. 460). This study is important because it reminds us of the powerful influence of *both* social and cognitive factors with respect to religious socialization. Furthermore, it emphasizes the critical role of parents in influencing religiousness and religious change in their offspring.

that parents are especially powerful influences in the religious socialization process. However, the influence of parents seemed more prominent for high school students than for college-age respondents, suggesting that parental influence may decrease as adolescents make the transition to adulthood.

Other studies have also indicated that parental religiousness is a good predictor of adolescents' and even adult children's religiousness. A survey investigation of Catholic high school seniors led to the conclusion that the three main factors predicting adolescent religiousness were perceptions of the importance of religion for the parents, positive family environment, and home religious activity (Benson, Yaeger, Wood, Guerra, & Manno, 1986). A national probability sample of more than 1,000 U.S. adolescents revealed that parental religiosity was a significant predictor of adolescent religious practice (Potvin & Sloane, 1985). The religious participation of Jewish parents was a powerful predictor of the religious beliefs and practices of their adolescent children (Parker & Gaier, 1980). Such influence may even extend into adulthood; a study of college teachers indicated that their parents' church attendance constituted the best predictor of their own religiousness (Hoge & Keeter, 1976).

Similarly, numerous studies have noted a strong tendency for children raised within a specific familial religious denomination to continue to identify with that denomination from childhood through adolescence and young adulthood (e.g., Altemeyer & Hunsberger, 1997; Bibby, 2001; Hadaway, 1980; Kluegel, 1980; see also Beit-Hallahmi & Argyle, 1997; Benson, Donahue, & Erickson, 1989). In general, several different parental religion variables seem to be reasonable predictors of the extent to which adolescents and young adults maintain the family religion.

Parent–Child Agreement Studies

During the 1960s and 1970s, the mass media and social scientists were very interested in a possible "generation gap"—"a kind of organized rebellion against parents by their teenagers, one component of which supposedly involves considerable discrepancy between teenagers' attitudes and those of their parents" (Hunsberger, 1985a, p. 314). Some researchers concluded that there was indeed a generation gap (Friedenberg, 1969; Thomas, 1974); others contended that parent–adolescent attitudinal differences were relatively minor (Lerner & Spanier, 1980) or virtually nonexistent (Coopersmith, Regan, & Dick, 1975; Nelsen, 1981b). Also, parent–child attitudinal agreement may vary from one issue to another, and religious attitudes in particular may involve more parent–child agreement than some other domains (Bengtson & Troll, 1978).

A study of university students and their mothers and fathers confirmed this latter tendency (Hunsberger, 1985a). In general, there was moderately strong agreement on core elements of religiousness, including scores on a scale measuring the orthodoxy of Christian beliefs (correlations were .43 between students and their mothers, and .48 between students and their fathers), and reports of frequency of church attendance (correlations were .58 and .57, respectively). Furthermore, there tended to be stronger parent–child agreement on religious matters than there was on some other issues (e.g., self-rated happiness, personal adjustment, political radicalism).

Other investigations of mother–father–adolescent triads have led to similar conclusions, though relationships are sometimes weak. A study of triads from Catholic, Baptist, and Methodist homes showed weak to moderate correspondence between parents and their offspring on religious measures (higher for mothers than for fathers), with endorsement of a specific creed revealing stronger relationships (Hoge, Petrillo, & Smith, 1982). These relationships remained significant when the effects of denomination, family income, and father's occupation were partialed out, though Hoge et al. emphasized that extrafamilial influences (e.g., denomination) were also important in religious socialization. In a study of mother–father–child triads from Seventh-Day Adventist homes, modest agreement emerged across a series of religious and nonreligious values, with generally stronger relationships between offspring and mothers than between offspring and fathers (Dudley &

Dudley, 1986). Glass, Bengtson, and Dunham (1986) carried out a study of three generations of family members, the youngest generation being between the ages of 16 and 26.
They concluded that there was substantial agreement on religious and political issues for
both child–parent and parent–grandparent dyads, suggesting that parental influence in
these areas may persist into adulthood.

Such findings of weak to moderately strong parent–adolescent agreement on religious
issues do not "prove" that parents are important influences in their children's religious lives,
of course. But such results are consistent with the data obtained through other approaches,
which suggest that parents are indeed influential in this regard. Certainly, if parents play an
important role in their children's religious development, one would expect to find at least
modest correlations between measures of adolescent and parental religiousness. Interestingly,
in Hunsberger's (1985a) study, parents were reasonably accurate estimators of the religious
beliefs and practices of their college-age children, *unless* those children had drifted away from
the family religious teachings. When the children had become apostates (i.e., had abandoned
the home religion), parents were significantly poorer predictors of their children's religious
attitudes than when they had remained in the family religion. This might suggest that parents are relatively unaware of adolescent shifts away from the family religion when they
occur—or, as argued by Bengtson and Troll (1978), that parents tend to minimize differences between themselves and their adolescent children.

There also seems to be a tendency for adolescents to perceive that their parents are more
conservative or traditional than the parents report themselves to be (Acock & Bengtson,
1980). Adolescents also perceive more attitudinal agreement between their parents than in
fact exists. Thus there seems to be a tendency for youths to view their parents as more conservative and in closer agreement than they really are; the impact of these misperceptions
on the socialization process is unknown.

It should be noted that the findings of these parent–adolescent agreement studies are
generally consistent with recent conceptualizations of adolescence as a time of reasonably
stable development and socialization, and a time when there is considerable similarity in
values and attitudes between parents and their adolescent offspring. This is in contrast to
earlier conceptualizations of adolescence as a time of turmoil and rebellion, resulting in a
sizeable "generation gap." This shift in our view of adolescence is reflected, for example, in
Petersen's (1988) review of the adolescent development literature, and in recent textbooks
on adolescence (e.g., Cobb, 2001).

Self-Reports of Religious Influence

A pioneering study carried out in the 1940s found that about two-thirds of a Harvard and
Radcliffe student sample reported having reacted against parental and cultural teaching
(Allport, Gillespie, & Young, 1948). However, these students indicated that the influences
underlying their sense of need for religious sentiment included the following (with the percentage of respondents mentioning each influence shown in parentheses): parents (67%),
other people (57%), fear (52%), church (40%), and gratitude (37%). Clearly, parents were
perceived to play a primary role in the development of religious sentiment.

More recent studies involving a wide variety of age groups in North America and elsewhere have confirmed that parents are perceived to be the most important influence on
religiosity. Hunsberger and Brown (1984) asked 878 introductory psychology students at
the University of New South Wales in Sydney, Australia to identify the three people who

had the greatest influence on their religious beliefs. Parents were clearly the "winners," being designated as the most important influence by 44% of all respondents (friends came next at 15%). In subsequent studies, Hunsberger asked several hundred students at a Canadian university (Hunsberger, 1983b) and 85 older Canadians (aged 65–88 years; Hunsberger, 1985b) to rate the extent of religious influence that 10 possible sources of influence had exerted in their lives. Both the students and the older persons ranked their mothers and fathers first and third, respectively. Church received the second highest ranking.

One striking thing about these two studies (Hunsberger, 1983b, 1985b) was the extent to which the students and senior citizens agreed in their rankings. Also, the senior citizens generally reported stronger absolute proreligious influence in their lives than did the students; this was consistent with findings from other cross-sectional studies (Benson, 1992a; Hunsberger, 1985a) and a panel study of Swedes (Hamberg, 1991), which all showed a general increase in religiosity across the adult years. Furthermore, the rankings for the Canadian university students were quite similar to those given by the Australian university students (Hunsberger & Brown, 1984).

Francis and Gibson (1993) explored parental influence on religious attitudes and practices of 3,414 secondary school students in Scotland (ages 11–12 and 15–16), with approximately equal numbers of males and females in each age category. Primary dependent measures included self-report of frequency of church attendance, and scores on a 24-item Likert-type scale[2] measuring attitude toward Christianity (Francis, 1989a). The authors concluded that parental influence was generally important with respect to church attendance, and there was a tendency for this influence to *increase* from the younger to the older age groups. Consistent with some of Hunsberger's (1983b, 1985a) and Acock and Bengtson's (1978, 1980; see also Dudley & Dudley, 1986) findings, they also concluded that mothers had more influence on children's religion than fathers overall, but that there was some tendency toward stronger same-sex influence for both mothers and fathers. Also, parental influence was greater for overt religiosity (i.e., church attendance) than it was for more covert religiosity (i.e., attitudes toward Christianity).

In two studies of attitudinal predispositions to pray, described in Research Box 5.2, Francis and Brown (1990, 1991) concluded that parental influence was of primary importance with respect to church attendance for adolescents attending Roman Catholic, Anglican, and nondenominational schools in England. Church attendance in turn was positively related to attitudes toward prayer. Also, as in the Francis and Gibson (1993) study, they found that mothers seemed to exert more influence than fathers, although parental influence was stronger when both parents attended church.

Influence of Mother versus Father

As noted above, some findings suggest that mothers are more influential than fathers in the religious development of their offspring; however, not all studies confirm this generalization. Kieren and Munro (1987) concluded that fathers were more influential than mothers overall. And the findings of some other studies have been equivocal in this regard (Baker-Sperry, 2001; Benson, Williams, & Johnson, 1987; Hoge & Petrillo, 1978a; Nelsen, 1980). But the

---

2. A "Likert-type scale" invites respondents to indicate the extent to which they agree or disagree with attitude statements. It might range, for example, from +3 ("strongly agree") to –3 ("strongly disagree").

Research Box 5.2. Social Influences on the Predisposition to Pray (Francis & Brown, 1990, 1991)

These two studies focused on predispositions to pray, as well as the practice of prayer, among two age levels of English adolescents. The first investigation involved almost 5,000 students aged 11, and the second about 700 students aged 16; all students attended Roman Catholic, Church of England, or nondenominational state-maintained schools. As well as self-reports of their own and their parents' religious behavior, participants completed a six-item scale assessing attitudes toward prayer (e.g., "Saying my prayers helps me a lot").

Results confirmed that the parents were powerful factors with respect to children's church attendance at both age levels, though mothers consistently exerted more influence than fathers. However, there were indications that parental impact on children's prayer had decreased somewhat, and that church influences (e.g., attendance) had increased, for the 16-year-olds. Attendance at Roman Catholic or Church of England schools did not seem to affect adolescent *practice* of prayer, after other factors had been controlled for; however, there was a slightly negative impact of Church of England schools on *attitudes* toward prayer.

The authors concluded their 1991 paper by stating that their findings "support the importance of taking seriously social learning or modeling interpretations of prayer. Children and adolescents who pray seem more likely to do so as a consequence of explicit teaching or implicit example from their family and church community than as a spontaneous consequence of developmental dynamics or needs" (p. 120).

---

weight of the evidence suggests that mothers are more influential than fathers (e.g., Hertel & Donahue, 1995; see also Benson, Masters, & Larson, 1997). Mothers may serve a primary nurturing role for religious socialization, since in Western cultures women are on average more religious than men (e.g., Donelson, 1999; Francis & Wilcox, 1998), and women also tend to assume more child-rearing responsibilities (Smith & Mackie, 1995). They may, for example, assume primary responsibility for taking children to church and teaching them basic religious views. Because of this, it is not surprising that people typically perceive that their mothers exerted the stronger influence on their religiousness.

However, it is quite possible that fathers also play an important role, especially to the extent that their religious views are consistent or inconsistent with those of mothers and the church. Fathers might serve as role models for continued religiousness, or for rejection of religion after initial religious socialization. Thus mothers and fathers may play somewhat different roles, and have influence in different ways or at different periods, in their children's socialization. For example, a study of more than 400 families in rural areas of Iowa found that the roles of both mothers and fathers were important in religious transmission to their offspring (Bao, Whitbeck, Hoyt, & Conger, 1999). But when adolescents perceived that their parents were generally accepting of their adolescent children, mothers' influence was reportedly stronger, especially for sons. Such subtle nuances could well contribute to seemingly contradictory conclusions in the literature concerning the relative importance of mothers and fathers in religious socialization.

Other Aspects of Parenting

Consistent with the Bao et al. (1999) investigation, a number of studies have suggested that the *quality* of young people's relationships with parents can also affect religious socialization. For example, in a panel investigation spanning the years 1965–1982, children who reported while in high school that they had a warm, close relationship with their parents were less likely to rebel against religious teachings (Wilson & Sherkat, 1994). Furthermore, longitudinal data led Wilson and Sherkat to conclude that "Lack of closeness and contact have created a religious gap between parents and children rather than religious differences creating a distant relationship" (p. 155). Others have come to similar conclusions regarding the importance of the emotional relationship between parents and adolescents (e.g., Dudley, 1978; Herzbrun, 1993; Hoge, Petrillo, & Smith, 1982; Nelsen, 1980; Okagaki & Bevis, 1999). Myers (1996) interviewed parents and their adult offspring, and concluded that the main determinants of offspring religiosity were parental religiosity, the quality of the family relationship, and traditional family structure.

Cause and effect are not always clear, however. Most authors seem to assume that higher quality of family relationships "causes" increased religiosity in offspring. Of course, if the parents are themselves nonreligious, the higher quality of family relationships may then "cause" decreased religiosity in offspring. But Brody, Stoneman, and Flor (1996) concluded that causality was in the opposite direction in their study of 9- to 12-year-old African American young people and their parents living in the rural southern United States. That is, Brody et al. felt that when the parents were more religious, this contributed to a closer, more cohesive family, as well as to less conflict between the parents. Additional research is needed to address the direction of cause-and-effect relationships in this area.

Similarly, more general parental values and behavior may affect some aspects of the religious socialization process. Research has shown that parental valuation of obedience is associated with theological positions of Biblical literalism, the belief that human nature is sinful, and punitive attitudes toward sinners (Ellison & Sherkat, 1993). Also, parental disharmony (e.g., arguing and fighting) seems to inhibit the transmission of religiosity across successive generations (Nelsen, 1981a). Moreover, as suggested in Chapter 4, adult parenting values, goals, and practices may have important implications for children's subsequent religious orientation (e.g., Danso, Hunsberger, & Pratt, 1997; see also Flor & Knapp, 2001).

Although it is clear that parents play an important role in the religious socialization process, the relationship is not always a simple one. The behavior, parenting style, goals, attitudes, and values of the parents, as well as the quality of their relationship with their children, may facilitate or inhibit their children's religious socialization. Unfortunately, there is a dearth of research on the subtle interplay between family life and religion (Cornwall & Thomas, 1990; D'Antonio, Newman, & Wright, 1982).

Parental Influence: Summary

All of the different approaches to studying parental influence in the religious socialization process converge on a single conclusion: Parents play an extremely important role in the developing religious attitudes and practices of their offspring. In fact, few researchers would quarrel with the conclusion that parents are *the* most important influence in this regard. Other reviewers of the related literature have come to similar conclusions (e.g., Batson,

Schoenrade, & Ventis, 1993; Benson et al., 1997; Brown, 1987; Cornwall, 1989). However, it has been pointed out that parental influence can sometimes be more indirect than direct (Erickson, 1992; Cornwall, 1988; Cornwall & Thomas, 1990). For example, parents to some extent are "managers" who control which "other influences" their children are exposed to (e.g., through church attendance, or selection of religious vs. secular schooling), and these in turn may have some influence on young people's religion. Furthermore, different aspects of the mother–father and parent–adolescent relationships can affect the strength of parental influence on young people's religion, and mother–father consistency and agreement also seems to enhance acceptance of the parental religious teachings (Benson et al., 1989).

The Influence of Peers

Some authors have concluded that peer groups play an important role in influencing adolescents generally (Allport, 1950; Balk, 1995; Sprinthall & Collins, 1995), but relatively few studies have investigated peer influence on religiousness. Those that have done so tend to report some relatively weak peer group effects. Such studies almost always rely on self-reports of peer influence, and the direction of the influence (positive or negative) is not always specified.

The impact of parents and peers were compared in a study of 375 Australian youths aged 16–18 (de Vaus, 1983). Consistent with some previous research (Bengtson & Troll, 1978), it was concluded that parents were more influential for religious beliefs, and that peers tended to have more influence outside of the religious realm (e.g., with respect to self-concept); however, de Vaus found that peers also influenced religious practice to some extent (see also Hoge & Petrillo, 1978a). Erickson (1992) similarly found that peer influence was relatively unimportant in adolescent religiousness. But he pointed out that peer influence might be hidden because of the way in which effects were measured, and also because it was difficult to separate peer influence from religious education, which itself involved "a social/friendship setting" (p. 151) that might constitute a kind of peer influence.

Similarly, Hunsberger's (1983b, 1985b) studies involving self-ratings of religious influences suggested that friends were well down the list of 10 potential influences for both university students (fifth) and older Canadians (ninth). Ozorak (1989) concluded that peers do influence adolescent religiousness, though this relationship is rather complex and is overshadowed by more important parental influences. Other researchers have confirmed the primary importance of parents in religious socialization, but have also found evidence that the religiosity of college students' current friends offers a kind of supplementary reinforcing effect (Roberts, Koch, & Johnson, 2001). In another investigation, both peer and family influences predicted adolescent religiousness (King, Furrow, & Roth, 2002).

Of course, peer influence may be stronger in some religion areas than in others. For example, peers may have little influence for core religion measures such as frequency of church attendance, but may be more important with respect to youth group participation and enjoyment of that participation (Hoge & Petrillo, 1978a). Also, peer influence is probably complex, especially with respect to dating and heterosexual friendships. For example, particularly for adolescents of minority religions, religiously based attitudes toward interfaith dating may initiate a kind of filtering process in partner selection (Marshall & Markstrom-Adams, 1995). This filtering may in turn affect dating partners' interactions and reciprocal influence regarding religion (i.e., a type of peer influence).

In an exception to the usual self-report studies in this area, an unusual field experiment (Carey, 1971) involved randomly assigning 102 Catholic school students in seventh grade to one of three groups: prorelision, antirelision, or no influence (control group). Confederates (boys who were "leaders" in the same classes as the other participants) urged their classmates to comply or not to comply with a nun's talk on "Why a Catholic should go to daily Mass." Actual attendance at Mass was then monitored, and an effect did emerge for the position taken by the male confederates to influence their peers, but only for girls. Of course, the peer influence assessed in this study was very specific and short-term; we should be careful not to confuse such transitory impact with more general, long-term, and complex peer effects.

Finally, we should not assume that peer influence is relevant only to child and adolescent religion. Olson (1989) found that in five Baptist congregations, the number and quality of friendships were important predictors of adults' decisions to join or leave a denomination. And Putnam (2000) has pointed out that people who belong to religious groups tend to have more social commitments and contacts in their lives; this increased social interaction may allow for greater peer influence. Unfortunately, there has been little investigation of possible peer influence on religiousness in adulthood, beyond friendship networks.

Does Education Make a Difference?

The Impact of College

The extent to which education affects religious socialization has been a controversial topic. Early studies generally concluded that education, especially college, tended to "liberalize" religious beliefs of students. For example, a review of more than 40 investigations led Feldman (1969) to conclude that these studies

> generally show mean changes indicating that seniors, compared with freshmen, are somewhat less orthodox, fundamentalistic, or conventional in religious orientation, somewhat more sceptical about the existence and influence of a Supreme Being, somewhat more likely to conceive of God in impersonal terms, and somewhat less favorable toward the church as an institution. Although the trend across studies does exist, the mean changes are not always large, and in about a third of the cases showing decreasing favorability toward religion, differences are not statistically significant. (p. 23)

Other reviewers (e.g., Parker, 1971) have similarly concluded that religious change may be considerable during the college years, especially in the first year. However, we should be cautious about such (average) trends toward decreased religiousness, because they may mask substantial change in the opposite direction for *some* students (Feldman & Newcomb, 1969). In addition, if change occurs, education itself is not necessarily the cause of the change. Shifts away from orthodox religion may be part of maturational or developmental change, or may result from the fact that some students are effectively away from parental control for the first time. Such shifts may also reflect peer influence or a tendency for less religious (or more questioning) students to attend (and not to drop out of) college, or at least to avoid campus religious involvement. Madsen and Vernon (1983) found a (not surprising) tendency for more religious students to be more likely to participate in campus religious activities. More importantly, those students who participated in campus religious groups tended to increase in religious orthodoxy, but nonparticipants became less orthodox at college. It is also possible that apparent effects of college are actually due to other factors, such as religious background (Hoge & Keeter, 1976). For example, Sieben (2001) found in a Dutch study that the influence of education on a variety of variables, including orthodox religious belief and church attendance, was considerably overestimated when the impact of family background was not controlled for.

Furthermore, studies began to appear in the 1970s that were not always consistent with Feldman's conclusion that there is a general shift away from traditional religion. For example, Hunsberger (1978) reported a cross-sectional study of more than 450 Canadian university students, and a separate longitudinal investigation of more than 200 students from their first to their third university years, including an interim assessment of about half of this longitudinal sample during their second year. His data offered little support for the proposal that students generally become less religious over their university years. The only consistent finding across both studies was that third- and fourth-year students reported attending church less frequently than did first-year students. Thus there was limited support for a decrease in religious practices across the college years, but this change did not generalize to some other practices (e.g., frequency of prayer), or to scores on a series of religious belief measures. Finally, measures of "average change" did *not* mask frequent or dramatic individual religious change in different directions.

Hunsberger speculated that college-related religious change may have been more characteristic of the 1960s, since other subsequent studies (e.g., Hastings & Hoge, 1976; Pilkington, Poppleton, Gould, & McCourt, 1976) also found little or no change. In fact, Moberg and Hoge (1986) concluded that the decade 1961–1971 had seen considerable shifts toward liberalism in college students, but that the following decade (1971–1982) involved a slight change in the opposite direction (toward conservatism and traditional moral attitudes). Finally, Hunsberger (1978) suggested that religious change may be more likely to happen in the high school years, and may be relatively complete by the time students reach college—a suggestion supported by the research of others (Francis, 1982; Sutherland, 1988). However, some authors have continued to conclude that higher education has at least indirect effects on young people's religiousness—by, for example, encouraging skepticism and a sense of religious and moral relativity (e.g., Hadaway & Roof, 1988).

Parochial School Attendance

Some investigations have compared public with parochial schools regarding the religiousness of their students. These investigations have generated rather muddy findings, possibly because of methodological shortcomings (Benson et al., 1989; Hyde, 1990). Although some early researchers (e.g., Lenski, 1961; Greeley, 1967) concluded that parochial school attenders were more strongly religious in some ways than their public school counterparts, the relevant research sometimes failed to take background factors into account. Some investigators apparently assumed that differences between parochial and public school students were *caused* by the environments of the schools involved, and they ignored possible self-selection factors. More than 30 years ago, Mueller (1967) found that when he held religious background constant, he could find no differences in the religious orthodoxy and institutional involvement of college students. He concluded that "high orthodoxy is a direct function of a strong religious background rather than specifically of parochial school attendance" (p. 51).

Other research has supported this finding, including studies of fundamentalists (Erickson, 1964), Jews (Parker & Gaier, 1980), Lutherans (Johnstone, 1966), Mennonites (Kraybill, 1977), and Catholics and Church of England adherents (Francis & Brown, 1991). For example, Francis and Brown (1991) argued that a positive relationship between Roman Catholic school attendance and positive attitudes toward prayer was really a result of "the influence of home and church rather than that of the school itself" (p. 119). Furthermore, as indicated in Research Box 5.2, their investigation even detected a small *negative* influence of Church of England schools on attitudes toward prayer, after other factors were controlled for (gender, home, church, private practice of prayer). This finding was consistent with Francis's (1980, 1986) previous work with younger children.

More recently, a study in the United Kingdom (Francis & Lankshear, 2001) similarly revealed very little impact of church-related primary schools on religiousness or religious activity in the local community. There was a tendency toward higher rates of religious confirmation in the preteen years (for voluntarily aided but not for controlled schools), but apparently no influence on older persons. However, these "minimal-impact" conclusions have been challenged by some authors (e.g., Greeley & Gockel, 1971; Greeley & Rossi, 1966), and Himmelfarb (1979) argued that church-related schools do indeed have a direct positive influence on the religiousness of their students.

In the end, there is probably variation across individual schools, different age groups (elementary, high school, and postsecondary students), and different religious denominations. Self-selection factors probably occur at many parochial schools, such that more religious students (or at least students with more religious parents) are likely to attend such schools. Findings may differ across studies, depending on whether they focus on religious beliefs or practices (Hunsberger, 1977). Effects may be unique to specific studies, or may depend on combinations of factors. For example, Benson et al. (1986) found that Catholic high schools with a high proportion of students from low-income families tended to have a positive influence on religiousness *if* those schools stressed academics and religion, had high student morale, and also focused on the importance of religion and the development of a "community of faith." There may also be effects for some specific measures of religiousness, such as an increase in religious *knowledge* (Johnstone, 1966). It is often very difficult to separate the influence of parochial schools from the effects of parents and the family generally (Benson et al., 1989).

In light of the findings available, and their many qualifications, we are led to this conclusion: The bulk of the evidence suggests that church-related school attendance has little direct influence on adolescent religiousness per se. The issue is not clear-cut, and the reader may wish to consult more comprehensive reviews of the relevant literature (e.g., Hyde, 1990).

Other Influences

Parents, peers, and education are not the only potential sources of influence on religiousness. Some studies have suggested that the particular church (or other religious institution) or denomination, as well as socioeconomic status, sibling configuration, city size, the mass media, reading, and so on, can also have some effect on the religious socialization process (see, e.g., Benson et al., 1989). For example, rural youths tend to be more religious than nonrural young people (King, Elder, & Whitbeck, 1997). However, self-reported ratings of influence (Hunsberger, 1983b, 1985b) and more indirect inferences (Francis & Brown, 1991; Erickson, 1992) suggest that factors related to the church (or to religious education, broadly defined) are the most important of various possible "other" influences on the religious so-cialization process. Francis and Brown (1991) have observed that church becomes a more important influence in middle adolescence, at roughly the time when young people are be-coming less susceptible to parental influence with respect to religion.

Erickson (1992) reported that religious education was of "overwhelming influence" (p. 151) in adolescent religious socialization. However, religious education was very broadly defined in Erickson's study, including involvement in religious activities, knowledge gained from religious instruction, and perceptions of religious education programs. In fact, as de-fined by Erickson and some others, religious education apparently has little to do with for-mal (school) education or educational institutions, but is more a measure of church involve-ment and activity. In this sense, church-related involvement clearly can be an important contributor to the religious socialization process.

But the term "religious education" is sometimes used to describe this area where church and education boundaries blur. In this context, articles that appeared in a special issue of the *Review of Religious Research* on adolescent religious socialization in the context of reli-gious education (Hoge, Hefferman, et al., 1982; Hoge & Thompson, 1982; Nelsen, 1982; Philibert & Hoge, 1982) are helpful.

In general, however, the various "other factors" discussed above have received scant em-pirical attention. There is a need for further investigation of attitudes toward the church, the role of the clergy, the influence of church-related peers compared to non-church-related friends, mass media effects, and so on, as well as the subtle interplay among these and other religious socialization factors.

The Polarization Hypothesis

Earlier we have mentioned Ozorak's (1989) social-cognitive model of religious socialization processes, which allows for the possibility of a "polarization" effect in religious development. That is, Ozorak noted a tendency for more religious adolescents to report change in the di-rection of greater religiosity, whereas less religious adolescents reported a shift away from religion (see Research Box 5.1). Tamminen (1991) found a similar religious polarization ten-dency among Finnish adolescents. This is consistent with the observation that more religious college students join campus religious groups, and also increase in religious orthodoxy while at college, but less religious students who do not join campus religious groups decrease in orthodoxy (Madsen & Vernon, 1983). In other words, the religious "distance" between these two groups increases at college. Similar self-reported polarization tendencies have been found among the most and least religious participants in a study of older Canadians (Hunsberger, 1985b). Reflecting back over their lives and "graphing" their religiosity across the decades, these senior citizens indicated that they had gradually become more religious across their lives since childhood if they were highly religious at the time of the study. However, senior citizens who were relatively less religious indicated that they had become progressively *less* religious across their lives, compared to their more religious counterparts.

These studies are limited by the retrospective, cross-sectional, and self-report nature of the data, as well as by the possibility that we are learning more about people's perceptions of reality than we are about reality itself. However, the findings are consistent with the pos-sibility that general trends toward greater or lesser religiosity may be established quite early in life, and that these trends may continue long after early developmental and socialization influences have had their immediate effects.

Gender Issues

Social influences (especially the influence of parents) in the religious socialization process can help to explain some important gender differences in adolescent and adult religiosity. For example, women have typically been found to be "more religious" than men (see Donelson, 1999; Francis & Wilcox, 1998). That is, they attend worship services more often, pray more often, express stronger agreement with traditional beliefs, are more interested in religion, and report that religion is more important in their lives. Batson et al. (1993) have proposed that such gender differences are probably attributable to social influence processes in sex role training, either through sex differences that have implications for religiousness (e.g., women are taught to be more submissive and nurturing—traits associated with greater religiosity), or through direct expectations that women should be more religious than men. Similar "socialization" interpretations have come from others (e.g., Nelsen & Potvin, 1981), though these are not the only possible interpretations of gender differences in religion (see Miller & Hoffman, 1995).

It is likely that religious socialization processes have important gender implications for other areas of people's lives, such as (nonreligious) attitudes, careers, and education. For example, national survey data from 19,000 U.S. women led to the conclusion that religious identification affects educational attainment more strongly than do other sociodemographic variables (Keysar & Kosmin, 1995). Women from more conservative, traditional, or fundamentalist backgrounds achieved less postsecondary education than did women from more liberal or modern religious backgrounds, on average. That is, "some gender inequality is indeed socially created by the influence of religion" (Keysar & Kosmin, 1995, p. 61). Although this was a correlational study, it does raise the possibility that religious socialization can ultimately affect "nonreligious" aspects of one's life.

There is also evidence that young men and women differ in their perceptions of God and in how they would react to a male versus female God. Foster and Babcock (2001) asked university students to write a story about a fictional interaction with a male or female God. Men's stories involved more action, whereas women were more concerned with feelings. There was also more skepticism, criticality, and surprise in reaction to a female God than to a male God. Such gender differences may well develop during childhood as part of the socialization process—an issue ripe for future research.

Influences on Religiousness: Summary and Implications

We must be cautious in drawing conclusions about religious socialization influences, since it is often difficult to isolate parental, church, educational, and other influences and their possible interactions. Many researchers simply ask people to report on the factors that influenced their, or their children's, religiousness. This approach assumes that (1) people do have a basic understanding and accurate memory of the forces that shape religiosity, and (2) they can clearly and honestly articulate these influences in a research context. However, these assumptions may be faulty. Also, relevant studies sometimes investigate very different samples. Some include a broad range of participants; others draw their samples from church or other religious sources; and still others focus on members of one specific religious group. Measures and data analysis techniques differ widely from one study to another, and the direction of influence (e.g., toward or away from religion) is not always assessed. However, given the large numbers of relevant studies and the convergence of some findings, we are able to offer some general conclusions.

Parents are potentially the most powerful influences on child and adolescent religion, though their impact becomes weaker as adolescents grow into adulthood, and some of their influence may be indirect. Mothers are often found to be more influential than fathers, though there is not complete agreement on this issue. Beyond parental impact, church is most often found to be a significant contributor to religious socialization, but there has been little investigation of the specific components of this relationship. Education, parochial school environment, the mass media, and reading have *not* been found to affect religious socialization to any great degree. It has been suggested, however, that when the parents and other potential influential agents (e.g., the church) reinforce the same religious perspective, the resulting combined religious socialization effects may be especially strong (Hyde, 1990). Furthermore, trends established early in life for people to become more or less religious may continue into adulthood (as predicted by the polarization hypothesis).

Finally, it is important that we not lose sight of possible implications of religious socialization for other aspects of people's lives. We have seen that religious growth processes can have a potentially powerful impact on gender issues. No doubt the effects of religious socialization extend into many other aspects of people's lives as well, as discussed throughout this book.

HOW RELIGIOUS ARE ADOLESCENTS AND YOUNG ADULTS?

Findings have usually confirmed that in general, adolescents and young adults are less religious than middle and older adults in North America and Europe (Dudley & Dudley, 1986; Hamberg, 1991). Moreover, religiousness is typically found to decrease during the 10- to 18-year-old period (Benson et al., 1989), at least for adolescents in mainstream religious groups. However, this should not be construed to mean that adolescents are nonreligious, or that religion has little impact on their lives.

In Allport et al.'s (1948) study of religion among college students, they found that approximately 7 out of every 10 students sampled felt they needed religion in their own lives (82% of the women and 68% of the men). Furthermore, only 6% of the men and 10% of the women reported a total absence of religious training. As might be expected, students trained in a religion reported that they needed religion more often than others, leading Allport et al. (1948) to conclude that early training is likely to be the principal psychological influence upon an individual's later religious life. Overall, 15% of Allport et al.'s sample denied engaging in any religious practices or experiencing any religious states of mind during the preceding 6-month period.

Other early studies also point to the importance of religion in the lives of university students. A 1962 study revealed that at entrance to college, about 90% of National Merit Scholarship winners felt a need to believe in a religion (Webster, Freedman, & Heist, 1962). At about the same time, it was noted that about 12% of college students had a critical concern about, or even an acute crisis because of, their religious conflicts (Havens, 1963). And Havighurst and Keating (1971) concluded: "The data indicate most youth are honestly and at times somewhat desperately trying to 'make sense' of their religious beliefs" (p. 714).

But these studies were carried out more than 30 years ago. Have times changed? Some countries have apparently experienced broad-based and substantial decreases in church attendance and religious belief in the last 50 years or so. For example, Bibby (1987, 1993) has estimated that about 6 in 10 Canadians were weekly church attenders in the 1940s. However, this figure dropped steadily until the early 1990s, when the comparable figure was just over 2 in 10 people. This 20% rate has continued to the year 2000 (Bibby, 2001), and is similar for Canada's teens and adults. Furthermore, the tendency toward decreased religious involvement has brought Canada more in line with Britain, France, Germany, the Netherlands, and the Scandinavian countries. Typically, in these European countries less than 10% of the population is involved in the churches (Bibby, 1993, p. 111), and regular attendance is correspondingly low (Campbell & Curtis, 1994). Francis (1989b) noted a progressive trend in the 1970s and 1980s for British adolescents to have less positive attitudes toward Christianity, and a general trend toward decreasing religious belief for British adults continued into the 1990s (Gill, Hadaway, & Marler, 1998). Also, religious involvement is much lower in Australia and Japan than in the United States (Campbell & Curtis, 1994).

This does not mean that young people do not care about the meaning of life. For example, although only 20% of Canadian teenagers are highly involved in religion, 75% of them identify with a religious group, and a similar percentage wonder "often" or "sometimes" about the purpose of life and what happens after death (Bibby, 2001, p. 120).

Figures for the United States suggest that there has *not* been a general disengagement from religion, at least not to the extent that has occurred elsewhere in the developed world. Religious involvement remains relatively high in the United States for both adults and adolescents, unlike the trends for many other Western countries. Some researchers have argued that self-reported church attendance may be substantially inflated, at least in the United States (Chaves & Cavendish, 1994; Hadaway, Marler, & Chaves, 1993; Marcum, 1999). However, other studies involving comparable data sources suggest that, relatively speaking, regular church attendance in the United States tends to be quite high, even when other factors are controlled for (see Campbell & Curtis, 1994). Overall, U.S. attendance rates for adults have remained relatively stable across recent decades (Chaves, 1989, 1991; Firebaugh & Harley, 1991; Inglehart & Baker, 2000), though the interpretation of this stability has been a source of some disagreement (see, e.g., Chaves, 1989, 1990, 1991; Firebaugh & Harley, 1991; Hout & Greeley, 1990). Similarly, belief in an afterlife was high (about 80%) and stable from 1973 to 1991, according to General Social Survey data from the United States (Harley & Firebaugh, 1993).

However, there have been some shifts for adolescents. Smith, Lundquist Denton, Faris, and Regnerus (2002) have provided a broad picture of the religious participation of U.S. adolescents, based on data from three separate major national survey organizations. Longitudinal data indicate that between 1976 and 1996 weekly religious service attendance for twelfth graders decreased by about 8% (from approximately 40% to 32%) and those "never" or "rarely" attending grew by about 4%. Just 44% of twelfth graders report *ever* being involved in religious youth group activities during their four years at high school.

Overall, it seems fair to conclude that "religious beliefs are an important aspect of adolescents' lives" (Cobb, 2001, p. 495) in the United States, and also that religion has a powerful impact on adolescents and their development (Benson et al., 1989). It is not clear why the United States should be a "more religious" society than other advanced industrial democracies (e.g., Inglehart & Baker, 2000). However, it has been suggested (Bibby, 1993; Finke & Stark, 1992) that cultural differences are important, particularly with respect to the role that religious groups have played in U.S. society over time. Perhaps it is the successful tendency for U.S. religious groups to "service the spiritual needs of Americans" (Bibby, 1993, p. 113). Perhaps in the United States disaffiliation is not simply indicative of a shift in religiousness; rather, disaffiliation is also symbolic in an important way, representing "a deep shift in outlook and lifestyles" (Hadaway & Roof, 1988, p. 31).

DOES RELIGIOUS SOCIALIZATION INFLUENCE ADJUSTMENT AND NONRELIGIOUS BEHAVIOR IN ADOLESCENCE?

So far in this chapter, we have examined the development of religion in adolescents' and young adults' lives, and have looked at how religion is a part of those lives. But to what extent does religion affect other aspects of young people's lives? A review of the literature on adolescence and religion led Benson et al. (1989) to conclude that religion has a powerful impact on adolescents and their development, and some research seems to confirm this assessment.

For example, adolescents who say that religion is important in their lives are more likely to do volunteer work in the community than are young people who say that religion is not important (Youniss, McLellan, Su, & Yates, 1999; Youniss, McLellan, & Yates, 1999). Also, it has been suggested that churches may serve a function of initiating youths into volunteer activity, and then sustaining this involvement (Pancer & Pratt, 1999). Some of this volunteering may result from church teachings about helping others and doing good. It is also possible that family religiousness is more generally linked to other group involvement, and that such effects may persist well into adulthood (see Putnam, 2000). For example, one study revealed that medical students' reports of family church involvement were positively associated with the number of group memberships they had some 39 years later (Graves, Wang, Mead, Johnson, & Klag, 1998).

Links have been found between stronger religiousness and decreased delinquent behavior for adolescents (e.g., Johnson, Jang, Larson, & Li, 2001), including lower rates of drug and alcohol use (e.g., Bahr, Maughan, Marcos, & Li, 1998; Corwyn & Benda, 2000; Francis, 1997; Lee, Rice, & Gillespie, 1997; see also Donahue & Benson, 1995) and less deviant behavior in general (Litchfield, Thomas, & Li, 1997). Also, religiousness seems to be associated with delayed onset of sexual activity (e.g., Benda & Corwyn, 1999; Lammers, Ireland, Resnick, & Blum, 2000; Miller et al., 1997; Paul, Fitzjohn, Eberhart-Phillips, Herbison, & Dickson, 2000), and less sexual activity but also less condom use in adolescents (Zaleski & Schiaffino, 2000). Some of these links are explored in greater detail in Chapter 13 on morality. For our purposes here, however, it is important to note that such associations between religiousness and decreased substance use, deviant behavior, and sexuality are relatively common in studies of adolescents and young adults.

Other research has investigated possible links between religion and personal adjustment. For example, Blaine, Trivedi, and Eshleman (1998) concluded that there is "a large research literature that has established that measures of religious commitment, devotion, or belief strength are associated with a range of positive mental health indicators, such as decreased anxiety and depression, and increased self-esteem, tolerance, and self-control" (p. 1040). Others have come to similar conclusions (see Koenig & Larson, 2001; Maton & Wells, 1998; Seybold & Hill, 2001), including some studies that have focused on adolescents (e.g., Moore & Glei, 1995; Wright, Frost, & Wisecarver, 1993), although some authors have pointed out that religion may be associated with maladjustment as well (see Booth, 1991; Ellis, 1986; Shafranske, 1992). This literature is discussed in more detail in Chapters 15 and 16.

Some authors are inclined to conclude that in light of the relevant research, religion must *cause* improved mental health, decreased deviance, more prosocial behavior, and the like, especially during the adolescent years. This is indeed plausible, but one must also consider other causal possibilities. For example, young people who live more moral and mentally healthy lives may be more inclined to attend church, where they may find other like-minded persons who have similar behavioral inclinations. Causality is difficult to study in this area, and possibly as a consequence, few researchers have tackled the issue head-on.

Furthermore, if there are indeed connections between religion and adolescent behavior and adjustment, we might wonder about the processes that could explain such connections. There is no shortage of potential explanations, and many of them rely on the socialization literature. Religion may aid adjustment by providing social support, assisting in value and identity formation, and teaching social control (Wallace & Williams, 1997). Forliti and Benson (1986) have emphasized the importance of value development in early religious socialization. Religious socialization may also teach children and adolescents coping techniques such as praying when anxious, or may show them how to choose alternate activities instead of engaging in delinquency or substance use (see Hunsberger, Pratt, & Pancer, 2001b). Religious training may contribute to a more positive self-concept (Blaine et al., 1998), which in turn may have benefits for adjustment and behavior. These types of suggestions imply that the religious socialization process either directly or indirectly produces the desirable outcomes related to adjustment and behavior.

Two studies were carried out by Hunsberger et al. (2001b) to test this possibility. They compared university students (Study 1) and high school students (Study 2) who were raised in "no religion" with three other groups—those raised in mainline Protestant, conservative Protestant, and Catholic homes—on various adjustment measures. But the students from nonreligious backgrounds did not differ from those from religious backgrounds on any of the main measures (scales assessing depression, self-esteem, dispositional optimism, and social support). Also, these adjustment-related scales were not related to scores on a more general measure of religious socialization (the Religious Emphasis scale). The authors also controlled for other variables that might have complicated the issue, such as family socioeconomic status and students' current religiosity, but this did not change the results.

These studies leave us scratching our heads a bit. Of course, other measures, or students from different geographical locations or of different ages, or the like, might have drawn out differences where Hunsberger et al. (2001b) found none. Or possibly religion's socialization impact is too subtle or complex for these rather broad investigations to detect. The researchers pointed out that most studies on related issues focus on degree of religiosity or extent of specific religious orientation, and that people with no religious background might either be excluded from such research or simply lumped in with weakly religious people. They recommended that more attention be devoted to the specifically nonreligious and those raised in nonreligious environments.

There is a need for researchers to refocus their efforts in this area. There is no shortage of studies of adolescents and young adults that reveal correlations between religiousness variables and (decreased) destructive behaviors such as substance use, as well as improved personal adjustment. We now need investigations of the mechanisms and underlying causal patterns that generate such correlations.

RELIGIOUS THINKING AND REASONING IN ADOLESCENCE AND YOUNG ADULTHOOD

Religious socialization processes clearly involve powerful influences during childhood and adolescence. In the past, these factors were characterized as affecting beliefs and practices, but little attention was devoted to the possibility that they might also alter *styles* of thinking about religion. In terms of Ozorak's (1989) social-cognitive model of religious development in adolescence, previous research has emphasized social aspects. Here we focus on cognitive change. It seems plausible that when individuals are being taught (directly and indirectly) about religion, they may be learning much more than simply what to believe and how to practice their faith. They may also be learning unique ways of thinking about religion and even about nonreligious issues.

As we have seen in Chapter 4, a developmental shift in thinking about religious (and other) issues occurs as young people move from childhood to adolescence. In Piagetian terms, this shift is from concrete to formal operations, which (especially for religious concepts) involves a move away from the literal toward more abstract thinking. It has also been suggested that this trend toward abstract religious thought may be linked with decreased religiousness, and possibly with a tendency to reject religion in adolescence. Possibly adolescents' emerging abstract thinking capability "complicates" their religious thought, and may even stimulate new styles of thinking in order to deal with "difficult-to-explain" religious concepts and existential issues.

Reich's Complementarity Reasoning

Reich (1991) has pointed out that there are "many perceived contradictions and paradoxes that characterize religious life" (pp. 87–88; see also Reich, 1989, 1992, 1994). He has suggested that "complementarity reasoning" may develop in order to deal with such religious contradictions. That is, people may develop rational explanations for specific perceived contradictions, which make the contradictions seem more apparent than real. Reich gives the example of a 20-year-old who attempted to explain the seeming conflict between creationist and evolutionary explanations of humans' origins and development as a species: "The possibility of evolution was contained in God's 'kick-off' at the origin . . . but God probably did not interfere with evolution itself . . . and perhaps so far not all of the initial potential has yet come to fruition" (Reich, 1991, p. 78). Reich has suggested that complementarity reasoning is crucial to religious development, though it does not emerge in fully developed form until relatively late in life, and sometimes not at all.

Reich proposes that five different levels of complementarity reasoning appear in developmental sequence. Essentially, these levels evolve from a very simplified (true–false) resolution of different explanations, through careful consideration of various competing explanations, to possible links between competing explanations and possibly even the use of an overarching theory or synopsis to assess complex relationships among the different factors. This analysis bears some resemblance to the "integrative complexity" analysis of religious and other thinking (see below), and the complexity approach has the advantage of an established scoring system tapping different levels of thinking. Possible links between religious orientation and complexity of thinking processes have been investigated in several studies of university students.

Integrative Complexity of Thought

Defining and Scoring Complexity

"Integrative complexity" is defined by two cognitive stylistic variables. "Differentiation" involves the acknowledgment and tolerance of different perspectives or dimensions of an issue, and "integration" deals with the extent to which differentiated perspectives or dimensions are linked. A manual for scoring integrative complexity (Baker-Brown et al., 1992) describes how such complexity is typically scored on a 1–7 scale. Lower scores indicate a person's tendency not to reveal (1) or reveal (3) differentiation; higher scores (4–7) indicate the extent to which people integrate these differentiated concepts into broader structures. Research Box 5.3 gives examples of responses receiving different complexity scores.

Are Religion and Complexity of Thought Related?

Batson and Raynor-Prince (1983) found that a measure of religious orthodoxy was significantly negatively correlated (–.37) with the integrative complexity of sentence completions dealing with existential[3] religious issues (e.g., "When I consider my own death . . ."). That is, people with a more orthodox religious orientation tended to think more simply about existential religious issues, as indicated by the sentence completion task. Also, the Quest religious orientation was significantly positively correlated (.43) with complexity scores for thinking

---

ঽ▲

Research Box 5.3. Religious Fundamentalism and Complexity of Religious Doubts (Hunsberger, Alisat, Pancer, & Pratt, 1996)

This interview study of university students provided examples of the integrative complexity anchor scores for content dealing with religious doubts. Students were asked questions about their religious doubts, and their responses were then scored for complexity of thought.

One question asked, "What would you say is the most serious doubt about religion or religious beliefs that you have had in the last few years?" The following response received a score of 1 (no differentiation), since it reveals just one dimension of religious doubt: "My only real doubt is why God could allow people to suffer so much in this world" (p. 207). Full differentiation (a score of 3) is illustrated by the following response, which outlines two different dimensions of doubt: "I have doubted why God allowed me to become seriously ill a few years ago. What was His purpose? Also, I could never understand why there is war and famine in the world if there is a God" (p. 207).

An example of a response showing integration of differentiated doubts (score of 5) is as follows:

> Over the years I have had various "little doubts." For example, I was bothered by the hypocrisy of some "religious" people, and the Bible seemed to not be very relevant to a lot of things happening today. After a while I sort of sat down and put all of these little things together and realized that in combination they made me doubt organized religion in general. (p. 207)

Scores of 7 are rare in this type of research, and no such score was found in this study. Scores of 2, 4, and 6 represent transition points between the odd-numbered anchor scores.

Results revealed a weak but significant correlation between the extent of one's religious doubts and the integrative complexity of thinking about those doubts. This finding is consistent with previous conclusions that complexity–religion relationships are restricted to domains involving existential religious content (Hunsberger, Pratt, & Pancer, 1994).

about existential content. For both orthodoxy and quest, comparable correlations involving *non*religious sentence completions were not statistically significant.

In a series of investigations, Hunsberger and his colleagues further specified the relationship between religious orientation and complexity of thinking about religious and nonreligious issues (Hunsberger, Pratt, & Pancer, 1994; Hunsberger, Alisat, et al., 1996; Hunsberger, Lea, Pancer, Pratt, & McKenzie, 1992; Hunsberger, McKenzie, Pratt, & Pancer, 1993; Pancer, Jackson, Hunsberger, Pratt, & Lea, 1995; Pratt, Hunsberger, Pancer, & Roth, 1992). They had their participants write brief essays on issues, or interviewed people to allow them to give full expression to their ideas. Although at first glance there appears to be some inconsistency in the findings of the various related studies, Hunsberger et al. (1994) reviewed the relevant investigations and concluded that

> religiosity does not seem to have a general (negative) relationship with integrative complexity across various domains. Rather, such relationships are restricted to content dealing with existential issues. . . . Further, religious fundamentalism and orthodoxy measures are apparently equally predictive of integrative complexity. (p. 345)

These authors also concluded that the unique relationship found between religious orientation and integrative complexity of thought about *existential* material adds substance to previous work suggesting that dealing with (or avoiding) existential questions does indeed have important implications for religion (see Batson et al., 1993; Altemeyer & Hunsberger, 1982). However, although we have apparently begun to fit together the jigsaw puzzle of how thought processes and religiousness may be linked, the issue of *why* the complexity–religion relationship is restricted to existential content must be left to future research.

Most of the research cited above involved adolescent and young adult populations, but it seems reasonable to expect that the obtained relationship between religious orientation or beliefs and the complexity of adolescent thought about existential issues would hold for adult samples as well. To date, there have been few investigations of this possibility for people in middle or older adulthood. The findings of one study (Pratt et al., 1992), involving integrative complexity in middle and older adults, are consistent with our speculation here. In a different context, somewhat similar findings were obtained by van der Lans (1991), who concluded that adults who were inclined to a literal interpretation of religious material also "gave evidence of a low developed structure of religious judgment" (p. 107).

Of course, the observed relationships between religiousness and complexity of thinking about existential religious issues are correlational, and one must be cautious in speculating about cause and effect. Thus, although our preferred interpretation is that the religious socialization process contributes to differential thought processes in dealing with existential content, other interpretations are possible.

There has also been interest in self-complexity theory (Linville, 1985) as it relates to religion. Self-complexity analyses focus on the various roles, activities, or other aspects of the self that are used in a self-description. Using this approach, Nielsen and Fultz (1997) found greater self-complexity in the religious domain when religion was important to people, and self-complexity was positively correlated with both Intrinsic and Quest scores. This might seem to conflict with Batson and Raynor-Prince's (1983) finding of a negative relationship

---

3. The term "existential" is defined by Batson et al. (1993) as involving "questions that confront us because we are aware that we and others like us are alive and that we will die" (p. 8).

between complexity and Intrinsic scores. However, as Nielsen and Fultz (1997) have pointed out, we must be careful not to confuse self-complexity and integrative complexity of thought; they are quite different, both conceptually and in their operationalization.

RELIGIOUS DOUBTS

Clearly, not all individuals simply copy their parents when it comes to religion. If the socialization process is as efficient as outlined previously in this chapter, how do people who grow up in religious families come to change their religious beliefs, or to reject religion entirely? Here we consider the origins, characteristics, and effects of religious doubting. In the subsequent section, we consider the factors involved in apostasy (i.e., abandoning one's religion entirely).

Of course, people are not completely passive recipients of social influence when it comes to the religious socialization process. They think about religious issues, and they may not be willing to accept all that they are taught. Almost everyone has questions related to religious teachings at some time. Questions may range from the relatively inconsequential (e.g., "Why does my minister insist that there be a long Bible reading to begin each worship service?") to the important (e.g., "Does God really exist?", "Should I abandon my religious faith?"). Many people apparently resolve their questions to their own satisfaction, and their underlying religious beliefs are not substantially altered. Others, however, may not resolve their questions so easily, and their questions may grow into serious doubts and concerns about religious beliefs. These doubts may eventually lead them to abandon some or all of their beliefs. Let us examine this process in greater detail.

Questions and doubts about religion seem especially common in adolescence. Nipkow and Schweitzer (1991) analyzed 16- to 21-year-old German students' written reflections about God, and concluded that most of their respondents had "challenging questions" about God. These primarily involved unfulfilled expectations of God; whether or not the students continued to believe in God was determined by the extent to which their expectations were fulfilled. Similarly, Tamminen (1991, 1994) noted an increase in early adolescence in doubts about God's existence and whether prayers were answered, among his Finnish students. Few psychological investigators ask about the religious questions and doubts of middle-aged and older adults, so until we have better comparative data, we should not conclude that such doubts are less prevalent in adulthood than in adolescence.[4]

Doubt: "Good or Bad"?

The personal tension, distress, and conflict implied by religious doubt were noted by numerous early authors (e.g., Allport, 1950; Clark, 1958; Pratt, 1920). Pratt (1920) further claimed that "The great cause for adolescent doubt is the inner discord aroused by some newly discovered fact which fails to harmonize with beliefs previously accepted and revered" (p. 116). Possibly because of the "distress" that sometimes accompanies doubt, but also because doubt has usually been perceived as antireligious, religious doubt has traditionally been considered

---

4. Bob Altemeyer (personal communication, October 31, 1995) gathered some unpublished data that support our conjecture. On a 20-item scale assessing religious doubts, 163 parents of university students reported doubt levels ($M = 39.4$) almost identical to those of over 1,000 students ($M = 41.8$).

"bad." "The official church attitude is that it is to be deplored as an obstacle to faith, at the worst a temptation of the Devil, at the best a sign of weakness" (Clark, 1958, p. 138). In this vein, Helfaer (1972) equated religious doubt with suffering, pain, and maladjustment, claiming that "religious doubt is in fact an example of the lack . . . of an integrated wholeness within the ego" (p. 10).

There is some empirical support for this stance, at least in terms of personal adjustment. An investigation of students making the transition to university revealed that the extent to which students reported doubting religious teachings was related to several adjustment variables (Hunsberger, Pancer, Pratt, & Alisat, 1996). Doubting was positively related to measures of stress, depression, and daily hassles, and negatively related to self-esteem, good relationships with parents, optimism, and adjustment to university life. These relationships were typically weak (ranging from .10 to .24) but statistically significant. A Religious Fundamentalism measure was significantly related (positively) to just one of these measures (optimism). Thus there seemed to be something unique about religious doubting that was weakly but consistently associated with poorer adjustment in first-year university students.

However, Batson's conceptualization of the Quest religious orientation (Batson & Schoenrade, 1991a, 1991b; Batson et al., 1993) as an open-ended, questioning approach to religion has cast religious doubting in a somewhat more positive light. Perception of doubt as positive is seen as one of three core characteristics of the Quest orientation, the others being complexity and openness to change (Batson & Schoenrade, 1991b). Furthermore, the Quest orientation is linked with some characteristics that many people feel should be encouraged, such as greater openness, lower prejudice, a tendency to help others in need, and some aspects of mental health (see Batson et al., 1993). Therefore, judgments about religious doubts' being "good or bad" depend on how one defines these terms, and probably also on one's personal religious orientation.

Doubts: Independent or a "Syndrome"?

Hunsberger et al. (1993) reported three studies in which they investigated the kinds of religious doubts that people have. The researchers suggested that previous authors had tended to characterize doubt as involving unique events or situations. That is, one person might doubt the existence of God because of certain educational influences; someone else might doubt the validity of religious teachings because of the despicable behavior of a previously respected religious person. However, Hunsberger et al. (1993) concluded that a series of doubts, having different sources, could often be found in the same people.

Initially, they categorized different kinds of doubting by building on Allport's (1950) and Clark's (1958) analyses of religious doubting as follows:

1. *Reactive and negativistic doubt.* There is a general reaction against religion, with anything religious being viewed negatively.

2. *Violation of self-interest.* Self-centered expectations have not been fulfilled (e.g., unanswered prayer).

3. *Shortcomings of organized religion.* The person questions such things as wars fought in God's name, commercialism, hypocrisy, dubious morality of some religious persons.

4. *God as a projection.* The person feels that God does not exist in reality and must be a "projection," since God's image changes across time and cultures.

5. *Religion as self-deception.* Religion is seen as fooling people—for example, serving merely to ease their fears and anxieties.

6. *Scientific doubt.* The person feels a need to verify statements before accepting them (a religion–science conflict).

7. *Ritual doubt.* This category involves questioning based on the apparent ineffectiveness of some religious rites (e.g., failure of faith healing in curing someone may lead to doubts about God's ability to cure people).

These categories were not intended to be exhaustive, but rather to represent a starting point for the investigation of religious doubting. Subsequent investigation of university students suggested that more orthodox religious persons reported lower absolute levels of religious doubting, and that doubting was associated with "apostasy, decreased church attendance, less agreement with religious teachings, and less family emphasis on religion" (Hunsberger et al., 1993, p. 431). That is, religious doubting seemed to be characteristic of disengagement from religion (see also Brinkerhoff & Mackie, 1993), rather than being an integral part of ongoing faith, as claimed by some (Allport, 1950; Tillich, 1957). Furthermore, varieties of doubting were moderately intercorrelated, leading to the conclusion that doubting typically did not involve just one or more independent doubts. Rather, Hunsberger et al. (1993) suggested that doubts "tended to 'hang together' quite reliably in a general 'doubt syndrome'" (p. 47). Finally, there was a correlation between integrative complexity of thinking about religious doubts on the one hand, and the extent of religious doubting on the other; this correlation suggests some relationship between ways of thinking about religious doubts, and the content and extent of those doubts.

Levels and Correlates of Doubt

The mass media's depiction of young people as rebellious and questioning of parental values might suggest that adolescents are boiling cauldrons of bubbling religious doubts. The evidence does not support this picture. Canadian studies of nearly 2,000 university students (Altemeyer & Hunsberger, 1997) and almost 1,000 high school students (Hunsberger, Pratt, & Pancer, 2002) revealed that average self-reported religious doubts were about 2 (a "mild amount" of doubt) on a 0–6 response scale. The greatest doubts in both studies were linked to (1) the perception that religion is associated with intolerance; (2) unappreciated pressure tactics of religions; and (3) other ways that religion seemed to be associated with negative human qualities, rather than making people "better." But even for these issues, the average doubt was less than 3 (a "moderate amount") on the 0–6 scale used. This mild to moderate level of doubt is not surprising, in light of evidence that adolescents' "reasoning is systematically biased to protect and promote their preexisting [religious] beliefs" (Klaczynski & Gordon, 1996, p. 317).

Is religious doubt unique to adolescents and young adults? One study did reveal a slight decline with age in scores on Batson's Quest measure ($r = -.19$), suggesting a decreased tendency among older adults to doubt, insofar as the Quest scale taps doubting (Watson, Howard, Hood, & Morris, 1988). However, we should be careful not to conclude that doubt is virtually nonexistent among older adults, as mentioned previously. For example, Nielsen (1998) reported that about two-thirds of his adult sample provided written descriptions of "religious conflict" in their lives, although it is not clear how many of these descriptions would be classified as religious doubts.

Also, although absolute levels of doubting tend to be mild to moderate, religious doubt-ing is apparently related to religious, personal, and social variables. Quite consistently, higher levels of doubt have been moderately to strongly associated with reduced religiousness, such as lower Christian orthodoxy (Altemeyer, 1988; Hunsberger, Alisat, et al., 1996; Hunsberger et al., 1993); with lower religious fundamentalism and less religious emphasis in the family home, and less acceptance of religious teachings (Hunsberger, Alisat, et al., 1996); and with lower Intrinsic religion scores and an inclination toward apostasy (Hunsberger et al., 1993). Moreover, religious doubting has been linked with such personality characteristics as greater openness to experience (Shermer, 2000), lower right-wing authoritarianism (Altemeyer, 1988; Hunsberger et al., 1993), and less dogmatism (Hunsberger, Alisat, et al., 1996). Finally, it has been associated with some aspects of social activism (Begue, 2000), increased complexity of thought about religious issues (Hunsberger et al., 1993), and some aspects of ego identity development (Hunsberger, Pratt, & Pancer, 2001a) as discussed later in this chapter.

Doubt and Personal Adjustment

Research has also suggested that religious doubting is related to personal adjustment. As noted earlier, doubts were weakly but significantly positively related to perceived stress, depression, and self-reported life hassles for college students, and significantly negatively related to ad-justment to college and relationships with parents, during students' first year in college (Hunsberger, Alisat, et al., 1996). Similarly, religious doubting has been associated with more psychological distress and decreased feelings of personal well-being in adult Presbyterians (Krause, Ingersoll-Dayton, Ellison, & Wulff, 1999). Krause et al. concluded that younger adults have greater difficulty with religious doubt than do older persons, since the associa-tion between doubt and depression scores was strongest at age 20 and decreased as age in-creased. These findings seem to support claims that religious doubt has negative implications for personal mental health, as suggested by earlier writers on the subject (e.g., Allport, 1950; Clark, 1958; Helfaer, 1972; Pratt, 1920), although supportive findings have not always been clear-cut (Kooistra & Pargament, 1999).

Why would religious doubting be associated with negative personal consequences? Sev-eral possibilities have been advanced (see Hunsberger et al., 2002; Krause et al., 1999). It has been claimed that there are positive mental health and adjustment benefits that derive from religiousness, possibly through coping mechanisms that are associated with religion (e.g., prayer, religious social support; Pargament, 1997). Because doubt is associated with decreased religious faith, it may be that the resulting decreased religiousness detracts from one's cop-ing ability, resulting in a less well-adjusted life. Also, doubt may be associated with feelings of shame or guilt, which in turn may adversely affect self-esteem (Krause et al., 1999). Doubt itself may be seen as a particular manifestation of Festinger's (1957) cognitive dissonance, and such dissonance is sometimes associated with psychological distress and negative affect (e.g., Burris, Harmon-Jones, & Tarpley, 1997).

Furthermore, Kooistra and Pargament (1999) found some (mixed) evidence that doubt-ing may be linked to conflictual family patterns. They suggested that this might result from the general negative consequences that family difficulties seem to have for children's and adolescents' religiousness, such as negative God images, alienation from and negative feel-ings about religion, and decreased religiousness. However, Kooistra and Pargament studied only parochial high school students in the U.S. midwest, and doubt was associated with conflictual families only for students at a Dutch Reformed school, not those at a Catholic school. Hunsberger et al. (2001a) were unable to replicate this difference between fundamentalist and Catholic students in Canada; rather, when they broke their findings down by major denominational groupings, relationships between doubt and poorer adjustment occurred only for mainstream Protestants.

Doubting may also have some positive associations. As noted earlier, religious doubting is an important component in the conceptualization of the Quest religious orientation (Batson et al., 1993), which has been linked with less prejudice, a tendency to help others in need, and some aspects of mental health (e.g., personal competence/control, self-acceptance, and open-mindedness/flexibility). Furthermore, Krause et al. (1999) have pointed out that doubt may be an important part of positive psychological development; this suggestion is consistent with research showing that doubt and uncertainty more generally might stimulate cognitive development (e.g., Acredolo & O'Connor, 1991).

Dealing with Doubt

Hunsberger et al. (2002) investigated ways in which young people attempt to deal with their religious questions and doubts, using two scales developed by Altemeyer and Hunsberger (1997). First, a 6-item Belief-Confirming Consultation (BCC) scale measured the extent to which their senior high school students consulted people and resources that were likely to push them in a proreligious direction (e.g., talking with one's parents, reading religious publications). Second, a 6-item Belief-Threatening Consultation (BTC) scale assessed the extent to which people consulted resources that would be more likely to give them nonreligious or antireligious answers to their questions (e.g., talking with friends with no religious beliefs, reading materials that go against one's religious beliefs). BCC scores significantly predicted increased religiousness 2 years later, beyond the variance accounted for by BCC scores in the original questionnaire and by the amount of doubt reported originally. Similarly, BTC scores significantly predicted reduced religiousness 2 years later. That is, people's inclination to seek "belief-confirming" or "belief-threatening" sources of information in dealing with doubts successfully predicted religiousness 2 years later.

Also, Hunsberger, Alisat, et al. (1996) found qualitative differences with respect to the nature of doubting, for respondents who were high and low in religious fundamentalism. "High fundamentalists" did not typically doubt God or religion per se; rather, their doubts were focused on others' failure to live up to religious ideals, or relatively minor adjustments that they felt should be made within the church (e.g., improving the role of women in the church). "Low fundamentalists," on the other hand, were more likely to be concerned about the underpinnings of religion, such as the existence of God, the lack of proof for religious claims, or the unbelievability of the creation account of human origins. Again, there was some evidence that people who reported more religious doubts tended to think more complexly about such doubts, and about existential material more generally. The results of this study suggested that

> high and low fundamentalists may actually perceive and deal with their own (and others') religious experiences in different ways. Our findings seem consistent with the possibility that religious cognitive processing is convergent among high fundamentalists, tending to confirm and reinforce religious teachings. Any divergence (e.g., active questioning of God or religion) seems to be resolved by interpreting information as consistent with one's beliefs, or at least by accepting the religious explanation for the doubt or concern. Low fundamentalists, on the other hand,

seem to respond to divergent thinking (i.e., critical questioning and considering alternatives to their beliefs) by changing their religious beliefs. . . . Overall, a picture emerges of low fundamentalists and high doubters as being more complex and critical processors of information related to religion. (Hunsberger, Alisat, et al., 1996, p. 218)

Little empirical work has been done to extend these findings, though it is important that we further clarify the nature of doubt and factors affecting it. There does seem to be a link between religious doubting and apostasy or religious defection, though it is possible that this link is moderated by other factors, such as developmental level or cognitive stage.

Secret Doubts

Altemeyer (1988) developed a "secret survey" technique that assures anonymity, allows people to respond in very private circumstances chosen by themselves, and encourages respondents to be especially truthful about themselves in a way analogous to the "hidden observer" technique used by Hilgard (1973, 1986) in studying hypnosis (see Research Box 5.4). Using this approach, Altemeyer was surprised to find that about one-third of his participants who were high in right-wing authoritarianism admitted that they had *secret* doubts about God's existence—doubts that they had *never* shared with anyone else. This suggests that many routine studies of doubting may not be tapping actual levels of doubt, but only what people are willing to admit to others.

We need more investigations of the frequency, nature, and implications of religious doubting, but we also need to be sensitive to the possible "secret" nature of some people's doubts. At least in some cases, doubt seems to be a precursor to abandoning one's religion. We turn next to an examination of this disengagement process, which is most likely to occur during late adolescence.

APOSTASY

Caplovitz and Sherrow (1977) concluded that apostasy (abandonment of one's religious faith) could be caused by secularization, alienation/rebellion, and/or commitment to the modern values of universalism/achievement. They proposed that four "germs" somehow infect young people, and that these germs predispose their "hosts" to become apostates. The germs were said to be (1) poor parental relations, (2) symptoms of maladjustment or neurosis, (3) a radical or leftist political orientation, and (4) commitment to intellectualism. Underlying all of these processes was the apparent assumption that apostasy represents a deliberate rejection of previous identification, and a conscious acceptance of a new identification. In fact, Caplovitz and Sherrow (1977) concluded that apostasy represents rebellion against parents and other aspects of society, as a result of familial strain. This thesis that apostasy results from adolescent rebellion against parents has also been suggested by other researchers (e.g., Putney & Middleton, 1961; Wuthnow & Glock, 1973).

The Caplovitz and Sherrow (1977) work has been criticized on theoretical, methodological, and data-interpretational grounds (see Hunsberger, 1980). Earlier findings (e.g., Johnson, 1973; Hunsberger, 1976) had suggested that religious socialization tends to follow a "straight line," such that lower levels of religiousness are related to lower levels of emphasis on reli-

---

Research Box 5.4. Religion and Right-Wing Authoritarianism (Altemeyer, 1988)

Altemeyer's book reports an extensive program of research on right-wing authoritarianism (RWA). Our interest here is in some aspects of the research involving religion. Altemeyer was intrigued by the fact that believing in an almighty God is a cornerstone of the belief system of high-RWA people. He suspected that doubts about God's existence probably arise for those high in RWA as they do for others, but that possibly because of the strong anxiety that these doubts arouse, high-RWA people do not acknowledge them. But if doubts do exist in the mind of a "true believer," how can we possibly discover them when the person involved does not want to admit to them?

Altemeyer decided to probe these doubts by using a variation of Hilgard's (1973, 1986) "hidden observer" research on hypnosis. Hilgard had found that even people who endure pain without seemingly noticing it while under hypnosis will admit that they did feel pain when they are cued to allow a sort of "inner self" to discuss these experiences. This supposedly involves a part of the person that knows things that are not available to the person's consciousness.

So Altemeyer gave some students the following instructions in a survey study, after they had heard about Hilgard's research in their previous introductory psychology classes:

> You may recall the lecture on hypnosis dealing with Hilgard's research on the "Hidden Observer." Suppose there is a Hidden Observer in you, which knows your every thought and deed, but which only speaks when it is safe to do so, and when directly spoken to. This question is for your Hidden Observer: Does this person (that is, you) have doubts that (s)he was created by an Almighty God who will judge each person and take some into heaven for eternity while casting others into hell forever? (pp. 152–153)

Five alternatives followed, allowing respondents to indicate the type and extent of secret doubts they had experienced. About half of the high-RWA students in this study indicated that they had *no* doubts about God's existence. But, remarkably, about one-third of these students said that they did have *secret* doubts, which they had never shared with anyone else.

We cannot be sure that Altemeyer's participants were being truthful about their hidden religious doubts; however, this investigation raises important questions about the meaning of responses in survey research. It also suggests that creativity may be required to tap into very personal information about such topics as religious doubting.

---

gion in the childhood home. That is, apostasy seems to represent *consistency* with a lack of parental emphasis on religion, rather than rebellion against parents and society, as characterized by Caplovitz and Sherrow.

This consistency may exist in spite of seemingly contradictory findings. One study reported that some people prefer to describe the development of their religious beliefs in terms of rejection of, rather than acceptance of, a belief system (Scobie, 1999); another found that a history of religious rigidity is linked with disaffiliation from the parental religion (Hansen, 1998). However, this does not necessarily tell us anything about rebellion against parents or society. That is, rejection of beliefs might or might not be accompanied by more general rebellion.

Three studies of university students, described in Research Box 5.5, were carried out to investigate this issue (Hunsberger, 1980, 1983a; Hunsberger & Brown, 1984). These investigations, from two different corners of the world, were consistent in finding that apostasy is most strongly associated with weak emphasis on religion in the home. Although this work involved Canadian and Australian university students, the essential findings have been replicated elsewhere in studies of Mormons (Albrecht, Cornwall, & Cunningham, 1988; Bahr & Albrecht, 1989) and Roman Catholics (Kotre, 1971), as well as in studies of more representative U.S. samples (Nelsen, 1981c; Wuthnow & Mellinger, 1978).

In Hunsberger's studies, no support was found for two of Caplovitz and Sherrow's hypothesized predisposing "germs"—symptoms of maladjustment, and a radical or leftist political orientation. In a study of more than 600 U.S. and Canadian college students, Brinkerhoff and Mackie (1993) found that apostates reported being less happy in their lives than did "converts" (people who grew up with no religious affiliation but who now identified with a religious group), "religious stalwarts" (people who maintained the same denominational affiliation from childhood to young adulthood), and "denominational switchers" (people who had changed denominational affiliation since childhood). However, apostates typically did not differ significantly from these other groups on measures of self-esteem or life satisfaction.[5] Although Brinkerhoff and Mackie (1993) concluded that apostates "are less satisfied in life, less happy and have lower self-esteem" (p. 252), the statistical evidence supports this conclusion only for the general happiness item mentioned above. Apostates did report a more liberal world view, in the sense that they were "less traditional" than the stalwarts.

Also, Hunsberger found weak evidence that apostates have poorer relationships with their parents; he suggested that the poorer relationships could be *either* a cause or a result of apostasy. However, others have argued that their data suggest that poor relationships with parents are more likely to precede disengagement from religion (Burris, Jackson, Tarpley, & Smith, 1996; Wilson & Sherkat, 1994). Therefore, it may be that such poor relationships contribute to disengagement, rather than vice versa. In a similar vein, there is some evidence that parental divorce (and possibly the accompanying poor family relationships) may make offspring more inclined to change religious identity or to leave religion altogether (Lawton & Bures, 2001).

One might wonder how apostates would respond if asked directly about the reasons for their disengagement. A large survey of Australian adults (Hughes, Bellamy, Black, & Kaldor, 2000) asked respondents to rate the impact of 17 factors that might discourage them from attending church. The top 5 choices of nonattenders (not necessarily apostates) were boring church services (42% indicated that this discouraged attendance), church beliefs (41%), "no need to go to church" (38%), church moral views (37%), and "prefer to do other things" (37%). In addition to the fact that there was no direct measure of apostasy, these participants were not asked about emphasis on religion in childhood, maladjustment, or intellectualism. Therefore, it is difficult to compare Hughes et al.'s (2000) findings with the literature on apostasy.

---

5. The only pairwise comparison between apostates and each of the other three groupings that was statistically significant for either the life satisfaction or self-esteem measures indicated that apostates were lower in life satisfaction than were denominational switchers.

&⬥

Research Box 5.5. Three Studies of the Antecedents and Correlates of Apostasy (Hunsberger, 1980, 1983a; Hunsberger & Brown, 1984)

In the first of his three investigations, Hunsberger screened about 600 Canadian introductory psychology students. He found 51 apostates (students who were raised in a religious denomination, but who currently were not affiliated with any denomination) who could be paired with 51 "matched controls" (people who came from the same religious background, and who were the same sex, approximate age, and year in university, but who continued to identify with the family religion). As one would expect, apostates obtained significantly "less religious" scores on a series of measures, including frequency of church attendance and prayer, and belief in God. But the two groups did not differ on a number of nonreligious measures, such as self-reports of parental acceptance, personal happiness and adjustment, and grade point average (contrary to what Caplovitz & Sherrow, 1977, would apparently have predicted). There was some tendency for apostates to report poorer relationships with their parents. Emphasis placed on religion in the childhood home significantly predicted apostate versus matched control status, but factors related to parental relationships and rebellion did *not* add to the explained variance in a factor analysis and subsequent multiple-regression analysis.

These findings were essentially replicated in a second study of 78 Canadian apostates and their matched controls, identified from a group of introductory psychology students. Again, the religious socialization process was the most important influence in determining apostate versus nonapostate status, with apostates reporting considerably less emphasis on religion in the childhood home than did their matched controls. The findings from these two studies of apostasy were interpreted as being consistent with social learning theory, such that increased parental modeling and teaching of religion were associated with increased acceptance of the family religion. Factors that did *not* seem to predict apostasy included political orientation, intellectualism, academic orientation, adjustment/happiness in life, scores on Minnesota Multiphasic Personality Inventory (MMPI) subscales, and general rebellion against parents. There was a weak tendency for poor relationships with parents to be associated with apostasy, but Hunsberger suggested that this could be a result rather than a cause of apostasy.

The third study in this series involved more than 800 Australian university students, for whom the apostasy rate (36%) was higher than in the Canadian studies (10–20%). This investigation confirmed the tendency for apostates to obtain much "less religious" scores on various measures, and to report considerably less emphasis on religion in the childhood home. However, these apostates also reported that they had a more intellectual orientation in their lives, consistent with Caplovitz and Sherrow's prediction.

In the end, these three studies all revealed that apostasy was most strongly related to weak emphasis on religion in the home. Caplovitz and Sherrow's claim that symptoms of maladjustment and a radical or leftist political orientation are related to apostasy was not supported. Nor was there any indication that apostasy represents rebellion against parents and society. Weak support was found for two other "germs" suggested by Caplovitz and Sherrow (poor relationships with parents and an intellectual orientation), though these were clearly weaker predictors of apostasy than was emphasis on religion in the childhood home.

How to Raise an Apostate

It would seem that if parents want their children to abandon the family religion, they can best encourage this by generally ignoring religion, or at least by communicating (through teaching or through example) that religion is unimportant. Recent research has confirmed the centrality of home influences in young people's decision to remain committed to the family faith or to abandon the home religion (e.g., Dudley, 1999). This is just what a socialization explanation of religious development would predict: Homes that emphasize the importance of religion and model religious behavior will generally produce children who remain religious later in their lives, whereas homes that pay little attention to faith and that model nonreligious behavior will generally produce children who pay no more attention to religion than their parents did. The concept of "drift" has sometimes been used to describe the tendency for apostates to have been only marginally involved with a religious denomination before defection (see Bahr & Albrecht, 1989).

This is not to deny the involvement of cognitive factors. Hunsberger and Brown's (1984) Australian study suggested that people who say they have an intellectual approach to life, enjoy debating or arguing with others about religious issues, and so on are more likely to be apostates. And, as discussed in the section on religious doubts, apostasy has been associated with questioning and doubting religious teachings. For example, Brinkerhoff and Mackie (1993) found that apostates reported more and earlier religious doubts in their lives than did nonapostates.

When does apostasy typically occur? Broad-based survey studies suggest that disengagement from religion is most common for people in their late teens and early twenties. For example, it has been estimated that about two-thirds of all dropping out among Catholics occurs between the ages of 16 and 25 (Hoge, with McGuire & Stratman, 1981)—essentially the same peak "dropping-out" years reported for Mormons (Albrecht et al., 1988), Presbyterians (Hoge, Johnson, & Liudens, 1993), and broader religious groupings (Albrecht & Cornwall, 1989; Caplovitz & Sherrow, 1977; Hadaway & Roof, 1988; see also Schweitzer, 2000).

Types of Apostasy

Some authors have attempted to define types of apostates, though the resulting groupings tend to focus on social and other characteristics of apostates (and some other disaffiliated individuals) rather than the underlying apostasy process itself. For example, Hadaway (1989) used cluster analysis to derive five characteristic groups of apostates: (1) "successful swinging singles" (single young people who apparently were experiencing social and financial success); (2) "sidetracked singles" (single people who tended to be pessimistic and had not obtained the benefits of the "good life"); (3) "young settled liberals" (those who were dissatisfied with traditional values but who had a very positive outlook on life); (4) "young libertarians" (people who rejected religious labels more than religious beliefs); and (5) "irreligious traditionalists" (somewhat older, conservative, married people who maintained some religious moral traditions in spite of their nonattendance and nonaffiliation).

Others have offered different typologies (Bahr & Albrecht, 1989; Brinkerhoff & Burke, 1980; Condran & Tamney, 1985; Hadaway & Roof, 1988; Hoge et al., 1981; Perry, Davis,

Doyle, & Dyble, 1980; Roozen, 1980). But no generally accepted categorization has appeared. These studies do indicate that we should not assume that apostates constitute a homogeneous group. The social characteristics of apostates may vary considerably, and the underlying processes of disengagement are not uniform.

Problems in Definition and Measurement

Caution is necessary when one is comparing the results of different investigations of apostasy. The terminology used to describe disengagement from religion varies considerably from study to study, involving such terms as "dropping out," "exiting," "disidentification," "leave taking," "defecting," "apostasy," "disaffiliation," and "disengagement" (Bromley, 1988). Furthermore, operational definitions of these terms have varied from one study to the next. Some authors (e.g., Caplovitz & Sherrow, 1977; Hunsberger, 1980, 1983a) have studied people who say they grew up with a religious identification or family religious background, but who no longer identify with any religious group. Others have focused on cessation of church attendance for a specified period of time (e.g., Hoge, 1981, 1988); have incorporated elements of loss of faith, as well as disidentification (Altemeyer & Hunsberger, 1997); or have focused on aspects of the organizational structure of the religious group a person is leaving (Bromley, 1998).

Such differences could potentially lead to divergent findings. It is important in relevant investigations to be clear about the criteria used to define apostasy operationally, and also to be sensitive to how this definition will affect the findings. For example, it has been estimated that in the United States, about 46% of people discontinue church participation at some point in their lives (Roozen, 1980). Whether this estimate is accurate or not, there are many reasons for cessation of church attendance that do not necessarily involve loss of personal faith (Albrecht et al., 1988). Studying all nonattenders could seriously inflate the seeming number of apostates. On the other hand, early studies may have underestimated rates of religious defection because of the wording of survey items (Wuthnow & Glock, 1973). And as we have noted earlier in this chapter, there may be differences in religiousness across countries, and these could have implications for apostasy (e.g., apostasy probably has different meanings in the "religious" United States vs. "less religious" European countries).

"Switching" religious denominations is apparently relatively common, especially in mainstream religious groups (Roof, 1989). Switching usually occurs across relatively similar denominations—for example as outlined by Kelley's "exclusive–ecumenical" continuum, described in Chapter 12 (Hadoway & Marler, 1993)—and it is often instigated by other life changes, such as marriage or moving to a new community (Babchuk & Whitt, 1990). In short, switching should not be confused with abandonment of religious faith and identification (Albrecht & Cornwall, 1989; Brinkerhoff & Mackie, 1993; Sandomirsky & Wilson, 1990). Greeley (1981) has referred to the switching process as "religious musical chairs" (p. 101)— a very different phenomenon from apostasy. Indeed, switchers tend to be more religiously involved than even people who simply remain in the same denomination (Hoge, Johnson, & Luidens, 1995).

We need greater precision and standardization of definition and measurement in research on apostasy, as well as careful consideration and integration of results of studies using different approaches and samples.

Is Apostasy Temporary?

Surveys often show that adolescents and college students are less religious than older persons. However, the disengagement from religion that is more common among adolescents and young adults is often characterized as a temporary phenomenon. Some "dropping out" may simply represent youthful exploration of alternative ideas and religions (e.g., alternate philosophies or belief systems, sects, cults) for a relatively short period in young people's lives. Gordon Allport (1950) suggested that after youthful disaffection with traditional religious values, many people return to religion by the time they are in their 30s. They may have children of their own and be concerned that their offspring should have some religious upbringing, or they may more generally have lost their rebellious tendencies and be settling down. In fact, longitudinal survey research has reported a significant tendency for religiosity to increase with age; the largest such increase occurs in young adulthood, between the ages of 18 and 30 (Argue, Johnson, & White, 1999). However, age-related increases in religiousness do not speak directly to the issue of whether or not apostates return to religion.

Some other evidence argues in favor of a "return to religion" tendency. Bibby (1993) claimed that many people who rejected religion in their teens eventually return to institutionalized religion, even if primarily to avail themselves of "rites of passage" (e.g., marriage or funerals), or to obtain some religious instruction for their children. Bibby showed that the percentage of Canadians claiming no religion was highest among younger adults aged 18–34. Furthermore, a cohort analysis suggested that almost half of the 16% of people aged 18–34 who claimed to have no religion in 1975 were reabsorbed into the religious realm, since in 1990 just 9% of the 35- to 54-year-olds (apparently many of the same people in the 1975 statistics) claimed to have no religion. This evidence suggests (albeit indirectly) that some people do return to religion after claiming "no religion" when they were younger. But of course we do not know how many of the 9% were the same people who claimed no religion 15 years earlier; individuals could not be followed longitudinally, and we do not know, for example, how many people might also have become apostates in the interim.

This is an important point: High church membership turnover may prevent a clear view of apostasy and "return to religion" trends. For example, the British Methodist Church experienced a net loss of 375,279 members from 1960 to 1998. However, this occurred within more than 1 million gains and more than 1.4 million departures from the church (Field, 2000). Such statistics, by themselves, tell us nothing about apostasy and return rates.

Not all research findings are consistent with the "return to religion" tendency. One study asked young people in rural Pennsylvania questions about religion when they were high school students in 1970, and again in 1981 when they were about 27 years old (Willits & Crider, 1989). Focusing on the 331 respondents who were married by 1981, the researchers concluded that these people were in fact *less* frequent church attenders at 27 than they had been in their middle teens. However, this study involved a relatively short-term follow-up, and it could be argued that the timing of the surveys (at ages 16 and 27, on average) might account for the unique findings. For example, a shift away from religion might well have occurred soon after the age of 16. Another follow-up when these people are in their 30s or 40s might be more informative.

An extensive longitudinal study of a U.S. national probability sample suggested that most religious dropping out probably occurs after age 16. Wilson and Sherkat (1994) followed the religious identification and other trends of people from 1965, when they were seniors in high school, to 1973 and again to 1983. In the third wave of their study, they managed to retain more than two-thirds of the original 1,562 participants. They focused their attention on those who reported a religious preference in 1965, but then reported no preference in 1973. For these dropouts, they found few differences between those who retained their apostate status in 1983 and those who had returned to religion. The returnees did report closer relationships with their parents in high school than did the continuing apostates. Furthermore, there was a tendency for early marriage and forming a family to be related to returning to religion, though this relationship was found only for men. Women were less likely to become apostates than were men, but women apostates were also less likely to return to the fold than were men. The researchers speculated that men are more likely to be religiously affected by transitions to marriage and parenthood: "Given the cultural understanding that the religious role is primarily allocated to women in the family, dropping out of the church is a stronger statement for women to make than for men, especially in a society where denominational affiliation of some kind is normative" (Wilson & Sherkat, 1994, p. 156).

The finding that marriage and parenthood are important factors in returning to the fold has been replicated elsewhere (Chaves, 1991; Hoge et al., 1993). This is consistent with our conclusion that parental religious socialization effects tend to weaken, and that other factors become more important as people move on through the life cycle and begin to live independent adult lives themselves. However, this does not necessarily imply that marriage and parenthood therefore are important contributors to stronger religiousness, generally speaking.

A methodical analysis of General Social Survey data from the United States from 1972 to 1991 revealed a trend toward increased religiousness with increasing age (Ploch & Hastings, 1994). However, there was no indication in these correlational data that either marriage or childbearing was associated with an increase in church attendance. According to Ploch and Hastings, researchers who have concluded that family formation is positively related to church attendance may have confused a long-term trend toward an age-related increase in religiousness with short-term events such as marriage and childbearing. The debate has continued, however, with other researchers finding that "family life cycle" attitudes and events (marriage, cohabitation, parenthood, divorce, etc.) *do* affect religion, though they may interact with age in complex ways (Stolzenberg, Blair-Loy, & Waite, 1995). This issue is a complicated one. However, we should be careful not to assume that church attendance and membership are ideal, accurate indicators of personal religiousness.

In conclusion, it seems likely that a substantial portion of apostates remain nonreligious for the rest of their lives. But evidence also suggests that some young apostates do return to religion later in their lives. We need additional data before we can make accurate estimates of the numbers of lifelong versus temporary apostates in different countries. It does seem clear that in most developed countries, the proportion of people claiming to have no religious affiliation increased steadily and sometimes dramatically in the 20th century. Even in the comparatively religious United States, the percentage of people saying that they have "no religion" jumped from 2% in 1967 to 11% in the 1990s (Putnam, 2000), and it is likely that a substantial part of this rise involved apostates.

Going against the Flow: "Amazing Apostates" and "Amazing Believers"

There is strong evidence that most people who become religious believers or apostates are behaving quite consistently with socialization theory predictions. That is, most apostates come from homes where religion was only weakly emphasized and parental modeling of religion was not strong. And most religious believers come from homes were religion was relatively strongly emphasized and modeling was readily available. There are exceptions to the rule, although they are rare. For example, just 2% of Canadian weekly church attenders in 1991 were going to church "seldom or never" as youngsters (Bibby, 1993), and just 10 of 631 Canadian and U.S. college students (1.6%) identified with a religious denomination after reporting that they grew up with no religion (Brinkerhoff & Mackie, 1993).

This is consistent with research on "amazing believers" and "amazing apostates"— people who seem to contradict socialization predictions (Altemeyer & Hunsberger, 1997; see also Hunsberger, 2000). Altemeyer and Hunsberger (1997) established strict criteria in an attempt to capture the exceptions to the socialization rule. Amazing believers scored in the top quarter of a scale that tapped the extent to which they now held orthodox Christian beliefs, but in the lower quarter of a scale that tapped the extent to which religion had been emphasized in the childhood home. That is, the amazing believers had come from relatively nonreligious backgrounds but now held orthodox Christian beliefs. Amazing apostates scored in the bottom quarter of the orthodoxy scale and the top quarter of the emphasis scale, indicating that they had come from highly religious backgrounds but no longer believed the basic tenets of their home religion.

The two researchers then interviewed as many amazing apostates (1.4% of the overall sample) and amazing believers (0.8%) they could find at their respective Canadian universities, after screening several thousand students across two separate academic years. The 46 amazing apostates who were interviewed confirmed that they had generally rejected family religious teachings, in spite of strong socialization pressures to accept religious beliefs. They were unique people whose "search for truth" had led them to question many things, especially religious teachings, often from an early age. Many of these people reported initial guilt and fear about dropping their religious beliefs (consistent with the findings of Etxebarria, 1992), but in retrospect they believed that the benefits of leaving their religion far outweighed any costs involved. Also, they held very tolerant, nonauthoritarian attitudes toward others, in contrast to more authoritarian views apparent among their highly religious counterparts.

Why did these people reject religious teachings when the majority of their peers accepted their religious backgrounds? The interviewees' own explanations typically revolved around their need to ask questions and get answers, their intellectual curiosity, and their unwillingness to accept responses that they felt did not really answer their questions. Most of these people had experienced conflict over their beliefs, and had spent considerable time and effort weighing different arguments for and against religious beliefs. In the end, they decided that the religious arguments and evidence simply did not make sense to them, and they very deliberately chose a nonreligious path for their lives. Clearly, these apostates were "amazing" in that they seemed to reverse socialization influences through an intellectual search for truth in their own lives.

But as rare as these amazing apostates were, they were still twice as common as amazing believers. And the 24 amazing believers interviewed by Altemeyer and Hunsberger (1997) did not take the same carefully considered route to their newfound religiousness. Rather, they were more likely to have had *some* religious training early in their lives (in spite of a general lack of religiousness in the home), to be influenced by friends or significant others, and to have "found religion" in an attempt to deal with crises in their lives. Emotional issues such as fear, loneliness, and depression seemed to drive their amazing conversion. For example, some were attempting to escape from a dependence on drugs, alcohol, or sex; others were grappling with serious illness or tragedy in their lives (e.g., one woman who became an amazing believer had had four close relatives and friends die tragically in 1 year).

In spite of the relatively small samples in this study, the findings are fairly clear and intriguing. A small percentage of people do seem to "go against the flow" and reject religion in spite of strong childhood religious emphasis and training; a smaller percentage of others become strongly religious in spite of having mostly nonreligious backgrounds. These exceptional cases do not necessarily fly in the face of socialization theory. Altemeyer and Hunsberger (1997) speculated that their amazing apostates may simply have acted on an important religious teaching from early in their lives: "Believe the truth." However, they pursued the truth in a critical, questioning way that led them away from their home religious teachings. Further research is needed to assess this interpretation. And the amazing believers usually did report some modeling of religion in their upbringing. In the end, as rare as these amazing apostates are, such "exceptions to the rule" can potentially help our general understanding of the religious socialization process.

RELIGION AND IDENTITY DEVELOPMENT IN ADOLESCENCE

In the past decade, some promising research has linked adolescent identity development with religion. Identity development has roots in Erikson's (1968, 1969) theory of psychosocial development, especially the importance of the appearance of a secure identity in adolescence (vs. the danger of role confusion). In theory, religion can be an important contributor to the process of establishing a secure identity (e.g., Erikson, 1964, 1965)—for example, by helping to explain existential issues, by providing a sense of belonging, and by offering an institutionalized opportunity for individuals to commit to a (religious) world view ("fidelity"). Four identity statuses have been proposed by Marcia (1966; Marcia, Waterman, Matteson, Archer, & Orlofsky, 1993), based on the extent to which crisis (exploring alternatives) and commitment (investment in a particular identity) are apparent in adolescent lives (see Table 5.1).

Evidence confirms that the emergence of identity is a progressive developmental process, with "foreclosed" and "diffused" statuses the least developed, and relatively immature. The most advanced or mature status is "achieved," with "moratorium" being intermediate (e.g., Waterman, 1985). That is, a "diffused" young person (who has done little or no exploring in the religious realm, and who has not made any firm religious commitments) would be considered to be relatively immature in terms of religious identity development. But someone who has done a lot of thinking about (exploring) religious issues and conflicts, and as a result has decided to accept (commit to) a particular religious ideology, would be accorded the more mature "achieved" identity status.

TABLE 5.1. Marcia's Classification of Identity Status Based on Crisis and Commitment

Crisis	Commitment	
	Present	Not present
Present	Achieved	Moratorium
Not present	Foreclosed	Diffused

It is surprising that in light of the theoretical intertwining of religious and identity development, there has been little research on this issue until the 1990s. Studies have indicated that more religious commitment, as measured by church attendance, tends to be linked with more general identity achievement and foreclosure—the identity statuses that involve ideological commitment (Markstrom-Adams, Hofstra, & Dougher, 1994; Tzuriel, 1984). But these findings have not always been clear cut, possibly because self-reported church attendance is not necessarily a good measure of religious ideological commitment (see, e.g., Markstrom, 1999). Also, since women are more likely than men to make a commitment in the religious realm (Pastorino, Dunham, Kidwell, Bacho, & Lamborn, 1997), failure to control for gender could contaminate results (see also Alberts, 2000). In spite of such gender differences in commitment, however, some evidence indicates that both genders use the identity process similarly in the religious domain (e.g., Archer, 1989).

Some studies have examined links between religious *orientation* measures and identity status. Markstrom-Adams and Smith (1996) found that the Intrinsic religious orientation was associated with achievement status (apparently because of the greater religious commitment of intrinsically oriented persons), and that the Extrinsic orientation was linked with diffusion identity status (apparently because of the lack of religious commitment and the lack of crisis or exploration for extrinsically oriented people). However, measurement of religious commitment and crisis was limited to the Intrinsic and Extrinsic religious orientation scales (Allport & Ross, 1967), and these might not be good measures of the extent of religious commitment and, especially, crisis.

In a study of college students, Fulton (1997) also found that Intrinsic orientation scores were linked with identity achievement (and Extrinsic orientation scores with foreclosure), as expected. In addition, scores on the Quest scale (see Batson et al., 1993) were associated with moratorium status, apparently because of the doubt exploration inherent in the Quest measure. However, a more recent investigation found no link between identity status and Quest scores (Klassen & McDonald, 2002).

Hunsberger et al. (2001a) attempted to improve on previous studies' limited measures of religious commitment, and especially of religious exploration/crisis. They carried out two studies, one of high school students before and after they finished high school, and another of university students. Their results generally confirmed the expected links between identity status and religion. For example, religious commitment was stronger for more achieved and foreclosed people, and commitment was weaker for more diffused and moratorium students. Also, religious crisis was positively correlated with moratorium (but not achievement) scores, and negatively related to foreclosure and diffusion scores. Finally, this research indicated that specific styles of religious crisis (belief-confirming vs. belief-threatening consultation for religious doubts) were also usually linked with identity status, as predicted (see Research Box 5.6).

In summary, recent findings suggest that the ego identity status is relevant to the study of religion and could help us to understand religious development, especially during adolescence. It is possible that variables such as right-wing authoritarianism affect both religious development and more general identity development in this regard, since high right-wing authoritarianism is linked with both greater religiousness (e.g., Altemeyer, 1996) and foreclosed identity status (Peterson & Lane, 2001); however, the exploration of such relationships is left to future studies. Also, because the resolution of religious doubt is potentially an important task in the development of a secure identity in adolescence and young adulthood, it is possible that information-processing styles contribute to young people's approaches to religious doubts, and ultimately to the ways in which such doubts are resolved.

Another issue that needs to be addressed is the extent to which identity status measures are "contaminated" by content that asks explicitly about religion, since one-third of the content of some identity status measures (e.g., Adams et al., 1989) is in the religious domain. That is, to what extent are the links reported between identity status and religion a result of common religious content in measures of these two supposedly different concepts? In this regard, it may be inappropriate to think in terms of overall identity status, since there is some indication that identity development can be quite uneven in different content domains. For

---

≥▲

Research Box 5.6. Adolescent Identity Formation: Religious Exploration and Commitment (Hunsberger, Pratt, & Pancer, 2001a)

These researchers used a Religious Doubts scale (Altemeyer, 1988) in order to tap religious "crisis" (see McAdams, Booth, & Selvik, 1981) more directly than had been done in previous studies. They also included several ways of looking at religious commitment (e.g., self-reported current religiousness, church attendance), to insure that any relationships found were not unique to a specific measure of commitment. Using the Objective Measure of Ego Identity Status (Adams, Bennion, & Huh, 1989) in two studies, they found that high school and university students revealed links between broadly defined identity status, and religious crisis and exploration generally, as expected. More achieved and foreclosed people did score higher, and more diffused and moratorium individuals did score lower, on measures of religious commitment. Also, moratorium status was related to more religious doubting, as expected, but achievement status was (surprisingly) not linked with doubting. The authors speculated that religious doubting may have occurred earlier in more achieved people's lives, and therefore may not have been adequately detected by the measures used. Finally, lower levels of doubting ("religious crisis") should be evident among more foreclosed and diffused people, but this was true only for foreclosed identity status. To summarize, these two studies then offer general (but not complete) support for hypothesized links between religion and identity status.

These same studies also investigated the ways in which people dealt with religious doubts by means of the Belief-Confirming Consultation (BCC) and Belief-Threatening Consultation (BTC) scales, discussed earlier in this chapter. The authors suggested that BCC and BTC scores would be related to identity status, based on Berzonsky and Kuk's (2000) finding that identity status is related to the ways in which people process information. The evidence generally supported their hypotheses. For example, higher achievement scores were linked with both higher BCC and higher BTC scores, and diffusion was associated with both lower BCC and lower BTC scores. Finally, longitudinal data in the second study allowed Hunsberger et al. to assess relationships over time. Again, relationships were generally (though not always) as expected. For example, foreclosure scores significantly predicted reduced BTC scores and less overall religious doubting 2 years later. These findings have been interpreted as partially supporting Berzonsky and Kuk's (2000) suggestion that identity status is linked with social-cognitive information-processing styles within the religious realm.

example, De Haan and Schulenberg (1997) concluded that covariation between religious and political identity was low and inconsistent. Skorikov and Vondracek (1998) found that religious identity development lagged behind vocational identity development. Possibly researchers should focus on *religious* identity development, with purer (religious identity) measures that are not complicated by content from other domains (e.g., politics, career).

OVERVIEW

In this chapter we have focused on a socialization approach to the development of adolescent and young adult religiousness. There are certainly other ways of conceptualizing religious development as children move into adolescence; as we have seen, however, much evidence is consistent with a socialization perspective, especially one based on social learning theory. Empirical work confirms that parents are the strongest influences on adolescent religiousness, though their influence seems to decrease as young people grow older. It is not entirely clear whether mothers or fathers exert the stronger influence on religious development, though the weight of the evidence suggests that mothers are more powerful. Certainly both mothers and fathers have some influence, and interactive factors also play a role (e.g., warmth of the family environment, mother–father consistency in religiousness). Other religious socialization agents have sometimes been presumed to be active, such as the church, peer groups, and education. However, with the possible exception of specific effects of religious education (e.g., increases in religious knowledge) and the church, these other variables apparently exert relatively weak effects on adolescent religiosity.

Some studies have suggested that early tendencies for children or adolescents to increase or decrease in religiosity may continue into adulthood. This "polarization" tendency needs to be explored further.

Generational effects occur, such that adolescents and young adults are "less religious" than older adults. However, although religiosity has apparently decreased substantially in many parts of the world, religion itself is hardly on the verge of disappearing. The United States seems to be an exception to the "decreasing religiousness" rule, since rates of regular church attendance have been relatively stable, with about 30–40% of high school seniors reportedly attending weekly.

Some evidence suggests that the religious socialization process may affect the ways in which people think about existential religious issues. Research on integrative complexity has indicated that more orthodox and fundamentalist persons think less complexly about such issues. Possibly these stylistic thought differences are related to the ways in which people resolve conflicts, questions, and doubts concerning religious teachings. The evidence suggests that questions and doubts about religion are common (though certainly not intense, on average) during adolescence and early adulthood, and that those with more doubts tend to think in more complex terms about religious doubts and conflicts. There is some tendency for more fundamentalist persons to resolve their questions and doubts in ways that support their religious beliefs, whereas less fundamentalist persons are more likely to achieve resolutions that change their religious beliefs.

Work on apostasy has suggested that leaving the family religion is generally consistent with socialization explanations of religious development. People who abandon the family faith tend to come from homes where religion was either ignored or only weakly emphasized. Thus apostates often simply "drift" a bit further away from a religion that was not important to the family in the first place. Apostates tend to have poorer relationships with their parents, and cognitive factors are probably involved in apostasy to some extent, since apostates are more likely to question, doubt, and debate religious issues earlier in their lives than nonapostates. This critical questioning approach to religion seems especially true of "amazing apostates"—people who become apostates in spite of considerable socialization pressure in their childhood to accept religious teachings. Finally, some apostates apparently return to religion in adulthood, but others become "apostates for life."

Recent research has linked ego identity status with religious exploration/crisis and commitment in predicted ways. Apparently religious development is associated with Erikson's hypothesized establishment of a secure identity, as opposed to role confusion, in adolescence. Moreover, evidence suggests that identity status can be moderately successful in predicting religious doubt levels and ways of dealing with doubts 2 years later; this is consistent with the suggestion that unique information processing styles may characterize different identity statuses.

The research reviewed in this chapter constitutes a considerable body of knowledge concerning religious socialization processes. We continue to learn more about how young people become religious, how they think about religion, and why they sometimes leave a religious background. However, research has tended to focus on description rather than explanation. It *is* important to understand the integral role of parents (and the relative unimportance of some other factors) in the religious socialization process. It *is* valuable to gain insight into the thought processes and correlates of religious doubt and apostasy. It *is* worthwhile to devise typologies of apostates. And so on. But it is also important that we generate testable explanations concerning *why* these processes occur as they do, and what the causative factors are with respect to religious development. Too much attention has been devoted to the social correlates of religious socialization and religious change, and not enough attention has focused on factors within individuals (e.g., styles of thinking, ways in which people approach and resolve information that challenges their beliefs). Correlational studies, which are the norm in this area, can help us to understand the processes involved, but do little to clarify cause-and-effect relationships. The issues discussed in this chapter therefore have considerable potential for future research.

Chapter 6

THE FORM AND CONTENT
OF ADULT RELIGION

> Among all my patients in the second half of life—that is to say, over thirty-five—there has not been one whose problem in the last resort was not that of finding a religious outlook on life. . . . none of them has really been healed who did not regain his religious outlook.
>
> Religion reveals itself in struggling to reveal the meaning of the world.
>
> Every serious life has that experience where the profundities within ask for an answering profundity. No longer do the shallows suffice. Life within faces some profound abyss of experience, and the deep asks for an answering deep. So when deep calls unto deep and the deep replies, we face the essential experience of religion.
>
> People will do anything for religion, argue for it, fight for it, die for it, anything but live for it.
>
> No creed is final. Such a creed as mine must grow and change as knowledge grows and changes.[1]

RELIGION IN ADULT LIFE

For 120 years, North American psychologists have constructed theories and conducted research in the psychology of religion (Booth, 1981). Following the pattern established by mainstream psychology, the psychology of religion did not explicitly focus on religion in adulthood at first; this was taken for granted when religious experience, beliefs, and behavior were studied. An emphasis on religion in childhood was established by G. Stanley Hall, who has often been viewed as a founder of our field. Hall extended his work to deal with adolescence, and wrote extensively on religion in the teenage years (Hall, 1904). His writings paralleled those of James Mark Baldwin, who has been called the father of North American child psychology. Adult psychology per se was generally overlooked, however, and was regarded as "new" as recently as 1970. It did develop rapidly in the last quarter of the 20th century, though (Botwinick, 1978). Unlike the situation in child psychology, there seem to be no giants in our psychological past who emphasized research and theory in *adult* development.

---

1. These quotations come, respectively, from the following sources: Jung (1933, p. 229); S. H. Miller, quoted in Simpson (1964, p. 204); H. E. Fosdick, quoted in Simpson (1964, p. 212); Caleb Colton, quoted in Edwards (1955, p. 535); and Sir Arthur Keith, quoted in Edwards (1955, p. 539).

Religion as a force in adult living was first recognized in relation to faith during one's closing years. Cumming and Henry (1961) looked on religious interest and activity as part of the process of disengagement from life prior to death. However, surprisingly little has been written on what is usually termed early and middle adulthood—roughly, the years between 18 and 50.

Our task in this chapter is to detail the nature and content of religion in adult life. We need to examine adult religious activity and beliefs in relation to such factors as gender and age. Here we set the stage for comprehending the meaning, influence, and function of one's faith in other areas of life.

THE COLLECTIVE EXPRESSION OF RELIGION

Many faiths in the United States and Canada are unrelated to the Judeo-Christian tradition. These include Native American, Near Eastern/Middle Eastern, and Asian religions. Many local cults and sects also exist. The representation of some major world religions (e.g., Islam) in North America is growing rapidly, in large part because of immigration. But little psychological research has been conducted to date on these other religious groups, as noted in Chapter 1. We therefore emphasize in these pages the Judeo-Christian heritage and its expression in contemporary North American (especially U.S.) culture. In addition, it is not unreasonable to theorize that similar psychological principles underlie all faiths. This has, of course, been our message in Chapters 1 through 3, where we have set forth our theory suggesting the universal primacy of needs for meaning, control, and relationships with others (sociality). Greeley (1972b) earlier emphasized the roles of meaning and social belonging in the formation and maintenance of religion. These themes are clearly helpful, but, given their largely theoretical and assumptive status, they have not stimulated much specific research (Mills, 1959).

The Judeo-Christian heritage is worldwide in scope, and national surveys show that U.S. residents in particular are among the most religious people on earth. Table 6.1 shows this for "belief in God" and "religious experience," two core elements in the Western religious tradition. These data further reveal that among the nations studied, the United States joins Ireland and Poland as strongest in its belief in God. The latter two countries have a long history of established Roman Catholicism. Interestingly, over 40 years of Communist negativism does not seem to have adversely affected the Polish people's belief in God. Over 70 years of Soviet rule in Russia may have had some effect, but its data are not very different from those observed for France, the Netherlands, and Sweden—lands with no history of formal opposition to religion. Greeley (2002) provides some additional insight into these findings.

Though the questions used by domestic pollsters versus those of Greeley's investigators may be a factor, the incidence of subjectively reported religious experience is much higher in the United States than for all the other nations studied, including Ireland and Poland. Is it possible that Irish and Polish Roman Catholicism is not congenial to the expression and/ or reporting of religious experience? The fact that belief in God is much higher and more variable across the countries compared in Table 6.1 suggests a need to search for influences that keep the experience rates so much lower in Europe, and also so much more similar in nations as diverse as Britain, Denmark, Russia, Ireland, and the Scandinavian countries. Again, we are confronted with the fact that researchers have studied the United States in particular (and North America in general) to such a degree that they may lose sight of the

TABLE 6.1. Percentages of the Population in Various
Countries that "Believe in God" and Have Had Religious
Experience

Country	Belief in God (%)	Religious experience (%)
United States	95	41
Czech Republic	6	11
Denmark	57	15
France	52	24
Great Britain	69	16
Hungary	65	17
Ireland	95	13
Italy	86	31
Netherlands	57	22
Northern Ireland	92	26
Norway	59	16
Poland	94	16
Russia	52	13
Spain	82	19
Sweden	54	12

Note. The U.S. "belief in God" data are from Gallup and Lindsay (1999) (in
the Hirsley [1993] data, this percentage was 94%). The U.S. "religious experience" data come from the General Social Survey (GSS) data for 1972–1998
(GSS, 1999). "Belief in God" data for other countries are from Hirsley (1993).
"Religious experience" data for other countries are from Greeley (2002).

necessity of comprehending faith in the rest of the world. Greeley's efforts to look beyond
U.S. borders are important for broadening our perspectives.

RELIGIOUS AFFILIATION AND BEHAVIOR
IN THE UNITED STATES

U.S. residents take their religion very seriously. Sociologists indicate that "upwards of 93%
of Americans have a religious preference" (Hadaway & Roof, 1988, p. 30). With regard to
religious affiliation, Table 6.2 indicates its current status in the United States. Even though
these findings only cover two decades, no notable changes in commitment over the last half-
century have been demonstrated. Religion is deeply ingrained in the U.S. milieu and mind,
and is therefore quite stable.

Nominal affiliation is buttressed by Moore's (2000) findings that 69% of U.S. adults said
in 1980 that they were church or synagogue members, and that in 1999 the number was 70%.
In 1999, 44% of adults also reported that they attended services within the preceding week—a
rise of 5% from 1950 (Moore, 2000). The stability of church attendance among U.S. residents
is further evidenced by a review of Gallup Polls in the 20th century, which indicates that church
attendance in 1939 and 1999 was identical, at 41% (Newport, Moore, & Saad, 2000).

Another behavioral sign of religious commitment is Bible reading. In 2000, 59% of
those surveyed stated that they read the Bible, at least occasionally; 16% claimed to read
the Bible daily, and 14% said that they participated in Bible study groups (Gallup & Simons,
2000).

TABLE 6.2. Religious Affiliation in
the United States for 1980 and 1999
(Percentages of the Population)

Affiliation	1980 (%)	1999 (%)
Protestant	61	55
Roman Catholic	28	28
Jewish	2	2
Other	2	6
None	7	8

Note. Data from U.S. Bureau of the Census (2000, p. 62).

Prayer is also a very significant expression of religious devotion. National data suggest that 88% of U.S. adults pray, but that only one-third pray once a week or more (General Social Survey [GSS], 1999; Poloma & Gallup, 1991).

The foregoing statistics are impressive testimony to the religious behavior of adults in the United States. This information is, however, premised upon the verbal statements of those surveyed, and thus may not always be accurate. Most Americans view religious activity in a very positive light; the notion that good people are religious people is widely held. When U.S. residents are questioned, some exaggeration of personal religious commitment is to be expected because of its socially desirable character. Responding in this manner is quite common, as a massive literature on social-desirability-based responding amply illustrates (Batson, Schoenrade, & Ventis, 1993; Epley & Dunning, 2000). Still, the issue is not so simple, as inclinations toward this type of responding are probably confounded with the values of a committed, intrinsic faith (Watson, Morris, Foster, & Hood, 1986). Both motivations are likely to be expressed: People want to look good both to themselves and others, and they often try to live in accordance with the tenets of their faith. This, of course, means that surveys are likely to produce higher rates of religious activity and belief expression than hard observational data might indicate.

Hadaway, Marler, and Chaves (1993) carried out a major study to compare survey data on church attendance with actual counts of those attending services. Their results strongly "suggest that Protestant and Catholic church attendance is roughly half" (p. 748) that reported in surveys. Citing earlier work, these researchers feel that "inflation errors are more serious for membership statistics than for attendance counts" (p. 743). Though we are usually forced to rely on questionnaire and survey data that may be subject to social desirability influences, such data are frequently all we have. We must therefore understand the direction of potential bias, and account for it wherever possible.

The discrepancy between membership and attendance statistics tells us that being affiliated with a religious institution should not be confused with the idea of being religious. For many people, joining a church is the "right" thing to do, and is not necessarily different from being a member of some fraternal organization or local service club (Demerath & Hammond, 1969). Many who are not affiliated with a specific institution could easily be seen as more religious than the average church member. A common self-identification is to say that one is "spiritual." Though this term is fraught with unclear meanings, it is (as noted in Chapters 1 and 2) amenable to a wide variety of interpretations, not the least of which is a search to locate oneself in the scheme of things—to find ultimate answers (Emmons, 1999; Roof, 1993).

The foregoing discussion shows that there does not appear to have been any significant decline in religion in the United States for a century or more, ever since formal data on religious devotion and commitment have been gathered.

RELIGIOUS BELIEFS IN THE UNITED STATES

Similar backing for the central role of religion in the life of U.S. adults comes from polls on religious beliefs. The simple question, "How important would you say religion is in your life?" has been asked by the Gallup Poll organization since 1952. At that time, 95% of respondents claimed that their faith was fairly or very important to them. Since 1980, this percentage has shown minor erratic fluctuations between 86% and 89%. Though it has declined slightly in the past 50 years, in March 2000 the response to this query was 88%—suggesting the relative constancy of the feelings of U.S. adults regarding their religion for at least the last 20 years (Moore, 2000).

When asked about the applicability of religion to "today's problems," those polled are less sure that faith is relevant to impersonal matters beyond their own lives. During the late 1990s, the percentage believing that religion has such practical value showed no real change, remaining largely between 66% and 68% (Moore, 2000). Even greater indecision is evidenced when the issue concerns the growth or loss of religion's "influence in American life": The vacillating character of responses to this query is revealed in numbers varying from 27% to 48% in the 1990s. This item may be particularly sensitive to national problems that exist at the time the survey is administered. The overall pattern suggests that the 36–38% range is most representative. In March 2000, 37% of those sampled believed that religion is increasing its national influence (Moore, 2000). We are also probably witnessing the normal variation one can expect from different national samples. A broader picture of the pervasiveness of religion may be gained from the Christian beliefs examined in Table 6.3. Clearly, a considerable number of U.S. adults testify to the truth of these aspects of Christianity.

Again, however, it must be remembered that survey research is fraught with pitfalls. Just as we have mentioned earlier that data may be biased by social-desirability-based response sets, there are many instances when we have to curb our desire to take large-sample survey findings at face value. The GSS, the Gallup Polls, and the National Opinion Research Center provide information on thousands of people over long periods of time. These names are

TABLE 6.3. The Percentages of U.S. Adults Subscribing to Various Christian Beliefs

Beliefs	%
Miracles	48.3
Heaven	64.1
Hell	52.2
The Devil	64.9
Life after death	56.1
Bible is the word of God	33.5
Bible is inspired word	49.8

Note. Data from GSS (1999).

household words for social scientists, and it is not unusual to read sample sizes in the thousands. We cannot fail to be impressed, but results are invariably presented in percentages. For example, some data presented above indicated that the personal importance of religion to U.S. adults dropped from 95% in 1952 to 88% in 2000. Before the flag of battle or surrender is raised, we must recognize that the U.S. population increased by 79% during this period. Whereas about 150 million claimed religion was fairly or very important to them in 1952, the comparable number in 2000 was approximately 248 million. Descriptive terms such as "fairly" or "very" offer some guidance, but their meanings may have shifted. The average religionist today could be more committed and involved than in past years. This is implied by Gallup Polls finding that 33% of those surveyed described themselves as "born again" or "evangelical" in 1986; in 1994, 39% felt similarly (*The Gallup Poll Monthly*, 1994). Translating these figures into population equivalents suggests that there were about 23 million more people who felt this way in 1994. There are obviously great strengths to employing percentages, but there are times when we need to think of the actual numbers behind these percentages.

GENDER AND RELIGION

Appreciating the many overt and subtle influences that affect adult religion necessitates a blurring of the frequently vague boundaries between sociology and psychology. Demographic factors, such as age, sex, and socioeconomic status, need to be addressed in relation to religious belief and behavior. These factors also must be translated from their collective character into individual psychological expression.

The Data on Gender and Religion

The data are clear: Women consistently demonstrate a greater affinity for religion than men. The national findings presented in Table 6.4 demonstrate both stronger beliefs and higher levels of religious activity on the part of females.

TABLE 6.4. A Comparison of Male and Female Religious Affiliation, Activities, and Beliefs

Question	Men (%)	Women (%)
Religion "very important"	53	67
Member, church or synagogue	63	73
Attend church, last 7 days	63	57
Believe in miracles	71	86
Cope with crisis by prayer	74	86
Cope with crisis by reading Bible	56	72
Taught religion as child	78	81
Want their children to get religious training	86	90
Describe selves as "born again"	37	41
Thought a lot about developing faith in last 2 years	41	58
Interested a lot in relations with God	48	66
Feel need for spiritual growth	79	84
Religion relevant to today's problems	60	69

Note. Data from Gallup and Lindsay (1999). Percentages indicate "yes" responses.

This has fascinating possibilities, not the least of which have the potential of involving biology. Whitney (1976), citing data from many mammalian species, shows greater social cohesiveness and cooperation among females than among males. The observation that religion and ingroup social cohesion go together has been well explicated by Durkheim and others (see McGuire, 1992). Arguments in favor of women's religion and spirituality stress cooperation and cohesion (Conn, 1986). Echoes of biology may thus be heard in the strong propensities of women for religion and social unity.

Explaining the Data

A number of theories have been proposed to explain the foregoing data. Anthropologists and sociologists suggest that male dominance means that females are socialized to be dependent and submissive. This is commonly translated into lower status for women, and has repercussions in terms of the division of labor. In many societies women are defined as homemakers and child rearers. Not being in the work force, they are regarded as having more time for religion, and this is cited as a reason for their greater church attendance and stronger religious beliefs and commitments. Women's greater religious participation is thus treated as a natural aspect of the overall female role within the social order (Miller & Hoffman, 1995).

Psychologically, Miller and Hoffman (1995) provide an opportunity to interpret the female social role in terms of risk taking. Being in a weaker position than men, women should therefore be lower in risk-taking behavior (more "risk-aversive"), and should tend to adopt culturally safe positions such as religion. In other words, women are expected to confront life stresses and ambiguities conservatively. The case can then be made that males are socialized to be independent and hence to become risk takers. This may explain gender differences in many aspects of life in which females take risks less often than do boys and men. As expected, the research does show that risk aversion is positively associated both with religiosity and with being female (Miller & Hoffman, 1995).

The lower status and power of women (McGuire, 1992; Pargament, 1997) has been analogized by Hinde (1999) to the "religion of the oppressed"—namely, the need of the powerless to turn to their faith when all other avenues fail. Hinde further appeals to a biological foundation that affiliates femininity with a greater propensity for social connections and relationships with others, as suggested above.

This greater attachment to religion on the part of women has some interesting implications. One is that religion is likely to possess more utility for women than for men, and the evidence suggests that this is true (Pargament, 1997). That is, the more religious people are, the more helpful religion is seen to be in coping with life's problems. In general, as will further be shown in Chapter 15, the use of religion as a psychosocial resource is positively associated with good outcomes. Religion may perform such functions to a greater extent for women than for men.

In most instances, women are the "religious culture carriers." A fascinating demonstration of this role across the centuries is illustrated by the work of Janet Jacobs (1996) on the function of women in the survival of "crypto-Jewish culture." Crypto-Jewish culture is a result of the 15th- and 16th century persecution of Jews during the Spanish Inquisition. Facing death or conversion to Catholicism, many Spanish Jews either left Spain or "converted." This frequently meant that their Judaism "went underground," but persisted in one form or another until the present day as a crypto- or concealed Judaism with largely hidden traditional Jewish practices. Crypto-Jews live primarily in the southwestern United States and

Mexico, though some are also found in the eastern states among Hispanic émigrés from the Caribbean.

Interviewing a sample of crypto-Jews in Arizona, Colorado, New Mexico, and Texas, Jacobs (1996) attributed the survival of crypto-Jewish culture to the women in these families. This framework of beliefs and behavior was historically and still is kept secret from outsiders, often beneath a veneer of Catholicism. Support for crypto-Judaism is associated with the maintenance of classical Jewish rituals, primarily by the women in the home. Among these, Jacobs observed the lighting of Sabbath candles; the enforcement of kosher dietary laws; and the celebration of Jewish holiday ceremonies for Passover, Purim, and Chanukah. Since these families were and still are often overtly Catholic, the Jewish festival of Purim might be practiced as the festival of St. Esther, and Chanukah masked as the festival of Las Posadas (a celebratory representation of the journey of Joseph and Mary). Often central to this Catholic–Jewish syncretic activity is the preparation of food, which in these families is strictly a female duty. The importance of secrecy plus the maintenance of classic Jewish rituals and practices endows the women in these crypto-Jewish families with both power and responsibility. The mothers must protect the family's religious integrity in each generation, and pass on to their daughters the heritage they have received from their forebears. In all likelihood, similar religious practices and perspectives are conveyed through the women in Christian families, especially among those who have changed churches. These possibilities do not say that the men in such religious settings play no role in preserving religious tradition, but rather that the women are the dominant force in teaching their faith to the children.

Women's Changing Roles in Relation to Religion

Though for hundreds of years a few exceptional women publicly expressed unhappiness with their position as underlings in virtually all aspects of life, effective large-scale change only began in the 20th century. The classical roles of women in relation to religion began to change radically in the 1960s. Subservience was often replaced by self-direction. Instead of following the paths set by males, many women decided on finding new ways of developing their own directions. Initially, this took two forms. Women spoke of their religious and spiritual struggles and aspirations (Meadow & Rayburn, 1985; Ware, 1985). Next came an attempt to realize these hopes and dreams by critiquing traditional religious institutional structures and their theological justifications (Christ & Plaskow, 1979; Plaskow & Romero, 1974; Ruether, 1974). Concurrently, resources were created to permit women to take long overdue leadership positions in churches and synagogues (Conn, 1986; Ruether & McLaughlin, 1979). Chaves (1997) argues that pressures for gender equality were a major force in spurring the ordination of women—a trend that has increased rapidly in several Protestant groups and in Reform Judaism over the past 30 years.

Religion and the Women's Movement

It is hard to believe that real concern about women's roles in regard to religion only developed with the women's movement of the last 40 years. There is no comparable line of questioning about the religion of men, as it was traditionally taken for granted that men should naturally dominate both women and religion. Historically, members of the clergy were males, and scripture has been used to validate the controlling role of men in both the family and the Judeo-Christian tradition. Even when women did serve the church, such as Catholic nuns, real power still resided in the hands of a masculine hierarchy. So, although individual women may have begun questioning their position in relation to religion well before the 1960s, this development was not widely articulated before that time.

Feminism and Religion: The Struggle

Cultural change is often slow and troubled. This is evidenced in recent work on the conflicted attitudes of women in conservative Christian and Jewish groups. While arguing for equality in self-expression and opportunity outside of their conservative faiths, they appear to be ambivalent regarding the liberalization of their roles in church and home. There is also a tendency to oppose feminism explicitly, while implicitly accepting its ideas when these are framed in appropriate orthodox/conservative terminology (Manning, 1999).

Studying the feminist identity of Jewish women, Dufour (2000) encountered a situation similar to that in Manning's study. Dufour perceives this process of coping with conservative religion versus change as one of "sifting." Judaism is examined, and doctrinal selection takes place in order to resolve the conflict between spiritual and religious identities. Beliefs and actions that do not satisfy feminist spiritual needs are "sifted" out. We need to know more about what is observed and what is removed from consideration, however. When is feminism challenged and/or threatened, and, conversely, when does one's religious identity become tenuous?

THE SIGNIFICANCE OF AGE

The Phenomenon of Adulthood

The psychological correlates and effects of age have been primarily examined with regard to childhood, adolescence, and old age. Research surveys on religion and aging seem exclusively devoted to work with elderly individuals (Fecher, 1982; Koenig, 1995). When one becomes a "senior citizen" or "elderly person" is unclear, ranging from about 50 to 65 years. Atchley (1977), however, points out the inadequacy of chronological age as a criterion for one's later years. Great individual variation exists in how people respond to the advances of time. There are very many physically and mentally active people in their 80s; others still in their 50s manifest the debilitating effects of what we regard as old age. Even though we generally treat adulthood and aging as reasonably well-circumscribed times in the life cycle, we must recognize the overwhelming significance of individuality and avoid engaging in age stereotyping.

At first glance, becoming an adult is simply defined chronologically. Sometime about the age of 18, there is a vague sociocultural transition to adulthood. A new image of maturity is invoked, with accompanying political and social responsibilities (for which adolescents are assumed to be unprepared). Still, for many young people, 4 years or more are taken up with continuing education before they enter the job market. Usually, without further ado, these young adults are expected to take on the burdens of adult life. Though these pose many new concerns, most can be subsumed under a few major problem areas. We explore these in Chapter 7.

Unfortunately, there are no agreed-upon divisions of the years constituting adult life. Even though Erik Erikson (1963) referred to "early," "middle," and "late" adulthood, he was not consistent with respect to their boundaries. In less than rigorous formality, early adulthood ranges from 17 or 20 years to about 45, with middle adulthood continuing to about 65 years of age (Levinson, Darrow, Klein, Levinson, & McKee, 1978). As conceptually appealing as this framework is, very little has been done to provide it with empirical verification. Some fine efforts have also been made to coordinate Erikson's thinking with religion, but the need for research to supplement these ideas continues (Browning, 1973; Wright, 1982).

We can gain a broad perspective on religion in adulthood by looking at the phenomenon known as the "baby boomer" generation. "Baby boomers" are Americans born immediately following World War II, during the years from 1946 to 1964—a time of high birth rates. An estimated 76 million children were born in the United States during this period. Currently, most boomers are middle-aged; some are now on the threshold of old age. With respect to faith, the noted sociologist of religion Wade Clark Roof (1993) has called them "a generation of seekers."

Religion and the Baby Boomer Generation

Many baby boomers have attempted to pursue spirituality outside of the religious mainstream, but their main direction has been much more mundane, which suggests that the future of organized religion in our nation is probably safe for some time to come.

In his major study of the baby boomers' religion, Roof employed a sample of 1,599 people in four states spanning the nation. He distinguished three groups: "loyalists," "returnees," and "dropouts." Loyalists, as the word implies, stayed with traditional religion; the returnees often deviated considerably in their personalized experiments with faith before coming back to the mainstream. The dropouts included those who either moved away from or were never affiliated with mainstream religious institutions. Table 6.5 offers some insight into the journey of those who were reared as Catholics, and as "mainline" and "conservative" Protestants.

The table suggests that orthodox Protestants and Catholics, the more conservative groups, were more successful in keeping their members as active religionists than mainline Protestants were. In addition, about twice as many of the mainline Protestants as of the other groups shifted to other faiths. These effects may be an expression of the power of conservative religious bodies. More mainline Protestants also became nonreligious than members of the other groups. Still, Roof (1993) found that before their possible return, over 60% of all the young adults with religious backgrounds had dropped out of their faith. When they did come back, 13% moved toward fundamentalism, and 21% were denoted as conservative (technically "evangelical moderates").

We see some possible contradictions when we look at attitudes toward churchgoing and actual weekly attendance among Roof's subjects. With respect to the latter, as we move from liberal to conservative groups, the attendance percentages for men ranged from 31% to 51%; for women, the comparable figures ranged from 30% to 80%. When subjects were asked, however, whether a person "can be a good Christian and not attend church," the parallel agreement percentages varied from 66% (conservative) to 94% (not conservative). Churchgoing has thus become an issue of personal determination and choice, which Roof (1993) has described as the "new voluntarism" (p. 110).

There is no doubt that exposure to the 1960s "revolution against the establishment" had a rather pervasive effect. For those minimally affected by this period, 56% dropped out. Where such influence was high, 84% left the institutional fold. Still, in terms of belief in a deity, the baby boomers essentially matched the overall population, with 94–95% of the total group affirming this stance. An interesting subtle shift may be inferred from the finding that,

TABLE 6.5. Religious Paths Taken by Baby Boomers Reared as Catholics, Mainline Protestants, and Conservative Protestants

Religious path taken	%
Reared as Catholics	
Loyalists (identify selves as Catholics)	33
Currently active as Catholics	50
Shifted to other faiths[a]	12
Currently religiously active	58
Initial dropouts	67
Returnees	25
Final dropouts	42
Inactive Catholic	31
Reared as mainline Protestants	
Loyalists (identify selves as mainline Protestants)	31
Currently active mainline Protestants	39
Shifted to other faiths[a]	24
Currently religiously active	56
Initial dropouts	69
Returnees	24
Final dropouts	45
Inactive mainline Protestants	26
Reared as conservative Protestants	
Loyalists (identify selves as conservative Protestants)	39
Currently active conservative Protestants	55
Shifted to other faiths[a]	13
Currently religiously active	64
Initial dropouts	61
Returnees	25
Final dropouts	36
Inactive conservative Protestants	25

Note. Adapted from Roof (1993, pp. 176–179). Copyright 1993 by HarperCollins Publishers. Adapted by permission.
[a]For Catholics, this includes shifts to conservative and mainline Protestant groups, with a variety of undefined faiths. For mainline Protestants, this includes shifts to conservative Protestant groups; for conservative Protestants, this includes shifts to mainline bodies.

as Roof (1993) has put it, "these intense seekers prefer to think of themselves as 'spiritual' rather than as 'religious'" (p. 79).

Perkins (1991) studied a subset of the baby boomers, called "yuppies" ("young, upwardly mobile, urban professionals"). On the average, religious commitment and yuppie values were negatively related, but many yuppies still identified themselves with religion. In addition, a religious stance was positively associated with a sense of happiness. Greater insight into the religious perspectives and needs of the yuppies would have nicely supplemented Roof's research.

Even though Roof's study appeared to include Jews, no data on Jews were offered, little discussion was provided, and only a few individuals were mentioned. It is therefore difficult to form an opinion regarding "religious seeking" on the part of Roof's Jewish respondents.

Using poll data, Waxman (1994) studied a sample of 801 Jewish baby boomers. Unfortunately, very few questions were employed, and it is very difficult to compare Waxman's findings with those of Roof (1993). On the surface, a quite different situation seemed to exist with this group than with those studied by Roof. If we assume some tenuous correspondence between Roof's category of "loyalists" (Protestants and Catholics identifying with their traditional faith) and Waxman's "personal importance" distinction, Jewish identification among Waxman's subjects appeared greater than traditional Catholic or Protestant identification among Roof's Christians. From 31% to 39% of Roof's groups were classified as loyalists, whereas Waxman found that 85% of his sample regarded being Jewish as important to some degree. (Keep in mind that this comparison may be challenged.)

Sometimes one hears the term "cultural Jew," which may be valid here. Christianity is tightly tied to religion, whereas Judaism often refers to both a faith and a culture, especially in the United States. One rarely if ever hears of "Christian Americans," but "Jewish Americans" is a common referent (Goldstein & Goldscheider, 1968). Also, though being Jewish was considered important, essentially half of Waxman's baby boomers (49.8%) were not married to Jews; by contrast, almost 80% of an older comparison sample of 46- to 64-year-olds had Jewish spouses. This favors the "cultural Jew" argument, rather than one based on conformity to Jewish religious principles.

Neither the work of Perkins (1991) nor that of Waxman (1994) approaches the depth of Roof's (1993) effort, and we can easily ask for more. Interview data are excellent for the development of hypotheses that can be quantitatively assessed. We can view the struggles of individuals, but as poignant as they are, they point to subgroups that need further exploration. Studies of background motivational and experiential factors are largely lacking. Among Jews, distinctions among Reform, Conservative, and Orthodox affiliations need to be examined. Whether Jewish or Christian groups are studied, there are seekers, rejecters, and those who are simply apathetic about religion. There is much more to be learned about the life histories of such individuals.

THE ACCEPTANCE AND REJECTION OF INSTITUTIONAL RELIGION

Adulthood is a time when people make decisions about how religion may affect their lives. Not the least among these is how people will relate as individuals to their faith. Will it be through the traditional avenues of church involvement in the style of their parents? Will there be a seeking of new paths and expressions, a turn to some alternative version of orthodoxy, a loosening of ties, a shift to a different faith, or a complete rejection of religion? These are questions that all individuals ask themselves at one time or another, but they become especially significant when raised in adulthood. What choices will be made and why? These concerns are dealt with, in part, in other chapters; however, let us look at a few of their manifestations in adulthood.

Becoming Involved with Religious Institutions

There are many reasons for people to affiliate themselves with religious institutions. These range from an automatic, habitual continuation of family tradition to deep personal struggles with understanding one's place in life and society. (See also Chapter 11 on conversion, since conversion is mainly an issue of adult life.)

A fine example of research in this area was carried out by Roberts and Davidson (1984). Recognizing the importance of psychosocial factors in church involvement, these researchers noted two major approaches to the problem: (1) the importance of religious meaning to the individual, and (2) religion as a social phenomenon (i.e., the significance of belonging to a church and relating to its members). Research Box 6.1 details this work.

This study shows that many factors may affect the choice to become involved with a church (or other religious institution). Meaning systems and social relationships are both very important and are probably not independent of each other. For example, both may relate to socioeconomic status, education achieved, the nature of the church under consideration, and a host of other sociocultural factors (Roberts & Davidson, 1984). Surprisingly, actual religious beliefs were shown to be least important in this complex array of motivations. In all likelihood, we are witnessing the effects of little variation in beliefs. Those involved in specific churches probably believe quite similarly, showing high agreement in their belief systems. Because this work is basically correlational, low variability works against obtaining the kinds of data (correlation coefficients) that might reveal the significance of reli-

---

ह▲

Research Box 6.1. The Nature and Sources of Religious Involvement
(Roberts & Davidson, 1984)

Seeking to answer the very basic question of why people become involved in their church, Roberts and Davidson studied 577 members of two Methodist and two Baptist churches in relation to four sets of possible predictors of involvement. These were (1) one's personal meaning system, (2) social ties to church members, (3) sociodemographic factors, and (4) religious beliefs. Specifically, these variables were assessed as follows:

Meaning: How one makes sense out of the world—theism, science, nonreligious materialism, social humanism.
Social relations: Connections to other church members, a sense of belonging to the church community.
Demographic factors: Age, gender, socioeconomic status (education, occupation, income), denominational affiliation.
Religious beliefs: Beliefs in existence of God, divinity of Jesus, miracles, virgin birth, life after death.

Using the statistical method of path analysis, Roberts and Davidson observed a complex set of associations among the measures. Meaning and social relations were positively correlated, which suggested that others confirmed and supported one's personal meaning system. These two factors directly contributed most to church involvement. Religious beliefs were weakly and indirectly influential. (One possible major reason for this is presented in the text.) Sociodemographic variables were also indirectly effective, largely through their influence on one's meaning system. Older members and women tended to be most involved, but the important factor was whether a respondent was a member of the liberal (Methodist) or conservative (Baptist) denomination being studied. Overall, meaning and social ties were the big determiners of church involvement. More research of this nature would help us understand further the connections among the predictor variables—in particular, the role of religious and social beliefs.

gious beliefs. This limitation in analysis masks the qualitative and quantitative importance of beliefs. Clearly, liberal churches have members whose views differ from the views of those in conservative churches; however, within each there is probably considerable similarity, and hence little variation.

Utilizing a slightly different theoretical cast, Cornwall (1987) asked two basic questions: "How do adults come to their religious perspectives?" and "What maintains these outlooks?" Her research answer to the first query was religious socialization by family and friends. Once this framework is established, a connection to a "personal community" of like-minded believers supports and strengthens the religious system.

O'Hara (1980) suggests some differences between Protestants and Catholics in why church participation persists from childhood to adult life. For Protestants, the dominant influence is "accommodation," or how one deals with the social pressures exerted by significant others. Second comes meaning or cognition—namely, the degree to which the faith that is embraced resolves basic questions about life, death, God, and the supernatural. Third is socialization—being part of a religious group that has established norms for religious belief and behavior. The order of these factors for Catholics is cognition, accommodation, and lastly socialization. This variation between Catholics and Protestants is probably a function of the historically conditioned practices and beliefs that distinguish these two broad patterns of faith.

The processes of becoming and remaining involved in religion are clearly complex. Sociocultural influences operate on a large scale. Psychologically, we contend that religious behavior, belief, and experience are gratifying to the individual. Basically, religion makes people feel good: It helps resolve conflicts, answers fundamental questions, enhances their sense of control in life, and brings like-minded individuals together. One meta-analysis of 28 studies concluded that among adults, subjective well-being and religion are positively correlated (Witter, Stock, Okun, & Haring, 1985). Apparently religious activity is more important than belief, but both contribute to the sense of self-satisfaction generated by religious participation. These positive feelings probably result from social integration, which, according to Durkheim (1915), makes life more meaningful. Note that in Chapter 3, the evolutionary/genetic theory of religion presented there relies on meaning and social integration as two of the three basic religious motivations. The third, control, could well be a natural development from these two foundations. It should also contribute to them.

Peter Benson (1988a, 1988b), a scholar known for studying the big problems in the psychology of religion, has undertaken extensive research on what he terms "mature faith." This concept has much in common with Allport's Intrinsic religious orientation—namely, a deep religious commitment that includes social sensitivity and "life-affirming values" (Benson, 1988a, p. 16). The latter constitute Saint Thomas Aquinas's classical duties to oneself, others, and God (Spilka, 1970). In mature faith, then, a healthy lifestyle is combined with an appreciation of human welfare, equality, personal responsibility, and what sounds like the role of faith in everyday life.

Utilizing thousands of respondents, Benson found religious maturity to be an outgrowth of literally being steeped in one's faith through family, early religious education, and affiliations throughout life with like-minded others. Maternal and spousal influence (which may be translated into support and reinforcement) also appeared to be central in maintaining strong attachments to religious principles and church doctrines (Benson, 1988b).

We can see that becoming deeply involved with religious institutions has many facets, among which are the need for personal meaning, identification with a like-minded community, and (probably most important of all) a family background and familial ties that stress the pertinence of religious faith to the way life is lived. Undoubtedly, there is room for utilitarian attachments to religion, as Allport's concept of Extrinsic religious orientation conveys.

Apostasy: Leaving the Faith

At the opposite end of the spectrum from involvement is apostasy, disaffiliation, or leaving the faith (which has been discussed in regard to young people in Chapter 5). This has two main facets: A person may join a different church, or may simply reject religion *in toto*, embracing either agnosticism or atheism. When we look at why individuals leave their church, the situation gets even more complicated. One study identified three kinds of "unchurched" Protestants (Perry, Davis, Doyle, & Dyble, 1980). Those regarded as "estranged" and "indifferent" held similar traditional beliefs, but differed in commitment: The latter just became inactive, whereas for the former, religion was no longer salient in their lives. This was also true for "nominal" Protestants, for whom traditional beliefs were irrelevant.

After interviewing respondents in six counties across the United States, Hale (1977) offered a scheme that demonstrates how complex the realm of unchurched individuals actually is. Table 6.6 details this framework. A system such as Hale's begs for rigorous, objective study, for there is a high likelihood that some of these categories overlap and/or may represent personality and social dispositions for which religion is a convenient scapegoat or expression.

Some of these factors are also present in a classificatory scheme for Catholic dropouts that has been proposed by Hoge (1988). There is some overlap with Hale's (1977) framework, but some new (more personal and familial) factors are described in Table 6.7. Hoge also noted that dropout type in his study was a function of age. Those under 23 were mostly in the "family tension" group; adolescent rebellion entered this picture. In contrast, "weary" and "lifestyle" dropouts were commonly found among those older than 23. Problems with faith may well represent personal and social needs that one struggles with in early and middle adulthood.

Simple institutional disaffiliation may occur for a number of reasons, not the least of which is the prevailing influence of secularization in modern society (Nelson, 1988). Some of these are implied in the labels researchers have applied to the various types of "dropouts" and "unchurched" individuals. Many such people remain personally religious, but churches, temples, and synagogues no longer seem relevant to their life in the modern world. Causes for this strain between persons and religious institutions also lie in the considerable level of physical, social, and economic mobility that prevails in much of early and middle adulthood. People are often "too busy" to consider questions of ultimate meaning or to feel the need to relate to a specific religious community. With respect to a wide variety of attitudes and beliefs, those who are religiously disengaged tend to be more liberal than churchgoers on many social, moral, and political issues (Nelson, 1988).

The Possible Role of Education

These observations raise questions about the possible role of education in disaffiliation from institutional religion. This relationship is by no means clear. Though a negative correlation between education and holding orthodox beliefs was found in the 1950s, by the 1980s this association had essentially disappeared (Wuthnow, 1993). Roof (1993) has commented that his baby boomers were exposed to more secular and scientific explanations for various phe-

TABLE 6.6. A Taxonomy of Unchurched Individuals

Unchurched type	Description
Anti-institutionalists	See themselves as truly religious, "better Christians" (Hale, 1977, p. 40).
The boxed-in	Church was too restrictive.
The constrained	Feel limited by doctrinal rules.
The thwarted	Feel suppressed from growing by church insistence on conformity and dependence.
The independents	Independent, nonconformists.
The burned-out	Feel exhausted, drained, emptied.
The used	Feel exploited, worked over.
Light travelers	Feel no need to continue a deep commitment, just "take it easy."
The cop-outs	Never really committed, involved.
The apathetic	Can "take it or leave it."
The drifters	Establish no real attachments.
Happy hedonists	Either utilitarian or leisure-oriented; seek gratification.
The locked-out	Feel rejected or victimized.
The rejected	Feel church has not accepted them.
The neglected	Feel church ignores them.
The discriminated	Feel church is biased against them.
The nomads	Religious vagrants, expect to move on and up; casually attached.
The pilgrims	Seekers and searchers who believe.
The publicans	Self-righteous; feel "better than others." Can't find their "true faith" in church.
The scandalized	See power seekers, factions, and divisiveness in church.
True believers	Hold alternative or antichurch positions.
Agnostics/atheists	Don't know if God exists, or fully reject the idea.
Deists/rationalists	Rely on reason, not revelation.
Humanists/secularists	Committed to human ideals outside of the church.
The uncertain	No reason for nonaffiliation.

Note. Data from Hale (1977).

nomena than earlier generations were. Though these perspectives were found among postgraduates, they do not appear to have adversely affected their belief in God. Roof has noted that "both uncertainty and belief in a higher power are more common among the better educated" (1993, p. 73). Greeley's (2002) multinational study also finds that current university graduates are likely to be theists. Atheistic propensities among these highly educated people have been declining for many years.

TABLE 6.7. Hoge's Classification of Catholic Dropouts

Dropout type	Description
Family tension	Rebellion vs. parents causes rejection of church and family.
Weary	Low religious motivation; church "boring and uninteresting."
Lifestyle	Lifestyle clashes with church's moral position and teachings.
Spiritual needs	These needs not met by church.
Antichange	Oppose church liberalization.
Out-converts after intermarriage	Marriage to a non-Catholic and shift to spouse's faith.

Note. Adapted from Hoge (1988). Copyright 1988 by Sage Publications. Adapted by permission.

In contradiction, Shermer (2000) cites large-sample data (over 2,000 respondents) showing a negative relationship between belief in God for either rational or emotional reasons and education. These results may be statistically significant, but they are rather weak. Other work on a sample of over 12,000 people revealed that the average educational attainment of church members fell 1 year below that of nonmembers (Caplow et al., 1983). Again, one should approach such small differences with caution.

Alternative Possibilities

Albrecht and Bahr (1983) describe some subtleties in the inclinations of those who either leave Mormonism or abandon their original church to become Mormons. Most ex-Mormons drop out of religion altogether; that is, they simply become nonreligious. The next largest group of leavers become Catholics, suggesting that they remain conservative religionists. Most converts to Mormonism come from mainline Protestant bodies, and possess rather orthodox outlooks that the Mormon faith can effectively satisfy.

An interesting hypothesis is offered by Albrecht and Bahr in regard to either dropping out altogether or switching to a new faith. Switching may be seen as more deviant than dropping out. It means going public with a rejection of the previous identification (in this case, Mormonism) in favor of a new group that, by implication, the switcher considers "better." The person who just drops out can be viewed as a "lost soul" who has not found any real alternative. The first action can stimulate hostility; the second, pity by former coreligionists. The dropout may be considered potentially salvageable; the switcher is not. One wonders whether pity might turn to rage and total ostracism if a dropout publicly denies the existence of God. This could add even more insult to injury than switching.

Hadaway (1980), using Gallup Poll data from national samples, also notes that switchers are mostly conservative religious seekers. The motivation to change is frequently associated with a religious experience, particularly among evangelicals. Apparently a period of integration of the meaning of the experience takes place during the process of reaffiliation into a group that values such encounters.

Though we discuss intermarriage in greater detail in Chapter 7, we briefly consider it here as a basis for switching and dropping out. Again there are a number of possibilities. First, religion may be unimportant to two people from different religious backgrounds. If they marry, religion may never be a problem. In many instances, however, the initial unimportance of faith changes for one or both spouses when children enter the family. Individually or together, they may become seekers, like many of the baby boomers. Community and family social pressures relative to religion also frequently enter the picture. U.S. society, with its high level of religiosity, makes independence from a religious or spiritual framework increasingly difficult with the passing years.

The most common intermarriage situation entails one spouse's switching to the faith of the other. Using national data on approximately 8,000 individuals, Musick and Wilson (1995) show least switching for marital reasons among Jews, Baptists, Mormons, and Catholics. The highest switching rates for intermarriage occur among Disciples of Christ, Lutherans, Presbyterians, and members of the United Church of Christ. With regard to the details of switching for marital purposes, Musick and Wilson suggest that liberal religionists tend to affiliate with conservative religious bodies, while conservatives move toward the liberal end of the spectrum. Interestingly, Catholics shift to the no-religion category when marriage is an issue. The need for a more in-depth analysis of factors that relate to marital switching is abundantly evident.

RELIGION AND ELDERLY INDIVIDUALS

It is widely assumed and often stated that people in late adulthood are more religious than their younger peers. This makes eminently good sense, but the data are often equivocal. Can we then say that people become more religious as they age? Despite Freud's and others' theories that the knowledge of death stimulates religious thinking and beliefs, and the fact that elderly people are approaching death, we cannot simply say that increasing age creates a need for faith. The alternative is simply that elderly persons were reared in a time when religion was more widely accepted and taught than it is today.

Some support for this latter position was found in a large-scale study of 11,000 people (Benson & Eklin, 1990). Those respondents aged 60–69 years had, when young, attended church-related or religious schools longer than younger respondents had. The same was true of coming from families in which devotions, Bible reading, and/or prayer were practiced in the home. When this work was undertaken in the late 1980s, these people in their 60s still demonstrated the highest frequencies for reading the Bible and other religious literature, plus engaging in prayer or meditation. Unhappily, the situation in this study was confused by the respondents aged over 70, who did not reveal a similar high level of background religion or current religious activity. Lack of data on this latter sample restricts our understanding of possible influences.

Survey data from different sources sometimes provide information that is difficult to reconcile. According to the U.S. Bureau of the Census (2000), church and synagogue membership increases with age. Sixty-four percent of those 30–49 years old report an institutional affiliation; this increases to 82% for those 65 and older. In contradiction, the GSS (1999) data show no clear pattern of membership with age (see Table 6.8). Still, the United Methodist Church reports that the average age of its members has been increasing for over 40 years (*Christian Century*, 1995). The Presbyterian Church (U.S.A.) further indicates that new members are younger than current members by 7 years (Marcum & Woolever, 1999). In some instances, church membership may be confounded with church attendance. There is reason to believe that the latter declines in old age, as illness and infirmity may make church-going increasingly difficult (Ainlay, Singleton, & Swigert, 1992; Atchley, 1977; Payne, 1988).

This inference may also be questioned, however, as Orbach (1961) found no patterning of age with attendance at services. Other research supports a decline in institutional religious activity, but suggests a corresponding growth in private religious behavior (Brennan & Missinne, 1980).

Table 6.8 illustrates the problem of too readily assuming that the religious beliefs and behavior of elderly individuals can be distinguished from those of younger people. The data in this table run counter to both popular and supposedly informed beliefs about religion among elderly persons. That is, a fairly consistent decline in religious beliefs and activities is evident from the 30s through the 70s. Could it be that the oldest decade sampled here was the least religious because those questioned were the healthiest in their age group, and possibly utilized religion the least? Finney and Lee (1977) have tied increased religiosity to the anxieties of old age. Benson and Eklin (1990) used some items identical to those in the GSS schedule; their oldest respondents likewise showed lower levels of religious activity and weaker beliefs than their younger cohorts did.

By contrast, two classic patterns emerged from a recent Gallup Poll (Gallup & Simons, 2000) when the data were analyzed by sex and age. First, among respondents who were frequent Bible readers, 43% were women and 29% men. Second, Bible reading increased with age in this overall sample, from 27% of those 18–29 years old to 50% of respondents 65 and older.

Given these observations, it appears that the expected pattern of high religiosity among elderly people is supported by the Gallup Poll data, but not by the findings of other researchers who also employed large samples. If we shift to studies of smaller samples, virtually everything is found. Hunsberger (1985) observed increased religiosity in old age. Others have shown essentially no change over many decades in adult life (Blazer & Palmore, 1976; Brennan & Missinne, 1980). Stark (1968) noted increases in belief in life after death with age, but no other evidence of growth in religious feelings. Blazer and Palmore (1976) revealed a decline in church activity, but no change in religious beliefs. Glamser (1987) has suggested

TABLE 6.8. Relationships between Age and Religious Beliefs/Behaviors from the GSS, 1972–1998 (Percentages in Each Age Category)

Belief/behavior	20–29 (%)	30–39 (%)	40–49 (%)	50–59 (%)	60–69 (%)	70–79 (%)
Respondent religiosity[a]	15.5	21.4	22.7	14.7	14.0	11.8
Church activities[b]	15.7	23.4	20.6	9.5	15.9	14.9
Church/synagogue member[b]	19.8	21.8	17.8	10.3	15.6	14.7
Frequency of prayer[c]	16.2	23.6	20.7	15.0	10.3	11.9
No doubt God exists[b]	18.3	24.3	20.0	14.1	12.4	11.0
Belief in miracles[b]	19.4	26.3	20.2	13.8	10.9	9.5
Life after death[b]	19.4	27.3	21.0	12.8	10.4	9.1
Belief in heaven[b]	20.5	26.1	20.1	13.2	10.8	11.4
Belief in hell[b]	20.4	26.9	20.6	12.8	10.6	8.6
Belief in Devil[b]	21.1	26.5	20.0	11.5	11.1	9.9

Note. Data from GSS (1999).

[a]Includes "very high" plus "extremely high" categories.

[b]Response is "yes."

[c]Several times a week or more.

that there may be a tendency for older people to move toward extremes in churchgoing—either to cease attending, or to increase attendance. This possibility needs corroboration. Moberg (1965b) concluded his fine review of this literature by noting that "religion as a set of extradomiciliary rituals apparently increases in old age, while the internal personal responses . . . decrease among religious people" (p. 87).

There is another lesson here about survey research that should be added to our earlier cautions; this also applies to research in general. That is, we need to know in detail how data are collected and from whom. Furthermore, different pollsters and researchers often employ different phrasings in conceptually overlapping questions. The comparability of results may thus become questionable. In addition, variance in age groupings and other demographic categories can be influential.

RELIGIOUS PURPOSES

We have examined the form and content of adult faith, and have suggested motivations for individuals' affiliating themselves with religious institutions, such as achieving meaning and becoming part of a supportive community. Collectively, Monaghan (1967) suggests three basic expressive needs: authority seeking, comfort seeking, and social involvement. Those in the first group want an authority upon whom they can be dependent, and to whom or which they can submit themselves for guidance. For these people, "the minister provides meaning for church members where none existed before" (p. 239). Is it possible that the baby boomers are primarily searching for authorities who offer ultimate meanings? There could, of course, be overlap with Monaghan's second type, in that comfort seekers are also looking for answers, particularly regarding death and its aftermath. It is generally believed that such concerns increase as people age. In contrast, Monaghan's socially involved individuals are really persons for whom the church becomes their life. Religion is primarily relational and interpersonal rather than ideological. This third group may be a rather small one.

Benson and Eklin (1990) speak of "horizontal," "vertical," and "integrated" faith. The first two forms, introduced earlier by Davidson (1972a, 1972b), refer to an orientation toward people or toward God and the supernatural, respectively. When both orientations are strong, one's faith is said to be integrated. Benson and Eklin note that the overall tendency for adults is for a vertical perspective to be dominant. The survey data we have presented in this chapter strongly testify to this stance.

Throughout history, theologians have promulgated doctrines that church and faith should both comfort and challenge believers. The comforting function is abundantly evident when personal tragedy strikes. People turn to their God in times of stress and loss, and clergy translate these circumstances into practices that bring solace to petitioners. Socially, this comforting function maintains the cultural status quo. The social order is not challenged.

Adherence to religious ideals has the potential of questioning and threatening both the individual and society. Becoming a better person may call attention to collective injustice, inequity, and suffering. Individual problems are often transformed into moral, social, economic, and political issues. Public authority and power are defied, and defiance commonly results in confrontation. When such challenge is legitimized by religion, the resulting conflict is especially bitter. Jensen (1989) has illustrated how belief in God and strong religious feelings can eventuate in improved medical care, aid to the needy, environmental action, stress reduction, nonviolent protest, actions to counter racism, and educational reform.

Generally, researchers who have employed fairly large samples to study the comfort–challenge issue in U.S. churches have overwhelmingly come out on the side of their comforting function (Davidson, 1972a, 1972b; Glock, Ringer, & Babbie, 1967). A number of scholars attribute this to religion's largely becoming "a private matter related to personal and family problems more than to social and community problems" (Davidson, 1972b, p. 65). (For more details on Davidson's work, see Chapter 7, Research Box 7.1.)

Even though the evidence is strong that U.S. religion is more concerned with personal comfort and satisfaction than with humanistic action, we will see in Chapter 13 on morality that there is a large potential for constructive and challenging social involvement.

OVERVIEW

In this chapter we have examined the content of adult faith, primarily stressing the U.S. situation. Through some international comparisons, it is evident that the United States is one of the most religious nations in the West. The faith of adults is by no means a simple affair. It frequently involves personal and social struggles. First, there is a need to bring meaning into one's life, to gain some insight into ultimate questions and issues, and to understand basic truths. Concurrently, adulthood confronts people with the tasks of relating to others and becoming part of a compatible community. Institutional religion offers pathways to solve both the personal and the social problems with which thoughtful adulthood is concerned. As Roof's (1993) research well illustrates, seeking satisfying answers often involves disaffiliation from churches or synagogues and a search for new anchors. Sometimes this occasions rejection of religion; more often, shifts to a new and more conservative stance occur. Not infrequently, there is a return to the faith in which one was reared. All possibilities are found, leading us to an awareness that we need to know much more about the psychology of seekers.

Demographic factors such as gender, age, and education enter the picture, but again answers are elusive. Theories are offered to explain why women find religion more congenial than men; these directions range from biology to culture. Definitive tests of such possibilities are lacking, however. Large-scale surveys from different sources often disagree because of methodological problems that need to be resolved.

Stereotypes about the association of religion with old age abound, but the assumptions that prevail do not find much support. Simplistic thinking is challenged at every turn.

Research on the role of religion for the individual shows that it is primarily directed at personal comfort and utilitarian goals, rather than at resolving sociocultural problems and issues.

The real meaning of adult religion may be found in the roles and functions of faith in other realms of life than just the religious. We look at these in Chapter 7.

Chapter 7

THE ROLES AND FUNCTIONS
OF RELIGION IN ADULT LIFE

> Therefore all things whatsoever ye would that men should do to you, do ye even so to them.
>
> Going to church doesn't make you a Christian any more than going to a garage makes you a mechanic.
>
> They that work not cannot pray.
>
> For as the body without the spirit is dead, so faith without works is dead also.
>
> God gives us love. Something to love He lends us.
>
> It is better to marry than to burn.
>
> My pollertics, like my religion, being of an exceedin accomodatin character.[1]

HOW ADULTS ARE INFLUENCED BY RELIGION

From both a psychological and a religious/spiritual perspective, the true meaning of faith is to be found in its consequences. We may therefore ask, "Does personal religion affect other aspects of life besides how one behaves religiously?" Our concern is to look for correlates and consequences of one's faith in the realms of personal, social, economic, and political life. Basically, we want to know whether religion influences how people regard and treat each other. This obviously takes us into such matters as morality and social adjustment—topics that will be treated later in this book (see Chapters 13 and 15).

According to Alfred Adler (1935), there are three great basic problems of adult life: "problems of behavior toward others; problems of occupation; and problems of love. The manner in which an individual handles these three problems, and their subdivisions—that is his answer to the problems of life" (p. 6). In a similar vein, Erik Erikson (1968) quoted Freud to the effect that a normal person should be able to do two things well—"*Lieben und Arbeiten*" (to love and to work) (p. 136). In this chapter we discuss Adler's three realms, and add a fourth one: politics.

---

1. These quotations come, respectively, from the following sources: Matthew 7:12; Anonymous, on the Internet (2000); Anonymous, quoted in Bartlett (1955, p. 583); James 2:26; Tennyson (1899, p. 77); I Corinthians 7:9; and Artemus Ward, quoted in Cohen & Cohen (1960, p. 409).

RELIGION AND SOCIAL RELATIONSHIPS

Adler's "problems of behavior toward others" covers an immense territory. Even though he may have been exclusively concerned with interpersonal relationships, this is really only one aspect of how people deal with others. Individuals also relate themselves to groups and to institutions.

Research suggests that religion performs many functions for people. Basically, these can be encapsulated in two categories: personal and social consequences. Before we examine the specifics of religion in social life, let us look at the insightful pioneering work of Davidson (1972a, 1972b), which is presented in Research Box 7.1.

Given the findings of Davidson (1972a, 1972b), let us turn first to religion and how we deal with others. Psychologists have studied interpersonal trust and faith in people (Bahr &

Research Box 7.1. Religious Belief as an Independent Variable (Davidson, 1972a, 1972b)

Recognizing that research on the consequences of religion often fails to distinguish among different types of religious beliefs, and also among the possible outcomes of holding these perspectives, Davidson decided to specify these domains in an exacting manner.

For his research, Davidson constructed questionnaires to assess "vertical beliefs" (religious other-worldly and supernatural beliefs), (2) "horizontal beliefs" (this-worldly social relationships), (3) "personal consequences" (the individual comforts and satisfactions people derive from their faith), and (4) "social consequences" (the community-oriented behavioral responses in which people engage). These questionnaires were administered to a total of 577 respondents from two Baptist and two Methodist churches. In each denomination, one church was primarily middle- to upper-class; the other was primarily lower-middle-class to working-class.

Scores on these scales defined four groups of believers: (1) "true believers" (those who scored high on both vertical and horizontal beliefs), (2) "mainliners" (those scoring in the moderate, middle range on both belief measures); (3) "fundamentalists" (those scoring high on vertical beliefs and low on horizontal beliefs); and (4) "humanists" (those scoring low on vertical beliefs and high on horizontal beliefs). An "unbeliever" category denoted those with moderate or low scores on both kinds of beliefs.

Vertical beliefs correlated negatively with the index of social consequences and positively with the index of personal consequences. Horizontal beliefs were associated with personal consequences in a more complex manner: In the low and moderate vertical belief categories, horizontal beliefs were tied positively to personal consequences, but in the high group, horizontal beliefs related negatively to personal consequences.

Most of the sample—in particular, fundamentalists, mainliners, and true believers—stressed the personal consequences of their beliefs. The humanists and unbelievers were moderate in the personal consequences realm, and fell mostly in the moderate and high categories of social consequences, whereas true believers, mainliners, and fundamentalists manifested low leanings toward social consequences. Davidson concluded that "religion today is oriented to personal and family matters more than it is oriented to social and community problems" (1972a, p. 74).

Martin, 1983), the breadth of one's social perspectives (Black, 1985; Lupfer & Wald, 1985), forgiveness (McCullough, Pargament, & Thoreson, 2000), intolerance toward patients with AIDS (Johnson, 1987), and interpersonal conflict (Pratt, Hunsberger, Pancer, & Roth, 1992), among other possibilities. Much of this work is treated in Chapter 13. For our present purposes, let us first look at a matter central to most faiths—forgiveness.

Forgiveness

Though religions may ideally make much of forgiveness, the concept encounters a classic problem—namely, the discrepancy between the word and and its realization in action. Forgiveness is most likely to apply to believers of religious systems, not to nonbelievers, to outgroup members, or to "alien" others. Throughout their history, Christians have practiced discrimination against those who have been different (variously, those denoted as heretics, pagans, or Jews). The religiously committed in many faiths have also enslaved outsiders or even backed inhumane indentured servitude of their own coreligionists. Forgiveness on the part of either the perpetrators or victims of such inhumanity has invariably been considered irrelevant. Frequently, with the approval of church authorities, deviation from religious norms has been treated as unforgivable sin, resulting in disenfranchisement, exile, torture, and murder (Bennett, 1966; Flannery, 1985; Quinley & Glock, 1979). Nevertheless, enlightenment, understanding, and forgiveness are extolled as virtues.

When we view forgiveness as an individual matter, it is regarded positively. Local churches and religious groups are perceived as aiding people to practice forgiveness, specifically through prayer, Bible study, and interpersonal sharing. The real key is the degree of emphasis placed on forgiveness in the religious setting. Its effects cover a broad range of social and self-improvement possibilities (Wuthnow, 2000). Forgiveness is favorably associated with countering guilt, providing support when one is depressed, helping to overcome bad habits and addictions, and increasing participation in voluntary activities for social and religious betterment.

Pargament and Rye (1998) conceptualize forgiveness as a form of transformational coping. One transforms both the methods one uses to attain goals and the goals that are sought. The end is peace, not simply rehearsing the pain and injustice that has been perpetrated on the victim. Anger and the sense of injury must be put aside. The situation must be reframed and understood differently. The offender is now seen in a new light—with empathy, and as human. Religion offers the teachings and resources to accomplish these ends. Spiritual figures such as Jesus may serve as examples for guidance and perceiving the problem with a constructive outlook.

One study of forgiveness among elderly Christians shows that the process of forgiveness is far from simple (Krause & Ingersoll-Dayton, 2001). Christianity may recommend unconditional forgiveness, but this message is qualified in a variety of ways. Selective cognitive processing often causes the notion of automatic forgiveness to drop out of the picture. Apparently the nature of the transgression implies the ease or difficulty of forgiving. The attitude and behavior of the wrongdoer is then considered. Other questions are implicitly present: Is the offender contrite and remorseful? Has an apology been tendered? Has an effort been made to effect restitution? Is the offender even aware of having committed an offense? One also wants to know whether the transgressor is a relative, friend, or stranger. Finally, the involvement of clergy or one's religious peers may affect the forgiveness process. In short, forgiveness is by no means easily conceived or undertaken.

A number of studies have found a positive relationship between religious beliefs and activity on the one hand, and the degree to which forgiving is valued on the other. Since these involve self-report measures, they limit us to the position that those who are religious know that forgiveness is an important aspect of faith, and *should* be highly regarded (McCullough & Worthington, 1999). In a rather sophisticated study, Gorsuch and Hao (1993) found that religious devotion is associated with the desire to forgive, whereas religious conformity is not. Self-report is still a potential influence, but this distinction could imply that personal commitment or devotion to one's faith is what really counts. On another dimension, there are indications that religious people also think and reason more about forgiveness than their less religious peers do (Enright, Santos, & Al-Mabuk, 1989). This sounds like what one would expect of those who are personally committed, as opposed to those who are simply conforming.

Even though the limited research data available on religion and forgiveness suggest a meaningful relationship, the distinction between personal involvement and social conformity needs to be explored with regard to the actual *practice* of forgiveness, not its social desirability, conformity, and self-serving verbal possibilities. A factor that may be overlooked in these relationships concerns the relatively weak ties between forgiveness and faith that have so far been demonstrated (McCullough & Worthington, 1999). These considerations have caused researchers to focus on measurement issues that have yet to be resolved. At present, there is more theory than substantive data in this area.

Another possibility that has been raised in the literature is that forgiveness is linked with better physical health. According to Thoresen, Harris, and Luskin (2000), "no evidence is available that forgiveness is associated with positive health outcomes" (p. 257). Witvliet and Ludwig (1999), however, report that forgiveness is related to reduced anger, fear, and sadness; lower diastolic blood pressure; lower mean arterial pressure; and reduced sweating. All of these effects are tied to health. The need for more research on this topic is abundantly clear.

Additional hints on the significance of forgiveness come from the work of pastoral counselors and therapists. In their practice, forgiveness is viewed as a possible antidote to destructive guilt. Psychological well-being is thus considered an outgrowth of the process of forgiving (McCullough et al., 2000; Paloma & Gallup, 1991). The pastoral experience of Patton (2000) has led him to believe that forgiveness reduces shame on the part of those who have been unjustly treated. He feels that it also allows victims to broaden their perspectives and see similarities between themselves and wrongdoers. Emmons (2000) supports this notion of links among forgiveness; personality integration; and positive relationships to oneself, others, and God. There is a wealth of research possibilities in these ideas.

Trust

There are few more important interpersonal necessities than trust. It appears to be founded in evolution and biology, and among humans its roots have been traced to the initial relationship between the mother or initial caregiver and the infant (Ainsworth, 1982; Bateson, 1988; Bowlby, 1969). Trust is also regarded as the foundation on which cooperative behaviors and social relations are premised, including those underlying institutional economics and politics (Gambetta, 1988; Good, 1988).

Attachment is the core concept here. The desired goal is secure attachment, which Myers (1998) asserts "nurtures social competence" (p. 98). Data support such an inference (Weiss, 1982). Lack of trust nourishes conflict on all levels from the interpersonal to the societal. The child's earliest attachment to the mother or the first caregiver is followed by many other attachments (to children, adults, peers, lovers, spouses, etc.), and as Kirkpatrick (1992) has clearly pointed out, God is a significant attachment figure for a great many people. Kirkpatrick notes that Jesus, Mary, the saints, the angels, and other supernatural beings may serve similar functions. Such attachment figures represent security and safety, as parents did when children were young.

On the average, secure infant and childhood attachments relate positively to secure attachments in adulthood (Waters & Cummings, 2000; Weiss, 1982). This finding may be extended to images of God. That is, a secure early attachment base is associated favorably with faith in self, others, and the deity; this pattern holds from the individual to the societal level (Benson & Spilka, 1973; Kirkpatrick, 1992). Phrased differently, trust is a correlate of secure attachment. We often hear religious people advising others to "trust in God." In U.S. culture, the assumed universality of this theme is illustrated by the phrase "In God we trust" on the nation's coins. Kirkpatrick (1992) shows how prevalent the theme of secure attachment is in the images of God that prevail in our society. These same personal protective, helpful, and loving concepts imply the basic trust that a secure attachment conveys throughout life.

We might assume that religious people accept these trusting images of God and apply them to their views of others. In support of this hypothesis, Schoenfeld (1978) related church attendance to increased trust in people. There is, however, other work indicating that this may not be true for extremely conservative, fundamentalist, and Pentecostal groups. Their view is that people are primarily sinners, and hence cannot be trusted (Ostow, 1990).

Trust is also implicit in the notion of a "just world" (Lerner, 1980). According to this concept, justice underlies existence, and so "people get what they deserve." In other words, things will always work out in a just and fair manner. Because religion fosters such an assumption, we can expect belief in a just world to correlate positively with religious faith, and indeed it does (Lerner, 1980). The more important faith is to people, the more they feel that suffering is justified and/or that a good person will eventually be rewarded (either in this existence or in an afterlife). This outlook is especially true among poor fundamentalists, whose religion teaches that justice will ultimately prevail, that their merits will be recognized, and that ultimate happiness awaits them (Lerner, 1980). The poet Robert Browning (1841/1895) put this concept well: "God's in his heaven—All's right with the world!"

Social Integration and Concern

Forgiveness and trust are basic elements of interpersonal relations that have deep roots in religion. Many other aspects of interpersonal behavior can be subsumed under such major issues as morality and coping behavior; these will be dealt with in later chapters. We also need to recognize that religion integrates people into society and teaches them to be concerned with the welfare of their fellow humans (although, unhappily, it can also be a source of conflict with others).

Charitable and voluntaristic behavior are integral to Christianity, Islam, Judaism, and other world religions. In the United States, aiding others economically has a strong grip on the collective conscience. In 1998, 45.2% of U.S. households contributed an average of $1,002 to charitable causes (U.S. Bureau of the Census, 2000). Over half of the population was engaged in at least one volunteer activity, while almost one-quarter volunteered to realize religious aims (U.S. Bureau of the Census, 2000). Financially, the amounts contributed to religious causes alone were prodigious, exceeding $75 billion.

The available data show that devout individuals are more concerned than their less religiously involved peers about the relationship of money to spiritual issues (Wuthnow, 1994). Wuthnow further points out that religious people justify wealth by associating it with hard work, generosity, charity, and helping others. This view is realized in church giving, where the main predictors are a strong religious commitment, theological conservatism, and church involvement (Donahue, 1994; Hoge & Yang, 1994). Insofar as intrinsic religiosity implies a committed religious perspective, it may well be a significant element in making religious donations. This perspective combines two orientations—strong personal religious involvement, and social awareness and sensitivity. This is seen clearly in Research Box 7.2, which briefly overviews the important work of Davidson and Pyle (1994).

What about volunteering for non-church-related activities in a local community? Some investigators claim that religion per se relates positively to such involvement; further research identifies the critical variable as participation in church activities (Park & Smith, 2000). Involvement in a church may represent a broader inclination to gain satisfaction from working with and contributing to others.

Our treatment of religion in relation to Adler's (1935) life task of "behavior toward others" clearly shows a meaningful pattern of associations. Religion is positively affiliated with forgiveness, trust, and social integration/concern in the broad sense of personal and financial contributions to both one's church and community. Still, the possible differential roles of the various forms of personal faith in these relationships need to be specified. Also, most of the research reported to date has been sociologically stimulated; the need is to evaluate further the place of psychological factors.

RELIGION, WORK, AND OCCUPATION

Achievement Motivation and the Desire to Succeed

The Protestant Work Ethic

> Waste of time is thus the first and deadliest of sins. . . . Loss of time through sociability, idle talk, luxury, even more sleep than is necessary for health . . . is worthy of absolute moral condemnation. . . . it is at the expense of one's daily work. (Weber, 1904/1930, pp. 157–158)

Although this Calvinist theme on the value of work and labor may seem a bit extreme by today's standards, the notion is well embedded in Western civilization. Labor and good works are regarded as inseparable. Historically, they have also been considered indispensable to personal salvation and success, as well as to the rise of the capitalist economic order (Rotenberg, 1978; Tawney, 1926).

Collectively, all of the characteristics cited above constitute what has become known as the "Protestant ethic" or, more specifically, the "Protestant work ethic" (hereafter abbreviated as PWE) (Furnham, 1990). Mueller (1978) has suggested a Catholic ethic that values "a steady state economy and society . . . cooperation, security, and authority" (p. 143), and hence support for the status quo. This may in part explain the relatively low achievement of Catholics in North America (Riccio, 1979; Stark, 1998), although this condition has been changing over the past 50 years (Porterfield, 2001; Roof & McKinney, 1987). A precursor to this change was offered by Greeley (1963), who found that Catholics and Protestants share similar economic aspirations.

ざ

**Research Box 7.2. Passing the Plate in Affluent Churches:
Why Some Members Give More than Others (Davidson & Pyle, 1994)**

Studying financial giving in a number of affluent churches in northeastern Kansas, the researchers tested two theoretical views: "social exchange" and "symbolic interactionism." The former stresses donations as a function of benefits to be gained in relation to costs; the latter looks at religious self-concepts and beliefs. Three independent variables were defined: "benefit orientation," "intrinsic religiosity," and "belief orientation." The dependent variable was the amount given to the church.

The biggest direct contributors to giving were income and participation. Since the details of this work are quite complex, we may briefly note that neither the benefits and costs per se, nor the beliefs by themselves, were primary independent predictors of giving. Participation and intrinsic religiosity, representing a linking of social exchange and symbolic interactionism, were both operative. Future research must therefore consider relationships between these frameworks and church giving.

Achievement Motivation and Occupational Success in Different Religious Groups

Underlying work and labor, in the perspective of the PWE, is the motivation to achieve. This has three components: activism, individualism, and a futuristic orientation (Riccio, 1979). A strong institutionally centered faith such as Catholicism is theorized to counter activism and individualism. In contrast, the history of Protestantism suggests the opposite, with the PWE spurring capitalism and individual strivings in all areas (Rosen, 1950; Tawney, 1926).

Judaism has no source of central control, and certainly no direct PWE influence. Even though local religious enforcement through Jewish families might have been stronger in the past than it is today, formal Talmudic learning has always stressed debate and argument, with the potential of new discovery. The scholar has thus been highly valued. Discrimination against Jews has also fostered action to escape the restrictions of prejudice, and secular intellectual achievement has paralleled religious knowledge in importance.

The need for freedom from bigotry and oppression stimulated Jewish immigration from Europe to North America. The United States in particular offered many opportunities, including education; Jews often gravitated toward security-enhancing professions such as medicine and law (Gorelick, 1981). New chances to succeed in business were rapidly adopted. Jewish families now saw learning and higher education as avenues to honor and economic success, and strongly inculcated achievement values in their children (McClelland, 1961).

Independence training of children in the home is a positive correlate of achievement motivation, and Rosen (1950) has shown earlier independence training among Protestants and Jews than among Catholics. He also found that independence training and achievement motivation go together, further supporting the underpinnings of the PWE. This is also realized in the vocational aspirations of Jewish and Protestant mothers for their children. The occupational goals selected by both groups are higher than those chosen by Catholics. In other words, until the late 20th century, Catholic mothers were more satisfied with lower-status occupations that offered stability and job security for their children than their Jewish and Protestant counterparts were (McClelland, 1961).

Lenski (1963) and Mayer and Sharp (1962) took the next step and compared religious groups in terms of socioeconomic status, using measures of income, self-employment, occupational positions, and education, among other associated variables. The patterns they found were in harmony with the findings of Rosen (1950): Jews and Protestants exceeded Roman Catholics in all of these indicators. Bronson and Meadow (1968) reported a similar finding when Catholic and Protestant Mexican Americans were studied; the latter also revealed higher achievement needs than the former. A review of such studies by Riccio (1979) showed that the majority of U.S. adults at that time supported the PWE; however, its acceptance was higher among Protestants and Jews than among Catholics.

Changes over Time in Achievement Motivation?

Considering the many changes that have occurred in North American society in the last three decades, there is a need for further comparative testing of religious groups. Riccio also concluded that the situation even in 1979 was far more complex than a surface perusal of this research would suggest. He felt that "these studies were plagued by serious conceptual and methodological deficiencies" (p. 226). Finally, though this research also needs updating and correction, Blackwood (1979) offered data showing a sharp decline in favorable attitudes toward the PWE between 1958 and 1971. This decline may have caused religious group differences to begin disappearing. Such findings could reflect the disruption and protest that prevailed in the Vietnam era (the 1960s and early 1970s). By the 1980s, a conservative calm had returned. In a more recent study, Wuthnow (1993) observed that hours spent working had increased while leisure time had decreased.

Furnham (1990) has examined the issue of change over time in the PWE, and found that arguments and conflicting data exist: Different studies contend that the PWE either hasn't really changed, has possibly weakened, or in some instances has actually strengthened in recent years. Problems of when, where, and how change has been measured cloud the picture. As is so often true, we must await more and better research before definitive answers are available.

When Is Work Considered a "Calling"?

A rather basic empirical question regarding the relationship of religion to work has been asked by Davidson and Caddell (1994). One assumption of the PWE is that work is not simply a career, but possesses religious significance and is therefore a "calling." Studying 1,869 respondents from 31 Catholic and Protestant congregations, these scholars found that about 15% of their sample did consider work a "calling." Overwhelmingly, however, secular cost and benefit factors dominated in how respondents viewed their own labor and occupation. Davidson and Caddell concluded that interpreting work religiously is most likely to occur when people are strongly committed, indicating that they are personally intrinsically religiously oriented. Such a perspective infuses all aspects of life with religious and spiritual significance, including work.

The Phenomenon of Jewish Achievement

As noted previously, Jews found that many new opportunities were open to them when they left Europe and came to North America. Again, their heritage had nothing to do with the PWE; in the "old country," achievement for most Jews meant the gaining of religious knowledge and then occupational success. In discussing the small Jewish communities of Eastern Europe, Zborowski and Herzog (1952) noted that "A Jewish community without a center of learning is unthinkable" (p. 71). This tendency translated well to the North American milieu. A Jewish subculture that adapted Old World values regarding knowledge and education to the New World environment now developed. If anything, the greater chances for advancement strongly reinforced family pressures to inculcate achievement motivation in children (Greenberg, 1960). The result is well stated by Stark (1998): "The Jews rapidly became the most highly educated group in North America . . . and have the highest average family income of any racial, religious or ethnic group" (p. 298). Stark notes, furthermore, that male Jews are overrepresented in the professions and among managers and proprietors, whereas they are underrepresented in blue-collar occupations.

Concurrently, a disproportionately high number of Jews have come to the forefront of North American society. For example, a study of the 1974–1975 edition of *Who's Who in America* revealed that Jews had a rate of inclusion two and a half times higher than expected for the overall population (Silberman, 1985). More recent work, on the 1992–1993 edition of *Who's Who*, indicates that this incidence increased for Jews to over four times their numbers in the United States; between 1930 and 1992, the percentage of Jews in *Who's Who* increased over 900% (Davidson, Pyle, & Reyes, 1995). Study after study further reveals the presence of Jews among the intellectual elite at 4 to 10 or more times their percentage in the U.S. population, the latter being less than 3% (Silberman, 1985). Similarly, among Nobel laureates, Jewish percentages have been for some time in the 30–40% range (Levitan, 1960). A strong attraction of Jews toward the sciences has been observed among applicants for the Westinghouse Science Talent Search (Datta, 1967), and Stark (1963) also noted that the percentage of Jews in arts and sciences graduate programs was three times greater than their presence in the general population.

In a society as complex as ours, explaining the continuing level of Jewish achievement in a number of areas requires more than the bare-bones theory presented above. Statistical analyses confirm that "the traditional emphasis on education among Jews is a dominant factor in their occupational and income levels" (Homola, Knudsen, & Marshall, 1987, p. 201). To explain this pattern further, a number of theoretical possibilities have been advanced (Stark, 1998). The dominant view stresses Jewish cultural norms in Europe that emphasized scholarship and intellectual achievement. These norms were easily transferred to America, and there stimulated educational and economic advancement. Another position with some support claims that the Jews who immigrated to North America, though they may have been poor, had worked in high status occupations in their largely eastern European societies. In other words, relative to other immigrant groups such as Italians, the Jews brought their greater sense of success and higher status with them from home. Stark (1998) also discusses research showing that a higher proportion of Jews than of other immigrants became self-employed and conveyed the individualistic values of personal achievement and success to their offspring. However, understanding religious, social, and familial factors that may have been significant 50–150 years ago is not enough. Again, research needs to be done today on the current generation and its immediate forebears.

Integrating Religion and Work

Religion and Vocational Choice

Koltko (1993) has proposed a theory that religious values may influence vocational choice. This may seem obvious when one decides to enter the ministry or a religiously related profession (see "Religion as a Profession," below). The question is whether religious values may be part of the background that spurs one to select certain interests and avoid others, thus affecting one's eventual choice of an occupation/profession. Koltko has selected four dimensions of religion as crucial in the process leading to vocational selection. These are belief structures (theology); the history of the religious group studied; its social structure and socialization (religious practices, organization); and lifespan milestones (standardized practices relative to life events).

Unfortunately, these rather interesting directions for research do not appear to have been taken up by psychologists of religion. Wuthnow (1994) points out that we really know very little about how people in the United States integrate their rather strong religious beliefs with their equally firm economic motivations. His impressive survey reveals that even though religion's role in U.S. economic life is muted, as a background variable it nevertheless exerts a subtle influence. For example, Calvinistic/Puritan ideas counsel morality in business dealings. Likewise, appeals to thrift and economic advantage probably find responsive ears, as they are purveyed in advertisements by banks, investment firms, stock brokers, insurance agencies, and other financial "movers and shakers."

When asked directly about the role of religion in choosing a job, about 22% of Wuthnow's (1994) sample felt that their faith might have been operative in their decision. A comparison of churchgoers with the total labor force on a wide variety of characteristics revealed none that really distinguished these two groups. With regard to their sense of personal worth, churchgoers placed considerably more weight on their relation to God than was found in the overall labor force. Slight differences showed churchgoers favoring familial, social, moral, and community values over personal pleasure and gain. These tendencies are in line with research revealing that intrinsic/committed leanings are associated positively with social, altruistic, and religious values. As Wuthnow (1994) theorized, those who subscribe to a utilitarian/extrinsic/consensual faith orientation are more concerned with status, materialism, achievement, income, and security (see also Spilka, 1977). The classical Calvinistic view that hard labor is pleasing to God still prevails; Wuthnow (1994) found that 53% of the total work force and 68% of weekly churchgoers affirmed this view.

Given the foregoing, one might reasonably ask about ties between religiosity and job satisfaction. Validating earlier research, Wuthnow (1994) found that religiosity was positively correlated with job satisfaction. He has suggested that religious beliefs and activities might also reduce job stress. From his data as a whole, it appears that faith endows work with meaning, and constructively helps integrate work into one's life.

Religion, Science, and Scholarship

A fair amount of work has been done on the religion of scientists. Some suggestive directions have also been identified for psychologists. Hardy's (1974) study of U.S. scholars and scientists distinguished religious groups and religious types. With regard to groups, he identified Unitarians, Quakers (Friends), and secularized Jews as "highly productive." Roman Catholics were categorized as exhibiting "very low productivity." Southern Protestants in general, Disciples of Christ, and Lutherans were said to be low in productivity. Hardy's notion of religious types provided a more inclusive perspective, with liberal, secularized Protestants and Jews being described as most productive, and fundamentalists and conservative Protestants being characterized as low in productivity. In Hardy's work, "productivity" appeared synonymous with "intellectuality"—namely, generating inventions, making discoveries, writing books and other professional publications, and engaging in other activities.

Religious belief in relation to science takes an interesting turn when we go back to a study by Leuba (1934). This revealed that physical scientists believed most strongly in God and an afterlife; next came biologists, with sociologists showing less belief, and psychologists showing the least acceptance. Apparently, as one gets closer to understanding the mental lives of people, it may become more and more difficult to maintain religious outlooks. Of course, we do not know whether the psychological study of religion counters a religious stance, or whether those who enter psychology are initially low in religious feelings. Still, Beit-Hallahmi (1977) has claimed that "Most psychologists of religion are religious" (p. 388). In a succeeding study comparing different kinds of psychologists, this position was partially confirmed (Ragan, Malony, & Beit-Hallahmi, 1980). Nevertheless, psychologists of religion were not found to be more religious than their fellow psychologists who did not study religion. Overall, psychologists are generally low in religiosity. Leuba did note that the numbers holding religious views declined between 1914 and 1933; though he showed this for his time, new research needs to assess this trend for today.

Religion and Ethics in the Workplace

Continuing his examination of the potential influence of religion in work settings, Wuthnow (1994) examined the possible role of ethics and found a number of differences that were related to faith commitments. In defining what work ethics entail, weekly churchgoers were more likely than the work force in general to stress honesty and fairness. There was also a tendency to see such concerns in a more absolutist than relativistic manner. With regard to making major work decisions, moral absolutism was again present, along with a theistically premised moralism and altruism. These inclinations countered an individualistic utilitarianism. In other words, Wuthnow's respondents felt that personal desires and benefits should give way to religious and humanitarian considerations. They also felt that moral concerns take precedence over individual ones; hence those who subscribe to absolutist moral and theistic perspectives were likely to adhere to ethical rules and regulations in the workplace. These positions were held most strongly by persons who were affiliated with religious fellowship groups, again revealing the behind-the-scenes role of religious involvements.

In summary, even though Wuthnow's (1994) work is generally in line with Koltko's (1993) recommendations, data on the specifics of the four dimensions identified by Koltko (see "Religion and Vocational Choice," above) is still lacking.

Social Change and New Considerations

The 20th century witnessed almost unbelievable events and developments in all aspects of life, and religion has not escaped these changes. In order to assess contemporary religious and spiritual views in relation to work, the impressive studies of Roof (1993) and Wuthnow (1993, 1994) may be considered models that require follow-up. Similar work detailing the beliefs of scientists is again necessary. We must keep in mind that beliefs in God and an afterlife can take many forms, so simplistic assumptions and generalizations about what highly intelligent and intellectually sophisticated individuals believe cannot be made lightly.

Much has been made of the role of socioeconomic status for understanding how vocation relates to religion (Roberts, 1984). Religious groups have frequently been ordered along status lines, and findings from the 1980s and later place Episcopalians, Congregationalists, Presbyterians, and Jews at the top, and Baptists, other Protestants, and sectarian groups at the bottom. Catholics have slowly been moving up the economic ladder (Porterfield, 2001; Roberts, 1984; Roof & McKinney, 1987). For our purposes in understanding the relationship of work to religion, socioeconomic status adds little, since we have looked at occupation and education (both of which correlate highly with income), and these same criteria denote socioeconomic status.

As noted earlier, Koltko's (1993) interesting theory has not been very thoroughly investigated to date. We have noted what might be termed broad social-structural variables, but possible psychological ties between vocation and religion have yet to be studied. There can, however, be no doubt about such connections when we look at religious careers in particular.

Religion as a Profession

The relationship between religion and work finds its fullest expression in the lives of those who dedicate themselves to their faith. There is little place in the modern world for idyllic images of the clergy. Seminarians and other aspirants with high hopes must eventually confront the many difficulties that plague the contemporary world. Rather than being above the fray, most clergy are participants in a struggle to aid their congregants, realize their spiritual ideals, and maintain decent lives for themselves.

A great deal of research has been conducted on religious professionals. Over 40 years ago, Dittes (1962) observed that most of this work focused on the Christian ministry. A few years later, Menges and Dittes (1965) annotated approximately 700 psychological research studies on clergy. Detailing this work further, Dittes (1971b) reviewed the literature and confirmed his earlier judgment (Dittes, 1962) that this sphere was plagued by a lack of organizing theory plus serious methodological problems. An increasing level of theoretical and research sophistication has been manifested from the 1970s on, even though the perennial problem of scattered studies still troubles students of the area.

Much energy has been expended on the mental health of seminarians and clergy, but the literature is confusing. One can make a case for a fair amount of mental disorder, or can suggest that many of the findings are attributable either to the stressful demands of the profession, or the inappropriateness or psychometric defects of the measures themselves (Dittes, 1971b). Again, one confronts the issue of methodology, in addition to the view that there is little to be gained from isolated studies on clerics with varying specialties in specific groups in certain geographic areas. The current need is to understand clerical effectiveness and coping efforts in the variety of functions that clergy perform.

Why Become a Religious Professional?

Dittes (1971b) suggested a "little adult" theory as directing individuals toward becoming clergy. Basically psychoanalytic in nature, this theory posits a continuation of childhood and adolescent roles in which approval and dependency needs are expressed by becoming a religious professional. Unfortunately, there is a dearth of research supporting this view.

Well over 40 years ago, the Ministry Studies Board of the National Council of Churches produced the Theological School Inventory (TSI), which assessed personal motives for becoming a minister (Kling, 1958, 1959). Two patterns were identified: "special leading" and "natural leading." Though both are grounded in the seeker's faith, special leading involves the perception of being "chosen" by God for a religious profession. In contrast, natural leading emphasizes issues of personal and social identity in order to meet the religious, spiritual, and psychosocial needs of oneself and others. In a rather rigorous study of preseminary college students, however, Embree (1964; Embree, Spilka, & Horn, 1968) explored a variety of religious variables and found the distinction between natural leading and special leading to be a weak contributor to motivation to enter the ministry.

One variation of this search is to determine whether there might be personality factors that dispose one to become a cleric. A plethora of older uncoordinated and isolated efforts largely imply that various personality inadequacies and shortcomings direct one to seek a clerical career (Meissner, 1961; Menges & Dittes, 1965; Summerlin, 1980). Much of this work is simplistic and questionable.

More recently, Francis and his colleagues (Francis, Jones, Jackson & Robbins, 2001) have asked whether the well-known inclination of females to be more religious than males might not provide a clue about the personality of Anglican clerics. Using the widely studied Eysenck Personality Profile, these researchers compared over 1,100 Anglican male clergy with the norms for males and females, and observed that the clerics showed a "feminine" profile on 16 of the 21 scales. The meaning of this gender orientation, particularly in terms of development, needs to be clarified.

The work of Embree, Francis, and their respective associates suggests a need to understand more fully what selective factors are active in directing individuals to become clergy. Programmatic research based on theory is essential. We hope that Francis et al. (2001) have begun a project that may counter the older scattered and often conflicting studies, which pose a dilemma for workers in this area.

The Effectiveness of Clergy

When we look closely at the duties and responsibilities of clergy, it is surprising to realize how complex they are, and therefore how much we are asking ministers, priests, and rabbis to do. Table 7.1 summarizes the roles identified and studied by two different research efforts.

Different theoretical emphases, measuring instruments, and statistical analyses result in some variation between the two approaches in Table 7.1. Each of the effectiveness factors listed in the table is further defined by those who evaluate the roles and functions of clergy. As can be seen, vocationally, the profession has many varied facets. Overviewing ministerial effectiveness research, Nauss (1996) suggested the possibility of using 65 variables; examining five inventories that were constructed using cluster or factor analysis, Nauss eventually identified 56 dimensions of ministerial effectiveness. Schuller (1980) found some 64 clusters of traits and behaviors that may be subsumed under the two frameworks presented in Table 7.1. Though each is further specified by a variety of subfactors, different religious groups evidence different degrees of emphasis on the various clusters. This diversity may be due to theological or sociocultural factors that distinguish among clergy from different religious bodies.

Evaluating Effectiveness

The Growth in Ministry Research Project of the Lutheran Church in America (Johnson et al., 1975) observed that pastors see themselves as less effective than their congregants see them. The meaning of "effectiveness" may be crucial here. Pastors could interpret effectiveness in terms of how "perfect" they are in performing their pastoral duties, whereas laypersons may be judging how faithful they think their pastors are to church doctrine.

TABLE 7.1. Two Frameworks for Assessing Clergy Effectiveness

Johnson, Lohr, Wagner, & Barge (1975)	Aleshire (1980)
Priest and preacher	Ministry to community and world
Community and social involvement	Ministry from personal commitment of faith
Enabler	Disqualifying personal characteristics
Office administrator	Open, affirming style
Teacher and visitor	Development of fellowship and worship
Personal and spiritual development	Privatistic, legalistic style
	Priestly, sacramental ministry
	Congregational leadership
	Caring for persons under stress
	Theologian in life and thought
	Denominational awareness, collegiality

Nauss (1983) employed the six effectiveness components denoted by the Growth in Ministry Research Project (see the Johnson et al. column in Table 7.1) and, by means of ratings, selected clergy who were considered highly effective in their various pastoral roles. A 30-element Job Diagnostic Survey (assessing such characteristics as motivations, job satisfaction, social skills, personal responsibility, and feedback) was then applied to discover the profiles for effective priests/preachers, administrators, teachers/visitors, and the other effectiveness categories. In the main, effectiveness was found to relate to positive considerations such as good feedback and high motivation. Though promising, these rather vague findings imply the need for more focused research.

Utilizing an attributional approach, Nauta (1988) studied how clergy responded to success or failure. The results were in line with the well-known theory and findings of Weiner et al. (1971)—namely, that clerics, like people in general, take credit for success and deny responsibility for failure. The reasons for success given by Nauta's respondents were internal, personal, and variable; for failure, they were external and stable. The variable or unstable success attributions referred to the notion that success was a function of the effort clerics put into their work. The stable (changeable) referents for failure were task difficulty and lack of ability. To some degree, successful outcomes were also attributed to divine influence—a finding previously observed, and one especially appropriate to ministers (Spilka & Schmidt, 1983). Overall, clerics were found to adopt a self-protective attributional stance.

Gender and the Religious Professional

Entering a Religious Profession. Traditional gender relations in religion have always reflected the prevailing cultural pattern: Males have dominated females, and religious authorities justify this pattern with reference to sacred sources. One can claim that sanctifying this relational pattern is a means of removing male dominance and female submission from potential debate. True or not, this archetypal paradigm elicited isolated instances of rebellion in such figures as the scriptural Deborah, Eleanor of Aquitaine, Mary Wollstonecraft, and feminists of the 19th century. The 20th century, however, witnessed women's suffrage, the entrance of women into the armed services in World War II, and finally a strong and continuing feminism from the 1960s on. The movement for gender equality had entered institutionalized religion by the 1970s, and has been increasing in strength ever since (Chang, 1997a).

Despite signs of progress toward gender equality among the clergy, a closer look shows that bias continues. A number of religious bodies are still conflicted regarding the ordination of women (Chaves & Cavendish, 1997). Where such opposition exists, it appears to be well organized and quite capable of resisting the efforts of women to enter seminaries or otherwise aspire to become ordained. Most Protestant denominations have resolved these difficulties, paving the way for women to serve their institutions effectively (Chaves & Cavendish, 1997).

Unfortunately, these indicators do not tell us that it takes 33% longer for a woman to obtain her first clerical assignment than for a man (Chang, 1997b). Studying the Unitarian Universalists and the Episcopalians, the fine analyses of Nesbitt (1997) reveal that women are likely to obtain lower-level jobs than those of their male competitors. Entrance into the higher church positions is also more difficult for women than men. Real power therefore still resides in the hands of men, and the evidence suggests that they are unlikely to surrender it easily (Nesbitt, 1997). Possibly as a function of these trends, when women enter the ministry or get their church jobs, their salaries are lower than those for men (McDuff & Mueller, 1999). McDuff and Mueller have also found that women tend to obtain posts in smaller, lower-budget churches. There is some social compensation, however, as they get greater support from colleagues and the church hierarchy than their male coworkers do.

Hard data are invariably impersonal when the need is for balance with the human side of the issue. Much good information can be obtained by skilled interviewers using relatively small samples. These idiographic approaches are often excellent sources of theory and hypotheses that can be further assessed by more objective and quantitative methods. The work of Martha Long Ice (1987) is a good example of such an effort. Her work is described in Research Box 7.3.

Sexual Issues. Sexual matters are often serious impediments to personal effectiveness as a cleric. A female minister may encounter considerable stress in her role as wife and mother, especially in conservative religious bodies. These groups emphasize the denial of sexuality, along with the notion that being a woman implies inferiority (Lawless, 1988).

One way such a problem may be manifested comes to the fore in Catholicism. Celibacy constitutes the major reason why priests leave their profession (Verdieck, Shields, & Hoge, 1988). This is probably a factor in the estimate "that at any one time 20 percent of Catholic priests are involved in a sexual relationship with a woman" (Chibnall, Wolf, & Duckro, 1998, p. 144).

RELIGION IN LOVE, SEX, AND MARRIAGE

Adler's third great task of adult life concerns love and marriage—topics that place the individual at the center of a matrix of biological, historical, sociocultural, and psychological forces. The biology of love, translated into sex and procreation, has been analyzed in relation to evolution (Ackerman, 1994; Fisher, 1983). The historical, cultural, and psychological aspects of love and intimate relationships have also been widely discussed and researched (Brehm, 1992; Hunt, 1959). Even though the modern world has seen a considerable liberalization of religion, there remains a fair degree of tension, ambivalence, and discomfort in the religious

---

Research Box 7.3. Clergywomen and Their World Views (Ice, 1987)

This in-depth study of 17 clergywomen demonstrates the rich variety of outlooks that exist among such women. In a sense, they are pioneers charting a difficult path for others who follow in their footsteps.

The women studied by Ice represented 12 denominations and spanned a broad range of ages, from the 20s to the mid-70s. Fifteen of the women were actively serving in congregations. Only one, a Catholic, was not officially ordained. There were 15 Protestants, a Catholic, and a Jew in the sample. Ice attempted to get as full an autobiographical perspective as possible, and to this she added concerns with gender orientation, views of authority, religious institutional administration, moral leadership, the issue of theological truth, and other related matters.

Though Ice's respondents felt comfortable with themselves as women, a flexible, androgynous orientation prevailed. Their situation called on a variety of characteristics that are sometimes regarded as stereotypically male and sometimes female; no gender limitations were evident. This does not mean that these women were not aware of gender differences in power, or that such differences could be ignored. Their preference was for equalitarian ideals and democratic relationships, and the women were confident in seeking to realize such goals. Evidence of struggle for personal growth was indeed present, marking many of these women as "transcenders"—those who grow above the difficulties and restrictions they have faced in life.

A holistic outlook stressing people, not things and mechanics, typified the faith and life of these women. This might be characterized as a form of Allport's Intrinsic religious motivation. A stress on moral modeling was also evident. The women further demonstrated an integrative theologizing that fit well with their moral and administrative leadership.

Of special significance is the fact that as a social scientist, Ice perceived her observations as contributing to a theoretical approach and hypotheses that could be assessed in future work.

---

context with regard to love, sex, and marriage. Historically, much of this is associated with institutional religion's sexist treatment of women (O'Faolain & Martines, 1973; Ruether, 1975). Furthermore, in recent years homosexuality has also "come out of the closet," and must be understood in contemporary life. The world now openly confronts established faiths with many love- and sex-related problems that in earlier times were suppressed or ignored. In addition to the ones already noted, we may think immediately of premarital and extramarital sex, spousal and child abuse, and divorce—all of which involve religion.

Religion and Heterosexuality

History and Context

The relationship between religion and sexual behavior has a long and troubled history. (This is particularly true for homosexual behavior, but we describe this in a later section; our present discussion is confined to heterosexuality.) One might even call this relationship "neurotic," but even that identification does not carry the extent to which conflict, ambivalence, and outright insensitivity have characterized the way organized religion has often dealt with sexual needs and expressions. In terms of one book title, religion and sexuality have been "intimate enemies" (Bach & Wyden, 1969). Indeed, at best, they have often been poor bedfellows.

Historically, studies of ancient peoples reveal the significance of sexuality and its circumscription and control by religion (Burkert, 1996). Hardy (1975) quotes a Church of England document that summarizes the matter succinctly: "In the long history of mankind religion and sex have been closely intertwined as forces of human nature" (p. 141). The Judeo-Christian perspective on sexuality fits into a broader context. In part, it reflects an earlier Greek view that placed pleasures of the mind above those of the body. This was sometimes equated with the notion that the body is corrupting, whereas the exercise of mind through reason reaches toward enlightenment. Early Christian ascetics often claimed that the body interferes with the attainment of a mystical union with the divine. In certain quarters, this translated into the association of the body with sexual activity, which soon united sexuality with evil (Bottomley, 1979). This kind of thinking was a step toward the justification of celibacy for those dedicating their lives to the church.

Another step in this process was to identify sexuality with women and to associate the two with evil, as in Tertullian's reference to woman as "the Devil's gateway" (O'Faolain & Martines, 1973). Although one could also selectively view scripture emphasizing the mandate to "be fruitful and multiply" as implying a positive and constructive purpose to sex, stress was often placed on the role of Eve in the fall of humanity, in order to generalize wrongdoing to all females. By the 3rd century A.D., elements of Manicheism filtered into Christianity (Mathews & Smith, 1923). This movement emphasized the conflict between good and evil, and regarded even marital sex negatively. Such views could have influenced Saint Augustine and other early church fathers to relegate sensuality, sexual relations, and women to a lower and more sinful realm (Ruether, 1972, 1974).

Contemporary Research on Sexual Behavior among Religious People

Although sexual activity can take many forms, we restrict our present discussion to male–female intercourse. In regard to premarital sex among people in general and religious people in particular, the data are often challengeable. One does not know about excessive denial or excessive admission of such experience. Gender may be a factor, with men trying to appear very experienced and women desirous of presenting images of chastity and selectivity. *The Janus Report* (Janus & Janus, 1993) claims that 67% of married men and 46% of married women engaged in premarital sex. Janus and Janus also note that the more religious people are, the less likely they are to be sexually active before marriage, or at least to admit it. Nevertheless, they report figures of 52% for "very religious" men and 37% for such women. Obviously, these findings are far from the religious ideal of abstinence prior to marriage.

Even though religious commitment reduces the probability of premarital sexual behavior, evidence of such activity has been repeatedly shown (in addition to Janus & Janus, 1993, see Reynolds, 1994, and Tavris & Sadd, 1977). However, Reynolds (1994) notes signs of a potentially serious error in such research—namely, a failure to identify and control for instances of forced intercourse or rape. She suggests that 20–30% of premarital involvement by young people, particularly teenagers, may involve coercion. If this is true, and such instances are statistically removed from the data, religious effects should become much more strongly negative.

Though the incidence of intercourse is lower among religiously active, currently un-married evangelical Christians than it is in the general population, some are nevertheless sexually active, contrary to their faith. In a study by Wulf, Prentice, Hansum, Ferrar, and Spilka (1984), 59% of such individuals reported no such involvement, while 18% were ac-tive once a month or more. These data were gathered on 365 respondents, and the predic-tion of who was engaged in these behaviors proved to be fairly reliable. Older men and women who had previously been married and currently had a close friend of the opposite sex were likely to be sexually involved. Though the relationships were not strong, high scores on Allport's Intrinsic religious motivation scale were negatively correlated with sexual activity, while high Extrinsic scores were positively related.

Another issue that has been examined concerns the extent of sexual pleasure reported by religious people. Masters and Johnson (1970) indict religion as adversely affecting sexual pleasure. Among the difficulties discussed, it is suggested that orgasm may be inhibited and sexual satisfaction diminished. These hypotheses have not been borne out by research. Re-ported sexual activity levels are higher for very religious respondents than those who are not religious. In addition, the frequency of such activity appears to have increased in the 3 years preceding the Janus and Janus (1993) study, and more for those who were "very religious" than for their nonreligious counterparts. Tavris and Sadd (1977) found no difference in fre-quency of orgasm between religious and nonreligious women. Mathews (1994) studied the sexuality of conservative, evangelical, submissive wives and found that "accountability to God for a wife's happiness and sexual satisfaction is part of exercising headship in the home" (p. 12). Fifty-seven percent of the men and 49% of the women in these marriages gave them-selves a 10 or 10+ on a scale of sexual fulfillment. Religion thus appears to be no barrier or impediment to sexually gratifying relations.

Some social scientists are reluctant to accept the positive testimony of religious women. Suggestions have been made that they probably "don't know what they are missing," or are responding to researchers in a socially desirable way. No evidence to support these interpre-tations has been forthcoming. Although Tavris and Sadd (1977) believed that such women may have lower sexual expectations and are less willing to believe widely purveyed popular fantasies about ecstatic sexual gratification, no data to back this belief have been produced. In short, efforts to cast religion in repressive or suppressive roles relative to sexual expres-sion have not gained support from research.

Religion and Marriage in Context

The noted anthropologist Bronislaw Malinowski (1956) claimed that "marriage is regarded in all human societies as a sacrament" (p.64). Whether the social order is called "primitive" or "civilized," the wedding or uniting ceremony is circumscribed by religious rites and sym-bols. Marriage is always considered a sacrament with religious and legal sanctions designed to continue its existence and confirm its rectitude. This purpose has become problematic in modern life. Despite these tendencies, Malinowski considered the marriage and family rela-tionship of such sociocultural value and personal importance that he felt it "has its roots in the deepest needs of human nature and social order" (1956, p. 72). Fundamentally, this same position was taken by both Adler (1935) and Freud (1943/1917). Adler treated a mutually satisfying marital relationship as the essence of his third great task of life. Freud viewed it as the necessary framework in which procreation should occur. This last stance has been the Judeo-Christian position for over two millenia. The prescription of intercourse only for producing children has, however, steadily given way to a more liberal treatment of sexual activity for both affectional and pleasurable purposes within marriage (Douglass, 1974; Janus & Janus, 1993; Tavris & Sadd, 1977). In addition, the traditional notion of the married woman as exclusively a homemaker is no longer true. In 1970, 43.3% of married women held jobs; by 2000, the number had increased to 61.9% (U.S. Bureau of the Census, 2000, p. 403). The role of wives in Western society is indeed changing.

Religion and Marital Adjustment

Dating precedes marriage, and singles are more willing to date than to marry someone outside of their religious group. Furthermore, the characteristics that are appealing in dating are different from those desired in a marriage partner (Udry, 1971). The choice of a potential marital partner entails a shift to more stable, lasting behaviors that are most appropriate to creating a successful marriage and home life. This includes a heightened emphasis on religion.

When both members of a married couple are religiously committed, they are also likely to be involved in a moral community. This helps explain many of the findings reported in Chapter 13 on religion and morality. It should therefore come as no surprise that in one study, marital happiness was positively correlated not only with agreement on religious matters, but also with the belief that love had continued to grow since the spouses were married. As might be expected, these findings paralleled increasing satisfaction with both oneself and one's mate (Hunt & King, 1978). Extrinsic religion was also operative here, suggesting that faith was performing a utilitarian function—one that was beneficial both to the marital union and to its members as individuals.

Evans, McIntosh, and Spilka (1986) found that spouses with similar religious orientations/motivations expressed greater marital satisfaction. Since this work was correlational, those with high Intrinsic and Extrinsic religion scores either acquired mates with similar perspectives or increasingly grew to share the same religious outlook, thereby enhancing the success of their marriages along with their personal happiness. Regardless of the process, the outcome was beneficial.

There is more to personal faith than attitudes and public observance, both of which were concerns of the two studies just described. Recognizing the lack of attention to private devotional practices, Gruner (1985) looked at the frequency of prayer and Bible reading, and found that both were related positively to marital adjustment. With respect to religious affiliation, the relationship between Bible reading and marital satisfaction was strongest for members of sects, somewhat less strong for evangelicals, and least strong for Catholics and members of liberal Protestant denominations. Of interest would be information on the degree to which members of such groups perceive prayer and Bible reading as pertinent to their marital state. Certainly, sects and evangelical bodies do emphasize Bible reading more than the other groups, but we know very little about the effects of such a private devotional practice on other aspects of an individual's life. An interesting possibility is that Bible reading may be more of a joint spousal activity in conservative than in liberal faiths. In sum, regardless of the measures used, religiosity and marital happiness have been found to go together (Filsinger & Wilson, 1984).

What about the other side of the coin—namely, those who describe themselves as having "no religion," or who conceive of their religion as outside of established faiths? The data suggest what the studies above imply: Religious independents are more likely to be unmarried, separated, divorced, or remarried than those who are affiliated. In addition, they reveal lower levels of satisfaction and of personal and social integration (Bock & Radelet, 1988).

The evidence is strong that marital adjustment and longevity are functions of the "sanctification of the family" (Mahoney, Pargament, & Swank, in press). This means that spouses who consider their marriage a sacred covenant are more satisfied with their union, and are more devoted to each other, than those who do not view their union in religious terms. Regarding a marriage as "made in heaven" is a powerful force in producing a happy family.

Religion, Marriage, and the Employed Woman

Virtually all of the major religious traditions—Buddhism, Christianity, Hinduism, Islam, and Judaism—have espoused the principle that the husband is the breadwinner and the wife is the homemaker (Bancroft, 1987; McLaughlin, 1974; Reineke, 1989). In the West, this pattern was shattered in the late 20th century. For instance, the number of women in the U.S. labor force more than doubled between 1970 and 2000 (U.S. Bureau of the Census, 2000, p. 403). To the extent that a woman is religious, she is likely to maintain established sex roles in marriage, to continue to be a homemaker and mother, and not to work outside the home (Bridges & Spilka, 1992). On the average, however, married working women demonstrate higher self-esteem than their stay-at-home counterparts (Messer & Harter, 1986), despite the fact that being a "superwoman" (i.e., holding a job, but still performing as a traditional wife and mother) can be a serious risk factor for depression (Basow, 1980). Religion can either increase this burden by arousing guilt, or act as a buffer against stress by enhancing a woman's sense of personal control (Bridges & Spilka, 1992; Messer & Harter, 1986).

Research on marital satisfaction in religious families with working wives over the past three decades has produced all possible findings, from depression through no effects to increased happiness (Johnson, Eberly, Duke, & Sartain, 1988). This apparent confusion is understandable, as many confounding factors are involved. Among these are degree of religiosity, educational level, the presence and age of children, and the relative conservatism of the religious group with which a family is associated. Such considerations hold for both husbands and wives. The unclear nature of findings in this area is illustrated in Research Box 7.4.

Religion and Gender Traditions

The situation of wives' employment when spouses are members of a conservative religious body raises the conventional argument about "woman's place." Classic Christianity denotes the man as head of the household. One survey of evangelicals (both males and females) indicated that approximately 90% affirmed the Biblical injunction of male domination in the family, and that about 40% would deny women any positions of power in the church (Kosmin & Lachman, 1993). Tradition has it that women should be subject to male control. The more orthodox a religious body, the more such a doctrinal view prevails.

However, Carolyn Pevey's (1994) study of a fundamentalist Southern Baptist church shows that tenet or theory is one thing, but practice may be another. Pevey found that wives were sometimes forced to submit, but that apparently, when necessary, these religiously conservative women subverted masculine claims to authority. Usually, though, husband–wife relationships seemed to be mutually supportive and cooperative rather than combative (albeit within an authoritarian framework).

Research Box 7.4. Wives' Employment Status and Marital Happiness of Religious Couples (Johnson, Eberly, Duke, & Sartain, 1988)

Mixed results have plagued research on marital satisfaction and the employment of wives. Theory has it that religiosity should correlate positively with the happiness of wives. Johnson and colleagues selected Mormon wives for study. Even though such women are members of a conservative religious group, they are as likely to work outside the home as members of any other denomination in the United States. Data were gathered for both husbands and wives on religiosity, education, age of children, the full- or part-time nature of wifely employment.

Johnson et al. found that marital happiness and religious commitment went together for both husbands and wives. The wives who were employed part-time were, however, less happy than those holding full-time jobs. Among the husbands, the most satisfied were those with full-time-employed wives. They were followed by husbands of traditional homemaking, nonemployed wives. Among the wives, the traditional homemakers were most happy, followed by the full-time-employed wives. The finding that both the part-time-employed wives and their husbands were least satisfied may be due to a number of factors. Part-time-working wives may be under stress by also remaining full-time homemakers. In addition, wives' part-time jobs may not provide enough income—another source of familial stress. In other words, the provider role may not be fully satisfied for both spouses. More work needs to be done to clarify the relative importance of traditional provider and homemaker roles among husbands and wives in this group.

Intermarriage and Religious Switching

Even though most people remain with the church in which they were reared, there is a fair amount of movement within the major religious bodies, and some of this results from marriages between people of different faiths. McCutcheon (1988) indicates a rather orderly increase in the number of "exogamous" marriages (i.e., marriages outside the religious group) among Protestants, Catholics, and Jews throughout the 20th century. The more conservative the faith in which people were raised, the less often switching occurs (Hadaway & Marler, 1993): Over 80% of conservative Protestants and Catholics maintain their original church affiliation. If a person is brought up within a specific religious tradition, and marries someone of the same persuasion, the probability of either spouse's changing affiliation is extremely low (Hadaway & Marler, 1993).

When it comes to switching because of marriage, Jews have been reported to have the lowest rate (3.4%; however, see below), with Catholics, Baptists, and Mormons reporting approximately 5% (Musick & Wilson, 1995). Still, intermarriage is the main route to religious change for Jews, Catholics, and Lutherans. When marriage prompts a shifting of religious affiliation, liberals usually move to moderate or conservative groups, while conservatives are inclined to adopt more liberal faiths. Catholics are most likely to reject religion altogether rather than adopt their spouses' faith.

There is a real problem in determining the actual percentages of people who marry outside their religious groups. This is most evident in Jewish intermarriages. Between 1900 and 1920, only 2% of Jews reportedly intermarried; between 1966 and 1972, 31.7% reportedly did so (Reiss, 1976). By the 1980s, Silberman (1985) suggested a rate of 24%, but noted that others put the rate as high as 60% The 3.4% rate given by Musick and Wilson (1995; see above) is suspect, but considering their use of national data, their findings must be noted. To suggest that the actual numbers range between 3% and 30% is not very informative. Some of this variation might be explained by noting where samples are gathered; in areas where there are few Jews, the rate of intermarriage is high. A distinction also needs to be made between first and second marriages, as the latter have an intermarriage rate about 50% higher than that for first marriages. This also means that older Jews are more likely to intermarry than their younger cohorts (Mayer, 1985). Despite these numbers, one study reported that in 1990, 94% of born Jews maintained their religious identification as Jews (Fishman, 2000).

Intermarriage usually occasions considerable unhappiness on the part of both parents and religious officials (Petsonk & Remsen, 1988; Stark & Bainbridge, 1985). A 1965 survey of Jews in Boston found that almost 70% felt that the Jewish community had "an obligation to urge Jews to marry Jews" (Geffen, 2001, p. 7); according to Geffen, a more recent survey still indicated that about 40% of Jews would be greatly distressed if their children married outside the faith.

Changing one's religious affiliation may involve a formal conversion; however, such switching does not often involve serious commitment. A convert for whom faith doesn't mean much may simply take on the affiliation of the more devoted spouse to please that spouse. Unfortunately, long-term discrepancies between spouses in terms of religious observance commonly result in conflict and divorce (Gordon, 1967; see "Intermarriage and Divorce," below).

There is another effect that merits study. What about the religious identification of the children of intermarried couples? A study of Jewish intermarriages in New York City showed that if the wife is Jewish, their children are raised as Jewish in three out of four families; if the husband is Jewish, the ratio is one out of four (Silberman, 1985). The noted sociologist Hart Nelsen (1990) studied this issue with regard to parents who were Catholic, Protestant, and unaffiliated. The last group is interesting, as the proportion of those who are unaffiliated with churches has been steadily increasing since the beginning of the 20th century. From about 1900 to 1965, their numbers grew from 3% to 13% of the U.S. population (Roof & McKinney, 1987). Nelsen's (1990) breakdown of the numbers of youths identifying their religion as "none" with regard to each parent's faith is presented in Table 7.2.

Even though the small samples where unaffiliated mothers are married to affiliated fathers is worrisome, the overall pattern for youth religion makes sense. When parents share the same faith, the percentage of unaffiliated youths is miniscule. When parents avow different churches, religious differences may cause some conflict and confusion in their offspring; hence the percentage of youths claiming no affiliation increases. The main difficulty occurs when one or both parents report "none" for religious identity. When fathers report no affiliation, the proportion of youths who are unaffiliated increases two to three times above the proportion when the intermarried spouses are either Protestant or Catholic. When mothers report "none," the rate of "none" among their adolescents again increases, now by at least three times. This supports the common finding that mothers are more important than fathers in affecting the religious inclinations of their offspring. Lastly, when both parents are unaffiliated, their combined potency is considerable; in this instance, 85.4% of their children also report "none." These findings make an important contribution to our understanding of the socialization of religious identification.

TABLE 7.2. Percentages of Youths Indicating No Religious Identity, by Parental Religious Identity

Religion of parents		Youths indicating "none" for religious identity	
Mother	Father	%	Sample size
Catholic	Catholic	1.5	3,919
Protestant	Protestant	3.1	4,985
None	None	85.4	398
Catholic	Protestant	5.6	303
Protestant	Catholic	9.7	288
Catholic	None	16.1	112
Protestant	None	17.2	221
None	Catholic	47.4	19
None	Protestant	57.1	21

Note. From Nelsen (1990, p. 130). Copyright 1990 by the Religious Research Association. Reprinted by permission.

Intermarriage and Divorce

The data are clear and consistent: Interfaith marriages have a much higher likelihood of ending in divorce than within-faith unions do (Lehrer & Chiswick, 1993; Levinger, 1979; Mahoney, Pargament, Tarakeshwar, & Swank, 2001). The problem is not only that intermarried spouses often have different backgrounds and expectations, but that they also may vary in degree of religiousness. When the "honeymoon is over," and the spouses face the realities of married life, religious issues can take on a new importance. This frequently occurs after children are born and the new parents clash over needs for religious identification and education. One estimate suggests that religious differences are mitigated through conversion, which takes place in about 50% of marriages (McCutcheon, 1988).

Even though we do not know the full extent to which intermarriage may be part of the divorce picture, Lawton and Bures (2001) have shown that the experience of parental divorce among those who intermarry commonly eventuates in religious switching. Since religious switching and intermarriage go together, one wonders whether a maladaptive marriage pattern might not be transmitted from parents to their children. Moreover, since religiousness and marital stability are positively related, it comes as no surprise that divorce adversely affects spiritual growth (Blomquist, 1985). Evidently intermarriages pose difficult problems and have a fair probability of ending in divorce. Needless to say, divorce by itself is a problem for those coping with religious difficulties (Shortz & Worthington, 1994).

Religion and Children

If there is one aspect of the marital union with which religions are concerned, it is, in the Western tradition, the scriptural prescription to "be fruitful and multiply." Every major world religion views the family as a childbearing and child-caring institution.

Birth Control. Though the classic Catholic stance against birth control is still officially on the books, it is overwhelmingly rejected by modern Catholics. Surveys in 1992 and 1996

found that from 80% to 91% of Catholics do not consider birth control to be wrong. In 1980, however, only 30% of priests supported birth control (Coffey, 1998). Given data like these, it is understandable why even devout Catholics consider the church's traditional stand hypocritical (Coffey, 1998, p. 24). In contrast to the official Catholic position, the Mormons have recently put aside the demand that procreation be the sole reason for sexual activity. Currently, they consider the purpose of sexual relations a personal decision, which may express love and marital commitment (Anderson, 1998).

In Western nations, religion exercises little authority when it comes to birth control and family planning. The controlling factors are primarily individual preference, socioeconomic status, and education.

Abortion. Obviously, abortion has become one of the most controversial topics in the last half century, but we cannot do more here than look at a few relevant considerations. Public attitudes toward abortion have been surveyed in the Gallup Polls for over 25 years, and considering the major changes that have occurred, it is surprising that the variation observed since 1975 has been so small and unpatterned (Bowman, 2000). As of 1999, 16% of U.S. residents felt that abortion should be illegal; 27% supported its legality in all circumstances; and 55% approved of abortion with qualifications (Bowman, 2000).

The endpoints of the main dimension underlying attitudes toward abortion have been termed "pro-life" and "pro-choice," with the former opposing abortion and the latter favoring it. Eighty-three percent of those who are pro-choice regard religion as unimportant in their lives, whereas only 9% of pro-life people feel similarly (Bowman, 2000). A comparison of pro-life and pro-choice women indicates that the latter are more educated and career-oriented than the pro-lifers. Birth control and possible abortion would be of potential benefit in realizing their ambitions. On the other hand, pro-life activists oppose birth control, and value highly having children and caring for them (McGuire, 1992). These radically different attitudes and behaviors represent broad social and psychological patterns.

Religion and Fertility. Despite the fact that religion has largely become irrelevant in relation to birth control and family planning, one still finds a few influences that represent the subsurface mix of culture and faith. For example, Lehrer (1996) notes that in an intermarriage, the husband's religion is more of a determiner of fertility than the wife's religion is. These interfaith unions, however, have fewer offspring than single-faith marriages do.

In a study of fertility and religious activity among conservative, moderate, and liberal Protestants (Marcum, 1988), the number of children under 6 years of age increased with church attendance for conservatives and decreased for liberals and moderates, but less so for the latter. When private devotional practices (Bible reading, prayer, saying grace before meals) were studied, the same pattern was observed for conservatives, but none was found for liberals and moderates (Marcum, 1988). Apparently conservatives buy into the "be fruitful" theology that supports fertility, but this is not true for more liberal Protestants. There is a need to consider class and education as possible controls in these analyses.

Religion and Homosexuality

The control and expression of sexual impulses have always been central issues for religion—not only in the West, but also throughout the world. This holds for both heterosexuality and homosexuality, as noted earlier. Historically, Western religion has been hostile toward homosexuals, citing scripture as the basis for its negative outlook. Many contemporary religious groups, particularly liberal ones, have challenged the traditional Judeo-Christian stance. Among others (Boswell, 1980; Cohen, 1990), Daniel Helminiak (1994), a Catholic priest and a noted psychologist of religion, has examined in depth the Biblical bases of antipathy and fear of homosexuals. He raises serious questions about the unfavorable scriptural heritage that has pervaded Western religious thought on this topic.

Placing homosexuality in a broader, anthropological light, Carlsson (1997) explains the great variation in the way homosexuals are regarded across cultures. He feels that one reason for this variation is the relative frequency of homosexuality. In societies where it is common, it seems to be treated in a positive manner; where it is rare, strong efforts to suppress homosexuality are common. Without question, the valuation of homosexuality is culturally defined. In one study of 76 societies, 49 did not treat homosexuality as negative, deviant, or abnormal (Farb, 1978). Furthermore, whether it is viewed as culturally normal or not, in many of these societies homosexuality is defined in supernatural and religious terms (Hoebel, 1966; Katchadourian, 1989).

The Judeo-Christian Tradition: An Extreme View

Pargament (1997) describes an extremely harsh religious view advanced by one Christian critic, who avers that AIDS is God's punishment for homosexual activity. As for those innocents who contract AIDS, "they, too, must pay the price for the moral depravity of a society that tolerates such abominations" (quoted in Pargament, 1997, p. 326). Stances like this can be exceedingly dangerous. Being homosexual and part of an orthodox religious community can eventuate in such a degree of shame and fear that not only does one remain "in the closet," but may deny being infected with AIDS, seriously jeopardizing life (Bieser, 1995).

Clerical Perspectives

A relatively early study of the attitudes of Methodist, Presbyterian, Roman Catholic, and Lutheran clergy toward homosexuality observed the expected relationship between orthodoxy and rejection of homosexuals (Wagenaar & Bartos, 1977). This position also related to what the researchers termed "a unidimensional approach to life" (p. 123). This refers to a polarized view of many issues in terms of simple dichotomies—good–evil, acceptance–rejection, and the like—which are premised on a fundamentalist Biblical literality. A much more recent research effort examined the attitudes of 1,100 pastors of the Evangelical Lutheran Church in America, and confirmed the earlier work (Taylor, 2000). Again, Biblical literality was the justification. Attempting to define the religion of these clerics further, Taylor found that only the Quest religious orientation made any distinction: High Quest scores correlated positively with favorable attitudes toward gays and lesbians.

Hochstein (1986) examined the stance of pastoral counselors, overwhelmingly clergy, relative to lesbian and gay clients. Though no distinction was made with regard to mental health between homosexuals and heterosexuals, 30% of the counselors scored high on a measure of homophobia. The main finding was that sex stereotyping was present. Interestingly, heterosexual males were seen as *less* masculine than heterosexual females, gays, or lesbians. Unfortunately, Hochstein provided no data that would distinguish the outlooks of male and female counselors.

The problem of homophobia in Western religion is not only individual but also institutional. Even relatively liberal churches maintain the biases of their more conservative peers. The United Methodist Church has very recently "ruled that practicing gays cannot be in the ministry" (Culver, 2001, p. 11A). In reality, this is largely translated into a "don't ask, don't tell" policy, but the burden is actually placed on local bishops and their politics. Homophobia remains official doctrine.

Conservative Views of the Bases for Homosexuality and Its "Treatment"

Arguments for and against various environmental, developmental, and biological causes for homosexuality are common throughout the psychological literature. The search for unidimensional and multidimensional possibilities is far from resolved, but this has not deterred partisans from believing that they know the answers and possess the truth.

The Argument for Celibacy. Cole (1995) has reviewed the evidence for a biological basis for homosexuality, and even though he accepts the data for biological causation, he takes the conservative Christian stance against such behavior and feels that churches can play a role in its change. Cole suggests that homosexuals adopt celibacy as an alternative. Apparently Lutheran churches will now accept lesbian and gay pastors if they remain celibate (*The Denver Post*, 2001). Although this approach seems insensitive, there is evidence that engaging in religious/spiritual activities is negatively correlated with participation in high-risk, unprotected homosexual behaviors (Folkman, Chesney, Pollack, & Phillips, 1992).

The Issue of Conversion Therapy. Regardless of the reasons for homosexuality, many conservative religionists believe in what has come to be known as "conversion therapy" (Haldeman, 1991, 1994, 1996). The intention is, of course, to convert homosexuals into heterosexuals (though, as noted above, celibacy seems acceptable to the proponents of this therapy). The notion of therapy implies that homosexuality is conceived of in orthodox circles as, at best, an illness. Neither the American Psychiatric Association nor the American Psychological Association holds such a view.

In an impressive effort to get past isolated anecdotal statements regarding the effectiveness of conversion therapy, Shidlo and Schroeder (2002), using rigorous selection criteria, were able to interview 202 recipients of conversion methods administered by a total of 308 therapists. The majority (66%) of the latter were licensed mental health practitioners, and 14% of these explicitly identified themselves with a particular religion. Of the unlicensed therapists, 55% were religious counselors. Two-thirds of the clients were religious. Eighty-seven percent of the respondents regarded their therapy as a failure; only 13% felt that it was successful to some degree. Approximately half of the "successes" experienced lapses or participated in alternative practices that implied continuing adjustment difficulties. There was also evidence that such therapy could eventuate in considerable psychological harm.

The landmark research of Shidlo and Schroeder is much more complex than this brief summary indicates. It spanned some 5 years, and provides very little support for those who consider conversion or reparative therapy a useful and productive alternative to homosexuality. Strong emotional biases cloud any serious attempts to evaluate all of the issues involved in changing homosexual behavior (Winfield, 2002). Shidlo and Schroeder offer the kind of solid scholarship that this troubled realm needs. In previous work, Haldeman (1991, 1994) simply concluded that there is no evidence that conversion therapy actually changes sexual orientation.

The Link between Right-Wing Authoritarianism and Antihomosexual Sentiment

The antipathy of fundamentalists and other religious conservatives toward gays and lesbians has been well established (Altemeyer & Hunsberger, 1992; Hunsberger, 1996). Even though scripture serves as its justification, one may ask whether an antihomosexual stance is simply another form of prejudice. Laythe, Finkel, and Kirkpatrick (2001) looked at this question with respect to personality/attitude characteristics that might foster bias. The researchers distinguished religious fundamentalism (RF) from right-wing authoritarianism (RWA), which is also part of fundamentalist ideology. Even though RWA and RF were positively correlated, RF was associated with antihomosexual feelings, but not with racism when RWA was statistically controlled for. RWA was tied positively to both forms of prejudice. After obtaining some contradictory findings in two additional studies, these researchers concluded that RF is at best weakly related to antihomosexual sentiment. The culprit really seems to be RWA.

Hunsberger (1996) extended the relationship among RF, religious RWA, and antihomosexual sentiment to Hindus, Muslims, and Jews. Even though the non-Christian samples tended to be small, the correlations showed that the same connection between RF and antihomosexual sentiment was found across all of the groups. Even when we restrict ourselves to the large Christian samples in four different studies, the connection is clear; Table 7.3 presents this information.

Even though there is variation among the coefficients in the table, these data show that RWA is indeed the problem, as four of the five partial correlations become nonsignificant when RWA is removed from the RF–RWA relationships. The .18 is of only borderline significance. Still, when RF is removed, all of the coefficients are statistically significant, further indicating that the RWA component causes the difficulty.

TABLE 7.3. Zero-Order Correlations and First-Order Partial Correlations among Right-Wing Authoritarianism (RWA), Religious Fundamentalism (RF), and Antihomosexual Sentiment (AHS) in Four Samples of Christians

	Altemeyer & Hunsberger (1992)	Laythe et al. (2001)		Wylie & Forest (1992)
		Study 1	Study 2	
Initial (zero-order) correlations				
RF–RWA	.68	.72	.68	.75
RF–AHS	.42	.48	.41	.56
RWA–AHS	.65	.52	.64	.72
Partial correlations				
RF–AHS/RWA	.04	.18	−.05	.04
RWA–AHS/RF	.54	.28	.52	.54

Note. The control variables are RWA and RF. The sample sizes are of such a magnitude to make virtually all of the zero-order and partial correlations statistically significant. They are: Altemeyer & Hunsberger, $n = 432$; Laythe et al., $n = 140$; Wylie & Forest, $n = 75$.

There is a more basic ethical question here—namely, whether sexual decisions are up to individuals as long as they are within the bounds of law. (Of course, the fact that laws against homosexual activity are still on the books in some U.S. states complicates this issue.) We hope that our readers will seek further knowledge in this highly controversial and emotionally charged area, so that their decisions are truly informed.

Alternative Religious Organizations and Approaches for Homosexuals

The rejection homosexuals encounter in mainline churches often causes them to reject those who spurn them. A common development is for lesbians, gays, and bisexuals to search for and/or actually establish their own churches and religious/spiritual organizations. A representative group is Dignity, a group for Catholic gays and lesbians (Wagner, Serafini, Rabkin, Remien, & Williams, 1994). Sometimes these organizations take unusual forms. Stark and Bainbridge (1985) describe a militant lesbian commune that organized as Wiccans, peaceful practitioners of contemporary witchcraft who pray to a "Great Goddess." One can view this and their other actions as a struggle to obtain a sense of power.

Helminiak (1995) speaks of the development of a nontheist spirituality, particularly among gays with HIV. He also notes that there are ministers who go beyond the traditional limits of their religious bodies to care for the spiritual needs of gay men and lesbians. Marshall (1996) details the problems of women who are in the process of developing lesbian identities. She specifies procedures and other considerations that pastoral caregivers can employ in their work with such women.

Effects of Religion-Based Hostility on Homosexuals

There is no reason to believe that the religious needs and desires of homosexuals are any different from those of nonhomosexuals (Goodwill, 2000; Haldeman, 1996; Lynch, 1996). In other words, faith may be of considerable importance to homosexuals, as it is to most people. The hostility of traditional religionists can therefore have extremely deleterious effects on lesbians and gay men (Clark, Brown, & Hochstein, 1989; Grant & Epp, 1998; Haldeman, 1996; Lynch, 1996).

But what are these effects? Quite often, homosexuals reject traditional religion (Clark, Brown & Hochstein, 1989; Goodwill, 2000). One study suggested that up to 50% of Catholic gays may leave the church. This is commonly associated with confused and contradictory images of God, as well as with negative self-concepts (Marcellino, 1996). The latter tendency may be one adverse effect of damaged identity development (Grant & Epp, 1998). Homophobia can also be internalized as part of a pattern of self-hatred (Wagner et al., 1994).

Influence of Religious Motivation in Heterosexuals' Views of Homosexuals

A number of researchers have looked at the influence of religious motivation or orientation in heterosexuals' views of homosexuals (Batson, Floyd, Meyer, & Winner, 1999; Fulton, Gorsuch, & Maynard, 1999). The results have been confusing.

Batson et al. (1999) undertook an experiment in which heterosexual subjects could monetarily help a same-sex peer who disclosed homosexual inclinations or gave no such information. In the case of the former, the gay respondent indicated that the money donated would go either to a cause that promoted homosexuality or to one that did not. Apparently devout heterosexuals with an Intrinsic religious orientation gave less to the gay discloser, regardless of where the money would go. This was seen as reflecting a bias against homosexuality. In order to resolve some of these difficulties with religious orientation or motivation, let us examine Research Box 7.5, which presents the work of Fulton et al. (1999).

Speculations on the Future

Though it is a slow process, there is reason to believe that the overall negativity toward homosexuals is decreasing in the United States. There is a growing understanding that this sexual orientation may have biological origins, although this point remains controversial. Psychologists and psychiatrists no longer consider homosexual inclinations to be pathological. In legal quarters, the process of decriminalization has been proceeding rapidly (Jennings, 1990). Since 1960, 26 states have repealed sodomy laws, and another 9 states have had such laws invalidated by the courts (American Civil Liberties Union, 2001).

Base estimates from survey data still indicate high antihomosexual sentiment, however (Newport, 2001). For example, concerning whether homosexuality "should be considered an acceptable lifestyle," 51% said yes in 1982 and 52% agreed in 2001. In other words,

---

Research Box 7.5. Religious Orientation, Antihomosexual Sentiment, and Fundamentalism among Christians (Fulton, Gorsuch, & Maynard, 1999)

This study attempted a systematic evaluation of the role of the major forms of religious motivation in fostering antihomosexual sentiment. Because of the complexity of the issue, measures of Intrinsic (personal) and Extrinsic (social) religious orientation plus their total, as well as scales assessing a Quest orientation and Fundamentalism, were employed. In addition, indices of antihomosexual sentiment and prejudice against black people were used, along with social distance and racism relative to blacks and a variety of other groups. A measure of social distance was also administered to evaluate attitudes toward practicing and celibate Christian and non-Christian homosexuals. Because Intrinsic faith has been confounded with religious orthodoxy, the Fundamentalism scores were partialed out to obtain a purer measure of Intrinsic motivation.

Intrinsic faith was associated with rejection of prejudice against blacks and antihomosexual sentiment. Even though homosexuals were not the object of Intrinsic bias, homosexual behavior was still regarded as a moral problem. Extrinsic motives correlated positively with antiblack and antigay indices. There were few significant correlations with the Quest scale; where present, these were weaker than, but similar to, those of Intrinsic religion with attitudes toward homosexuality. The Fundamentalism scale was independent of antiblack measures, but those with high Fundamentalism scores were rather strongly negative toward homosexuals. As a rule, distinctions were not made between active and celibate homosexuals.

Clearly, different religious motivations need evaluation when feelings about homosexuality are studied. The authors concluded that "not all negative sentiment toward homosexuals by Christians should be interpreted as prejudice, while not all committed Christians are bound to express negative sentiment toward homosexuals" (p. 21).

essentially half the U.S. population has consistently rejected such an alternative over the past two decades. Nevertheless, there has been a slowly growing acceptance that homosexual relations between consenting adults should be legalized. In 1977, 43% agreed; in 2001, this number increased to 54% (Newport, 2001). A much more significant change occurred in the approval of equal rights in terms of job opportunities: In 1977, 56% approved; in 2001, 85% agreed. Interestingly, in 2001, only 54% felt that homosexuals should be hired as clergy (Newport, 2001).

According to a recent Kaiser Family Foundation (2001) study, 76% of lesbians, gays, and bisexuals indicated that they feel more accepted. Concurrently, 74% still reported encountering verbal abuse, and one-third reported physical abuse (Kaiser Family Foundation, 2001). Table 7.4 details how religion relates to some of these issues. As can be seen, a rather high level of antihomosexual sentiment continues to prevail in the United States, and too often religion supports such views.

We need research that focuses more on educational efforts and their effects within the churches. Even though the more liberal religious institutions appear to be making some efforts to enlighten the public, gay and lesbian groups and their supporters still need to be heard more clearly, both within the overall society and in religious circles.

RELIGION AND POLITICS

Adulthood is more complex than the three great tasks of Adler (1935) imply. We are individuals nested in ever-larger communities—families that can be defined in relation to cultural variables, such as education, socioeconomic status, religion, and politics. The relationship between religion and politics is especially fascinating. It has also been extensively studied by psychologists and social scientists. Mahatma Gandhi is quoted as saying that "those who claim religion and politics don't mix understand neither" (see Coffin, 1990, p. 18). This is a

TABLE 7.4. Selected Recent Attitudes toward Lesbians, Gays, and Bisexuals in Relation to Religion

Attitude	Evangelicals %	Nonevangelicals %	Catholics %	No affiliation %
Homosexual behavior is morally wrong.	74	48	40	20
Homosexuality is a normal part of some people's sexuality.	50	73	72	88
Sexual orientation cannot be changed.	42	56	57	68
L, G, B couples can be as good parents as heterosexual couples.	47	60	59	63
Support laws to protect L, G, B couples from discrimination in:				
Employment.	—	69	78	77
Housing.	—	65	76	75
Health insurance.	—	61	77	70
Social Security benefits.	—	58	71	72
Oppose L and G marriages.	—	75	52	50

Note. L, lesbian; G, gay; B, bisexual. Data from Kaiser Family Foundation (2001).

challenge we dare not ignore. It is a realm of strong emotions and motivations that we should examine.

Civil Religion

Robert Bellah (1967) adopted Jean Jacques Rousseau's phrase, "civil religion" to describe the pervasive influence of religion in U.S. public life. Despite the constitutional separation of church and state, Greeley (1972a) has stated that "there is an official religion, if not an official church in the American republic. This religion has its solemn ceremonials such as the inauguration, its feast days, such as Thanksgiving, Memorial Day, the Fourth of July, and Christmas" (pp. 156–157). Many public figures have identified our national religion as Christianity or have referred to the United States as a Christian nation. The Judeo-Christian heritage, with emphasis on the Christian aspect, is the prime source of the religious elements we observe in our national holidays.

The power of using religious themes and language has long been known to politicians. Franklin Roosevelt is reported to have said that every major presidential address should have some of that "God stuff" in it (Lerner, 1957, p. 704). Bellah (1967) observes that only one inauguration speech—George Washington's—did not cite the deity and faith in terms designed to make the public feel good. Even Washington, however, included religion in his Farewell Address. Such expressions of civil religion in the U.S. political context led Marty (1976) to conclude that "Civil religion is the *real* religion of the American people by the mere fact of their being American people" (p. 182). It pervades U.S. cultural life; it is the context for much more of U.S. residents' thinking than they are aware.

The Christian Right

The drive to keep religion in U.S. political life and to influence the government in ways favoring religion has for over two decades been variously labeled the "Christian right," the "new Christian right," "Christian conservatism," the new "religious/political right," the "Christian crusade," and the "fundamentalist new right." All denote the conservative end of the political–religious tradition, and are essentially interchangeable. At least two specific organizations—the Christian Coalition and the Moral Majority—have also represented or continue to represent this tradition in the U.S. political arena.

Throughout U.S. history, religious groups have attempted to elect candidates who would support their programs (Marsden, 1983). These efforts have usually been limited and poorly organized, and, as a rule, have not lasted long. The situation began to change in the early 1900s with the rise of fundamentalism and evangelicism. These movements first gained a national audience in the early 1920s, and local and regional groups achieved largely transitory successes that were rapidly followed by electoral rejection. With the rise of anti-Communism in the 1950s and 1960s, the Christian right gained new strength; it became noteworthy with the 1980 election of Ronald Reagan, who freely used the movement's language and ideas, but seldom attended church (Wilcox, 1996).

The chief issues that concern the Christian right and many political conservatives have been the separation of church and state, prayer in the schools, abortion, evolution versus creationism, "big government," immorality, gay rights, gays in the military, and related topics. In essence, none of these issues has been resolved, and are unlikely to be handled in a manner that will satisfy the Christian conservative movement. The Christian right has been heard loud and clear in the political arena, and has continued to make gains throughout the 1990s (Wilson, 2000). The infusion of civil religion into all aspects of public and political life is strongly supported by Christian conservatives (Wilcox, 1996).

The Christian Right and the Political Process

Green (2000) has accurately pointed out the complexity of religion relative to the U.S. political landscape. He notes that the Christian religious right is primarily composed of white evangelical Protestants, who account for 13% of the U.S. adult population. The membership of these religious right bodies is about 4 million, with a few hundred thousand real activists (Wilcox, 1996). In 1994, the Christian right also exercised substantial to dominant influence in the Republican Party in 28 states (Wilcox, 1996). The positions taken by these conservatives are not restricted to a narrow audience. Depending on the issue, they have the support of many millions of voters throughout the country.

As indicated above, Christian rightist groups are, as a rule, affiliated with the Republican Party. One study of four states (Virginia, Minnesota, Washington, and Texas) shows that the process involves both confrontation and consolidation (Green, Rozell, & Wilcox, 2001). When access to power within the Republican hierarchy is easy, confrontation is common. The slightly variant perspectives of the different factions become overly important. The result is conflict among the party subdivisions. This seems to hurt the party at election time. If access to power is controlled, a more constructive consolidation occurs that apparently benefits the party in elections. The limitations imposed by party controls make the Christian right minimize its internal differences, coordinate its intentions, and focus its energies to attain specific goals. This results in well-designed programs. An example of the degree to which Christian right positions have been mainstreamed is evidenced by the treatment they received from Ronald Reagan. In important speeches, he publicly approved six of the eight top Christian right agenda items, but exercised considerable restraint in enacting legislation to support these positions. Needless to say, little action was taken on issues that would arouse strong opposition (Moen, 1990).

Some Individual Concerns

Over the years, different Christian right leaders and issues have taken center stage. One may ask whether any individual patterns of traits and characteristics distinguish among allegiances to certain issues or candidates. Studying the religious identifications of over 600 Republican contributors to Republican presidential candidates, Jelen and Wilcox (1992) found that in one instance, self-definition as a fundamentalist was important; in another, charismatic identification was most significant. The authors feel that different facets of religion may be influential with different candidates and groups. There does not appear to be any single or simplistic motivation underlying Christian right orientations.

Another approach to understanding the appeal of the Christian right has examined two popular theoretical stances. One theory claims that adherents are religiously and politically socialized to embrace conservative values in both spheres (Elms, 1976; Stone, 1974). The other avers that people who are deprived and under stress gravitate to extreme positions to solve their problems (Glock, 1964). Indirectly approaching these theories, Wilcox (1989) sought explanations in geography, religious beliefs, social status, political beliefs, alienation, and symbols. Wilcox found that political stance was strongly associated with evangelical doctrines (socialization), as opposed to any signs of deprivation or stress.

Catholics and Political Conservatism

Even though the Christian right calls to mind Protestant evangelicals and fundamentalists, the appeal of this conservative program among Catholics has been studied. Examination of the Catholic data in the same four states studied by Green et al. (2001) shows that Catholic conservatism falls between that of mainline Protestants and Christian right evangelicals. Conservative Catholic Republicans take their stance less from their faith and more from social issues than Protestant rightists do (Bendyna, Green, Rozell, & Wilcox, 2000). With data similar to those analyzed by Wimberly (1978; see below), Welch and Leege (1988) have looked at Catholic beliefs, participatory styles, closeness to God, and religious imagery in relation to political attitudes. Apparently the image of God as judge is tied to political conservatism. The same is true of expressing an evangelical devotional style. One conjecture advanced by Welch and Leege is that changes in Catholicism since the Vatican II conference of the early 1960s may play a role in these conservative associations.

Religious–Political Factors and Relationships

Psychologically, how does one get from religion to politics? In order to understand this correlation, Wimberly (1978) measured religious and political dimensions with items assessing beliefs, behavior, experience, social interactions, and knowledge in both areas. He found that the two realms are related in many ways. Political and religious liberalism, knowledge, and social behavior are positively related. Political belief, knowledge, and private behavior are associated negatively with religious experience, behavior, and social interaction. The positive correlations are easier to interpret than the negative ones. Liberals and conservatives in religion tend to hold similar political views, and to respond accordingly. This work also shows that people are averse to integrating certain aspects of religious life with politics—most likely their personal and private religious and spiritual concerns. Research of this nature bears repetition and extension, in order to clarify further how these domains are related.

How Religion Influences the Political Person

Psychologically, the infusion of faith into the public domain often functions to control thinking and stifle debate. The high valuation of religion introduces a "stop-thinking" quality to pronouncements that associate the deity and faith with freedom, flag, family, and political issues that may be masked under such labels as "traditional values." This conveys a moral essence that is not to be questioned. The topic in question is now endowed with a sacred quality, and it is strongly implied that we must correct what is religiously wrong. In addition, the affiliation of religion with politics gains validation, so that it is viewed as natural and appropriate.

Extending this identification of faith with politics may activate people to enter into public discussion or justify inaction and withdrawal from the political arena. Specifically, one's faith can act as a source or sanction for political loyalty or conflict; it can also offer opportunities to avoid, or even to reduce, conflict and dissension (Geyer, 1963).

Religion as a Source and Sanction for Political Loyalty and Conflict

Both religion and politics are categorical domains. Religion has its major faiths, all of which are subdivided into formal and/or informal denominational and sect forms. Islamic authorities, for example, might deny the multiform nature of their faith, but recent experiences with Islamic groups have demonstrated how different degrees of orthodoxy may be combined with various ethnic identities and traditions. It is not clear whether these are sects or should be denoted cults (see Chapter 12). In like manner, political parties are commonly fractionated by geographical and socioeconomic identifications and concerns. In the United States, it is normal to think of breakdowns by north, east, south, and west, or by agricultural or industrial interests. In local areas, tourism, ranching, or fishing may be significant. Loyalties to the values and needs of the different people and groups to which such matters are important imply the potential for conflict. The probability that institutional religion will enter the battle is considerable. Nevertheless, the label "Christian" is no guarantee of similarity on any specific topic. If pressed, Christians are usually arrayed on all sides of political issues—and, of course, they do not find it theologically difficult to justify their stances.

For many people, the presence of religious language endows the item in question and its supporters with the aura of doing "God's work." It was thus politically astute for both Ronald Reagan and Bill Clinton to close their partisan speeches with the phrase "God bless you and God bless America" (quoted in Fowler & Hertzke, 1995, p. 244). This conclusion commonly followed other religious allusions throughout their presentations. The media are reticent about calling such uses of religion to the attention of the electorate, as it might have adverse effects on their audience and sponsors (Wills, 1990).

One may look upon the uses of religious language and concepts in politics as types of control systems. The intention is to direct and focus thinking and behavior. Faith thus selects and reinforces political ideas. Terms like "moral," "truth," "evil," and "good" are not open to negotiation. This primitive moralism blurs the actual complexity of issues (Lane, 1969). The result is enhanced loyalty both to church and to certain political ideologies (Kelly, 1983).

These devices are often attempts to pit liberal religionists and their conservative counterparts against each other. Different concepts of human nature and different interpretations of scripture come into play. Such arguments also keep the underlying considerations of social and economic stratification and power out of the picture. The skillful manipulation of religious–political ideas in sermons, church publications, and radio and television programs have their effects both at the ballot box, and in establishing faith as a source and a sanction for political loyalty.

Issue loyalties get transformed into group identifications, and ingroup–outgroup distinctions are described in alienating terms. The rhetoric can become "Christians versus secular humanists." The question "Who opposes prayer in the schools?" may take on an anti-Semitic (or anti-Muslim, anti-Hindu, etc.) tint. "True believing" dispenses with boundaries, especially when religion is an organizing force. Conspiracy fantasies theorize who is behind pornography, evolutionary theory, women's rights, and many other controversial issues. The approved answers often excite bigotry. Purity of purpose is distorted into a group purity advocating a separatism that ruptures the social fabric. Religion thus becomes a source and sanction for political conflicts.

Religion as a Sanctuary from Political Conflict

To many others among the faithful, the church, synagogue, or mosque should stand above the fray. Such people feel that seeking God and transcendence is the goal of religion, and that the sacred and divine must not be sullied with the mundane and commonplace. Politics and politicians often connote something worse—a lower realm where bad people "make deals," where corruption and opportunism prevail, and where the realm of the spirit is ignored and demeaned. Within this perspective, true faith is translated into rejection of the world. In wartime, pacifism may be embraced; in peace, the call may be for isolation and separation (Geyer, 1963). The saving Puritan graces are honesty, cooperation, thrift, sincerity, good will, mercy, forgiveness, truth, beauty—all that is good in the world, all that is God's due. There are still many people who feel that the only way these high aims can be achieved is by the fullest devotion to one's faith. This clearly entails estrangement from the world and alienation from politics. A considerable literature suggests that the prime element in alienation is powerlessness, and that this results in political apathy (Finister, 1970; Roelofs, 1972; Seeman, 1959). In other words, the role of religion as sanctuary may sometimes be less a positive striving than a retreat from a world in which people feel powerless and alienated.

This perspective has a surprisingly strong following in the United States. One study of 1,580 California clergy revealed that over one-third had never given a sermon on a political topic. The more traditional the cleric, the less likely it was that mundane, worldly matters would be presented. Moreover, due to a sampling bias, the authors of this work felt that they actually *underestimated* the aversion of ministers toward politics (Stark, Foster, Glock, & Quinley, 1970).

Conflict between being "in the world" and being "out of the world" varies greatly among conservative religious groups. A few, like the Amish, work hard to maintain their separation from all aspects of the broader community (Hostetler, 1968). Fundamentalists frequently oppose "things of the world" and explicitly take stances to combat modernism as defined by the Christian right (Lawrence, 1989). Political involvement may, however, be taken as creating a value system that competes with religion; this implies that politics must be resisted unless it is subsumed under the categories of faith, where its influence can be limited and made acceptable. In the last two decades, however, several countries have had radical political regimes replaced by radical religious regimes that exercise governmental power all too enthusiastically.

Religion as a Reconciler of Political Conflict

Paradoxically, religion both exacerbates conflict and also works to reduce it. The seriousness with which established faiths currently take the importance of peace may be gained from a simple Internet search. One conducted in December 2002 turned up over 1,130,000 sites dedicated to the furtherance of peace by the world's great religions.

Probably the largest religion-based peace organization is Religions for Peace (RfP). Founded over 40 years ago, it has sponsored the World Conference on Religion and Peace for the past 30 years. This conclave of hundreds of major world religious figures takes place every 5 years. RfP (2001) defines itself as "the largest international coalition of representatives from the world's great religions who are dedicated to achieving peace" (p. 1).

Recognizing the many foundations for group conflict, RfP has developed an extensive list of programs and projects. These deal with peace education, human rights, disarmament and security, women, children, poverty, ecology, humanitarian aid, and attempts to transform conflict into peaceful resolutions of differences. Over the years, RfP has been active in bringing warring factions together for dialogue in such troubled areas as west Africa and the former Yugoslavia, and have coordinated its efforts with various divisions of the United Nations.

In the 19th and 20th centuries, many religious institutions and groups tried to find means of countering war and domestic and international strife. The World Council of

Churches currently sponsors a program on Justice and Peace that stresses the basic unity of peoples. Recently, a Parliament of World Religions meeting was held in Chicago and attended by over 8,000 representatives of a wide sampling of world faiths. The outcome was a Declaration of a Global Ethic, designed to "promulgate a set of 'irrevocable, unconditioned ethical norms' for the entire human community" (Skidmore, 1993). The Catholic Worker Movement, founded by Dorothy Day, has a long history of taking stands on a wide variety of economic and political issues. Its supporters assert that their aim is "to live in accordance with the justice and charity of Jesus Christ," and this has spurred many social and political actions (*The Catholic Worker*, 1991, p. 5).

Religion and Legislation: Individual Dimensions

We have already described the efforts made by pressure groups, particularly the Christian right, to influence governmental processes. An unintended implication of this description may have been that politicians rationally weigh the various forces that may affect reelection, consider the ramifications of potential laws, and choose either to support or to reject what comes before the legislative body. Granted that the public does not have a high opinion of politicians, it also knows surprisingly little about the statute-making process. The 19th-century British prime minister Benjamin Disraeli is reported to have said that "you should not know too much about what goes into your sausage and your legislation." In part, he may have been referring to the nature of those who enact laws. An impressive project that attempted to unravel influential intraindividual factors in religion among members of the U.S. Congress was conducted by Benson and Williams (1982). This is summarized in Research Box 7.6.

&

Research Box 7.6. Religion on Capitol Hill: Myths and Realities (Benson & Williams, 1982)

This study was designed "to chronicle the religious beliefs and values held by members of the United States Congress, and to track how they connect with the legislative decisions of the Congress" (p. 2). Eighty senators and representatives were interviewed. On a variety of pertinent demographic variables, this group closely matched those not interviewed. Seven categories of beliefs were assessed: (1) "the nature of religious reality," (2) "religious reality's relationship to the world," (3) "means of apprehending religious reality," (4) "salvation and paths to salvation," (5) "about the last things," (6) "people and society," and (7) "values and ethical principles" (p. 24).

Eighty-six percent of the participants affirmed a belief in God, and described images of a transcendent, loving deity. Their religion addressed the lack of meaning and purpose in life. They viewed salvation as possible through good works, faith, and a virtuous life.

Ninety percent of the respondents were formally members of churches and synagogues; 74% attended services once a month or more, and also reported praying at least once a week; and 37% read scripture weekly. Ninety-seven percent considered religion to be moderately to very important in their lives. The authors concluded that Congress reflects the dominant religious beliefs and behaviors of the U.S. public.

continued

Research Box 7.6. *continued*

Benson and Williams distinguished six types of religionists in the Congress:

1. *Legalistic religionists* (15%) placed "very high value on rules, boundaries, limits, guidelines, direction, and purpose" (p. 126). They also stressed self-discipline and self-restraint.

2. *Self-concerned religionists* (29%) were articulate, and regularly and genuinely practiced their faith. However, they were "almost entirely concerned with the relationship between the believer and God" (p. 128); they exhibited little concern for fellow humans.

3. *Integrated religionists* (14%). "These people's beliefs work[ed] to liberate them . . . to speak and act. . . . God not humankind [was] their audience" (p. 129). They were likely to vote in terms of religious principle.

4. *People-concerned religionists* (10%) emphasized the connection between faith and action, and possessed well-examined religious concepts and images of God.

5. *Nontraditional religionists* (9%) were intellectually perceptive members of Congress who held abstract concepts of God and many individualized religious ideas. They also shared a secular-humanist orientation.

6. *Nominal religionists* (22%) rejected most traditional religious ideas and held rather superficial church attachments. Their rather vague, unanalyzed religion was concerned primarily with solace; it was unlikely to affect daily life and thought.

Ninety-nine percent of the sample felt that there were connections between religious outlook and voting behavior; 24% saw a strong association. Political conservatives held images of God as omnipotent, strict, guiding, protective of social institutions, and playing an active role in life. They believed that an afterlife is assured, and that the path to salvation is personal and accomplished by doing good. Liberals stressed justice, love, and the social nature of salvation.

Studying eight political issues on which the Congress had voted, Benson and Williams found noteworthy associations between the various religious types and voting records. These data are summarized in the table below. Most conservative votes were cast by the legalistic and self-concerned religionists, whereas the majority of liberal votes were cast by people-concerned and nontraditional religionists.

	Percentage of votes cast, by religionist type					
Voting behavior	Legalistic	Self-concerned	Integrated	People-concerned	Non-traditional	Nominal
Pro- . . .						
Civil liberties	32	30	60	80	81	51
Foreign aid	21	26	63	97	88	55
Hunger relief	30	29	78	90	83	60
Abortion funding	23	28	71	87	86	44
Anti- . . .						
Government spending	47	45	25	23	22	34
Pro- . . .						
Strong military	84	78	44	19	26	58
Private ownership	50	54	29	19	18	37
Free enterprise	65	61	35	23	20	42

Note. Adapted from Benson and Williams (1982, p. 161). Copyright 1982 by the Search Institute. Adapted by permission.

The Benson and Williams research demonstrates how psychologists of religion can conduct creative studies of ties between faith and politics.

OVERVIEW

We have covered a massive amount of information on the roles and functions of religion in adult life. Even though each section could easily be expanded, we hope that the essential issues and data have been identified. Our selected age range of 18 to 80-plus years for "adulthood" leaves much room for innovation and experimentation in life, and there can be no doubt that theorists and researchers have attempted to circumscribe virtually every major possibility. Although we look at collective data, we know each person introduces a uniqueness that research can never fully limit or describe. The individual integration of religion is truly a lifelong task.

Chapter 8

RELIGION AND DEATH

&

O death, where is thy sting? O grave, where is thy victory?

I am a frightened child in the presence of death.

Death is an endless night.

Let me die the death of the righteous.

It is impossible to experience one's death objectively, and still carry a tune.

Achieving immortality is surprisingly simple. . . . To reach human immortality we must follow Rule No. 1 of anti-aging medicine: *Don't die.*[1]

DEATH AND RELIGION: A FRAMEWORK

We humans do not take kindly to death. Shakespeare (1604/1964, p. 81) called it "a fearful thing," and Matthew Arnold (1853/1897, p. 288) viewed death as "a hideous show." One may speak of "noble deaths," "death with dignity," "eternal paradise," or "ultimate rewards," or may state that "nothing can happen more beautiful than death" (Whitman, 1855/1942, p. 18), but its immediate reality is terrifying to virtually all of us. We lament those who die, and dread the awareness that we too, in time, will confront the end of our own existence. Many of us refuse to come to terms with death. We repress, deny, shun, and withdraw where possible from reminders of death, and above all, we fight to delay death. If there is a basic purpose to medicine, it is to reduce mortality and increase longevity. And when we die, the customary North American way of death includes embalming, which Aries (1974) interprets as a "refusal to accept death" (p. 99). In other words, we wish to keep our bodies unchanged. Furthermore, our faiths inform us that we do not simply die; we move to another realm— heaven, hell, limbo, purgatory, or life with God. Finally, there is resurrection: We return to everlasting life. In sum, we never die; our destiny is immortality. Religion guarantees it.

Theologian Paul Tillich (1952) championed such an inference by claiming that "the anxiety of fate and death is the most basic, most universal, and inescapable" (p. 40). Reasoning further, the noted anthropologist Bronislaw Malinowski (1965) maintained that "Death, which

---

1. These quotations come, respectively, from the following sources: I Corinthians 15:55; Maeterlinck (1912, p. 4); Paul Theroux, quoted in Andrews, Briggs, and Seidel (1996, No. 57808); Numbers 23:10; Woody Allen, quoted in Peter (1977, p. 134); and McFatters (2002, p. 1W).

of all human events is the most upsetting and disorganizing to man's calculations, is perhaps the main source of religious belief" (p. 71). In one study of clergy, only 2% felt that concern about death was not a factor in religious activity (Spilka, Spangler, Rea, & Nelson, 1981).

Even though Western religion assures us of our continuation, it often treats death as a correlate of evil. Scripture is replete with references to death as the appropriate punishment for sin. We are told that it all started with Adam and has been our heritage ever since: "Wherefore, as by one man sin entered into the world, and death by sin; and so death passed upon all men, for that all have sinned" (Romans 5:12). Through death, therefore, religion engenders hope, guilt, and fear.

Wheeler (1971) cites what he terms the "complaint" of the philosopher and poet Unamuno (1921/1954), who somewhat pessimistically opined:

> We require God to exist because we must die. Death is not only unacceptable, it is insulting. It makes life absurd. Because death exists God must also exist in order to eliminate the absurdity of life. Of course, if things were different among men—if men ceased to die—then the ontological existence of God would no longer be necessary. (quoted in Wheeler, 1971, p. 11)

Relative to the theory of religion presented in Chapters 1 through 3, we recognize death as the ultimate threat to our sense of control, and religion has historically been our culture's dominant means of coping with the inevitability of our own demise. Religion makes death meaningful. Death is a mystery that we must unravel. As an unknown, it belies meaning and demands explanation. We do not tolerate ambiguity easily. We have questions, and religion offers us the desired answers. Taken at face value, death implies a simple, final termination. Understandably, we do not easily accept the prospect of ultimate extinction; it is not just that we want to live on indefinitely, but that we desire certainty that this will occur. Religion provides assurance that this will eventually take place. Unamuno (1921/1954) further asserted that the theme of "immortality originates and preserves religions" (p. 41).

Institutionalized faith, as we have seen, plays many roles in life, but the issue of death lies at its core. Kearl (1989) gets to the heart of the matter when he points out that "religion has historically monopolized death meaning systems and ritual," and helps "create and maintain death anxieties and transcendence hopes as mechanisms of social control" (p. 172). Social control easily translates into personal control, another major function of religion (see Chapters 1–3). Expectations of judgment in an afterlife can prompt socially conforming behavior and give people the feeling that they are in charge of their final destiny. Underlying this perspective is the obvious fact that death is the ultimate challenge to our sense of personal control, or, as Langer (1983) puts it, the "illusion of control" (p. 59). Especially in individualistic, achievement-oriented U.S. society, this means, as the historian Arnold Toynbee observed, that death is "un-American, an affront to every citizen's inalienable right to life, liberty, and the pursuit of happiness" (quoted in Woodward, 1970, p. 81). Religion, therefore, stands as the only major bulwark against the threat of death.

RELIGION, DEATH, AND IMMORTALITY

Belief in an Afterlife

Table 8.1 indicates that beliefs in an afterlife, heaven, and hell have a strong grip on the minds of U.S. adults. Whereas the General Social Survey (GSS) in the United States indicates that 81.9% of its respondents believe in an afterlife (GSS, 1999), the International Social Survey

TABLE 8.1. Beliefs in Afterlife, Heaven, and Hell by Religion, Gender, Age, and Education

	Afterlife (%)	Heaven (%)	Hell (%)
Religion (25,190)			
Protestant	84.0	73.2	61.2
Catholic	78.6	63.0	47.7
Jewish	39.7	18.6	10.4
None	54.1	24.2	17.9
Gender (25,190)			
Male	76.3	57.4	48.2
Female	81.5	70.1	55.5
Age (24,737)			
20–29	77.7	60.5	49.0
30–39	80.5	62.4	50.4
40–49	81.1	62.9	53.4
50–59	78.9	68.4	53.5
60–69	78.4	66.5	55.8
70+	79.1	72.1	55.1
Education (9,123)			
0–8 years	77.0	86.1	63.0
High school graduate	80.0	70.1	58.9
College graduate	79.5	50.0	40.2

Note. Data from the General Social Survey (GSS) (1999). Numbers in parentheses at left indicate the total number of valid cases for each domain. Belief in afterlife is indicated by a simple "yes"; beliefs in heaven and hell are given as "definitely yes."

Program data for 1998 reveal no European country with such a high proportion of its population holding these views (Greeley, 2002). Cyprus with 80% and Ireland with 79% are close, but most of the other nations are in the 30–60% range. Since the mid-1950s, however, the general tendency has been toward an increase in such beliefs among Europeans (Greeley, 2002). Morin (2000), utilizing data from the National Opinion Research Center (NORC), has recently reported a similar pattern in the United States. This finding holds for Jews in the GSS, but not for Protestants and Catholics (Harley & Firebaugh, 1993). According to the NORC, between the 1970s and 1990s, belief in life after death increased from 19% to 56% among Jews and from 74% to 83% among Catholics (Morin, 2000). A satisfactory explanation for these findings has yet to be offered. There is need to understand such considerations further, in the light of the rapid rate of technological development, national and international stresses, and a certain tenuousness to life (as shown by terrorist activities such as the World Trade Center tragedy). In a sense, we might hypothesize that for many people, the world has "gotten away from them." The personal sense of control may be increasingly threatened, and the search for immortality may be one effort to regain the security that the "illusion of control" confers.

There are a number of other patterns in Table 8.1 that should be noted. First, belief in an afterlife does not mean that one accepts notions of heaven or hell. Considerable room exists for other beliefs. It would be of interest to define these possibilities and discover their origins and correlates.

Second, people are less inclined to believe in hell than in heaven. Given the religious criteria for being consigned to either realm, self-examination might prompt a considerable aversion on the part of most people to recognizing the potential for a postlife hell. A Harris

Poll (Taylor, 1998) supports this hypothesis: 79% of this poll's respondents believed they would go to heaven, and less than 2% felt that their final destination would be hell.

Third, the distribution of afterlife beliefs by faiths is more or less what one might expect. These ideas have a long history within Christianity, but not within Judaism. In the latter, an undefined eschatology essentially prevails. Note that the 39.7% of Jews accepting an afterlife observed by the GSS (1999; see Table 8.1) is considerably less than the 56% reported by the NORC (Morin, 2000; see text above). Such discrepancies call to our attention the methodological problems one faces in survey research.

Considering the evidence that women are more religious than men, it comes as no surprise to note that they believe more strongly in an afterlife, heaven, and hell. As regards age correlates, there is a slight tendency for beliefs in heaven and hell to increase with age. The youngest age grouping (those in their 20s) are furthest from expected death, and show least belief in an afterlife, heaven, and hell. Sampling variation might account for the highest beliefs in an afterlife for those in the 30–50 age range. Though not truly striking, these higher percentages could also reflect the typical concerns at these ages with supporting a family and raising children. Further verification of these observations is necessary, as well as hypothesis testing to explain such findings.

An interesting earlier study of church members revealed that only 46% of Protestants and 71% of Catholics claimed that "what we do in this life will determine our fate in the hereafter" (Stark & Bainbridge, 1985, p. 53). In addition, there seems to be considerable reluctance to change one's ways to avoid hell (Litke, 1983; Stark & Bainbridge, 1985). Since over half of the Protestants and almost a third of the Catholics surveyed by Stark and Bainbridge agreed that heaven and hell are our destiny for reasons other than the way we live, one wonders whether we are seeing a return to Calvinistic predestination. Again, further detailed investigation into afterlife beliefs is warranted.

A certain vagueness attends these beliefs, since personal continuation is usually viewed as applying to the spirit rather than the body. Still, for many believers, the afterlife is succeeded by resurrection of the body. Contemporary Christianity prefers to conceptualize this as a "spiritual" body rather than a physical one (Badham, 1976). Those desiring further details are often referred to faith and "trust in the Lord." Under such circumstances, this imagery becomes individualized. Nevertheless, the promise that one will not simply and totally cease to exist is present and is widely believed.

Transcending Death

"Transcending death" means overcoming its existence as a simple and final termination of further life in any form. Afterlife beliefs interpret transcendence as simple transformation from one realm to another—a transition from predeath life to a postdeath form.

Lifton (1973) speaks of a universal need to keep in contact with life, to transcend death. Utilizing the rubric of "symbolic immortality," he suggests five ways of accomplishing such a goal. "Biological immortality" lets one live on through offspring and descendants. This potential is further realized in a broader framework in which the person continues through contributions to larger biosocial units, such as attachments to groups ranging from one's family to the human species. "Theological immortality" or "religious immortality" stresses spiritual attachment, implying the triumph of spirit over bodily death. "Creative immortality" is attained through one's works and achievements, the lasting contributions one hopes to make to the future. "Nature immortality" deals with our continuation as part of an undying, enduring, permanent nature. Lastly, there is a state of "experiential transcendence" or a mystical kind of immortality, "a state so intense that in it time and death disappear. . . . the restrictions of the senses—including the sense of mortality—no longer exist" (p. 7).

Modern science, especially medicine, has extended the notion of biological immortality. Males have preserved their sperm in "banks" for use after they have died. In a number of instances, widows have been artificially impregnated with their deceased husbands' sperm.

A few research efforts have related these modes of immortality to personal faith. Gochman and Fantasia (1979) found, as might be expected, that the religious form is strongest among devout persons, while the remaining types appear to be independent of religion. Religious immortality is also associated with short- and long-term life planning, implying a flexible time perspective—a tendency also noted in the positive relationship between time perspective and religion found by Hooper and Spilka (1970).

Utilizing a cognitive theoretical framework, Hood and Morris (1983) constructed a more rigorous quantitative assessment of Lifton's modes, relating these to forms of personal faith and death perspectives. This work is described in Research Box 8.1.

Research Box 8.1. Toward a Theory of Death Transcendence
(Hood & Morris, 1983)

With sensitivity to the necessity of theoretically guided research, Ralph Hood and his associate Ronald Morris denoted what they termed "transcendent" and "reflexive" facets of the self. The former is conceptually associated with immortality, in which the person "survives" this world. The reflexive self or selves, which exist in this world in a real sense, can also survive after bodily death. Cognitive issues come to the fore in thinking about transcendent–reflexive relations and the various forms of the latter. Robert Lifton's (1973) modes of biological, creative, and nature immortality/transcendence, which have been cited in the text above, fall into the reflexive category.

Applying these ideas, Hood and Morris developed reliable measures of the Lifton modes from interviews with 39 persons averaging 65 years of age. Independent judges agreed 94% of the time on classifying the responses to the modes. In terms of their presence or absence, 27 people were identified with nature transcendence, 30 with biological (now viewed as biosocial) transcendence, 31 with religious transcendence, and 33 with the creative mode. These people were then administered scales assessing death anxiety and death perspectives, as well as the Allport–Ross scales for Intrinsic and Extrinsic religious orientations. Patterns of meaningful relationships were obtained, suggesting the usefulness of both the Lifton modes and Hood and Morris's transcendent–reflexive distinction with elderly persons.

Hood and Morris found that the religious mode was associated with perceptions of death as (a test of) courage, and with belief in an afterlife of reward. It further prevented not only fear of death, but perceptions of death as pain and loneliness, failure, the unknown, or a loss of experience and control—tendencies not found with the other modes. The experiential/mystical mode negated the idea of death as a natural end. The biological (now biosocial) mode shared the positive religious correlation with courage and an afterlife of reward, but added death as failure. The creative mode was tied to perceptions of death as pain and loneliness, the unknown, forsaking dependents, and failure, as well as with indifference toward death. These findings suggest that personal achievement is antithetic to ideas of death—which, of course, terminates individual accomplishment.

Using a broader range of samples, Vandecreek and Nye (1993) redeveloped the Hood and Morris measures, but did not relate them to religious variables.

The Search for Evidence of Immortality

The idea of total termination is rightfully terrifying to most people; hence the need to convince oneself that life never really ends is intensely pursued on all fronts, from the humanistic to the scientific. Most people take the religious promise of immortality very seriously.

A massive psychological literature testifies to how perceptions and cognitions are influenced by our beliefs, values, expectations, and desires. When motivation is extremely high, we seek information to buttress our convictions, usually making inferences that go beyond the pertinent data. This is probably nowhere more true than in the way we deal with death. We desperately want to believe that life must continue after death, and grasp at every possible sign that this supposition bears the mark of absolute truth. An excellent illustration of this tendency may be seen in making a leap of faith from near-death experiences (NDEs) and possible contact with the dead to the existence of an afterlife. Even though these phenomena pose interesting theological problems, they are compatible with religious thinking in this sense: They imply that people do not simply die and cease to exist, but are transformed and have the potential of remaining connected to the living.

Near-Death Experiences

What we call an NDE has been formally studied since 1882, when the Society for Psychical Research was founded. Undoubtedly, this phenomenon has fascinated people since antiquity (Blackmore, 1991).

The concept of the NDE was greatly popularized during the 1970s. Rather easily, many people transformed the idea of "near death" to "after death." It was commonly believed that those undergoing NDEs had really died, entered an aspect of the afterlife, and then returned to tell about what occurred to them. Little does more to legitimate extraordinary occurrences than to have such events backed by experts. The volume *Life after Life* by psychiatrist Raymond Moody (1976) performed such a function, and, in the process, Moody became quite celebrated. Criticality, logic, and alternative explanations were acceptable only in limited quarters.

The noted pollster George Gallup, Jr., and his associate William Proctor (1982) point out that NDEs (which they term "verge-of-death experiences") have much in common with mystical and religious experiences, in that all may be triggered by extreme threats to life. They even suggest seven different situations that can elicit these episodes. (Keep in mind, as we indicate elsewhere in this volume, that at least a third of the U.S. population reports having had mystical experiences, and that among religious persons the percentage is far higher.) According to Gallup and Proctor, 15% of their respondents claimed to have had NDEs. The possible identification of religious encounters with NDEs suggests that those who report the former may be inclined to have had the latter, and this appears to be true. Gallup and Proctor (1982) found that 23% of those claiming religious experiences also stated that they had had NDEs—a percentage 8 points above that for the general populace. Another variation on this theme is apparent in consistently found correlations between NDEs and belief in other extraordinary phenomena, such as UFOs, reincarnation, and the likelihood that the living can contact the dead.

Turning to a specific group that is likely to question NDEs—namely, scientists—Gallup and Proctor (1982) reported that 10% admitted personal involvement in an NDE. Though 32% believed in an afterlife, only 3% felt that they had actually had a supernatural encounter. The overall tendency of scientists was to separate NDEs from the idea of an afterlife, and many attempted theoretical explanations of these phenomena in terms of physiological changes related to brain chemistry and function under oxygen deprivation, anesthetic effects, or the operation of endorphins. It is also significant that many religionists are also reluctant to claim that NDEs represent proof of an afterlife.

Even though one reads of NDEs in relation to terminality and the appearance to the experiencer of having "died," there is evidence that what occurs in an NDE is also found when drugs have been taken, or even in the normal course of everyday life (Blackmore, 1991).

Further doubt is cast on the supernatural origins of NDEs by the fact that these seem to have changed over time, and are also affected by place (Osis & Haraldson, 1977; Zaleski, 1987). In addition to much individuality entering the picture, cultural influences are obviously present (Osis & Haraldson, 1977; Kastenbaum, 1981). To some religionists, the rather general absence of religious content in NDEs raises questions about their authenticity. The claim has also been made that NDEs often profoundly affect the lives of those who have these perceptions (Ring, 1984). Suggestions of increased social concern and compassion, less materialism, improved self-esteem, and greater internal control have been reported (Ring, 1984).

One may ask whether certain characteristics of the experiencers may dispose them to have NDEs. Kastenbaum (1981) notes that many persons who have "died" and been resuscitated report no NDEs. In addition, various kinds of NDEs have been identified; some people indicate that they perceived one type, whereas others describe different forms. Though most of these are considered positive, frightening or otherwise negative NDEs are also endured. Lastly, people who report NDEs are also apt to have had other paranormal experiences (Kastenbaum, 1981). This last work suggests an avenue for further exploration with regard to personality, suggestibility, and reality contact, among other possibilities. The cross-cultural work of Osis and Haraldson (1977) is widely cited. Even though its findings are in line with other observations on NDEs, there is a "softness" to this effort that is representative of much of the research in this area. Research Box 8.2 presents a number of the issues raised, along with the findings.

The initial enthusiasm that greeted NDEs in the 1970s and 1980s has subsided. Interpretation of these experiences varies widely—from their acceptance as proof of an afterlife, to the concept of NDEs as "spiritual experiences," to analyses in terms of consciousness and brain function. Our psychological perspective assumes that the last possibility may prove of greater importance to a scientific approach than the first two.

Contact with the Dead

The idea of contact with the dead is very popular in Western society. One Internet browser listed 2,040,000 Web sites pertaining to this topic in January 2002, but this appeal to electronics may have originated in 1928, when Thomas Edison unsuccessfully attempted to build an electrical device that would permit one to contact the dead.

To be able to communicate with the deceased means that they are still somehow "alive," existing in a state that is "connected" to our life realm. Death thus means transformation, not termination. For some years, approximately 40% of U.S. adults have believed that they had some degree of contact with a deceased person (GSS, 1999). In 1973, a NORC survey

---

Research Box 8.2. At the Hour of Death (Osis & Haraldson, 1977)

These researchers have presented their work as the culmination of three major surveys: a pilot study, a U.S. survey, and a survey conducted in India. The last two efforts constituted the final comparative study. The pilot study, which was undertaken in 1959, sampled 5,000 physicians and 5,000 nurses. We read that "640 medical observers returned their questionnaires. These reported a total of 35,540 observations" (p. 27). In other words, there was a 6.4% return rate, which was not further defined by the nature of the "medical observers." Still, an effort is made to imply validity with reference to over 35,000 pieces of data, but these themselves remain largely undefined. In any event, a respondent return rate as small as the one obtained here casts considerable doubt on the generalizability of the information. Apparently 190 cases "of interest" were followed up with questionnaires and phone interviews, but again vagueness prevails. Given the use of questionnaires and the low return rate, one also wonders about the completeness of the returned forms. This is not discussed.

The real "meat" of the work by these researchers consisted of the further studies in India and the United States. In the United States, mail questionnaires were sent to 2,500 physicians and 2,500 nurses. The return rate was 20%, or 1,004 responses. A more personal procedure was used in India; 704 medical professionals responded, which the authors indicate comprised almost all who were approached. Unhappily, again, an unscientific lack of precision is present in the descriptions of both the sampling and responses. Still, an attempt is made to provide data, some of which are interesting and possibly useful.

If we concentrate on the India–U.S. comparisons relative to religion, the categories employed often lack the necessary exactitude. It makes good sense to see that only Indian respondents viewed the apparitional figures of Shiva, Rama, and Krishna, and a grouping of Mary, Kali, and Durga. If we interpret this latter grouping correctly, it mixes Christian and Hindu beings. The same is true of "saints and gurus" and of "demons and devils." Of special interest to us is the finding that there were 418 apparitional figures seen and only 140 religious beings. Of the figures seen by the U.S. respondents, only 12% were religiously identified. The comparable proportion witnessed by the Indian sample was 37.5%.

This work is more useful for hypothesis construction and testing than it is for making reliable and valid inferences. Its subjectivity demands rigorous cross-checking. Considerable room is left for the expectations and values of researchers and interpreters of NDEs to introduce bias, while giving the impression that such work is scientifically rigorous. A door has been opened to understanding a fascinating phenomenon. To date, however, there has been much more talk than solid research (Bailey & Yates, 1996).

---

indicated that 27% of the U.S. population felt they had participated in such an interaction; this number increased to 42% by 1987 and has been fairly steady since (Greeley, 1987; Morin, 2000). If this represents a real trend between the 1970s and the 1990s, we need to understand what has been happening.

Kalish and Reynolds (1973) found that 44% of those they interviewed claimed contact with someone who had died. A study of widows (Glick, Weiss, & Parkes, 1974) revealed that 64% still thought a great deal about their deceased husbands a year after their deaths. In this work, almost all reported that they frequently experienced a sense of the presence of the departed one. The descriptions often fell into an intermediate category between thinking about the dead spouse and a sense of actual contact. In all likelihood, the dividing line between perceived contact and obsessive thinking is often quite tenuous, and it is difficult to know how to distinguish the two. The combination of desire, need, hope, and other factors may create the conditions necessary for one to experience some alteration of consciousness that leaves the impression of contact with the dead. If someone has died recently, thoughts about that individual can be expected to occupy one's mind for some time to come. Many environmental cues may stimulate such ideas, along with anniversaries of birth, death, marriage, and other important events.

With its emphasis on an afterlife, religion may be influential in reports of contact with the dead. Sixty-six percent and 68% of Catholics and Mormons, respectively, feel that "religious observances by the living" (Kearl, 1989, p. 185) may actually benefit those who are deceased. All other Christian groups are considerably less likely to feel this way; nevertheless, such ideas keep alive the idea of a connection between the living and dead. In general, however, religion's effects do not appear to be major. This is seen in Table 8.2, which presents national survey data.

If religion is not a major influence, are those who report having contacts with the dead different in any other way from those denying such experiences? Data suggest a number of possible influences. On the sociological level, race and gender are significant. Specifically, blacks report more contact than whites, and females are more responsive in this regard than males (Kearl, 1997; MacDonald, 1992). The cultural circumstances of women and blacks are suggested as the reasons for these findings. Psychologically, the tendency of individuals to perceive contacts with the dead increases when they have had more recent experience with friends and relations dying; MacDonald (1992) inteprets these associations as functions of stress and change.

As with those who report NDEs, propensities to claim paranormal encounters are more common among those who state that they have had contact with the dead (Kearl, 1997). The possible role of religion in these observations has not been explored, though the influences of both extremely conservative faiths and New Age orientations are worthy of investigation.

People appear to seize on virtually anything in order to maintain a belief in immortality. The final possibility, which may have mental health ramifications, is simply to believe that someone has not died. Most people probably toy with such an idea immediately after a death. The problem comes when someone refuses to give up these convictions. In a less serious mood, we may ask what can be done to help those who claim that Elvis Presley or other

TABLE 8.2. Responses to the Question "How Often Have You Felt as Though You Were Really in Touch with Someone Who Died?"

Religion	Percentages reporting contact with a deceased person			
	Never	Once or twice	Several times	Often
Protestant	61	23	11	4
Catholic	56	26	12	5
Jewish	65	26	7	2
None	68	23	6	4

Note. Data from GSS (1999), based on 40,933 cases.

deceased notables still walk the earth in disguise. Happily, one's faith is not likely to be implicated directly in such notions.

RELIGION, DEATH ANXIETY, AND DEATH PERSPECTIVES

North American culture has a religious heritage that affirms ideas such as resurrection and life after death in the strongest terms. In one form or another, these views also seem to be worldwide. Such beliefs offer much gratification and help to alleviate a basic source of fear and anxiety. This last concern has been central to much work on the association of religion and death, for it deals with the immediate issue of how people conceptualize and confront death.

Death continually surrounds us. The mass media reveal its presence in daily news accounts of accidents, crimes, natural disasters, and war, and more specifically in ever-present obituaries, death notices, and funeral announcements. However, we tend to be inured to the impersonality of death and dying, because death is usually distant from our everyday lives. The front page is easily put aside; young people ignore everyday reports of death. Their elders increasingly attend to this information, not so infrequently seeing the names of those they have known. Nevertheless, we all must personally encounter death—beginning in childhood with the loss of pets and the demise of elderly relatives. And we often seek explanations and solace in afterlife notions that family, friends, and religious authorities reinforce.

We are suggesting here that we all know from childhood that death is inevitable, and that we don't like it; it is to be feared, and therefore elicits from us a pervasive underlying anxious awareness of death. Many psychologists have attempted to comprehend this phenomenon, and have found that it consistently correlates with religious beliefs and behavior.

Religion and Anxiety about Death and Dying

The principal death-related variable that has been studied in relation to faith has been variously termed "fear of death," "death anxiety," or "death concern."

Research Problems

Certain problems attend this research. First, the domains of religion and of death fear/anxiety have been confounded by measures from both areas containing similar items (e.g., belief in an afterlife). Second, a number of scholars have commented on such deficiencies as poor experimental designs, weak measurement indices, inadequate controls, inappropriate statistical analyses, and the use of questionable samples (Lester, 1967, 1972; Martin & Wrightsman, 1964). With respect to the last issue, most researchers have examined college students—a young population with limited experience of death. Other workers have studied children, elderly persons, psychiatric patients, student nurses, medical students, terminally ill individuals, seminarians, and regular churchgoing community members. Finally, we have described in Chapter 2 how measurement in the field of religion has gone from simple unidimensional scales to more refined and complex multidimensional instruments. A parallel development has occurred in efforts to assess death anxiety. Unitary approaches once dominated the field; now measures are usually multiform in nature.

Despite all these problems, it has been claimed that "one of the major functions of religious beliefs [is] to reduce a person's fear of death" (Groth-Marnat, 1992, p. 277). There has been a great deal of research on this issue; hence we may reasonably ask, "Does faith lessen concern about death?" Initially, we find inconsistency. Our own survey of this literature in the first edition of this book (Spilka, Hood, & Gorsuch, 1985) found that of 36 studies, the majority, 24, evidenced negative relationships between death fear on the one hand, and faith and afterlife beliefs on the other. Seven studies suggested that these domains were independent of each other, while three showed an unexpected positive association. Two others, which were more complex (e.g., assessing different levels of death fear, such as conscious and unconscious expressions), demonstrated two of the three possible relationships. Another examination of 16 studies conducted in the 1980s indicated that six evidenced a negative relationship, three a positive association, and five no affiliation between religion and death concern (Gartner, Larson, & Allen, 1991); there were also two studies with curvilinear patterns. These inconsistencies may be a function of the shortcomings noted above, plus other factors such as cultural influences (Pressman, Lyons, Larson, & Gartner, 1992). Again, we feel the necessity of appreciating the complexities of the religion and death fear realms, which unfortunately are sometimes ignored. Despite a minority of discrepant findings, our overview of this literature suggests that the more exacting research, particularly in terms of samples and instruments, argues for the reduction of death anxiety when religious commitment increases. We are not foreclosing other options, but feel that the best case can be made for this alternative, theoretically and operationally.

The general label of "religiosity" may mask certain factors that reduce death anxiety. Even though religion and afterlife beliefs correlate positively, especially among Christians, we need to consider the degree to which institutional faith in general includes belief in an afterlife as significant. Thorson (1991) further points out that belief in an afterlife correlates more strongly in a negative direction with death anxiety than does religiousness. Others confirm the centrality of afterlife ideas in resisting death distress and related depression (Aday, 1984–1985; Alvarado, Templer, Bresler, & Thomas-Dobson, 1995). Confounding may well occur between religion and belief in an afterlife.

Rasmussen and Johnson (1994) bring another issue to the fore—namely, the question of spirituality versus religiosity. Their research showed no relationship of death anxiety with religiosity, but a noteworthy association with scores on a Spiritual Well-Being scale. Because of the often great overlap between spirituality and religiosity (see Chapters 1 and 2), this relationship needs to be explored further, particularly with regard to afterlife beliefs.

Experimenting with Death Fear

We know that belief in an afterlife correlates negatively with death anxiety, but can we say that increasing concern with death might actually influence one's belief in an afterlife? In an ingenious study, Osarchuk and Tatz (1973) posed this question, and found that inducing death fear could affect one's afterlife beliefs. This work is described in Research Box 8.3.

When significant research findings such as those of Osarchuk and Tatz are obtained, their findings should be confirmed before congratulations are offered. Too often in psychology—or, for that matter, in all of the sciences—initial findings are later contradicted. This is suggested by another, more recent study (Ochsmann, 1984). Differences in method call for more research with new controls, in order to resolve the discrepancies between these studies.

꽈

Research Box 8.3. Effect of Induced Fear of Death on Belief in an Afterlife (Osarchuk & Tatz, 1973)

To test their hypothesis that making fear of death more salient would increase belief in an afterlife, these researchers constructed two equivalent and reliable 10-item scales of belief in an afterlife (Forms A and B). Two groups were created. Half of the people in each group received Form A initially; the other half received Form B first. From each group, 10 members were assigned to a death threat subgroup; 10 were assigned to a shock threat group; and 10 were designated as controls. Six subgroups were thus formed—three with high belief in an afterlife, and three with low belief. To the death threat subgroups, a taped communication was played giving an exaggerated estimate of the probability of an early death for individuals aged 18–22, due to accident or to disease caused by food contamination. The tape contained a background of dirge-like music. A series of 42 death-related slides was coordinated with the communication, including scenes of auto wrecks, realistically feigned murder and suicide victims, and corpses in a funeral home setting.

The members of the shock threat group were informed that they would receive a series of painful electric shocks (to which, of course, they never were subjected). The control groups engaged in ordinary play for the same amount of time that the other groups underwent the death or shock threats. All were then given the alternate form of the belief-in-afterlife scales that they had not taken earlier. The results were partially as predicted. Those with low belief in an afterlife, regardless of what group they were in, revealed no changes in their beliefs. In contrast, only those initially holding strong afterlife beliefs who were exposed to the death threat manifested a meaningful increase in these views. It appears that heightening one's concern with death can influence belief in an afterlife. It would have been interesting to see whether other religious views (such as belief in God) were also similarly affected, but this was not done here. The question is one of focus— for, as the 18th-century man of letters Samuel Johnson put it, "when a man knows he is to be hanged in a fortnight, it concentrates his mind wonderfully" (quoted in Boswell, 1791/n.d., p. 725).

The Influence of Circumstances

The Threat of War. It is a far cry from assessing death anxiety among college students and healthy adults to examining such concerns among those who have dealt with, or are likely to confront, life-threatening situations. Even though we are, in a sense, all born "terminally ill," death is rarely "real" to most of us. Among such groups as the military, terminally ill persons, or gays and bisexuals in proximity to HIV/AIDS, awareness of death is far more than an intellectual exercise.

With regard to military experience, Florian and Mikulincer (1992–1993) focused on Israeli involvement in Lebanon during the 1980s. They were able to study religious and non-religious participants who (1) were not in Lebanon; (2) were in Lebanon, but had no death-related experiences; and (3) were in Lebanon and had death-associated experiences. Fear of death was highest among those in the last group, but the researchers could not distinguish between the religious and nonreligious subgroups within this group. Still, of six fear-of-death factors, the nonreligious respondents scored higher in five. Florian and Mikulincer discuss the surprising complexity of trying to control for all of the relevant variables in work like this. Despite their creative effort, it is unfortunate that they could not deal with all confounding possibilities.

The Iran–Iraq war of the 1980s offered another opportunity to deal with the influence of confronting death. In a study of almost 1,200 Iranian Muslims, it was found that death anxiety and depression was highest among those exposed to war trauma who were least religious. Religion apparently performed a buffering role, it was felt through its support of belief in an afterlife (Roshdieh, Templer, Cannon, & Canfield, 1998–1999).

The Threat of AIDS. Another type of life-threatening situation is found primarily among gays and bisexuals. In this population in particular, the threat of AIDS is ever-present if one is sexually active. Research Box 8.4 details one significant study in this troubled area.

The Bivens et al. study charts a path to even more complex and insightful work regarding how religion may be employed as a resource to reduce fear of death by individuals suffering from a chronic, life-threatening disease. Concurrently, religion may play a negative role. One can also read the punishment motif of orthodox Christianity in Bivens et al.'s findings. This last theme may also be seen in other work, which found that the more men with AIDS attended church, and the more similar this church was to the one in which they were reared, the more death anxiety they showed (Franks, Templer, Capelletty, & Kauffman, 1990–1991).

In Franks et al.'s work, the greater death fear associated with religious activity in patients with AIDS does not necessarily point to the external stigmatizing role that religion may

---

Research Box 8.4. Death Concern and Religious Beliefs among Gays and Bisexuals in Variable Proximity to AIDS (Bivens, Neimeyer, Kirchberg, & Moore, 1994–1995)

A sample of 167 gay or bisexual men was obtained; 24 were HIV-positive and 19 had full-blown AIDS. These 43 were termed the "HIV+" group. The remaining men were HIV-negative ("HIV–"). Sixty-nine of the latter were defined as the "AIDS-involved" group, as they helped patients with AIDS in a variety of settings. The remaining participants were denoted "AIDS-uninvolved." All participants were administered a multidimensional scale that yielded eight measures of death fear/concern. An index of personally perceived threat from the potential of one's death was also used. This instrument yielded three factors plus a total score. Intrinsic and Extrinsic religious orientations were assessed by the Allport–Ross scales. Also included were a scale assessing Christian orthodoxy, and a more general inventory of religious beliefs and practices.

The HIV+ group displayed greater fear than the other two groups with respect to the likelihood of a premature death. No difference on this measure was found between the AIDS-uninvolved and AIDS-involved groups. The AIDS-involved participants, however, (1) manifested less global threat and less threat regarding meaningfulness and survival concerns, and (2) were significantly more religious, than the AIDS-uninvolved participants. Intrinsic faith, belief in God, and church attendance also associated with less global threat, threats to meaningfulness, survival concerns, and negative emotional appraisals. Literal Bible interpretations correlated positively with greater death fear, fear of personal destruction, and fear of consciousness in death.

perform. Churches are purveyors of community social values, and the prevailing levels of fear and rejection of AIDS and patients with AIDS are often internalized by these patients (Gilmore & Sommerville, 1994; Kegeles, Coates, Christopher, & Lazarus, 1989). The motivation to keep distance between oneself and AIDS is illustrated by the Muslim denotation of AIDS as a Western disease that can be best negated by complying with Islamic views and practices (Gilmore & Sommerville, 1994). Similar pronouncements by Christian ideologues are common.

The foregoing studies portray a negative role for religion in relation to AIDS, but there is research that indicates the opposite. Over the years, scientific progress has increasingly worked against the notion that AIDS is an automatic death sentence; newer treatments have provided hope. Moreover, the work of Hall (1994) with patients who have end-stage HIV disease shows that a major source of hope is religion. Hope is generated through religious beliefs and faith-related rituals that reduce death anxiety and depression on the part of those facing AIDS, as well as friends and relatives of those who have died from AIDS (Jull-Johnson, 1995).

As we have just seen, death threats from different sources may relate differently to religion in general. Belief in an afterlife is comforting to soldiers who encounter dangerous situations, but may be distressing to homosexuals with Christian inclinations who contract AIDS. Death in war usually has a religiously approved character to it, but traditional, conservative religion frowns on homosexuality.

Multidimensional Possibilities

In all of the above-described research on death anxiety, religion has been treated as a unidimensional phenomenon. One may simply speak of "religiosity," "religiousness," "religious importance," "religious beliefs," "religious practices," and "spirituality," among other conceptualizations. Each of these is treated as unitary—as one well-defined "thing" that somehow includes everything significant in the domain. By the mid-20th century, however, the complexity of personal faith became evident. The field was now faced with identifying the various forms of personal religion. This multiform approach currently dominates research in the psychology of religion.

As noted in Chapter 2, the first effort to understand religion in multidimensional terms was made by Gordon Allport. By the 1960s, his approach was operationalized into Intrinsic and Extrinsic religious orientations, a scheme that has essentially dominated religious measurement ever since (Allport, 1959; Allport & Ross, 1967).

Batson, Schoenrade, and Ventis (1993) have done yeoman service by surveying studies utilizing the measures of Intrinsic and Extrinsic faith in relation to death anxiety/fear. In this work, religion was multiform in character, while the death concern realm remained unidimensional. The findings are quite clear: An Extrinsic religious orientation was usually associated with death fear, concern, or anxiety (variously described), while an Intrinsic outlook opposed such negative outlooks. Even when controls were present for considerations such as guilt and personality, death anxiety maintained its positive tie to Extrinsic tendencies (Swanson & Byrd, 1998). A more recent effort has examined the idea of being obsessed with death, and, as above, found it to be negatively correlated with Intrinsic faith but positively correlated with an Extrinsic religious orientation (Maltby & Day, 2000).

Dimensionalizing Fear of Death

The next step in this research was to develop dimensionalized measures of fear of death. A number of schemes resulted in anywhere from five to eight forms. Minton and Spilka (1976) suggested five components: (1) lack of death fear; (2) sensitivity to death; (3) fear of the dying process; (4) awareness of the nature of death; and (5) loss of experience and control. Focusing on Christianity, Clark and Carter (1978) implied that different features of death anxiety might distinguish among persons varying in religious commitment—specifically, in Intrinsic versus Extrinsic perspectives.

Additional efforts to dimensionalize the fear of death were advanced by Leming (1979), Nelson and Nelson (1975), and Hoelter and Epley (1979); though there is a fair amount of conceptual and operational overlap among these instruments, they have proven useful in research. Nelson and Nelson (1975) identified four death anxiety factors that they labeled Death Avoidance, Death Fear, Death Denial, and Reluctance to Interact with the Dying. Scales were constructed to assess these areas, but important information was lacking, and these measures do not appear to have been used in other research. Pandey (1974–1975), also using factor analysis, found four components that he called Escape, Depressive Fear, Mortality, and Sarcasm. Again, serious questions may be raised about this work, which was not followed up. Not only are such aspects of death anxiety differentially related to religion, but curvilinear associations have also been demonstrated (Florian & Mikulincer, 1992–1993; Hoelter & Epley, 1975; Nelson & Cantrell, 1980). For example, Leming (1980) observed such relationships between overall religiosity, religious belief, experience, and ritual on the one hand and fear of death on the other. He suggested "that religiosity may serve the dual function of afflicting the comforted and comforting the afflicted" (p. 347).

In an effort to correct the shortcomings of the instruments described above, Stout, Minton, and Spilka (1976) factor-analyzed the responses of 221 people on 41 death anxiety items. Three reliable instruments somewhat similar to those of Nelson and Nelson (1975) were constructed. These were termed Lack of Death Fear, Experience in Death and Dying, and Awareness of the Potential of Death. Surprisingly, and in contradiction to other work, Intrinsic religiosity was independent of all three death anxiety scales; however, Extrinsic faith related (as expected) to death fear, to death experiences implying anxiety about how one will die, and to what being dead means.

A different approach to the issue of the complexity of death anxiety was introduced by Feifel (1974), who pointed out that both conscious and unconscious considerations should be evaluated when the death realm is examined. In other words, one's fear may be either conscious, unconscious, or both. Initially, Feifel was unable to find differences between religious believers and unbelievers with respect to these levels of death fear among persons who were either physically healthy or terminally ill. Expanding this work to three degrees of awareness, the deepest level (most unconscious) failed to relate to religion, but a midlevel fantasy approach did contribute markedly to associations with religious indices (Feifel & Tong Nagy, 1981). Employing different measures, Rosenheim and Muchnik (1984–1985) observed the influence of religion on the unconscious level, but found that it was less significant than the personality trait complex of repression–sensitization.

Other Death Perspectives

There are various other perspectives on death, which may or may not overlap with the various dimensions of death fear. This approach was initiated and refined by Hooper and Spilka (1970). Research Box 8.5 illustrates a later development of this work.

**Research Box 8.5. Death and Personal Faith: A Psychometric Investigation
(Spilka, Stout, Minton, & Sizemore, 1977)**

Early research on attitudes and feelings toward death focused on the main emotion people express toward death. Simply put, this is fear, even though some have called it death concern or death anxiety. It soon became evident, however, that different facets of the death and dying process were being emphasized. A simple positive–negative response had to give way to more complex cognitions regarding this inevitability. Hooper (1962) originally conceptualized 10 different ways of looking at death. One could view it (1) as a natural end, (2) as pain, (3) as loneliness, (4) as an unknown, (5) as forsaking dependents, (6) as failure, (7) as punishment, (8) as an afterlife of reward, (9) with courage, and (10) with indifference. A rigorous analysis of statements in these 10 perspectives resulted in the following eight reliable scales:

1. *Death as Pain and Loneliness.* Death is viewed as painful, and is associated with loss of mastery, consciousness, and isolation.

2. *Death as Afterlife of Reward.* Death leads to eternal reward and personal justification.

3. *Indifference toward Death.* Death is of no consequence, a trivial occurrence in the scheme of things.

4. *Death as Unknown.* The end of life is an unfathomable and ambiguous mystery.

5. *Death as Forsaking Dependents.* Death involves guilt over leaving one's dependents.

6. *Death as Courage.* Death is a final test of one's highest values, strength of character, and courage.

7. *Death as Failure.* Death is personal failure and defeat—the ultimate in frustration and helplessness.

8. *Death as Natural End.* Death is the simple natural conclusion to life, with nothing beyond it.

A number of studies related these death perspectives to scales assessing overlapping religious orientations (i.e., Intrinsic vs. Extrinsic faith, and Committed and Consensual religious forms). The table below shows the differential pattern of correlations between the death perspectives in the Spilka et al. (1977) study, and a later confirmatory one by Cerny and Carter (1977). In further work, Clark and Carter (1978) obtained similar findings.

	Personal religion scales							
	Committed		Consensual		Intrinsic		Extrinsic	
Death perspective scales	Spilka	Cerny	Spilka	Cerny	Spilka	Cerny	Spilka	Cerny
Death as Pain and Loneliness	−.08	−.19**	.13	.18*	−.26**	.21*	.36**	.41**
Death as Afterlife of Reward	.35**	.77**	.20*	.51**	.37**	.72**	−.07	.05
Indifference to Death	−.09	−.38**	.18*	−.14*	−.25**	−.38**	.39**	.14*
Death as Unknown	−.24**	−.41**	.12	−.23**	−.18*	−.47**	.21**	.14*
Death as Forsaking Dependents	−.11	−.07	.14	.12	−.13	−.13*	.31**	.31**
Death as Courage	.20*	.45**	.14	.35**	.12	.41**	−.01	.10
Death as Failure	−.18*	−.15*	.17	.25**	−.23**	−.17**	.49**	.41**
Death as Natural End	.04	.11	.19*	−.03	−.13	.04	.29**	.04

Note. The higher coefficients were probably a function of the broader range of religious activity and belief observed in Cerny and Carter's (1977) larger sample.

*p < .05. **p < .01.

continued

Research Box 8.5. *continued*

It is noteworthy that this table shows only one instance of disagreement in the direction of a relationship where both correlations were statistically significant. Full agreement in both direction and significance occurred in 22 of the 32 coefficients. In addition, of the nine correlations that attained significance in only one of the studies, eight occurred in the Cerny and Carter research. As the table footnote indicates, this could have been a function of the larger sample, as well as the use of less stringent criteria to denote religiosity. These would have permitted greater meaningful variance, and hence more significance.

The pattern of correlations was as expected. Scores on the scales for Intrinsic and Committed religious orientations related positively to scores on scales indicating favorable outlooks on death (e.g., Death as Afterlife of Reward and Death as Courage). Negative associations were obtained with scales indicating undesirable death perspectives, with one exception (Intrinsic religion with Death as Pain and Loneliness). The latter may simply have been an "artifact" (a chance occurrence). Again, we note that religious commitment endows the individual with strength and reason not to fear death. There is obviously considerable potential to understanding both death and religion in multidimensional terms.

RELIGION, DEATH, AND AGE

When we look at death, our understandings primarily encompass the period from adolescence to old age—in other words, young and middle adulthood. There is a popular aversion to associating death with children; although children do encounter death, and sometimes even die themselves, we acknowledge these facts with reluctance. In contrast, old age and death naturally seem to go together. Religion, however, is pertinent to both extremes of the age continuum.

Religion and Death in Children

Children's Views and Knowledge of Death

Before religion can exercise its influence on children, we need to know something about their views and knowledge of death. Using primarily Piagetian developmental concepts, a number of researchers have made efforts to determine how children learn about death and conceive of it as they develop (Anthony, 1940; Nagy, 1948; Wass, 1984). Even though possibilities of death awareness are implied as early as the age of 2, by the time children reach age 5 or so, they no longer regard death as a temporary and reversible phenomenon. For about the next 4 years, death is embodied as a person, and a child may feel that this personification can be avoided. After ages 9 or 10, death becomes understood as a universal and inevitable process that affects everyone (Nagy, 1948).

Also at about the age of 5, religious ideas become associated with death. Concepts of God, angels, heaven, and the like are introduced, probably reflecting the influence of parental faith, and instruction in church and Sunday school. For example, 5-year-olds are well acquainted with the deaths of animals and elderly people, particularly grandparents

(Goldman, 1970). Religious explanations of such experiences are commonly provided by teachers and parents, in an effort to reduce the anxiety and fear that may result as children attempt to comprehend what has occurred.

During these early years, religious language is anchored in tangible, concretistic notions. For example, Tamminen's (1991) young subjects generally stated that dead people and possibly pets go to heaven, which is located in the sky, and that they remain there with God. The relationship between death and religion follows Piagetian developmental concepts quite well (Hyde, 1990; Wass, 1984).

Employing galvanic skin responses (GSRs) with a word association test, Alexander and Adlerstein (1958) attempted to determine emotional correlates of death-related terms among children ranging in age from 5 to 16. The middle group (those aged 9–12) displayed the lowest GSRs. The youngest group (aged 5–8) came in second, while the oldest respondents (aged 13–16) evidenced the highest GSRs. Death-related words elicited significantly longer response latencies than neutral terms did over all ages, implying that death concepts do arouse emotion. This effect was greatest for the youngest children and least for the oldest group.

Childhood Spirituality and Death

Even though he recognizes the pervasive influence of religion in the lives of children, psychiatrist Robert Coles (1990) feels that the notion of "spirituality" better describes the holistic quality and innocent purity of how children treat religious ideas. Death is one of those realities that affect children deeply. Using primarily interview methods, Coles has simply inferred that "death has a powerful and continuing meaning" (p. 109) for children. Both actual death and potential death are profound mysteries that often call forth images of God and Jesus in children. Death is a puzzlement, an awesome phenomenon, a challenge to understanding, a stimulus for contemplation, and a source of emotional turmoil. Formal religion is put aside as children seem to marshal their defenses against death's finality. However, personal prayer is frequently employed as death is largely concretized in specific experiences and observations—the loss of grandparents, the accidental deaths of strangers, the death of friends, and thoughts of personal death. The idea that heaven is nearby mutes the fear and horror of dying. When one reads what Coles's children say, an individuality shines through, making his attribution of spirituality most appropriate. This is rich material, and even though we would like to analyze it in a more objective manner, it shows that our generally preferred method has limits.

Death apparently becomes increasingly important as individuals leave childhood and adolescence. Still, there is a dearth of solid research relating faith to death fear, anxiety, and attitudes among children and young people. The role of specific religious forms has also been overlooked. Anecdotal descriptions are useful, but objective research is necessary.

Religion, Death, and Elderly People

Death is too far from young persons and too near elderly people, both in fact and perception—but not always, as one might expect. As of 1997, persons over the age of 65 did account for 75% of the deaths in the United States; therefore, the reality of death grows as one ages, and this invariably becomes a coping issue (Kearl, 1989; U.S. Bureau of the Census, 2000). The average U.S. resident actually lived 75.4 years in 1991, the last year this information was presented (U.S. Bureau of the Census, 2000). Preliminary data for 1998 show that life expectancy at birth for the U.S. population was 76.7 years. The projection for 2010 is 78.5 years (U.S. Bureau of the Census, 2000). This number has increased 5.9 years since 1970; the process of increasing longevity is thus apparently slow but sure.

Death Concern among Elderly Persons

Erikson and his associates have claimed that "those nearing the end of the life cycle . . . [struggle] to balance consequent despair with the sense of overall integrity that is essential to carrying on" (Erikson, Erikson, & Kivinick, 1986, p. 8). The expectation of an association between increasing age and despair is probably overdone, however, and may be a view held by more younger people than older people. In one study of those over the age of 65, only 4% were troubled by their own relative temporal proximity to death (Munnichs, 1980). Other research reported that only 10% of an older sample indicated fear of dying, while 45% claimed a "forward-looking attitude toward death" (Swenson, 1965, p. 108). The same percentage were said to be evasive, preferring not to think about death; this does imply some degree of death anxiety.

Regardless of age, death anxiety may be essentially irrelevant when a person is healthy. A study of patients suffering from terminal cancer and heart disease plus a healthy control group found that most of those who were ill denied fears about death (Feifel, Freilich, & Hermann, 1973). No differences were observed between the patients with heart disease and those with cancer. Since clinically sophisticated interviewers gathered the data, conscious and unconscious indicators of death fear were distinguished. The results just described applied only to conscious fears; significant evidence of differences between the healthy and ill groups in unconscious fears were noted, with both ill groups revealing higher levels of unconscious death fears.

Another possibility is that thoughts of death and dying are replaced by "more optimistic life-affirming involvement" (Munnichs, 1980, p. 63). In a personal contact, a centenarian responded to a question about whether she thought about death with the response, "Of course, but I'm too busy to die."[2] She was indeed, and survived for another 3 years. Hers is not an isolated perspective. The notion of not wanting to die because of "unfinished business" may be quite common (Tobin, Fullmer, & Smith, 1994). This view challenges the most popular social science perspective on aging—namely, "disengagement" theory, which suggests that people are supposed to lead themselves toward death when they are old by slowly withdrawing from their worldly attachments (Kearl, 1989). In cases where such withdrawal occurs, it is usually accompanied by health problems.

The question of what constitutes "withdrawal" is controversial. The recent proliferation of senior centers and senior housing with exercise programs and a variety of intellectually stimulating courses is working increasingly against disengagement. In addition, older people are also often involved with religious institutions, and to regard such involvement as "disengagement" may be more pejorative than accurate. The constructive aspect of this behavior is most evident: Elderly persons who are religious generally reveal low levels of anxiety and concern about dying (Koenig, 1988). Though a minority of studies show no relationship between these variables, none show a positive association (Koenig, 1994a).

---

2. This response was given by Dr. Ruth Underhill in a 1977 course on the psychology of death and dying, which was taught by Bernard Spilka. Dr. Underhill was then almost 100 years old, and was still both mentally and physically active.

Faith apparently buttresses older people against the idea of impending death; it may accomplish this protective and beneficial function not only by its assurance of an after-life, but also by currently affirming one's worth and dignity. Koenig (1988) suggests that religion plays a buffering role against death anxiety, because it offers hope that death is not a final end. As in Swenson's (1965) study, highly religious people may perceive death as a doorway to a future life of reward. Koenig further reinforces the idea that religion may support the mechanism of denial—a kind of cutting off of such negative emotions as fear and anxiety. Lastly, we should not underestimate the role of the church in bringing together groups of elderly devout individuals, so that anxieties about death may be lessened through discussions and social reinforcement of doctrines and beliefs that neutralize concern about death.

Even in cases where aging people do reduce their social and occupational roles (i.e., where disengagement occurs), religious involvement may be substituted for other lost po-sitions. Church activities offer a number of social possibilities by sponsoring the acquisi-tion of new contacts and opportunities, to demonstrate that one is still effective and has worth. Blazer and Palmore (1976) thus noted that "religious activities . . . were correlated with happiness, feelings of usefulness, and personal adjustment" (p. 85) among those over 70 years of age. The emotion-controlling and directive roles that ritual plays should also be considered here. Not a few of the elderly regard religious ritual as reassuring (Erikson et al., 1986).

Old age is a time, as Erikson et al. (1986) have put it, of dealing with the issue of basic meaning. As we have noted in a number of chapters, this is one of the most fundamental of religious purposes. Facing death implies the attainment of integrity and what Erikson and colleagues call "wisdom." The task for the individual is to gain a sense of place in the uni-verse—a religious function if there ever was one. The last years of life are thus a period of taking stock, coming to terms with the past, and looking into a questionable future. In a rather straightforward study, Jeffers, Nichols, and Eisdorfer (1961) interviewed 269 community volunteers 60 years of age and older about their afterlife beliefs and fear of death. Table 8.3 summarizes the main findings in relation to religion. The data in the table are simple and clear: Religion negates fear of death among older persons.

TABLE 8.3. Fear of Death and Belief in an Afterlife in Relation to Religious Variables in an Older Sample

Fear of death was associated significantly with . . .
Less belief in life after death.
Less frequent Bible reading.

Belief in an afterlife was associated significantly with . . .
Less fear of death.
More frequent church attendance.
More frequent Bible reading.
Involvement in more church activities.
More favorable attitudes toward religion.
Greater personal importance of religion.

Note. All of these relationships attained statistical significance at the .05 level. Data from Jeffers, Nichols, and Eisdorfer (1961).

Religion, Elderly People, and Longevity

In the late 19th century, Francis Galton rejected the idea that piety and longevity may be positively correlated. Focusing on individuals who prayed the most or who were prayed for the most, he showed that neither group benefited from prayer (Mccullough, 2001). People have often been reluctant to accept such a judgment. Where research has dealt with this issue, either directly or indirectly, the results have not been either clear or consistent. A. H. Richardson (1973) studied over 1,300 octogenarians and found religion to be unrelated to 1-year survival rates. More recent work by Koenig (1995) confirmed this finding. Idler and Kasi (1992) also found that neither public or private religiousness predicted mortality; however, for both Christians and Jews, there were significantly fewer deaths in the 30 days prior to a major religious holiday than for the same period afterward.

Other research on a sample of institutionalized, chronically ill elderly people claimed that those who die within the year were less religious (Reynolds & Nelson, 1981). This picture is muddied by the fact that they also had poorer prognoses and were more cognitively impaired. In a similar vein, Zuckerman, Kasl, and Ostfeld (1984) reported that religion was positively correlated with longevity, but only among elderly individuals who were in poor health.

McCullough (2001), in a truly major effort, has attempted to resolve the many contradictory investigations in this area. He and his associates undertook a meta-analytic review of the research in this area, and came up with 42 independent estimates of the relationship between religion and mortality. ("Meta-analysis" is basically a methodological/statistical procedure in which one gathers together a great deal of data that are thought to be comparable, and analyzes these data in order to resolve discrepancies, disagreements, and conflicting findings). Even after considering some 15 possible confounding factors, McCullough (2001) found that religious involvement and longevity were positively related. The association was, however, rather weak. For example, if we had two groups of 100 people each—one group being high in religiosity, the other less religious—we could expect to find in a later follow-up that 53 people in the less religious group had died, while only 47 in the more religious group had died. This outcome would apparently hold for public religious activity (e.g., church attendance), but not for private devotions. The association between religion and mortality was also found to be stronger for women than men. McCullough (2001) offers a number of possibilities to account for these observations, opening the door to further research. This is an area that merits more rigorous study, along with theory that offers reasons why faith and mortality should be related, especially among elderly people.

RELIGION AND EUTHANASIA

Euthanasia is a troubled realm. Not a few seriously or terminally ill patients have appealed to be euthanized, and have even sought relief through the courts. Behind the scenes, however, such desires are surprisingly common.

This is an issue that is often simplified and euphemized by such terminology as "mercy killing," "assisted suicide," "right to die," and "death with dignity." A distinction must, however, be made between "passive" and "active" euthanasia. The former usually implies the withholding of heroic measures to sustain life when death is imminent and the quality of life is very poor. In contrast, active euthanasia is the intentional termination of life under the same conditions, especially when great pain and suffering are present. This is probably practiced more often than we think when the patient makes impassioned pleas to die.

Support for Euthanasia: Medical and General

Though active euthanasia is illegal in most jurisdictions, the overwhelming majority of medical professionals favor passive euthanasia. Surveys reveal that from two-thirds to over 90% of health care practitioners approve passive approaches, whereas only 17% of physicians and 36% of nurses take positive views of active euthanasia (Carey & Posavec, 1978–1979; Hoggatt & Spilka, 1978; Lavery, Dickens, Boyle, & Singer, 1997; Rea, Greenspoon, & Spilka, 1975). It should not come as a surprise that in 1993, a Gallup Poll reported that 43% of U.S. residents approved the "assisted suicide" actions taken by Dr. Jack Kevorkian (*The Gallup Poll Monthly*, 1993, p. 47); a slightly greater number (47%) disapproved. The Gallup Poll organization has taken a sophisticated view of the euthanasia issue, revealing how attitudes are dependent on a number of factors. Table 8.4 illustrates some of these considerations.

TABLE 8.4. Attitudes toward Euthanasia in the United States

Do you think a person has the moral right to end his or her life under these circumstances?[a]

	Yes	No
When the person is suffering from incurable disease	58%	36%
When the person is suffering great pain with no chance of improvement	66%	29%
When an otherwise healthy person wants to end his or her life	16%	80%

A terminally ill person wants treatment withheld so that he or she may die. The patient has the right to stop treatment . . .[a]

	Yes	No
If the doctor agrees	75%	22%
If the person is in great pain	78%	18%
If the family agrees	76%	22%
Under any circumstances	59%	4%
Under no circumstances	11%	87%

If you yourself were on life support systems and there was no hope of recovering, you would prefer to . . .[a]

	Yes
Remain on life support	9%
Have treatment withheld	84%

Do you think a doctor should be allowed by law to assist a person to end his or her life?[b]

	Yes	No
When the person is suffering from incurable disease	52%	42%
When the person is suffering great pain	64%	31%
When the person is a burden on the family	22%	71%
No reason	8%	88%

[a]Data from Gallup (1992, p. 4).

[b]Data from *The Gallup Poll Monthly* (1992, p. 34).

Religious Perspectives on Euthanasia

Though scripture and theology are usually interpreted as opposing euthanasia, there is much deviation from such a position. If euthanasia is approved by a physician, 61% of Protestants, 62% of Catholics, and 78% of Jews agree with such a stance (Kearl, 1989). The strength of one's religious position affects these findings, as the comparable data for "strong" Protestants, Catholics, and Jews are 49%, 51%, and 67%, respectively (Kearl, 1989). It is abundantly evident that euthanasia under certain circumstances is supported widely regardless of religious affiliation, but that this support decreases with an increasing degree of religiosity. In addition, for the last 50 years, the tendency has been for approval of euthanasia to increase slowly and steadily among moderate and liberal religionists (Kearl, 2002). Such approval is also a positive function of belief in an afterlife (Klopfer & Price, 1979).

Religion and Physician-Assisted Suicide

A conceptual variation on active euthanasia is "physician-assisted suicide" (PAS). Needless to say, sometimes the distinction between the two is tenuous. PAS takes one of two forms: (1) The physician may offer the individual the means (pills, injections, or equipment) to induce death; or (2) the doctor may accede to the patient's wish to die by actively causing the person's death (Koenig, 1994a). Though PAS is against the law in the Netherlands, the law is evidently not enforced, and it is estimated that up to 10,000 persons utilize PAS annually in that country. Despite the fact that these procedures are also illegal in the United States, there is much tacit approval of their use, and in a number of states efforts to pass laws permitting PAS are pending. Illustrative of this trend, in 1994, a federal district court in the state of Washington struck down the state's 140-year-old law that made assisted suicide illegal (Kearl, 2002). In states where the electorate has acted on such proposals, they have usually been narrowly defeated (Koenig, 1994a). Oregon, however, did pass such a law in 1997, and a number of terminally ill people have utilized their right to die under this statute. It is currently being challenged in the courts.

Opposition to PAS has come more from formal religious organizations than from their individual members. Still, the more liberal Christian and Jewish groups are slowly increasing their support for PAS. The United Church of Christ already formally backs such action (Koenig, 1994a).

Indications that it is probably just a matter of time before more religious bodies justify euthanasia and PAS come from the increasingly favorable positions taken by clergy. In one investigation, Carey and Posavec (1978–1979) found that 96% of the clerics they sampled advocated passive euthanasia, and that 21% espoused its active form. Support for passive euthanasia varies with the reasons advanced for such action, however (Nagi, Pugh, & Lazerine, 1977–1978). Depending on the justification, Carey and Posavec (1978–1979) found that support was offered by anywhere from 34% to 73% of Protestant clergy; for Catholic priests, the comparable percentages ranged from 30% to 69%. In regard to active euthanasia, the percentages were significantly lower: Only 13–25% of the Protestant clergy, and only 1–3% of the Catholic priests, countenanced such action. Even though Carey and Posavec's investigation failed to designate the Protestant denominations sampled, approval of euthanasia grows with liberality of a cleric's theological position and group. Conservative clergy balance their opposition with strong beliefs in a rewarding afterlife (Spilka, Spangler, & Rea, 1981).

Despite the fact that a study by Gillespie (1983) did not bear directly on the question of euthanasia, he demonstrated clerical differences on a variety of death perspectives across religious groups. This research implies that pastoral outlooks on euthanasia may be dependent on other factors than denominational conservatism and afterlife beliefs. It opens a significant door to further study.

A word is in order regarding why there is religious opposition to euthanasia and PAS. In brief, a position derived from scripture simply avers that both life and death are in "God's hands." That is, life can only be given and taken away by the deity. Other considerations are that the pain and suffering of the ill person is supposed to be experienced by that individual, and may benefit all concerned in the long run.

RELIGION AND SUICIDE

The tragedy of suicide is usually difficult to understand. In nations such as the United States and Canada—with so much to offer, with medicine making almost unbelievable progress, and with science and technology opening a future that points toward an easier and better life for all—suicide remains a mystery for most people. Psychological explanations such as depression abound, but these often mean little more than that a word has been substituted for a reality that can't be grasped. Death itself is enigmatic, but suicide remains the ultimate conundrum.

In 1998, 29,300 people in the United States committed suicide; the National Institute of Mental Health tells us that approximately another half million people entered hospital emergency rooms as a result of attempting suicide (Hoyert, Kochanek, & Murphy, 1999; U.S. Bureau of the Census, 2000). Though women attempt suicide more often than men, the latter "are four times more likely to die than are females" (U.S. Office of the Surgeon General, 1999, p. 1). Among whites, depending on age, male suicide rates range as high as six times those for women (U.S. Bureau of the Census, 2000, p. 93). The incidence of suicide is fairly level until age 59, after which it sharply increases from 23 per 100,000 to 65.3 per 100,000 for men 85 years and older (U.S. Office of the Surgeon General, 1999). After age 65, men account for 84% of all suicides. The suicide rate for elderly divorced or widowed men is 2.7 times that for their married peers and over 17 times the incidence for married women (National Center for Injury Prevention and Control, 2003). The fact that 85 people commit suicide each day in our country portrays a true national tragedy (U.S. Public Health Service, 1999).

Views of Suicide in Institutionalized Religion

Institutionalized religion has rather uniformly treated suicide in negative terms. The Judeo-Christian tradition has taught that suicide is immoral and therefore sinful (Kastenbaum, 1981). Those who commit suicide may not be allowed burial with the faithful in religiously sponsored cemeteries, and may be consigned to certain sections that imply severe condemnation and rejection. Because of the stigma that has traditionally been (and often still is) attached to suicide, medical, religious, and civil authorities commonly identify a death as a suicide with reluctance. The more modern religious perspective is to consider these individuals as mentally disturbed—a diagnosis that removes the burden of sin, and mitigates the opprobrium that members of the surviving family have often received from the religious community. The influence of religion on attitudes toward suicide has lessened considerably in the contemporary world, especially in the United States (Wasserman & Stack, 1983).

That institutionalized faith can affect the incidence of suicide has been well documented for over a century (Dublin, 1963; Kastenbaum & Aisenberg, 1972). Cross-national studies suggest a weakening of the impact of religion, such that the inverse relationship between faith and suicide may no longer hold for men, but this is questionable. It continues to exist among women (Stack, 1983). The classic finding that religious commitment and conservatism oppose suicide nevertheless persists; hence church attendance remains negatively correlated with suicide rates (Martin, 1984).

Religion and Suicide among Elderly Persons

We have noted above that people over 60 are at much greater risk of suicide than younger cohorts are. Kearl (1989) suggests that "for some elderly individuals, suicide is preferable to loneliness, chronic illness, and dependency" (p. 145). This may be especially true for physically ill older men, the group with the highest suicide rate in the United States. Again, however, among elderly individuals, religion plays its traditional role in opposing self-destruction. Koenig (1994b) suggests that faith suppresses suicidal thinking in this group. He found that 18% of his sample of physically ill older men experienced suicidal thoughts, and that these were negatively related to religious coping.

This last observation may reflect a generation effect. Elderly religious individuals were reared at a time when religion was a stronger cultural influence than it is today. Because of this, they may identify with their faith's opposition to suicide, as well as with the promise of a happy afterlife. A related finding is that the recovery from bereavement of those who lose a loved one via suicide is enhanced by high belief in an afterlife (Smith, Range, & Ulmer, 1991–1992). We need to know whether this is true for those who committed suicide. Also, were they more isolated prior to their action? Direct research relating suicide to belief in an afterlife with this group would make a noteworthy contribution to this literature. Obviously, such information would have to be obtained indirectly.

Another answer may lie in being socially integrated into the community, especially a religious community. The data tell us that the highest suicide rates are among older, single, socially isolated men (Dublin, 1963; Stengel, 1964). Dealing with suicide ideology—namely, attitudes toward suicide—Stack and Wasserman (1992) have noted three possibilities: (1) Religion fosters general social integration, which opposes suicide; (2) specific religious views, such as belief in an afterlife, may contravene self-destructive impulses; and (3) religious organizations foster networking and social support, which should thwart suicidal inclinations. Using sophisticated statistical techniques on national data, these researchers found evidence supporting all three views, especially for conservative religious bodies. Focusing on church attendance, Stack and Wasserman concluded that the social connections a common faith may create and reinforce could be the main elements hindering suicide.

Apocalyptic Suicide

Recent years have witnessed a spate of mass suicides among members of religious cults. The cases of the Jonestown People's Temple, the Branch Davidians, and Heaven's Gate (among others) have shocked the world, and have left most of us without a satisfying explanation for these tragedies. There is a considerable literature on doomsday cults, and the classic study

When Prophecy Fails (Festinger, Riecken, & Schachter, 1956) offers an entry into this topic, even though it does not deal with death except as a fantasy possibility.

The rather bizarre forms religion took in several cults in which there were mass suicides has been analyzed by Dein and Littlewood (2000). The inclination of scholars who have studied these groups has been to examine their leadership and group structure. Searching for common personality factors or various forms of mental disorder has not been productive. The lack of hard data—specifically, too much clinical subjectivity and a dearth of confirmatory efforts—makes inferences in the realm of the individual rather tenuous. Vague allusions to paranoid traits, poor reality contact, or distressing early life conditions also do not appear useful. Previous work on mental disorder among cultists indicates the incidence of such problems to be no higher in cults than in the population at large (Needleman & Baker, 1978; Richardson, 1980; Wright, 1987).

If generalizations can be offered, a number of possibilities seem in order. Cults are groups that center about charismatic leaders who work to see that their members are separated from society in general, from family members, and from anyone who might offer divergent views. Absolute devotion to the leader's beliefs and teachings is reinforced in every manner possible. These doctrines may include the notions that death is invariably a door to a future life; that the physical body is a hindrance; and that even if people commit suicide, they never truly die in the sense of total termination, but continue on toward an ideal realm, a heavenly existence. These groups create the conditions that make suicide appear to be the only means of achieving ultimate happiness. The chapters in this volume on conversion and religious organizations (Chapters 11 and 12) go into these considerations in much greater depth.

Religion and Suicide: A Cross-Cultural Note

In Chapter 1, we have regretted the fact that little research has been undertaken on other than Western societies and cultures. However, comparisons are possible between Hindus and Muslims in regard to religion and suicide. Though Ineichen (1998) points out that Hindu religious writings are ambivalent about ending one's life, ultimate salvation is denied those who commit suicide. Strongly contrasting with this stance, the Koran and Islamic interpretations explicitly condemns suicide. The result is that Hindus manifest much higher suicide rates than Muslims (Ineichen, 1998). A very recent survey of national suicide statistics reveals a much higher rate of suicide for India than for Muslim nations that report such data (World Health Organization, 2001).

These data may be questioned, however. It is often difficult to be sure that a deceased person committed suicide, and, as noted earlier, there is great resistance to making such an identification in a cultural/religious milieu that strongly opposes suicide. When nations such as Jordan claim that no suicides at all took place in 2001, and Egypt gives a rate of 0.1 per 100,000 (World Health Organization, 2001), there is good reason to question these reports.

RELIGION, GRIEF, AND BEREAVEMENT

Living means that we will experience the deaths of loved ones, for there must always come that time when a beloved person "goeth to his long home, and the mourners go about the streets" (Ecclesiastes 12:5). When someone dies, the likelihood is high that family and friends will turn to religion for solace and understanding. Faith is often a basic part of the coping process, and death is frequently confronted and conceptualized in religious terms.

The process of grief and bereavement is surprisingly complex. "Grief" is an emotional process. "Bereavement" is not unambiguously defined as separate from "grief," though it emphasizes the sense of loss that leads to grief. Another overlapping concept is "mourning," which refers to the combination of cognitive, emotional, and behavioral responses that one manifests in bereavement.

The literature offers discussions about stages of grief, models of grief, degrees of grief, ritual in grief, religion as a resource in bereavement, the grief of parents and grandparents for deceased children and grandchildren, the grief of spouses for deceased mates, and grief for other family members and loved ones. In all of these areas, the role of faith is significant. For example, Flatt (1987) suggests some 10 grief stages that range from "initial shock" to what he terms "growth." In most of these stages, God is given a role—whether it be a questioning of how the deity could let someone die or how the divine actively brings about a death, to a place for "God's grace" in recovery from the depression resulting from grief. Another possibility is that the recovery from grief may move the person along to new stages and tests, such that the deity is seen to care as the person is reintegrated into "God's world." This means that the bereaved gains new strength to realize "God's purpose" in his or her remaining life (Flatt, 1987). Here we observe how significant attributions to God may be when death is confronted.

The central issue is "making sense" out of the loss, and religion seems to be the main source of meaning available to the survivors. Whether it is the loss of a spouse, a child, or another loved one, religious/spiritual commitments, doctrines, and ideas offer the meanings that reduce symptoms of distress and engender hope (Dahl, 1999; Golsworthy & Coyle, 1999).

Though the majority of research on religion and bereavement points to the beneficial role of faith in such distressing circumstances, it should be noted that not all work in this area supports such inferences and observations (Sanders, 1979–1980). This is indeed an involved realm—one that requires more sensitivity to theory and the possibility of confounding factors.

Sanders (1979–1980) undertook an interesting study in which she compared grief reactions to the death of a spouse, a child, and a parent. Though the most intense responses occurred when a child died, church attendance was related positively to optimism, less anger, and a better appetite. When church attendance and family interaction were treated together, the findings even more graphically favored the religion–family combination. This may imply the significance of religion not only in terms of meaning, but in regard to a broader beneficial basis for social support from one's kin.

There is evidence that bereavement may vary as a function of the kind of death that occurred—in other words, whether the death was natural, accidental, a result of violence, or a suicide (Morin & Welsh, 1996; Sheskin & Wallace, 1980). Morin and Welsh (1996) interviewed urban and suburban adolescents. The urban adolescents were in a facility for adjudicated youths, and had experienced more violent deaths than the suburban groups had. Their views of death involved violence and religion to a greater degree than those of the suburban teens did. The latter emphasized the experience of suffering, while the urban youths were more concerned with the loss of loved ones. Both groups found that their grieving benefited from talking about their feelings and concerns.

Sheskin and Wallace (1980) studied widows, and observed that, regardless of the nature of their husbands' deaths, they usually needed to "unburden themselves" to good listeners.

Theoretically, one might expect clergy to fulfill such a role, but this was not found. According to the studies reviewed by Sheskin and Wallace (1980), the clergy were found to be particularly unhelpful by widows whose husbands committed suicide. The implication is that since organized religions strongly oppose suicide, their representatives (i.e., the clergy) will have difficulty counseling the survivors of those who have committed suicide. Accordingly, the clergy, who should be highly knowledgeable, understanding, and sympathetic regarding death, may not be very helpful in such cases. Clerics could be responding like others who relate to the surviving Family members of those dying by suicide. This group feels that they are less accepted by their communities than others whose relatives died accidental or natural deaths (Smith et al., 1991–1992).

Another consideration brings us back to the issue of meaning. Even though the meaning of death in the religious/spiritual sense is enhanced by devotion to one's faith, suicide poses additional explanatory problems, compared to accidental or natural deaths. We may try to play word games and attribute the death to depression or some "psychotic break," but then we face the question of why this mental state was present. We struggle to make sense out of the tragedy, for our social order stresses individual worth and dignity, and taking one's own life often poses a deep and troubling dilemma.

Religious Schemas and Bereavement over Child Loss

A creative and useful theoretical treatment of bereavement has been advanced by Daniel McIntosh and his colleagues (McIntosh, Silver, & Wortman, 1993). McIntosh (1995) has also extended this approach to religion in general and its role in life. Noting that "a schema is a cognitive mental structure or representation containing organized prior knowledge about a particular domain, including a specification of the relations among its attributes" (1995, p. 2), McIntosh further notes that "people have different schemas for many domains." Schemas influence what is perceived, speed up cognitive processing of information, and offer meaning in difficult situations by filling in the gaps in our knowledge. In sum, they orient us to the world and to the problems with which we must cope; they therefore influence our behavior, and can help us adapt to problematic circumstances. With respect to death and bereavement, one salient aspect of a religious schema might be belief in an afterlife. Apparently such belief is "associated with greater recovery from bereavement regardless of the cause of death" (Smith et al., 1991–1992, p. 222). In contrast, bereaved persons with low belief in an afterlife evidence less well-being in general, and poorer recovery from the bereavement in particular. Such people also make greater efforts to avoid thinking about the death in question.

For many reasons, primarily culturally based, most people possess religious schemas that are often called into play when ambiguity and threat become troublesome. In their significant work on how parents cope with the death of an infant from sudden infant death syndrome (SIDS), McIntosh et al. (1993) demonstrated how parents' faith, through the use of religious schemas, indirectly facilitated their adjustment—both cognitively and behaviorally. The schemas both made the death meaningful and also supported efforts to come to terms with the loss. Religious participation and social support promoted the acquisition of helpful religious explanations. Cognitively, religious importance contributed to constructive mental processing and helped reduce distress.

McIntosh et al.'s work explains similar findings in other studies that have dealt with parental and grandparental bereavement (Bohannon, 1991; De Frain, Jakub, & Mendoza, 1991–1992). Studying the influence of church attendance, Bohannon (1991) was able to show that it was inversely related to anger, guilt, helplessness, obsessive thoughts about a child's death, somatic complaints, and death anxiety on the part of the grieving mothers. Similar effects were found for paternal anger, guilt, and death anxiety. De Frain et al. (1991–1992) found that religious beliefs were strengthened for 46% of the grandparents of children who died of SIDS, and 90% felt that their faith aided them in coping with the SIDS death.

Further work by Gilbert (1992) stressed the perceived role of God in this situation. She found that when religion was employed as a resource, bereaved parents felt that (1) God did not do bad things; (2) God was in control and could be relied on to make the wisest decision; (3) God had good reasons for the child's death; (4) God inflicted this tragedy upon the parents because they had the strength to deal with it; (5) God wanted them to appreciate life more; and (6) God desired that they change their lives for the better. Interestingly, those who claimed that religion was not initially helpful acquired a more positive outlook over time. Lastly, those who claimed that religion was irrelevant tended to be extrinsically oriented. The implication is that for faith to be of significance in this kind of tragedy, it must have an intrinsic, not superficial or utilitarian, quality. An excellent example of theoretically guided and methodologically sophisticated work in this area is presented in Research Box 8.6.

Conjugal Bereavement

The demise of a spouse is extremely distressing to the widow or widower. No one has yet assessed all of the factors that may affect the surviving mate. For an older couple, separation

---

Research Box 8.6. The Stress-Buffering Role of Spiritual Support: Cross-Sectional and Prospective Investigations (Maton, 1989)

Maton has theorized that religion may mitigate the effects of stress through the use of cognitive and emotional pathways. Specifically, he has defined these as "cognitive mediation" and "emotional support." The former implies a positive reframing of negative life events, while the latter comprises perceptions of God as valuing and caring for the distressed individual. Treating these as independent, Maton assessed the contributions of each with two samples: (1) bereaved parents who had lost a child, and (2) college students. In the first sample, 33 parents who had been bereaved within the preceding 2 years constituted a high-stress group, and 48 whose child had died more than 2 years previously made up a low-stress group. Measures of spiritual, social, and friendship support plus depression were completed by the respondents.

Spiritual support correlated negatively with depression and positively with self-esteem for the high-stress group, but not for the low-stress sample. A similar pattern was noted for support provided to the high-stress group, but not to the low-stress group. A prospective study with college students ruled out the likelihood that spiritual help followed rather than contributed to well-being. Maton concluded that "spiritual support may influence well-being through directly enhancing self-esteem and reducing negative affect ('emotional support' pathway) or through enhancing positive and adaptive appraisals of the meaning of a traumatic event ('cognitive mediation' pathway)" (p. 320). He went on to theorize various forms of spiritual support, and to suggest various research possibilities for exploring this domain further.

after a half century or more of living together may be the most wrenching and distressing factor. (Often we read that the passing of an elderly husband or wife is shortly followed by the death of the other, as if their link in life must continue indefinitely.) The issue of an expected death versus an unexpected one must also be considered. If a wife's death is not anticipated, the level of somatic symptoms and depression is greater in the husband than if the death has been expected for some time (Winokuer, 2000). In the latter instance, anticipatory grieving may take place and reduce the overall amount of physiological disruption that occurs.

The classic work of Glick et al. (1974) stresses the benign effects of faith on bereavement when a spouse dies (see also Parkes, 1972). In this research, to the extent that the widows were devout, they were described as turning "to the formal doctrine of their religions for explanation" (Glick et al., 1974, p. 133). Again we see the significance of spiritual meaning and understanding in alleviating depression and the sense of loss. In other work, social and religious support appeared to operate independently, both working to counter depression and subjective stress (Levy, Martinkowski, & Derby, 1994). Study after study confirms these findings: Personal adjustment and religious commitment and activity go together. As might be expected, religious involvement is likely to increase following the death of a spouse (Bahr & Harvey, 1980; Haun, 1977; Loveland, 1968).

The Significance of Ritual

In Chapter 3, we have shown that ritual has roots deep within our human and animal past. It performs many functions, not the least of which is to establish and maintain control over our personal world and ourselves, especially when we feel pressured. Rites and ceremonies are integral to religion; they bring us psychologically closer to others and to our common cultural heritage. These confirm our oneness with the perceived source of all good and strength, and allow us to feel that we can overcome even death. Ritual is a core aspect of faith that plays a constructive role in grief. Variously said to create a sense of safety and impart new constructive meanings, it may also be "constructively self-alienating." In other words, ritual distances a person from emotions and permits him or her to return to the world—a process that obsessive self-concern hinders. Reeves and Boersma (1989–1990) thus maintain that "rituals can provide a sense of positive personal power for an individual who is feeling out of control and clarify and provide meaning to an issue so that it is easier to work on" (p. 289).

On another level, rituals introduce structure, elicit social support, and not infrequently serve as a distraction from the grief itself. Formal ceremonies allow bereaved individuals to work through the pain of loss. Death is a disruption in the survivors' lives, and religious ideology and ritual can function to restore stability to those who are bereaved (Honigmann, 1959).

Illustrative of this principle is the Jewish practice of *shiva*, a 7-day, repetitive set of mourning rites that evokes community support in the form of a group. Group members often bring food to the griever's home and participate in a well-established set of ceremonies. It has been compared to group therapy (Kidorf, 1966). Gerson (1977) describes in depth the formalized mourning process in Judaism, and notes how it is designed to thwart the development of pathological grief by specifying degrees of return to normal social interaction. For these reasons, the symbolic power of religious rituals has recently become part of the psychotherapeutic armamentarium of pastoral counselors.

Memorial rituals frequently follow the more immediate funeral ceremonies. This is particularly true of highly regarded community members, or of great and famous individuals who may be formally remembered through rites on their birth or death days for years following their demise. These rites may also be incorporated into one's faith. On the anniversary of the death, specifically for family members, specific prayers are often mandated. In Catholicism, there are votive Masses to aid the deceased in the afterlife. Judaism has its *Jahrzeit*, the time of year on the Jewish calendar for remembrance. In Japanese Buddhism, there is a kind of ancestor worship, *mizuko kuyo*, that allows one to maintain a ritualistic interaction for 35 or 50 years with those who have died. A variation of this ceremony has been created for abortions (Klass & Heath, 1996–1997). Women who have aborted fetuses use this rite to achieve a number of goals (to resolve guilt, maintain connections with the spirit of the aborted child, express regrets over having had the abortion, ask for forgiveness, apologize, etc.).

The San Francisco gay community has recently created a set of rituals to commemorate those who have died of AIDS (Richards, Wrubel, & Folkman, 1999–2000). Though many of these ceremonies are privately designed, the majority (69%) contain formal or informal religious content. Multiple rituals may be carried out over a number of months, and possibly years.

All known societies have their death rituals. Whatever biological resonances these represent, their significance is buried in cultural practice. Rituals do, however, reflect much elemental psychology—communication, emotional control, and the fostering of group cohesion (Lorenz, 1966; Wulff, 1997).

DEATH AND THE CLERGY

Unlike the rest of us, the clergy are commonly called upon to deal with death and dying. They are also trained in pastoral skills to deal with terminally ill patients and their families. Furthermore, once death has occurred, the clergy conduct the final rituals that consign the souls of those who have died to their ultimate divine destiny. Concurrently, they turn their attention to grieving family members and friends, attempting to bring solace to them. This may include such practices as praying with bereaved individuals, reading Scripture with them, interpreting theology, discussing spiritual and practical matters, conducting home visits, and whatever else may help to situate death in ultimate perspective. The pastoral goals are to engender hope in the face of death, and to assist the bereaved persons through the process of recovery from their loss.

Given these responsibilities, it is understandable why White (1991) perceives clerics as "primary caregivers" (p. 4). Leane and Shute (1998) define the aiding clergy as "gatekeepers," a first line of help to those who grieve.

The relatively recent development of the modern hospice program or facility has greatly extended the role of clergy in the predeath period. In the hospice context, a cleric provides friendship, and becomes a good listener to the patient and to visiting family members and friends (Dubose, 2000). The need for psychological understanding and clinical skills is overwhelmingly evident in these situations.

Three aims may be posited in work with dying persons and their survivors: (1) to make the death meaningful in terms of the perspective of a religious or spiritual system; (2) to transform the distress of the death and dying process into a vista of personal strength, self-identity, and a natural closing to an existence in which one has contributed to a better future; and (3) to attempt to convince all that death is not an end, but a new beginning, a doorway to immortality, a personal permanence, a new kind of life (Cook & Oltjenbruns, 1989). We have already shown how clergy may do these things by strengthening spirituality, offering hope, and enhancing the sense of death as meaningful beyond the immediate situation.

Training the Clergy to Deal with Death

The years since 1970 have witnessed a new sensitivity to death and dying that has profoundly affected clerical education. Programs to develop pastoral skills in this area have proliferated, along with a plethora of books and articles that detail the complexities of the tasks the clergy must confront (Bendiksen, Hewitt, & Vinge, 1979; Clemens, 1976; Jernigan, 1976; Kalish & Dunn, 1976; Malony, 1978; O'Brien, 1979; Wood, 1976).

Even though the clergy overwhelmingly feel that they have a responsibility to deal with those who are dying (91%) and bereaved (89%), they find performing these duties difficult and anxiety-producing (White, 1991). The fact that many clerics also feel deficient in this area is illustrated by one study of priests, ministers, and rabbis, which revealed that only 15% felt themselves educationally prepared to deal adequately with death and dying. Forty percent considered themselves poorly trained to do death work (Spilka, Spangler, & Rea, 1981). Though there is much variation in these feelings, more recent surveys continue to find that one-third to two-thirds of ministers still question their education in regard to dealing with terminally ill patients and their families (Missoula Demonstration Project, 2001).

In contrast, an increased emphasis on death education for prospective clergy has sometimes imparted a heightened sense of competence in dealing with terminality. In one study, 64% felt moderately to well educated in this area (Spilka, Spangler, & Rea, 1981). In contrast, older clergy had to learn about death and dying through direct experience in the pastorate. Today, these important skills can be acquired both in seminaries and through internships prior to ordination. Opportunities are currently provided for neophyte clerics to model themselves after mentors who have been engaged with dying people and their families for long periods of time.

With relatively little variation, those to whom the clergy provide their services are pleased with the pastoral efforts of hospital chaplains and "home pastors" (i.e., people's regular clerics making home visits) (Brabant, Forsyth, & McFarlain, 1995; Johnson & Spilka, 1991; Spilka, Spangler, & Nelson, 1983). An interesting exception occurs for patients with breast cancer: Both male and female clerics usually avoid discussing some of these women's central concerns about their identity as female and the surgical mutilation of their bodies (Johnson & Spilka, 1991). Obviously, there is still a need for pastoral training to deal with such sensitive personal issues.

Another approach revolves around the concept of a "good death." Utilizing focus groups of clergy and congregants, Braun and Zir (2001) found agreement on a number of criteria that pastoral education might emphasize for a terminally ill patient to have a "good death." The implication is that clerics should (1) be involved in pain management; (2) see that the dying process is not inappropriately prolonged; (3) work to encourage a supportive family atmosphere at the bedside; (4) try to resolve conflicts and introduce the potential of forgiveness, when desirable; (5) aid not only the terminally ill patient, but grieving family members; and (6) where proper, bring in theology and rituals to lighten the burden of mourning and bereavement.

Other troubling areas for which clergy feel unprepared are infants' deaths and youth suicides (Strength, 1999; Thearle, Vance, Najman, Embelton, & Foster, 1995; Leane & Shute, 1998). With regard to adolescent suicide, an Australian study revealed low levels of knowledge about risk signs for such an eventuality. This is believed to handicap clerical efforts to counteract such suicidal inclinations (Leane & Shute, 1998).

Pastoral education might also look more closely at the problems children have when loved ones die. The problem of inaccurate, distorted, and troubling magical fantasies needs to be confronted in order to resolve a child's grief (Fogarty, 2000).

Clerical Feelings about Death and Dying

Even though most clergy appear to buffer themselves against death and dying with strong beliefs in a life after death, the more theologically liberal they are, the more they see death as a natural end to life or simply as a mystery (Spilka, Spangler, & Rea, 1981; Spilka, Spangler, Rea, & Nelson, 1981). None of these perspectives implies that the clergy are not afraid of death. The evidence is that, like everybody else, they too manifest anxiety about death and dying (Kierniesky & Groelinger, 1977; Yudell, 1978). The theory has been proposed that this is one of the reasons why individuals become clerics. If this is so, the evidence suggests that the clergy's considerable personal experience with death does not help them come to terms with the prospect of their own deaths (Angelica, 1977).

A more serious and immediate likelihood is the development of clergy burnout or post-traumatic stress disorder. Echterling. Bradfield, and Wylie (1992) conducted a 6-year follow-up on the effects of a major disaster, a flood. This work is detailed in Research Box 8.7.

୬♠

Research Box 8.7. Six Years after the Flood: Clergy's Long-Term Response to Disaster (Echterling, Bradfield, & Wylie, 1992)

For 16 months after a major flood, these researchers gathered data on 44 clergy who were deeply involved in all aspects of flood relief, including rescue, cleanup, and offering both physical and emotional aid to the victims. Six years later, extensive follow-up interviews were conducted with 42 of the original clerics.

Even though considerable time had elapsed since the flood disaster, almost three-quarters of these 42 clerics were still discussing it in their sermons, and close to half held memorial services for the losses experienced. The dominant images of God presented by the clerics were of a loving deity rather than a punitive one: God wanted to provide an opportunity for those affected by the flood to re-establish basic human values and concerns. There was considerable evidence that the impact of the flood was a continuing issue to be resolved, however. A positive relationship was observed between a congregation's losses and the amount of flood relief in which its cleric was involved.

The authors interpreted many clerical responses as symptoms of posttraumatic stress disorder. From 10% to 25% cited continuing worries about the weather, illness, guilt about surviving, poor concentration, changes in appetite, dreaming about the flood, somatic complaints, avoidance, and reexperiencing the flood. Fewer than 10% showed signs of more serious disturbance. On the positive side, more than 90% of these clergy felt that their congregations had become more capable of handling similar crises in the future.

This study shows that the effects of a major disaster may persist and have religious repercussions for far longer than one might imagine. The researchers concluded, "In their struggle to face and meet the needs of a traumatized community, the clergy themselves became wounded healers" (p. 6).

Clerical Involvement and Effectiveness in Death-Related Situations

Spilka has participated in a number of workshops designed to aid clergy (and others who work with death) in their interaction with dying persons and their families. The growing hospice movement has also undertaken such training. Unfortunately, the proliferation of similar efforts has not been accompanied by research to evaluate the effectiveness of these programs. Still, in two studies of over 400 clergy, about 60% claimed that they deal often or very often with terminality; only 1% were not involved in this kind of work (Spilka, Spangler, & Rea, 1981).

But what do home pastors and hospital chaplains do when they interact with dying people and their kin? Over 90% of the clerics surveyed by Spilka, Spangler, and Rea (1981) claimed that they made two or more calls to the home of a bereaved family in the year following a death. Table 8.5 gives us some idea of the variety of actions that may take place in both home visits and hospital encounters.

Table 8.5 reveals a number of interesting differences between home pastors and hospital clergy, some of which may be due to the longer personal history of contact between the recipients and their regular clerics. In most instances, especially for patients with cancer, hospital chaplains were not likely to be as pastorally involved with the patients as home clergy were. This was less true when the clerics were dealing with the families of children with cancer. Still, for both groups, there was considerable reluctance to discuss the future. There may be a number of critical interactive subtleties in this process that call for additional research. Certainly, we still need to know the characteristics and behavior of successful pastors—that is, successful from the recipients' viewpoint.

Theology, Personal Faith, and Clergy Effectiveness

Spilka, Spangler, Rea, & Nelson (1981) found that among clergy dealing with death and dying, two-thirds claimed that the theology of their church was "very helpful," while only 2–3% felt it was of little or no use. Surprisingly, these numbers held whether the clerics were affiliated with a conservative or a liberal religious body. An interesting variation on this theme

TABLE 8.5. Activities of Home Clergy and Hospital Chaplains, According to Patients with Cancer and the Families of Children with Cancer

Activity	Patients with cancer		Families of children with cancer	
	Home clergy	Hospital chaplains	Home clergy	Hospital chaplains
Offering to pray for	43%	47%	42%	44%
Offering to pray with	42%	35%	51%	44%
Actually praying with	46%	22%	56%	48%
Reading religious material	17%	14%	20%	20%
Counseling	21%	16%	20%	24%
Talking irrelevancies	21%	18%	34%	36%
Seeming to understand	44%	28%	44%	44%
Talking about church matters	15%	6%	7%	12%
Talking about family	47%	12%	46%	40%
Discussing the future	15%	8%	15%	12%
Other	9%	22%	17%	8%

Note. Data from Spilka and Spangler (1979). Percentages add to more than 100, because clergy engaged in more than one activity per contact.

suggests that clerics' own personal faith is of greater importance than their church's theology, as 83% regarded the former as providing them with the most support in their death work (Spilka, Spangler, & Rea, 1981). Apparently, as important as formal theology is, the crucial issue may be the degree to which a cleric identifies with the official position.

There is little doubt that working with terminality is a very trying experience for clerics. Almost 70% of those surveyed by Spilka, Spangler, and Rea (1981) were less than "very satisfied" with their efforts, and 11–14% were quite unhappy with themselves. Some 43% of these pastors described themselves in this work with qualifying adjectives such as "frustrated," "inadequate," "apprehensive," and the like. In addition, Parkes (1972) observed that clergy "are often embarrassed and ineffectual when face-to-face with those who have been or are about to be bereaved" (p. 169).

At least in work with the families of the dying, however, theological conservatism implies more personal satisfaction; this may be a concomitant of afterlife beliefs that are more strongly held and more clearly defined by orthodox than by liberal institutions. Research further suggests that clergy from the liberal end of the theological spectrum are usually more concerned with their own psychological state than with that of patients and families when they are doing death work. (Spilka & Spangler, 1979). In these circumstances, the more conservative clerics emphasize religious, scriptural, and spiritual referents, and convey such to those to whom they minister. It is not amiss to note that terminally ill patients and their kin prefer these kinds of support, rather than what might be taken as strictly psychological pastoral actions. As important as the latter are in these situations, the appeal is clearly to God, not to psychotherapy (Spilka & Spangler, 1979).

That bereaved people consider the clergy helpful at this troubled time is abundantly evident. Carey (1979–1980) compared the satisfaction of widows and widowers with physicians, nurses, chaplains, social workers, and family members. Although family members were viewed as most helpful, the hospital chaplains came in a close second.

Like virtually everyone who confronts death, the clergy probably never become immune to the feelings that death and dying engender. They have entered a profession in which they must continually confront these hard realities. Undoubtedly, pastoral effectiveness is a function of experiences that force clerics to face their own mortality while expressing the empathy and humanity these situations call for. Fortunately, most clergy acquire the skills, compassion, and understanding to handle these trials. Additional comprehension of these difficulties from the consumers' viewpoint is offered in Research Box 8.8.

DEATH IN THE RELIGIOUS–SOCIAL CONTEXT

Though we emphasize the psychological aspects and influence of religion, we have also stressed the idea that individual behavior is embedded in various contexts—biological, social, and cultural. This principle is nowhere clearer than when death is confronted. People's perceptions and responses are commonly shaped by their group's heritage and ceremonial practices. For example, in the Jewish custom of *shiva* (see above), friends and relatives gather in the home of the deceased for 7 days following a funeral to offer their prayers, and family members are given emotional and social support. The idea that they are part of a long tradition is dutifully conveyed. Efforts are thus made to short-circuit deleterious mental and physical possibilities. In fact, Judaism exactly defines the mourning process with regard to time, stages, and duties.

**Research Box 8.8. Spiritual Support in Life-Threatening Illness
(Spilka, Spangler, & Nelson, 1983)**

In the last analysis, the effectiveness of clerics must be determined by those to whom the clergy demonstrate their skills. This was assessed in a study of 101 patients with cancer and 45 parents of children with cancer. All were questioned about their interactions with home pastors and hospital chaplains. The participants were generally quite religious. All respondents were administered a 45-item questionnaire, in which 6 items were open-ended, permitting a free response.

Twenty-nine percent of the patients were visited at home by their pastors, and 66% received hospital visits. With regard to the families of the children with cancer, 42% had home visits and 56% hospital visits. About 55% of both the patients and parents saw hospital chaplains. From 78% to 87% of the patients and parents were satisfied with the home and hospital visits. (Table 8.5, earlier in this section, has indicated what went on during these contacts.) The respondents expressed most satisfaction with situations where the home clergy actually prayed with the patients and the family. Engaging in religious reading was also positively regarded. In the hospital, the families approved discussions of the future by the chaplain. Finally, the willingness of a cleric simply to be present and to devote time to this troubling situation was considered most desirable.

As is so frequently true, the respondents were often clearer about the undesirable characteristic of clerics than about those they found positive. Most that was displeasing was broadly attributed to poor communication and lack of understanding by a pastor. Specifically, conveying the impression of visiting out of a sense of duty alone, or failing to appreciate or to be sensitive to the pain of the circumstances, was upsetting to these people. Extremely distressing were efforts (fortunately rare) to effect "deathbed conversions." For example, one cleric harangued a patient to "change his pagan ways." Much more common were indications of the pastors' own discomfort—looking at their watches, acting "nervous," verbalizing clichés, standing at a distance from patients, being painfully silent and unresponsive, and finally being in a rush to leave.

Pastoral identity was also a problem. A fair number of patients reported difficulty discovering who was and was not a chaplain. This resulted from the wearing of informal sports clothes, the absence of a badge that defined one as a chaplain (or the use of a badge too small to read at any distance), and/or a person's failing to state that he or she was a chaplain.

The many things pastors do and may represent can bring comfort and solace to those greatly in need of such aid. In most instances, this is what takes place. Still, clergy sometimes convey a lack of feeling and compassion without intending to do so. There is clearly a need for "on-the-job" training in these critical situations.

When cultural settings and religious rites are coordinated, their combined power is often quite compelling to all who are affected by the loss of a loved one. Death has always been circumscribed by rites that are usually quite meaningful to believers. The Mormons and the Amish offer excellent illustrations of the power of religious regulations and traditions concerning death.

The Mormons: Religion, Health, and Death

It is no accident that the lowest death rates in the 48 contiguous United States are found in Utah, the "Mormon state." These numbers hold for deaths from cancer, cardiovascular problems, and a variety of other diseases, as we have discussed in Chapter 3.

The Church of Jesus Christ of Latter-Day Saints possesses an extensive theology associating health and life with doing good, and evil with illness and death (Hansen, 1981; O'Dea, 1957; Vernon & Waddell, 1974). Kearl (1989) further tells us that "the Mormons baptize the dead, procreate to provide bodies for spirits caught in preexistence, and theologically reinforce the physical fitness ethos . . . to minimize premature deaths" (p. 171). This is an excellent example of how a strong and pervasive religious system that is well integrated with the sociocultural context can influence nutrition, health, and longevity.

The Amish: Religion and Family Support

Like the Mormons, the Amish have been able to blend the social setting in which they live with their religious ideology. To do so, they have been quite successful in preserving their religious and cultural unity by creating relatively isolated communities. Under such conditions, daily life is often inseparable from one's spiritual existence.

The Amish illustrate well what occurs when a distinctive faith group maintains its separation from others with variant beliefs and practices. Similar behavior is found among Orthodox Jews, Mormons, and a variety of sects and cults. A situation is created in which people rely primarily on their relations and close neighbors, and death is first a familial–religious obligation that is rapidly and willingly embraced by the community (Bryer, 1979). In essence, illness and death are community events. A dying person and a bereaved family are the recipients of extensive visits not only by friends and relations, but by any and all church and community members (Hostetler, 1968). This kind of support continues through the funeral, the burial, and thereafter, formally concluding with a meal that signifies the necessity of a return to everyday life. Hostetler (1968) uses the German term "*Gemeinsamkeitsgefuele*" (p. 188), which conveys the sense of a general community feeling of togetherness. A semiformal organization develops to provide mutual support and to perform various ceremonial functions, such as preparing the deceased for burial. In this way, the Amish view of "death as a spiritual victory over temporal life" is reinforced (Bryer, 1979, p. 259). Other families who have also lost members visit and aid the newly bereaved family to work through the grieving process. Death is not denied, but openly accepted as a necessary and essential fact of life, every aspect of which is encompassed by theological doctrine and meaning.

Under such circumstances, one may reasonably hypothesize that death, rather than diminishing the community and family, strengthens its ties and enhances religious commitment. In addition, this kind of religious–social support may be very effective in resolving the grief process, so that the likelihood of developing undesirable psychological aftereffects may be low.

Other Groups

The foregoing examples of how the Mormons and Amish deal with death can be easily extended to other, primarily nonmainstream religious groups. In 18th and 19th Century North America, for example, the Shakers developed their own unique theology relating to dying and the afterlife. To some degree they modeled themselves after the Quakers, circumscribed the care and dressing of the deceased, and denoted who might or might not attend funerals and burials (Andrews, 1963).

Scheffel's (1991) research on the Old Believers of Alberta describes the burial process, and specifies in great detail every aspect of body preparation, clothes, symbols, artifacts, body position, and activities that must take place at various times following the burial. The important thing is that the role of ceremony is made very clear, and ritual can be viewed in its structuring and emotion-controlling function. Considerations of meaning and control are ever-present, and one can easily see how well religion performs these functions. A similar situation exists in Hutterite society (Hostetler & Huntington, 1967) and undoubtedly in many other faiths. Death is thus an individual concern and a cultural matter—both of which are important to the psychology of religion, which recognizes that the person must always be understood in sociocultural context.

The fundamental factor here is group culture, but quasi-religious elements may go beyond religious bodies, as noted earlier in the practices of those who mourn the deaths of individuals from AIDS (Bivens et al., 1994–1995).

OVERVIEW

This chapter tells us that death and its relation to religion are far more complex than one might initially believe. Behind every obituary there is a life, and in some way this existence has included religious beliefs, experiences, and behavior. They may have also influenced the way the person died, and also what took place afterward.

With respect to religion, the psychology of death has not resolved the problem of theory—basically, how people explain and handle death and dying. Florian and Kravetz (1983), stating that this is an area that "may require a theoretical model that is more descriptive than valuative" (p. 602), suggest an attributional approach in which one searches for causal explanations that both reflect and shape thinking and behavior. To what do people attribute death? Is it simply the way nature works, or should they invoke faith-based notions of "original sin" or the penalty for not living a good life? Psychological coping theory also looks as if it may be quite productive, for death is, without question, a problem with which people must deal many times in life (Maton, 1989; Park & Cohen, 1993; Park, Cohen, & Herb, 1990; Pargament, 1997).

Sociological thinkers may have an advantage over psychologists as they can relate individual responsivity to sociocultural referents and to the social construction of ideas and attitudes about death. Leming (1980) thus utilizes the sociologist Homan's notion that religion both creates and resolves death-related anxiety. Another sociologist, Emile Durkheim (1897/1951), integrated suicide into the social order, recognizing bases for variation in suicide rates as a function of the primary religion in a society.

Overall, we have seen a major development in research in this area—namely, from the use of simplistic and unitary notions of death fear and religiousness to multidimensional conceptualizations in both domains. Even though more sophisticated instrumentation is now available, it does not seem to be employed as much as it should be in current research. Too much work still relies on unidimensional measures of death fear/anxiety. Part of this may be due to the fact that researchers are much more knowledgeable in the coping realm than they are with advances in the psychology of religion. Convenience samples in which testing must be kept to a minimum may also be impeding the use of more sophisticated measurement of religious perspectives However, we now see multidimensional trends in work on religiosity in relation to coping with AIDS, bereavement, and euthanasia.

Our position is that the deaths of others and the prospect of one's own death raise for each individual two very basic coping issues we have often referred to in this volume—that is, the issues of meaning and control. Death arouses these concerns in their most intimate and ultimate forms. It is here that faith probably makes its greatest adaptive contributions.

The contemporary world has united death more strongly with moral and religious considerations than ever before. Vacuous platitudes such as "God works in mysterious ways" and "The good die young" are highly likely to elicit rapid and vehement rejection in a time of AIDS, high suicide rates for adolescents and elderly people, the delaying of death indefinitely by leaving mortally ill individuals in an almost permanent vegetative state, and many calls for active euthanasia. Simple, easy, dichotomous yes–no answers must give way to deeper, more thoughtful considerations in which institutionalized religion plays a significant and central role. Death in the modern world has been become increasingly complicated; it challenges faith and the role of the clergy more and more, on both the individual and societal levels.

Chapter 9

RELIGIOUS EXPERIENCE

The very beginning, the intrinsic core, the essence, the universal nucleus of every known high religion . . . has been the private, lonely, personal illumination, revelation, or ecstasy of some acutely sensitive prophet or seer.

Belief, ritual, and spiritual experience: these are the cornerstone of religion, and the greatest of them is the last.

Therefore, let's consider the proposal that when our volunteers journeyed to the further bonds of DMT's [*N,N*-dimethyltryptamine's] reach, when they felt as if they were *somewhere else*, they were indeed perceiving different levels of reality. The alternative levels are as real as this one. It's just that we cannot perceive them most of the time.

I'd see serpent handling, and . . . I thought, "Oh, Lord, I'd like to feel that. I'd like to feel what they're feeling."

If humans were no longer taught any religions, they would, I think, spontaneously create new ones from the content of ecstatic experiences, combined with bits and pieces transmitted by language and folklore.[1]

The study of religious experience can be perplexing, partly because so much time and effort can be wasted on defining precisely what is meant by "experience." Gadamer (1986, p. 310) argues that the concept of experience is "one of the most obscure we have." At a commonsense level, we are aware that experience is something other than mere action or behavior. Yet it would be odd indeed to think of experience without any action involved—for even to do nothing is to do something. Similarly, experience is not simply thought or belief, even though we are often thinking when we have an experience. Finally, many people try to equate experience with emotions or feelings. Yet feelings and emotions are only part of what we sometimes mean by experience; they cannot be equated with the experience. Experience refers to a total way of reacting or being and cannot be reduced to its parts, even if such parts could be identified. To experience is to identify some totalizing aspect of life—an event or episode that is "experienced." Perhaps we can say of experience what Saint Augustine is reputed to have said of time: We know what it is until we are asked to *say* what it is.

---

1. These quotations come, respectively, from the following sources: Maslow (1964, p. 19); Lewis (1971, p. 11); Strassman (2001, p. 315; emphasis in original); Rachelle ("Shell") Martinez Brown, quoted in Brown and McDonald (2000, p. 73); and Goodman (1988, p. 171).

What then of *religious* experience? It often is opposed to being dogmatic in the negative sense of the mere insistence of particular beliefs. Gadamer (1986) argues that

> the experienced person proves to be . . . someone who is radically undogmatic; who, because of the many experiences he [or she] has had and the knowledge he [or she] has drawn from them is particularly well equipped to have new experiences and to learn from them. The dialectic of experience has its own fulfillment not in definitive knowledge, but in the openness to experience that is encouraged by experience itself. (p. 319)

Although Gadamer speaks of experience in general, it would appear that religious experience identifies something particular. Religious experience distinctively separates, from the vast domain of experience, that which is perceived to be *religious*. Thus we psychologists are free to identify religious experience as experience that is identified within faith traditions as religious. This tautology need not disturb us. Religious traditions define the distinctively religious for the faithful. What is religious within one tradition may not be so within another. With the possible exception of mystical and numinous experiences (discussed in Chapter 10), it is probably not fruitful to define religious experiences by their inherent characteristics. Whether an experience is religious or not depends upon the interpretation of the experience. It is in this sense that even if what is experienced is both immediately present and unquestionable to the experiencing subject, the epistemological value of the experience is dependent upon discursive meanings that entail public interpretations (Sharf, 2000). Interpretations provide meanings not inherently obvious to those who stand outside the tradition that provides the context for meaningfully identifying any particular episode as a religious. As psychologists, we often study retrospective accounts of experience that are linguistically framed as religious. Almost any experience humans can have can be interpreted as an experience of God (Leech, 1985). As Yamane (2000) notes, narration is dependent upon a loose relationship between experience and its linguistic representation, so that an experience not initially described as religious may be so described on subsequent reflection. However, it is within a linguistic community that claims to religious experiencing are ultimately judged (Williams & Faulconer, 1994).

CONCEPTUAL CONSIDERATIONS IN DEFINING RELIGIOUS EXPERIENCE

As we have noted in Chapter 2, James's (1902/1985) classic work *The Varieties of Religious Experience* has continued to influence psychologists since it was initially delivered as the Gifford Lectures at the beginning of the 20th century. Although one can speculate as to the varying reasons why this book has remained in print since its first publication, the simple fact remains that James set the tone for contemporary empirical work in the psychology of religious *experience* that is nonreductive (Hood, 2000a).

James's Formula for Religious Experience

James's definition of religious experience for the purposes of the Gifford Lectures clearly revealed his sympathy for the extreme forms of religious experience. James defined "religion" as "*the feelings, acts, and experiences of individual men, in their solitude, so far as they appre-*

hend themselves to stand in relation to whatever they may consider the divine" (James, 1902/ 1985, p. 34; emphasis in original). The presence of something divine within all religious traditions can be debated. Buddhism is often cited as an example of a faith tradition without a god (Hong, 1995). However, one need not equate something divine with belief in God or in supernatural beings. James's clarification of what he meant by "divine" makes the case for the near-universal application of this concept. As he saw it, the divine is "such a primal reality as the individual feels compelled to respond to solemnly and gravely, and neither by a curse nor a jest" (James, 1902/1985, p. 39). James's divinity is close to what we term a "foundational reality" in Chapter 10—that is, what each tradition finds most basic and foundational to its existence. Thus, influenced by James's notion of divinity, religious experience— ultimately, the experience of the solitary individual—is placed at the forefront of the psychology of religion. Culling from a wide variety of written and personal testimonies, James's Gifford Lectures minimized belief and behavior, focusing instead upon experience. Yet in these justly famous lectures, James was parsimonious in his conclusion regarding the value of religious experiences in general. As he perceived it, the infinite variety of religious experiences can be subsumed under a simple formula: discontent and its resolution. Placed in the context of individual lives, responses to the divine are resolutions. Studies derived from documents similar to those solicited and used by James support this sweeping generalization. However, as we shall see, the issue may be confounded by the methodology of focusing upon personal declarations of religious experience. As noted in Chapter 15, the resolution of discontent is an appealing formula that can mask the often complex relationships between religion and coping.

Varieties of Religious Experience: Research from the Hardy Centre

Perhaps most congruent with the Jamesian tradition of the use of personal documents to understand religious experience has been the work associated with what was originally known as the Religious Experience Research Unit of Manchester College, Oxford University. This unit continues as the Alister Hardy Religious Experience Research Centre in Watlington, Oxfordshire, England. Alister Hardy achieved scientific accolades as a renowned zoologist. Yet his lifelong interest in religious experience led him upon retirement from his career in zoology to form a research unit in 1969 devoted to the collection and classification of religious experiences. For this work, he was awarded the Templeton Prize for research in religion. Hardy's basic procedure, stemming from his zoological training, was to solicit voluntary reports of religious experiences and to attempt to classify them into their natural types. Typically these reports were solicited via requests in newspapers, as well as newsletters distributed to various groups, mostly in the United Kingdom. Requests were not simply for the more extreme and intense types of experiences favored by James, but for the more temperate variety of religious experiences as well. Often individuals simply submitted experience unsolicited. In *The Spiritual Nature of Man*, Hardy (1979) published an extensive classification of the major defining characteristics of these experiences from an initial pool of 3,000 experiences.

Hardy's major classifications included sensory or quasi-sensory experience associated with vision, hearing, and touch; less frequent, but still fairly common, were reports of paranormal experiences. Most common were cognitive and affective episodes, such as a sense of presence or feelings of peace (Hardy, 1979). Not surprisingly, other surveys of a more scientific nature, such as Greeley's (1975) survey of 1,467 people, show some overlaps with

Hardy's classifications (especially with the cognitive and affective elements) but also many differences. It seems that there is little agreement about exactly what might constitute the common characteristics of religious experience. Perhaps the term is simply too broad for agreement to be expected across diverse samples and investigators. There may be no common elements that all religious experiences share. The focus, then, must be upon not simply religious experience, but the varieties of experience that are interpreted as religious. It is better to think of religious experiences in light of Wittgenstein's (1945–1949/1953) notion of "family resemblance." We can identify the family resemblance among experiences we classify as religious, but not by finding a single criterion they all must share. What makes an experience religious is clearly not the discrete, isolated components that can be identified in any experience. As Leech (1985) has argued, hardly any experience could fail to qualify as "religious" or "spiritual" under some framework.

Are Anomalous Experiences Religious?

What is "religious" for some is merely "anomalous" for others. Earlier investigators identified anomalous experiences within a fiercely reductionistic frame, often attributing them to "magical" (e.g., erroneous) thinking (Zusne & Jones, 1989). However, more recent work keeps open the possibility of nonreductionist views of even the more extreme anomalous experiences. For instance, the editors of a book recently published by the American Psychological Association (Cardeña, Lynn, & Krippner, 2000b) identify anomalous experiences as those that, though perhaps experienced by a substantial segment of the population, are nevertheless believed to deviate from ordinary experience or from the usually accepted definitions of reality (Cardeña, Lynn, & Krippner, 2000a, p. 4). These experiences need not be identified as religious, but clearly many often are. Examples include out-of-body, near-death, past-life, mystical, and paranormal experiences. These experiences often gain added meaning when they are embedded in religious discourse that both explains and legitimates them. This applies even to hallucinatory experiences, as the recent history of modifications in the American Psychiatric Association's *Diagnostic and Statistical Manual of Mental Disorders* (DSM) shows.

Despite the fact that the DSM is suspect both theoretically and scientifically (Kirk & Kutchins, 1992), it is in widespread normative use in at least North America. In its last several revisions, moreover, it has included cautions about identifying hallucinations and possession experiences as pathological if there is normative support for these practices. This was made especially clear in DSM-III-R:

> When an experience is entirely normative for a particular culture—e.g., the experience of hallucinating the voice of a deceased in the first few weeks of bereavement in various North American Indian groups, or trance and possession states occurring in culturally approved ritual contexts in much of the non-Western world—it should not be regarded as pathological. (American Psychiatric Association, 1987, p. xxvi)

In DSM-IV, a hallucination is defined only as "a sensory perception that has the compelling sense of reality of a true perception but that occurs without external stimulation of the relevant sensory organ" (American Psychiatric Association, 1994, p. 767); it is not automatically deemed to be an indication of mental illness. The most recent edition of this manual (DSM-IV-TR) simply cautions that "a clinician who is unfamiliar with the nuances of an individual's cultural frame of reference may incorrectly judge as psychopathology those normal varia-tions in behavior, belief, or experience that are particular to the individual's culture" (Ameri-can Psychiatric Association, 2000, p. xxxiv).

Williams and Faulconer (1994) have persuasively noted the fallacies involved in defi-nitional efforts to determine the "pathology" of religious beliefs. The consequences are im-mense once one realizes that religious beliefs are less characteristics of an individual and more cultural or subcultural ways of interpreting experiences. If so, psychological processes, even "pathological" ones, cannot be used to reductively explain away religiously interpreted phe-nomena. Perhaps one of the most controversial examples is illustrated by responsible inves-tigators' refusing to dismiss reports of alien abduction experiences (hereafter abbreviated as AAEs) out of hand. Clearly, AAEs are likely to raise problems for those who think that the umbrella of religious discourse opens too wide when it legitimates such experiences. Yet Research Box 9.1 shows how even claims to unidentified flying object (UFO) sightings and AAEs are difficult to explain exhaustively by psychological processes if one simply frames experiences in a manner suggesting that they might be true. Such experiences are beginning to gain significant subcultural support (Appelle, Lynn, & Newman, 2000; Skal, 1998). As such, it is less profitable to ask what causes these experiences then to try to understand the experi-encing of the world from within a tradition, culture, or subculture that validates and finds meaningful what others can only describe as anomalous experiences from within their own perspective.

Exhaustive efforts to classify religious experiences would not have appealed to James, who preferred to let the experiences speak for themselves, unfettered by what he would prob-ably have seen as the tyranny of classification schemes. However, Hardy's conclusions (reached ostensibly independently of James) are interesting, as they are precisely what James concluded much earlier. Both James and Hardy affirmed the evidential value of religious experiences as at least hypotheses suggesting the existence of a transcendent reality variously experienced. As for the psychological consequences, the power of prayer is acknowledged; early childhood experiences are considered significant; and feelings of safety, security, love, and contentment are regarded as concomitants of religious experience. Few religious expe-riences are negative. By the very understanding of religion, at least in the West, experiences attributed to God must be ultimately positive (Spilka & McIntosh, 1995).

Other studies of voluntarily submitted reports of religious experience are not inconsis-tent with either James's or Hardy's claims (Ahern, 1990; Hardy, 1966; Hay, 1987, 1994; Laski, 1961; Maxwell & Tschudin, 1990). However, much of this research favors a methodology that probably biases the simple conclusion that religious experiences are resolutions of dis-content. This research probably solicits reports of religious experiences congruent with a simple, if not naïve, view of religion. These reports are often evaluated by persons commit-ted to a positive assessment of religious experience. Few negative experiences are reported, and almost none that were inconsequential or failed to produce positive fruits are volun-teered. In this sense, asking persons to report religious or spiritual experiences may be tap-ping general cultural views (especially in cultures heavily influenced by the Judeo-Christian tradition) that religious experiences are "good" and resolve problems. For instance, Lupfer and his colleagues have demonstrated that attributions are likely to be made to God only for events with positive outcomes (Lupfer, Brock, & DePaola, 1992; Lupfer, DePaola, Brock, & Clement, 1994). Although their research applies primarily to conservative Christians, other research suggests the general tendency among all believers to attribute to God only experi-ences with positive outcomes (Spilka & McIntosh, 1995).

꒰꒱

Research Box 9.1. Do Certain Paranormal Experiences Have Religious Import, and Could They Be True? (Various Studies)

A controversial issue in the study of religious experience is the persistent finding that individuals who report various religious experiences also report various paranormal experiences (Zollschan, Schumaker, & Walsh, 1995). Furthermore, studies employing survey data reveal that the reports of paranormal experiences have antecedents and structures similar to those in the reports of other ecstatic experiences commonly accepted as religious (Fox, 1992; Yamane & Polzer, 1994). Among paranormal experiences, the perception of unidentified flying objects (UFOs) and their more recent elaboration into "alien abduction experiences" (AAEs) have begun to generate a considerable body of scientific curiosity. Jung (1958/1964), while referring to the citing of UFOs as "visionary " (p. 315) or "symbolic" (p. 387), nevertheless cautioned that psychology alone cannot exhaust the explanation for such sightings. More recently, investigators such as Strassman (2001) have suggested that certain chemicals affecting brain receptor sites for serotonin may elicit awareness of dimensions of reality in which reports of AAEs become possible as actual events. However, as with many religious experiences, psychologists are more likely to be comfortable with explanations within the mainstream of realities that other psychologists are likely to accept. For instance, Skal (1998) has noted that the term "flying saucer" came into vogue only after newspaper headlines in June 1947, when a Boise, Idaho pilot named Kenneth Arnold described nine strange objects flying near Mount Rainier as moving "like a saucer if you skipped it across the water" (quoted in Skal, 1998, p. 204). Newspaper headlines reported "flying saucers," and quickly individuals began to reporting sighting of them. Thus cultural expectations based upon journalistic headlines that actually were in error might have played a role in shaping what have become common sightings of "UFOs." Instead of moving "like saucers," they became identified as "flying saucers."

Apparently even less plausible than the existence of UFOs are claims to AAEs, which typically include being captured and taken aboard a UFO and being subjected to physical, mental, and spiritual examinations before being returned to earth (Bullard, 1987). Other more extreme claims may include the taking of tissue samples, the implantation of objects into the body, and even the birth of alien-hybrid babies (Jacobs, 1992). As fantastic as these claims appear, explanations must accept the fact that the reports of such experiences are no more frequent among mentally ill people than among those without mental illness (Jacobson & Bruno, 1994; Parnell & Sprinkle, 1990). Among the most plausible and least controversial explanations for these reports are fantasy proneness or boundary deficits; using culturally available scenerios derived from film and other media sources; confusing subjective experiences with objectively real events; suggestibility and hypnosis (especially when such reports are "recovered" in therapeutic encounters using hypnosis); sleep disorders; and various possible psychoses in at least a minority of cases (Appelle, Lynn, & Newman, 2000). However, the fact that AAEs often contain "theophanies" (the receipt of explicit religious or spiritual messages) links them to other experiences that are more common within mainstream faith traditions. Lest skeptics too quickly consider these experiences to be simply bizarre manifestations that are exhaustively explainable by the social sciences, they might be cautioned that those who have studied these experiences in depth have found that the dismissal of their truth or reality, as with many claims to more mainstream religious experiences, is more difficult than one might at first think

continued

Research Box 9.1. *continued*

(Appelle, 1996; Strassman, 2001; Skal, 1998). It has been more than half a century since Jung said of UFOs (much less AAEs), "If military authorities have felt compelled to set up bureaus for collecting and evaluating UFO reports, then psychology, too, has not only the right but also the duty to do what it can to shed light on this dark problem" (1958/ 1964, p. 416).

However, not all religious or quasi-religious experiences may be positive in nature, and not all may be entirely culturally determined. For instance, Hufford (1982) has extensively investigated the "Old Hag" phenomenon common to Newfoundland. According to Newfoundland folk legend, what some might be tempted to dismiss as merely a nightmare is in fact a direct supernatural encounter with the Old Hag, a being who produces night paralysis and terror. This experience occurs in at least 15% of the population (Hufford, 1982, p. 245). One succinct description of the experience was given by a 20-year-old university student Hufford interviewed: "You are dreaming and you feel if someone is holding you down. You can do nothing, only cry out. People believe that you will die if you are not awakened" (quoted in Hufford, 1982, p. 2). Hufford notes that although culture affects the way the experience is described, it does not determine the experience itself. The experience is likely to occur in hypnogogic sleep states and is not associated with pathology (Hufford, 1982). Table 9.1 shows that while cultural knowledge about the Old Hag is related to having the experience, people unfamiliar with the cultural knowledge about the experience neverthe-

TABLE 9.1. The Old Hag Experience: The Relationship between Cultural Knowledge and Personal Reports of the Experience, and a Description of the Experience

Report of personal Old Hag experience as a function of accurate cultural knowledge in a sample of 93 Newfoundland students

	Reporting experience	Not reporting experience
Accurate knowledge	15.1% ($n = 14$)	24.7% ($n = 23$)
Inaccurate knowledge	7.5% ($n = 7$)	52.7% ($n = 49$)

Description of the Old Hag experience
Primary features (definitive)
   1. Subjective impression of wakefulness
   2. Immobility variously perceived (paralysis, restraint, fear of moving)
   3. Realistic perception of actual environment
   4. Fear
Secondary features (experiences contain at least one of these, often more)
   1. Supine position
   2. Feeling of presence
   3. Feeling of pressure
   4. Numinous quality
   5. Fear of death

Note. Data from Hufford (1982, pp. 25, 30).

less also report it. Thus cultural knowledge does not alone account for the report of this experience. After 10 years of study, Hufford concluded: "The content of the experience cannot be satisfactorily explained on the basis of current knowledge" (1982, p. 246).

Theoretical Orientations

Hufford's (1982) sympathetic study of the Old Hag phenomenon, as well as research on AAEs, suggests that the study of religious experiences is moving tpward careful descriptions of such experiences from the perspective of those who have them—and toward the possibility that even the reality claims of seemingly bizarre experiences may have validity. Hood (1995a) has identified 13 theoretical orientations, each of which organizes the empirical literature in a clearly identifiable if not unique manner. In addition, which empirical literature is relevant is largely determined by what theory, orientation, or philosophical assumption one adopts. The more distant theories are from one another in terms of basic assumptions and orientations, the less likely they are to appeal to congruent research literatures. Table 9.2 presents a listing of major theoretical orientations in the study of religious experience and the most typical methodologies favored by each.

Given our commitment to empirical psychology, largely defined by orientations that are measurement-based, our theoretical affinities can be readily surmised from an inspection of Table 9.2. However, even phenomenological and depth psychologies have influenced the empirical literature on religious experience. Thus we do not exclude any theoretical orientation; rather, we seek to illuminate religious experience from a variety of perspectives. Our test of any perspective is simply whether it generates empirical research.

TABLE 9.2. Theoretical Orientations in the Study of Religious Experience

Theoretical orientation	Most common research methods
Depth psychologies	
Freudian theory	Clinical case study; Oedipal interpretations
Jungian theory	Clinical and literary case studies; interpretation
Object relations theory	Clinical case study; pre-Oedipal interpretations
Major psychological orientations	
Developmental theory	Experimental; correlational studies; measurement
Affective theory	Experimental; correlational studies; measurement
Behavioral theory	Experimental studies (often with small sample sizes)
Cognitive theory	Experimental; measurement
Specific psychological perspectives	
Attachment theory	Experimental; correlational studies; measurement
Attribution theory	Experimental; correlational studies; measurement
Role theory	Correlational; participant observation; measurement
Specialty concerns	
Feminist theory	Correlational; interpretative; qualitative
Phenomenological theory	Descriptive; introspective reports
Transpersonal theory	Interpretive; correlational; experimental

Note. Adapted from Hood (1995a). Copyright 1995 by Religious Education Press. Adapted by permission.

There is no perspective listed in Table 9.2 that has not generated some interest among empirical researchers. Yet it is equally true that no theory has sufficient empirical support to be presented as *the* theory of religious experience. Indeed, in light of a postmodern perspective on the social sciences, perhaps it is fruitless to seek a single best orientation (Rosenau, 1992; Roth, 1987). Still, we must organize the richness and vastness of religious experience in some fashion. We have chosen James's formula as a guide, and we broaden its reference to include contemporary discussions of limits and their transcendence as the most general framework within which to discuss religious experience. We then add considerations from role theory, particularly as developed by Sundén, to add the specific influence of religious traditions and texts to the understanding of experience that is interpreted as meaningfully religious.

Limits and Transcendence: The James–Boisen Formula

Before looking at particular studies of religious experience, we are going to suggest the wisdom of James's simple formula for religious experience. For while James is most often noted for his insistence on the richness and diversity of religious experience, he also suggested that a resolution of a previously experienced uneasiness is the thread from which all religious experience is woven. James is not alone in this.

Boisen (1936, 1960) noted that what distinguishes religious experience from otherwise intense, but pathological, experience is that religious experience is a resolution of what would otherwise be a devastating defeat. For Boisen as for James, it is not the nature of the experience that defines it as religious, but its results. Religious experiences, like some pathological experiences, force a confrontation with great personal disharmony. But there is a difference: the outcome. A religious experience marks the successful resolution of an inner conflict defined in transcendental terms. A limit has been reached and meaningfully transcended.

This James–Boisen formula meshes nicely with both theological and psychological perspectives in which the concepts of limits and transcendence are related (Corssan, 1975; Johnson, 1974). In the simplest sense, a total involvement and awareness of limits produce the discontent and disharmony (James's uneasiness or discontent) that creates the possibility of transcendence. It is the very confrontation with limits, however conceived, that can produce despair and the tragedy of defeat if such limits are oppressively interminable—or joy and the ecstasy of transcendence when such limits are overcome. This is the sense in which Bowker (1973) has emphasized that the psychological origin of the sense of God must be rooted not in the particulars of experience, but rather in terms of content that meaningfully points to limits to be surpassed. In this sense, God is always "beyond," and the psychology of religious experiencing is the experience of this "beyondness" through the transcendence of previously experienced limits.

We have a rather basic perspective within which to organize the empirical literature on religious experience. It can be traced back to James's notion of discontent and resolution, but only if we keep in mind the fact that both discontent and resolution are *interpretations* rooted in James's definition of religion. In a fundamental sense, religious experience is the meaningful transcendence of limits of the resolution of discontent, rooted in a sense of the divine. Not surprisingly, then, religious experience is almost infinite in its varieties. It is the *understanding in a religious vocabulary* of the process of discontent and its resolution that makes an experience religious (Taves, 1999).

Sundén's Role Theory

If there is a typicality to religious experience, it comes from the uniformity of interpretation found within particular traditions. Traditions define what are relevant religious experiences. The experience of being religious varies across traditions. Perhaps most compatible with this perspective is the work of the Swedish psychologist Sundén (see Holm, 1995; Holm & Belzen, 1995). His theory of religious experience is truly social-psychological in nature. Most important for our present purposes is Sundén's conclusion that religious traditions, particularly in the form of sacred texts, provide the templates or models that make *religious* experience possible. In other words, the interpretation or perception of events in terms modeled by stories from sacred texts is what makes experience religious. Without knowledge of a religious tradition and its sacred texts, religious experiences are not possible. For example, many would not associate the handling of serpents with religion. However, in some southern Appalachian churches, serpent handling is a religious experience perceived to be in obedience to God's will as one of the five signs specified in Mark 16:17–18. These "sign-following" churches obey what they perceive to be God's will. Signs of obedience include speaking in tongues, casting out of demons, laying hands upon the sick, handling serpents, and the drinking of poisonous substances (Brown & McDonald, 2000; Burton, 1993; Hood, 1998; Kimbrough, 1995; Pelton & Carden, 1974).

Serpent Handling as a Religious Experience

In 18th-century North America, "rattlesnake gazing," or staring at snakes in the wild, was a common practice. Settlers, strongly informed by Biblical narratives, found in rattlesnake gazing a significance that attributed supernatural powers to this "agent of Satan." As one historian of popular religiosity (Lippy, 1994, p. 79) notes, "a people familiar with the biblical story of the serpent's tempting of Eve might well be predisposed to assume that the rattlesnake and other serpentine creatures did indeed possess supernatural power." However, rattlesnake gazing was never practiced as a religious ritual or acknowledged by any formal religious denominations.

At the turn of this century, Holiness sects in Appalachia emphasized numerous Biblical texts (e.g., Mark 16:17–18; Luke 10:19) by which the handling of serpents gained a religious significance. In its early history, the Church of God championed serpent handling as one of the "five signs" (Williamson, 1995). In obedience to their interpretation of scripture, believers handled serpents, or (with reference to Luke 10:19) walked upon them. Serpent handling was popularized by George Hensley, who modeled the handling of serpents in churches. Later abandoned by the Church of God (whose members continue to practice some of the signs, such as speaking in tongues), the practice persists in Holiness sects throughout Appalachia. In Sundén's role theory, both the scriptural text and the modeling of this text in actual practice permit believers to handle serpents as a religious act (Hood & Kimbrough, 1995). In addition, in terms of our notion of limits and transcendence, the actual handling of serpents in services permits a transcendence of the real possibility of death that lies at the rational basis of the fear of handling rattlesnakes and other vipers (Hood, 1998; Hood & Kimbrough, 1995). Whether serpent handlers are bitten or not, whether they live or die, they believe that they live and act in obedience to God's word based upon their understanding of the Bible (Hood, 1998). Research Box 9.2 presents a study that focuses upon the experience of serpent handling from the believers' own perspective.

ॐ

Research Box 9.2. What Is It Like to Handle a Serpent?
(Williamson & Pollio, 1999)

Williamson and Pollio taped sermons by serpent handlers, delivered spontaneously immediately after the handling of serpents. Eighteen sermons were analyzed for their basic thematic contents. Five themes emerged, all understood within the context of a powerfully embodied experience of handling serpents in obedience to the believer's understanding of such passages in the Bible as Mark 16:17–18 and Luke 10:19.

Theme I: The experience of anointment or feeling moved by God to handle the serpent.

Theme II: The reality of being in the presence of death. A common phrase that preachers use is "There is death in these boxes" (the serpent boxes in which serpents are carried to church and contained when not being handled).

Theme III: Feeling of uniqueness and of separation between "us" (believers who handle serpents) and "them" (others who do not handle serpents or even ridicule believers who do).

Theme IV: The power of true knowing. The experience of being special, of understanding truly God's word and of living what they often identify as "the good way."

Theme V: Intense joy and affective pleasure, most typically identified as "joy unspeakable."

As Williamson and Pollio note, if one simply assumes truth to be perspectival, their phenomenological approach and the identification of meaningful themes in the experience of serpent handling allow a researcher "to see the world as the religious practitioner sees it, unaffected (as far as possible) by theories external to the practitioner's belief and experience" (1999, p. 216).

Note. Adapted from Williamson and Pollio (1999, pp. 208–213). Copyright 1999 by the Society for the Scientific Study of Religion. Adapted by permission.

The example of serpent handling illustrates one criticism of the study of religious experience in North American psychology. It is a criticism leveled against James and to some extent inherent in the appeal to "experience." In general, it would appear that the demand to describe "experience" is a plea to identify something unique, intense, or exceptional in one's life. "What did you experience?" is one of those questions that focus on extremes, much as the expletive "What an experience!" is likely to identify something exceptional in one's life. In one of the early critiques of James's *The Varieties of Religious Experience,* Crooks (1913) bemoaned James's fascination with the extreme and unusual in religious experience, at the expense of the more common experiences characteristic of religion. In a similar vein, Starbuck (1904) urged other psychologists of religion to avoid a focus upon the extremes in religious experience. The echoes of such criticism are still heard today, but largely fall upon deaf ears. It would appear that for many social scientists, ordinary piety and the commonplaces of religious experience are as James saw them—the duller religious habits. What fascinated James most were the more passionate expressions of the extremes of religious experience. Little has changed in this regard since the *The Varieties.* The empirical literature has a Jamesian focus, if not in method, in terms of the topics that have elicited interest and study.

THE BODY IN RELIGIOUS EXPERIENCE

In her presidential address to the Society for the Scientific Study of Religion, Meredith McGuire (1990, p. 284) posed this interesting question: "What if people—the subjects of our research and theorizing—had material bodies?" McGuire answered her own rhetorical question by noting three broad themes in which the social sciences might better appreciate what she aptly termed the "mindful body" (p. 285): in the experience of self and others; in the production and reflection of social meanings; and in the body's significance as the subject and object of power relations. Although McGuire's concern is more sociological than psychological, her appeal to reconsider the body is useful for psychologists who tend to reduce the body to the study of physiological processes. This is a particularly pernicious tendency in the psychology of religion.

Perhaps one of the most shortsighted views of religious experience is to assume that such experiences are merely emotional. The "merely" here has a negative connotation; it suggests that since what is perceived as religiously meaningful is physiological in origin, it can be discounted. James (1902/1985) identified such disclaiming views as "medical materialism":

> Medical materialism finishes up Saint Paul by calling his vision on the road to Damascus a discharging lesion of the occipital cortex, he being an epileptic. It snuffs out Saint Teresa as an hysteric, Saint Francis of Assisi as a hereditary degenerate. George Fox's discontent with the shams of his age, and his pining for spiritual veracity, it treats as a disordered colon. (p. 20)

The point, of course, is not that physiological processes may not be involved in religious experience, but that some psychologists think the identification of the physiological processes involved in religious experience "reduces it away." Yet no experience is identical to the processes involved in its occurrence. This is not to say that physiological processes such as arousal may not be involved in some aspects of religious experiencing. What is crucial is that such arousal be appropriately identified as part of a broader context, which is identified as religious because of other than merely physiological processes. The consideration becomes not simply arousal, but arousal contextualized and interpreted.

Taves (1999) has shown that from Wesley to James, North American Protestantism has struggled with evaluating the legitimacy of experiences based upon what is known about how they can be elicited. Her basic categories involve two dimensions: supernatural versus natural origins, and religious versus secular interpretations. Those who interpret experience religiously and attribute it to a supernatural origin are essentially religious apologists doing religious psychology. Those who interpret experience in secular scientific terms and attribute them only to natural causes are doing what she calls the psychology of religion. The interesting effort to interpret natural experiences in religious language is what Taves (1999, p. 348) refers to as the "mediating" tradition—an effort that can be linked to William James and the desire to establish a comparative scientific study of religion in general.

Physiological Arousal and Religious Experience

It has long been noted that when persons describe their experiences, there are often large physiological components to their descriptions. It appears that as embodied selves, human beings must have feelings to claim to have experienced something. Yet in a critical survey of current psychological theories of feeling, Hill (1995, p. 355) flatly states that "there are no general overarching theories of affect guiding research on religious experience." However, in the conceptual literature on religious experience, there is a broad-based theory that has generated considerable discussion. It is essentially a social-constructionist theory, which argues that there are no natural emotions. Emotions are constructed, interpreted, and recognized according to cognitive interpretations of physiological arousal. Much of this theory is based upon the psychological research of Schachter (1964, 1971) and his two-factor theory of emotion.

Within the conceptual literature on religious experience, Proudfoot (1985) has focused upon Schachter's two-factor theory of emotion as providing a conceptual critique in support of constructionist theories of religious experience. Schachter's theory essentially argues that the identification of an emotional experience requires both physiological arousal and a cognitive framework within which to identify the meaning of the arousal. Neither alone is sufficient to determine an emotional experience. In other words, persons tend to know how they feel or what they experience in terms of two quite different processes: (1) what the arousal circumstances were (external, perceptual, or cognitive factors), and (2) what internal physiological processes the persons are aware of. Hence the labeling of physiological arousal is not due just to physiological arousal per se, but to the specific circumstances in which the physiological arousal occurs. In this view, otherwise unanticipated physiological arousal may be labeled as "fear," "awe," or "anger," depending upon the circumstances in which it occurs. Proudfoot (1985) relies upon Schachter's theory to defend the thesis that experience cannot be religious until and unless it is identified and interpreted to be religious. Thus, consistent with Sundén's role theory (discussed above), without religious training and instruction to provide a context for interpretation, one cannot have a religious experience.

In a now classic study, Schachter and Singer (1962) injected a drug, epinephrine (adrenaline), into persons participating in an experiment they were told was intended to test the effects of a vitamin compound on vision. In fact, half the participants received an injection of epinephrine, which reliably produces increased respiration and heart rate, slight muscle tremors, and an "edgy" feeling. The other participants received a placebo (saline solution), whhich produces no physiological feelings. Hence the experimenters could be fairly assured that only the experimental group would experience physiological arousal. The participants in the experimental group were further divided into three groups: One group was told truthfully what physiological effects to anticipate; one group was misinformed and told to anticipate numbness, itching, and perhaps a headache; one group was given no information.

Contextual cues were then provided for all persons in the experiment. The cues were provided by "stooges" of the experimenter, who were in the room with the real subjects, presumably as participants in the experiment. The stooges acted either euphoric or angry.

Results of the experiment were generally as predicted and support a cognition-plus-arousal theory of emotional experience. Persons who experienced no physiological arousal (the placebo [saline solution] group), or who were given correct information as to expectations, did not use environmental cues to label their emotions. On the other hand, those with incorrect information or no information tended to interpret their emotions to be congruent with the cues—as euphoric when the stooge acted euphoric, and as angry when the stooge acted angry. Both observation (through one-way mirrors) and self-report measures were used in this study. In both experimental groups physiological arousal was generally properly identified (e.g., change in heart rate). The placebo group reported no physiological changes. Hence Schachter and Singer argued that, given a situation of unanticipated physiological arousal, external cues (in this case, the stooges' feigned emotional behavior) influence the labeling of what emotion is occurring. Whether it is labeled as angry, happy or sad depends upon the context for unanticipated physiological arousal. Specific emotions are thus socially constructed.

Since its inception, Schachter's two-factor theory has generated much debate (see Kemper, 1978; Marlasch, 1979; Plutchik & Ax, 1967). Despite major methodological criticisms of the Schachter and Singer (1962) study, its importance for a theory of religious experience is that physiological processes per se cannot account for emotional experiences; cognitions must also occur, at least in ambiguous circumstances (Hill & Hood, 1999b).

It is important to note that Schachter's theory gives a place to both cognition and physiological arousal. More recently, theorists have begun to champion more extreme views that minimize the role of physiology in emotions. For example, the almost purely cognitive view of Lazarus (1990) is that emotions are organized psychophysiological reactions. The organization requires cognitive appraisal. Thus, without cognition or appraisal, emotions are impossible; they are merely unspecified physiological activation. However, the relevance of cognition–arousal theories such as Schachter's, and the more cognitive appraisal theories such as Lazarus's, is that the articulation of experience gains religious relevance from the tradition within which experience gains its validity. As Taves (1999) argues, language matters. How an experience is described and narrated is an integral part of what it means to have this experience, rather than some other. The more one is knowledgeable about a tradition, the more one can experience what it is the tradition defines as religious. Sundén's role theory meshes nicely with the cognitive aspect of these theories, insofar as familiarity with religious texts and traditions is the rich source for appraisals that a situation is religiously relevant. Traditions provide the relevant cognitions.

In our own view of limits and transcendence, cognition–arousal and appraisal theories suggest that physiological arousal may be a factor initiating feelings that become meaningfully religious only if other appropriate conditions are met. The relevant question is this: Under what conditions will physiological arousal be interpreted religiously? Modern research suggests what James long ago insisted: When a person interprets an experience as religious, one must in the end look at the immediate content and context of religious consciousness. However, much of the research literature on religious practices has been more concerned with aspects of arousal than with the context in which arousal is interpreted. Both prayer and meditation have been studied in terms of the state of the brain's arousal during these practices.

Brain Waves and Meditation

The activities of prayer and meditation have in common an effort to withdraw from normal waking consciousness and a concern with attention to another reality, often considered to be transcendent. Of course, we must be careful with language here: Prayer and meditation are affirmed by devout individuals to be meaningful confrontations with a "deeper" or "higher" reality, or perhaps, as in the case of Zen, simply a full appreciation of reality as it is. For instance, Preston (1988) has shown how converts to Zen are socialized into an interpretation of reality that is based upon nonconceptual meditative techniques, which demand attentiveness to reality presumably as it is, in and of itself.

Naranjo and Ornstein (1971) distinguish between "ideational" and "nonideational" mediation. The former encourages and utilizes imagery that is common within a tradition; the later seeks an imageless state and avoids attention to unwanted imagery that may occur during meditation. The fact that much imageless meditation is widely recognized as a spiritual practice has contributed to the psychophysiological study of meditation. Rather than assess either verbal reports or behavior, investigators have focused upon physiological measures, particularly of brain activity. This has proven a particularly useful technique for studying persons who are otherwise apparently "just sitting."

We have noted in Chapter 3 the preliminary status of any strong claim to have identified bodily determinants of religious experience. Seeking a precise physiology of either prayer or meditation may be one of those chimerical tasks that serve to satisfy those who will accept the reality of spiritual things only if they can identify their bodily correlates.

Yet is it is well established that there is at least a gross relationship between brain wave patterns and modes of consciousness. Table 9.3 reveals that within various brain wave frequencies, typical modes of consciousness can be identified. However, it is also obvious that despite physiological correlates of consciousness, the mere fact that a person is "in" a particular brain state as measured by frequencies does not tell us much about what is being experienced. Reading a book, playing baseball, and watching a great movie would all probably register as "beta" states; yet this equates them only in a trivial sense with all activities a person engages in when awake and attending to something external. Not surprisingly, prayer and meditation states can be either alpha or beta states. Imageless states are more likely to be alpha; image states may be alpha or beta, depending upon the degree of focused awareness on specific imagery. However, even these conclusions are qualified generalizations.

Specific studies of meditative traditions have focused upon the brain wave correlates of those learning to meditate and those adept at meditation. Kasamatsu and Hirai (1969) have identified four stages that occur as one progresses in *zazen* (Zen meditation): (1) alpha waves in spite of eyes being opened; (2) increase in the amplitude of alpha waves; (3) decrease in alpha wave frequency; and (4) the appearance of rhythmic theta waves in some adept meditators. Furthermore, dividing 23 Zen disciples into three groups according to years of training revealed a difference in typical brain wave patterns during meditation for these groups. Kasamatsu and Hirai also found that Zen disciples appeared to pass through stages (defined by brain wave patterns) as they became more adept at *zazen*. Those practicing *zazen* for over 20 years had increased alpha amplitude (assumed to measure intensity), but some also developed rhythmic theta waves.

In an important aspect of their study, Kamatsu and Hirai linked these advanced stages to the Zen master's evaluation of the mental states achieved by the 23 disciples. Importantly, the Zen master made his evaluation of the quality of the mental states (low, medium, or high) without knowledge of the brain wave data. Brain wave patterns were reliably associated with

TABLE 9.3. Modes of Consciousness Associated with Identifiable Brain Wave Frequencies

Brain wave frequency	Mode of consciousness
Beta (>13 cps)	Active thought; focused attention with eyes opened. Oriented toward "external world."
Alpha (8–12 cps)	Relaxed yet aware. Eyes closed. Oriented toward "internal world."
Theta (4–7 cps)	Drowsiness. Fluid, dream-like (hypnogogic) images.
Delta (<4 cps)	Deep sleep. Conscious but unaware.

Note. See Johnston (1974). cps, cycles per second.

advances in *zazen*. Furthermore, the Zen master's independent ratings of those most adept at *zazen* were clearly associated with brain wave patterns assumed to be indicative of the higher stages of *zazen*. It is also worthy to note that these objective electrophysiological correlates of the quality of meditative stages support the claims within the Zen tradition that advancement in *zazen* can be identified appropriately by Zen masters. They also support earlier research by Maupin (1965), who found that those most adept at *zazen* had higher tolerances for anomalistic experiences and were able to take advantage of what, in psychoanalytic terms, were regressive experiences. Maupin noted that if meditation is considered to foster such regression, each stage of meditation, successfully mastered, permits further adaptive regression. More recently, a sophisticated and comprehensive effort to develop a neurophysiology of meditative states within the Zen tradition has been provided by Austin (1998).

Associated with efforts to meditate or pray is the difficulty of attending to one's prayerful or meditative activity without not being disrupted by external stimuli. Research with yogis suggests that those with well-marked alpha activity in their normal resting states show a greater aptitude and enthusiasm for practicing *samadhi* (yoga meditation) (Anand, Chhina, & Singh, 1961). In laboratory studies, external stimuli can be introduced while persons meditate, and the effects of these on their alpha activity can be examined. In terms of brain wave patterns, external stimuli force attention so that alpha states are disrupted or blocked (alpha blocking), and beta waves are noted. Mediators must then attempt to return to their inward states, characterized by alpha waves. It has been postulated that those adept at meditation are less likely to exhibit alpha blocking when external stimuli are introduced. Investigators have confirmed this prediction, both with Zen meditators (Kasamatsu & Hirai, 1969) and with those who practice yoga (Bagchi & Wenger, 1957). Likewise, in their now-classic study, Anand et al. (1961) documented the ability of yogis in a laboratory setting to exhibit high-amplitude blocking during *samadhi*, as well as the ability to show no response to pain.

Although brain wave correlates of meditative states present a fairly consistent gross pattern, they can be misleadingly interpreted to carry more weight than they should in terms of documenting religious experiences. Experience is no more "real" because one can identify its physiological correlates than it is the case that identical physiological correlates of meditative states mean that the experiences are necessarily the "same." For instance, numerous differences exist between *samadhi* and *zazen*, not to mention varieties of prayer. These difference are not necessarily reflected in brain wave patterns (though they may be). A person's exhibiting alpha activity may not tell us whether the is practicing *zazen*, *samadhi*, or Christian contemplative prayer. The experience of mediation and prayer is more than its physiology.

Sundén thought that his role theory was particularly useful in addressing the question "How are religious experience at all psychologically possible?" (Wikstrom, 1987, p. 390). Jan van der Lans (1985, 1987) utilized Sundén's theory in a study of students selected to participate in a 4-week training course in Zen meditation. They were told simply to concentrate on their breathing for the first 14 sessions. Then they were told to concentrate without a focus upon any object—a method called *shikantaza* in Zen. Participants were divided into those with ($n = 14$) and those without ($n = 21$) a religious frame of reference, based upon intake interviews. Instructions varied for each group: The religious group was told to anticipate experiences common in meditation within religious traditions, and the control group was told to anticipate experiences common in meditation used for therapeutic purposes.

Dependent measures included writing down every unusual experiences after each daily session, and by filling out a questionnaire on the last day of training that asked subjects specifically whether they had had a religious experience during meditation. The daily experiences were content-analyzed according to a list of 54 experiences categorized into five types: bodily sensations; fantasies, illusions, and imagery (hallucinations); changes in self-image; new insights; and negative feelings. Responses per category were too low for any meaningful statistical analyses. However, the number of persons reporting a religious experience during their Zen meditation varied as a function of presence or absence of a premeditative religious frame. Half of the religious participants reported a religious experience during meditation, while none of the control group (those without a premeditative religious frame) did. In addition, all participants were asked a control question at the end of the study: Had their meditations made them feel more vital and energetic? The groups did not differ on this question.

The conclusion we may draw from this research is that the actual practice of meditation elicits a specifically religious experience only for those with a religious frame of reference. If we assume equivalent meditative states in both groups (e.g., achievement of alpha states), the meaningfulness of such a state is dependent upon the interpretative frame one brings to the experience. Of course, a paradox is that within Zen, interpretative frames are minimized; hence this research employed a technique more compatible with prayer within the Christian tradition, in which interpretation plays a more significant role (Holmes, 1980). Still, it is clear that experience, meaningfully interpreted, is dependent upon whatever framework for interpretation can be brought to or derived from the experience. Sundén's role theory simply argues that familiarity with a religious tradition is the basis from which religious experiences gain their meaningfulness—and without which *religious* experiences are not possible.

Whereas Zen mediation emphasizes contemplation without an object, Deikman (1966) empirically investigated contemplative meditation, in which the emphasis is upon focused concentration upon a single object. What is important about Deikman's work is that contemplative meditation is often associated with the mystical tradition, in which the goal is a state of unity that is devoid of content or imagery. This is introvertive mysticism, as discussed in Chapter 10. However, it is also known that various experiences are likely to occur as one concentrates, including imagery of various sorts. Much of this imagery is readily understandable in the psychology of perception as afterimages, stabilized retinal images, and hypnogogic imagery. If not interpreted as meaningful, such imagery is largely irrelevant; it is left as minimal experience without meaning. However, if such experiences are specifically interpreted to be distractions and not part of one's meditative goal, such experiences have no inherent religious meaning and are only clues that one has yet to reach the desired imageless state. Furthermore, to focus upon such imagery will distract achievement of the imageless, introvertive mystical state.

Deikman's study was unusual, in that it reported the results of a prolonged series of meditative sessions derived primarily from two subjects. They simply sat in comfortable chairs and for 30 minutes focused attention upon a blue vase. Contemplative meditation requires that one simply contemplate the meditative object, without attention to thoughts or peripheral sensations. In Deikman's study, no religious object was used as a meditative object; hence, in term of Sundén's theory, religious frames of reference were unlikely to be elicited. Deikman's study was thus phenomenological—that is, an effort to provide a clear description of whatever appeared to the subjects' consciousness. Wulff (1995) notes that phenomenological studies try to reclaim for psychology the preeminence of experience. Deikman's (1966) study and the Williamson and Pollio (1999) study of serpent handlers (see Research Box 9.2) are among the few studies that have attempted to reclaim experience for psychology. Each provided careful descriptions and documentation of phenomena that were not all expected by the subjects or easily interpreted as *merely* subjective phenomena. These studies have left open the possibility that contemplative meditation and serpent handling allow an openness to experience that permits other aspects of reality to be revealed.

Other descriptive studies of meditation and of serpent handling likewise reveal a rich variety of experiences, many of which cannot simply be dismissed as subjective states (Goleman, 1977, 1988; Hood, 1998; Naranjo & Ornstein, 1971). It may be that phenomenological methods are the most appropriate for descriptively exploring experiences that often have religious importance (Hood, 2002). As Wulff (1995, p. 197) has stated, "Indeed, systematically appropriated and developed by even a handful of investigators, phenomenological psychology could revolutionize the field."

Altered States of Consciousness

At the other extreme from phenomenological and introspective description of consciousness are studies that focus upon neurophysiological states. Part of their appeal is the obvious scientific legitimacy of "hard" data—the pure descriptive facts of identifiable physiological processes. Three areas have gained some considerable influence among those interested in the psychology of religion.

The catchall phrase "altered states of consciousness" rapidly emerged in the 1960s for what has become a loosely knit area in which the focus is upon the empirical study of experiences previously assumed to be pathological or anomalous (Berenbaum, Kerns, & Raghavan, 2000; Reed, 1974; Zusne & Jones, 1989). Included in this area are such phenomena as hypnosis, dreaming, meditation, drug experiences, and a number of other "fringe" topics (e.g., parapsychology and near-death experiences). Much of this literature is more popular than academic. Until recently, the serious academic study of such experiences has assumed that such experiences have no objective validity. However, among sympathetic researchers there has been a shift in attitude: The experiences themselves are positively valued and assumed to have ontological validity. In other words, previous efforts to provide reductive explanations of such experiences are now overshadowed by descriptive efforts to explore the meaning and validity of such experience, including their objectivity (Berenbaum et al., 2000). Much of this is incorporated into modern "transpersonal psychology"—an area yet to be clearly defined or to have general academic and research support among mainstream psychologists (Greenwood, 1995). However, it is apparent that investigators are beginning to study empirically a wide variety of experiences that are immensely relevant to religion. Much of this research promises to enliven the psychology of religion by including within the discipline phenomena that religious traditions take seriously.

Tart (1975a) has been extremely influential in linking transpersonal psychology and altered states of consciousness. Basically, an altered state of consciousness is characterized by an introspective awareness of a different mode of experiencing the world. Loosely speaking, for example, everyone experiences dreaming as an altered state of consciousness relative to the normal waking state. Each altered state of consciousness has a typical pattern of functioning, recognized as such by the person. Hence things that might seem strange or bizarre are not really so when they are recognized as normal for that particular state of consciousness. Furthermore, persons move in and out of various states of consciousness. In Zinberg's (1977) view, there are alternate states of consciousness, not simply one normal and appropriate state of consciousness. Generally, it is assumed that the more open to experience one is, the more states of consciousness one can experience. More controversial is Tart's claim that knowledge is state-specific—in other words, that it is derived from, and appropriate to, a particular state of consciousness and may not be applicable to other states. Thus many religions are seen as state-specific sciences, with knowledge claims that are valid only within the parameters of the experiences and interpretations provided by these traditions. This parallels the concept of "ideological surround," discussed in Chapter 12. In a sense, new religious movements represent the sociological counterpart to the psychology of alternate states of consciousness.

Although much of transpersonal psychology (especially the claim to state-specific knowledge) is controversial, the concept of altered states of consciousness is often supported by a physiological base. Most typically, this consists of identifying alterations in neurophysiology that are assumed to be associated with altered states of consciousness. None of these models have achieved any degree of consensus, and most are at best speculations, in neurophysiological terms, of processes assumed to underlie various altered states of consciousness. Perhaps most often cited is Fischer's (1971, 1978) cartography of mental states linked to a continuum of arousal. This continuum ranges from hypoaroused tranquility, to normal everyday consciousness, to arousal, to hyperarousal and finally to ecstasy. Although extensive discussion of the neurophysiology of consciousness is beyond the scope of our concerns, the important point is that neurophysiological corrrelates (verified or not) have given altered states of consciousness a respectability within mainstream science, especially insofar as consciousness is studied as a brain process. This respectibility comes at the same time that others are affirming the much more controversial claim that the objects revealed in such altered states of consciousness cannot be dismissed as merely subjective phenomena.

As new technologies emerge to allow noninvasive neurophysiological measurement of ongoing experience, neurophysiological correlates of more typical religious experiences can be identified. One technique measures changes in cerebral blood flow via positron emission tomography (PET) imaging. One suggestive study using this technique matched six self-identified religious subjects of a Free Evangelical Fundamentalist Community in Germany with six nonreligious subjects (Azari et al., 2001). The religious subjects believed the Bible to be the literal word of God, and had had conversion experiences in which the 23rd Psalm was significant. In various conditions all subjects read and recited in randomized orders the 23rd Psalm, a well-known German nursery rhyme, or material from a telephone book. Self-ratings were used to assure that the religious subjects felt they had achieved a religious experience while reading the 23rd Psalm, whereas the nonreligious subjects did not. The PET results indicated that the subjects having a religious experience exhibited significantly more cerebral activity associated with cognitive processes (i.e., activity in the dorsolateral prefrontal and medial parietal cortex) when having their religious experience than they did in the comparison conditions, or than the nonreligious subjects did in any condition. This study provides additional support for the claim that religious experience is a cognitive attributional phenomenon that often includes a causal claim as to its origins (Proudfoot & Shaver, 1975; Proudfoot, 1985). It also demonstrates that much of the speculation regarding the neurophysiological correlates of religious experience (see Chapter 3) is likely to be effectively tested in laboratory conditions with a variety of new technologies.

The Split-Brain Hypothesis

Closely related to altered states of consciousness research is the discovery of the perplexing duality of the human brain. It has long been noted that the cortex of the human brain is apparently doubled, with the two cortical halves connected by a structure known as the corpus callosum (Segalowitz, 1983; Springer & Deutsch, 1981). What is of interest to psychologists of religion about this fact of brain anatomy is the claim that it underlies a dual mode of human consciousness—a mode of direct relevance of religious experience (Ornstein, 1986).

The lateral specialization of the cortex is particularly relevant to issues involving language and the ability to describe experience, which are largely left-hemispheric functions. The right hemisphere is more involved with tactile and visual memories, but, lacking high linguistic capabilities, cannot allow descriptions of tactile and visual experiences. This has led Ornstein (1986) to argue that people have two distinct minds: the left, logical, analytical, and linguistic mind, and the right, creative, intuitive, and ineffable mind. In this view, many religious experiences—including those difficult to express or verbalize—are due to right-hemispheric activity, which is dominant in some persons. On the other hand, the ability to articulate experience clearly and in logical terms is a left-hemispheric capacity. An individual's primary mode of experiencing the world is assumed to be a function of the individual's dominant hemisphere. Although extreme claims to lateralization are inaccurate, the fact of dichotomies in both language and human experience is obvious (Kolb & Whishaw, 1990). People often contrast religion with science, verbal with nonverbal expression, rationality with intuition, and poetry with prose. The list of dichotomies seems endless, causing H. Gardner (1978) to bemoan the emergence of "dichotomania" among contemporary scientists. Many scholars have leaped to the inference that religious experience is essentially a right-hemispheric phenomenon, whereas the articulation of that experience is essentially a left-hemispheric phenomenon. Few theories are as provocative in this sense as Jaynes's bicameral theory of religious consciousness.

Jaynes's Bicameral Theory

In a provocative theory that postulates a neurophysiological basis for religion, Jaynes (1976) links modes of human consciousness with forms of culture that have emerged through evolutionary history. He speculates that reflexive consciousness (including the sense of a personal "I") is a recent evolutionary phenomenon, rooted in the earlier failure of "bicameral consciousness"—a God-centered consciousness that increasingly became dysfunctional and was unfavored by natural selection.

Jaynes argues that early persons were "bicameral," in that their left and right hemispheres functioned independently. The effect of this lack of interconnection between hemispheres was that persons acted unconsciously; they simply did what they were commanded to do by unseen "gods." These commands came from "inside" their heads via the right hemisphere, as a complex of visions and voices from gods who could not "speak" but could command and be understood (Jaynes, 1976). As such, obedience to an inarticulate will of the gods was assured by those whose consciousness was dominated by the right hemisphere. Jaynes speculates that even today a residual function of the right hemisphere would be an organizational one, "that of sorting out the experience of a civilization and fitting them together into a pattern that could 'tell' the individual what to do" (Jaynes, 1976, p. 118). Of course, the left hemisphere remains neither passive nor silent. Rather, it confronts and attempts to articulate the meaning of the experiences it receives from the right hemisphere. Here then are the well-known dichotomies of religion: its ineffable experiential base (rooted in the right hemisphere), and its rational attempt to articulate the meaning of experience (rooted in the left hemisphere). Often it appears that one has little direct relevance to the other. However, in Jaynes's bicameral model, these differences are but reflections of the hemispheric difference between persons and gods. Often overlooked in discussions of Jaynes's theory is that the more fully one articulates the meaning of an experience, the more the left hemisphere becomes involved and probably inhibits the actual experience being articulated. Thus religious experience often requires an "abandonment" or "letting go," which can be facilitated by left-hemispheric acceptance of a safe set or setting within which right-hemispheric actions can be facilitated. In this sense, Sundén's role theory remains relevant: Familiarity with text and traditions facilitates experience based upon right-hemispheric activity (often assumed to be a religious trance state), and sanctions it interpretively through left-hemispheric activity.

Jaynes further speculates that when the stable world order broke down, bicameral consciousness was less effective and no longer favored by natural selection. A more rational, reflectively directed consciousness emerged, typical of modern consciousness and associated with the inevitable silence (if not death) of the gods. The powerful visions/voices and ineffable experience of the gods survive as isolated religious experiences, probably elicited by stress, or as aspects of the traumatic experiences involved in mental illness. Jaynes proposes a general bicameral paradigm that incorporates the logical structure of his theory and yet remains relevant to modern inductions of experience based upon the neurological structures (as yet unspecified) assumed to operate in the bicameral mind. This paradigm is presented in Table 9.4.

One merit of Jaynes's admittedly speculative theory is that it represents a creative effort to relate religious experience to the neurophysiological and anatomical structure of the human brain. As noted above and in Chapter 3, new technologies make the study of the neurophysiological correlates of religious experience possible. Newberg and D'Aquili (2000) properly argue for research that compares and contrasts the phenomenology of various experiences with their neurophysiological correlates. Not only does Jaynes's theory do this, but it also links to cultural considerations—for instance, the idea that historical patterns of social control are maintained by left-hemispheric ideological justifications for the commanding imperatives of the voices/visions of the right-hemispheric gods or God. Yet this leaves pitifully little comfort for modern religiously devout individuals, whose religious experiences seem to lose their ontological validity in the curious neuroanatomy of the gods. Indeed, the appeal to evolutionary theory leaves the validity of the gods to a previous history, and leaves the content of their experience to those contemporaries who now are woefully inadequate

TABLE 9.4. Jaynes's General Bicameral Paradigm

1. *Collective cognitive imperative:* A culturally agreed-on expectancy or prescription that defines the particular form of a phenomenon and the roles to be acted out within that form. This is essentially a belief system.

2. *Induction:* A formally ritualized procedure whose function is the narrowing of consciousness. The major technique used is similar to contemplative meditation, but attention is focused upon a small range of preoccupations instead of a single object.

3. *Trance:* An altered state of consciousness characterized by a restriction of consciousness or its loss. The sense of "I" is diminished or lost. In this state one adopts a role accepted or encouraged by the group.

4. *Archaic authorization:* The individual (god or person) to whom the trance is related. This authority is accepted by the group and within its belief system is attributed the power to produce the trance state.

Note. Adapted from Jaynes (1976, p. 324). Copyright 1976 by Houghton Mifflin Company. Adapted by permission.

to the modern world. However, even this claim is tempered by those to whom the gods continue to speak, as noted in Research Box 9.3.

Speaking in Tongues (Glossolalia)

"Glossolalia," or speaking in tongues, is a universal religious phenomenon (May, 1956). Jaynes (1976) asserts that it is always a group phenomenon and that it fits well into the general bicameral paradigm, including the strong cognitive imperative of religious belief in a cohesive group, the induction procedures of prayer and ritual resulting in the narrowing of consciousness (trance), and the archaic authorization of the divine spirit in a charismatic leader. Whereas Jaynes (1976) asserts the musical and poetic nature of glossolalia, Samarin (1972) finds it to be merely a meaningless, phonologically structured human sound. Lafal, Monahan, and Richman (1974) dispute the claim that glossolalia is meaningless. Hutch (1980) claims that glossolalia aims to amalgamate the sounds of laughing and crying—signs of both the joy and pain of life. Early psychologists attributed glossolalia to mental illness, but modern researchers have made a strong conceptual case for distinguishing glossolalia

---

Research Box 9.3. Jaynes's Theory Applied in the Contemporary Netherlands (Romme & Escher, 1989, 1996)

Romme and Escher investigated the long-term consequences of the direct experience of the gods, as proposed by Jaynes's theory of the bicameral mind. A patient diagnosed with schizophrenia, who heard voices and who had read Jaynes's (1976) book, was intrigued with the fact that there once was strong cultural support (as in ancient Greece) for what psychiatrists often dismiss today as mere hallucination. Appearing on Dutch television with this patient, these investigators invited those who heard voices to contact them.

This sampling procedure, like that of Hardy as described earlier in the text, was far from scientific. Yet it did reveal how a self-selected sample of persons (450) described coping with what some might dismiss as only auditory hallucinations.

Some of the people who responded to Romme and Escher's invitation were interviewed in depth concerning their process of adaptation to the voices they heard. For the approximately one-third of persons who successfully coped with voices, the general process of successful adjustment followed a clearly identified pattern that fell into three main phases:

Phase I (*startle*): Voices appear suddenly, often following stress. Persons may panic. They often feel confused and powerless. Persons struggle, try to avoid the voices, or try to make the voices disappear.

Phase II (*organization*): Persons begin to adjust to voices. There are great individual differences. Some common techniques of adjustment include ignoring negative voices or deciding to listen to them only at certain times. Positive voices are listened to more frequently, and a person may even respond to them.

Phase III (*stabilization*): Persons accept voices, and often find that they can have positive influences. Voices are integrated into an otherwise normal life.

from what are only superficial clinical parallels (Kelsey, 1964; Kildahl, 1972). Empirically, glossolalia is normative within many religious traditions, including some Pentecostal and Holiness denominations in the contemporary United States. Thus it is not surprising that empirical studies comparing glossolalic with nonglossolalic controls have consistently failed to find any reliable psychological differences, including indices of psychopathology, between the two groups (Goodman, 1972; Hine, 1969; Malony & Lovekin, 1985; J. T. Richardson, 1973). However, it is also true that, as Lovekin and Malony (1977) found in their study of participants in a Catholic charismatic program of spiritual renewal, glossolalia per se may not be particularly useful in fostering personality integration.

The real focus of research has been on whether or not glossolalia occurs only in a trance or altered state of consciousness. The anthropologists Goodman (1969) has documented the cross-cultural similarity of glossolalic utterances. She attributes this similarity to the fact that glossolalia results from an induced trance. The trace state itself, for neurophysiological reasons, accounts for the cross-cultural similarity of glossolalia (Goodman, 1972). Her model of the induction of a trance state follows closely Jaynes's general bicameral paradigm (Goodman, 1988). She argues for induction techniques generated by religious rituals in believers. This trance state produces an altered perceptual state in which previous limits are transcended. One participant in her research stated the case for limits and transcendence quite succinctly: "At first you feel that you have come to a barrier, and you are afraid. All of a sudden you are beyond it and everything is different" (quoted in Goodman, 1988, p. 37). This altered perceptual state is identified by Goodman as the "sojourn." It is followed by dissolution, or the return to ordinary perceptual states, and by the joy and euphoria of having had this sacred experience.

Samarin (1972) has challenged Goodman's cross-cultural data on the grounds that all her samples were from similar Pentecostal settings, even though the data were collected within different cultures. Samarin also points out that patterns identified in typical Appalachian Mountain setting are similar to those found in glossolalia. This is the case, even though such preaching does not occur in a trance state; hence there is no reason to infer that glossolalia can only be elicited in trance states. This view is also supported by Hine (1969). More recently, however, Philipchalk and Muller (2000) demonstrated increased activation of the right hemisphere relative to the left in a small sample of participants who allowed infrared photography before and after speaking in tongues. The opposite was found before and after reading aloud. These data suggest the activation of the right hemisphere in glossolalia, and not necessarily the existence of a trance state.

Obviously, the outcome of the debate on whether or not trance states are necessary for such religious experiences as glossolalia or serpent handling is partly conceptually clouded. It would require a clear operational definition of glossolalia at one level and a clear operational definition of trance at another level to test whether the two covary, much less to see whether glossolalia can only be elicited in a trance state. Although such research has yet to be done, the debate has been useful as another instance of religious experience's gaining a foothold in mainstream social science by raising issues of possible physiological correlates. It is assumed that since such physiological processes can be identified in hard scientific terms, the experiences they facilitate have at least that validity. Of course, once again, for religiously committed individuals, such faint praise is less than sufficient. Experience attributed to the gods or to one's God must have more reality than the physiological conditions that facilitate them. A participant observation study of glossolalia, conducted over many years in Scandinavian countries and presented in Research Box 9.4, suggests that trance is not a necessary condition for glossolalia to occur.

Research Box 9.4. Sundén's Role Theory and Glossolalia (Holm, 1987b)

Holm is among the foremost researchers who have focused upon the social and contextual factors that facilitate glossolalia. He collected recordings of hundreds of Pentecostal meetings in Scandinavian countries over several years. He thus studied speaking in tongues within religious contexts where it was normative. He found that there were few linguistic impediments to producing glossolalia, and thus that a trance state was not necessary for one to speak in tongues. However, he also noted that a trance state could remove social inhibitions and hence facilitate glossolalia in some Pentecostalists.

Relying heavily upon Sundén's role theory, Holm conducted in-depth interviews with 65 Pentecostalists. Glossolalia is modeled both by relevant Biblical texts regarding the Pentecost story, and by others in services who speak in tongues. Individuals must wait for this experience to occur as a true "baptism of the Holy Spirit" and not attempt to produce the experience themselves. Holm noted that approximately two-thirds of his sample first spoke in tongues at some kind of religious meeting. Other believers' speaking in tongues, combined with an initiate's readiness to have this experience as a model in text and practice, produces the "gift of tongues." The emotional excitement that accompanies this experience is a function of a true "baptism of the Holy Spirit" and a religious sense of its presence. Subsequent doubts as to whether or not the glossolalia was perhaps self-produced are allayed by church members and authorities who assure its validity. Repeated glossolalic experiences confirm and solidify what can now be routinely experienced. It is important to note that in Holm's sample, 12 persons never spoke in tongues. Personality factors such as inhibitions (and perhaps neurophysiological factors as well) suggest that even with appropriate readiness and both textual and actual modeling, the experience is not available to all.

Note. See also Holm (1991, especially pp. 142–145) and Hood (1991).

The issue of whether or not trance states are required for glossolalia is paralleled in participant observation studies of serpent handlers. Williamson (1995) has emphasized that serpent handlers have historically been associated with denominations such as the Church of God, which once sanctioned *both* serpent handling and glossolalia. Based upon extensive participant observation on serpent handlers, Hood (1998) noted that some handlers believe that faith alone is sufficient for handling serpents, while others argue that only when "anointed" should one handle serpents. Anointing is the case that most closely parallels the claim to trance. That believers can handle serpents through either faith or anointing supports the claim that trance is not necessary for serpent handling, as it is not necessary for glossolalia. In one unique study, a serpent handler in an anointed state agreed to be videotaped and have his electroencephalogram taken. Research Box 9.5 presents the result of this study.

RELIGIOUS IMAGERY: THE RETURN OF THE OSTRACIZED

It has been almost 30 years since a distinguished psychologist prophesied the "return of the ostracized" to psychology (Holt, 1964). The "ostracized" that Holt spoke of was imagery, and

---

Research Box 9.5. Electroencephalogram of a Believer When Anointed
(Woodruff, 1993)

In Holiness sects, as in many Pentecostal groups, anointment by the Holy Ghost is believed to occur when the spirit of God possesses an individual. Anna Prince, a member
of a serpent-handling Holiness sect, partly defined anointing as follows: "It's a spiritual
trancelike strand of power linking humans to God; it's a burst of energy that's refresh-
ing, always brand new; it brings on good emotions. One is elated, full of joy" (quoted in
Burton, 1983, p. 140). The famous serpent handler Pastor Liston Pack stated, "The anointing is hard, real hard to explain; and 'cause if I was to tell you that you had to feel just
like me, I might tell you wrong, you see, but if you didn't know me, you would think I
was havin' a stroke or somethin' tremendous was takin' place" (quoted in Burton, 1983,
p. 140).

   At researcher Thomas Burton's request, Liston Pack agreed to be videotaped and to
have electroencephalographic (EEG) recordings taken while he was in an anointed state.
Michael Woodruff did the recording and interpretation of the recordings. His four major
conclusions were as follows: (1) Liston Pack's EEG showed no abnormal clinical signs; it
was neither a self-induced epileptic seizure nor brought on by some unknown state.
(2) Liston Pack had a great deal of control over his mental state, given his ability to prepare for anointment in a laboratory setting among skeptical scientists. (3) There was a
sudden conversion from alpha to beta when anointment began, with beta predominant
throughout the experience. The EEG was that of an aroused individual, but was accompanied by observations of an individual having a religious experience. It was *not* similar
to that of a Zen monk in contemplation. (4) Overall, the EEG patterns of Liston Pack were
more similar to patterns found in hypnosis than in meditation. However, Woodruff cautions that self-hypnosis is only a hypothesis worthy of further study and ought not to be
confused with self-delusion.

---

its return has fostered the development of the psychology of religion in two ways. First, as
Bergin (1964) has emphasized, it has helped shift the emphasis from psychology as the study
of behavior to psychology as the study of inner experience. Second, it has fostered interest
in religious experience, given the unquestioned centrality of imagery within the world's great
faith traditions (LaBarre, 1972b). Imagery as a central fact of much human experience often
gains unique relevance when interpreted religiously. The spontaneous presence or cultivated
facilitation of imagery is central to many religious traditions. However, before we discuss
religious imagery, we must briefly consider the issue of hallucinations.

Hallucinations

Recent studies question the existence of hallucinations as a unique phenomenon. Fischer's
(1969) identification of a perception–hallucination *continuum* is supported by a massive literature suggesting that hallucinations are not simply characteristic of organic deficiencies and
are not necessarily psychopathological (Bentall, 1990, 2000). DSM-IV defines a hallucination simply as "a sensory perception that has the compelling sense of reality of a true perception but that occurs without external stimulation of the relevant sensory organ" (Ameri-

can Psychiatric Association, 1994, p. 767). There is some debate as to whether or not to include as hallucinations perceptions that are felt to be internal rather than external in origin; DSM-IV does not make a distinction between these (American Psychiatric Association, 1994, p. 767). In many cultures, hallucinations are positively valued and are understood as meaningful. Al-Issa (1977) argues that the effort to classify experiences as "real" or "imaginary" is a preoccupation of Western psychiatrists, while Bourguigon (1970) has documented the meaningfulness of hallucinations in more than 60% of her sample of 488 societies worldwide. Thus whether or not an image is hallucinatory depends upon cultural and social factors, not simply neurophysiology. Furthermore, hallucinations are common in normal or nonhospitalized populations. Tien (1991), using DSM-III-R criteria for the lifetime presence of hallucinations, found that between 11% and 13% of a randomly selected general population had experienced them at some point. This percentage range corresponds closely to that found in a survey done over 100 years ago in Great Britain (Sidgewick, 1894). Thus, as critical reviews of the literature by Bentall (1990, 2000) clearly show, hallucinations are neither inherently pathological nor uninfluenced in either content or evaluation by culture. Psychologists have most typically studied auditory hallucinations, and as Research Box 9.6 notes, a consensus has been reached as to their explanation.

Research Box 9.6. Are Auditory Hallucinations
Misattributions of Inner Speech? (Bentall, 1990, 2000)

Bentall (2000) has summarized what he refers to as a "widespread consensus" about the nature of auditory hallucinations. Basically, auditory hallucinations are identified as misattributions of inner speech. "Inner speech" has long been identified as a normal psychological process; it refers to the internal dialogue people use to regulate or evaluate their own behavior. At about 3 years of age, children begin to regulate their behavior by talking out loud to themselves in the same fashion they have been talked to by their primary caregivers. Children then learn to talk to themselves quietly—a form of subvocalization. Subvocalization is a common part of normal development.

Bentall (1990, 2000) summarizes much physiological research indicating that the onset of self-reported auditory hallucinations corresponds to identifiable subvocalizations, regardless of whether subvocalizations are recorded by measuring muscle movements or by using sensitive electromyographic measures. Bentall summarizes other research indicating that the areas in the brain involved in speech are activated during the report of auditory hallucinations. Furthermore, the content of auditory hallucinations has been shown to match the content of actual recorded subvocalizations. Since the onset and content of auditory hallucinations correspond to those of subvocalizations, an individual who hallucinates may be making a misattribution—attributing to an external source what in fact is produced internally.

A psychologist of religion might hypothesize that religious belief influences not only the content of hallucinations, but perhaps their form as well. For instance, Catholics may be more likely to report visual hallucinations, while Protestants may be more likely to report auditory hallucinations. In any case, the study of hallucinations among religiously devout individuals within a cultural context is much needed and should help clarify the role of belief and expectations in legitimating, if not offering ontological options for, what otherwise are simply misattributions.

Cultural and social processes facilitate the reporting of imagery, whether or not it is defined as hallucinatory (Al-Issa, 1977, 1995; Bentall, 2000; Bourguigon, 1970). One major influence on the content of hallucinations is religion. For instance, as Kroll and Bachrach (1982) have documented, visions in the Middle Ages had almost exclusively religious content. Religions have also long been noted for their interest in fostering such activities as prayer and meditation, which either are aimed at or indirectly facilitate the elicitation of religious imagery (Clark, 1983; Larsen, 1976; Pelletier & Garfield, 1976). Similarly, apparently spontaneous experienced imagery possesses great significance when it is sanctioned as meaningful within religious traditions. For instance, Catholicism makes a distinction between a "vision" and an "apparition" that parallels psychological distinctions between "imagery" and "hallucinations." Volken (1961) notes that apparitions are perceived as "exterior" and are a special case of visions within Catholicism. A purely secular person would be tempted to call an apparition a hallucination, suggesting that it therefore has less objectivity than a "real" perception. However, social scientists have gained some insight into factors influencing the reports and sanctions of images of both Mary and Jesus, two dominant figures within the Christian tradition—whether these reports are considered apparitions, hallucinations, or simply images.

Images of Mary within the Catholic Tradition

Several investigators have focused attention upon reports of images of the Virgin Mary associated with the Catholic faith tradition. We use the term "image" in a neutral sense, to cover both the possibility that such occurrences are hallucinations (nonveridical perceptions) or apparitions (veridical perceptions accepted with the Catholic tradition). In either case, social-psychological factors clearly determine both the frequency of the reports of such experiences, their acceptance as authentic by the Catholic Church, and the differential appeal of the cult of the Virgin Mary. Much of the current research has been stimulated by the work of Carroll (1983, 1986).

Catholics have long accepted the worship of Mary as part of their faith tradition. Included in this worship is the recognition by the Church of apparitions of the Virgin Mary throughout history. Modern apparitions have ranged from the Miraculous Medal of the Immaculate Conception in France in 1830 to the visions at Medjugorje in the former Yugoslavia in 1981 (Perry & Echeverría, 1988). Sociological studied have focused upon the factors that influence the Catholic Church to accept only *some* reported apparitions of Mary as legitimate. For instance, Warner (1976) provides critical historical documentation in support of her claim that sanctioning apparitions of the Virgin Mary has often been linked with official support for sexual suppression. Perry and Echeverría argue that apparitions have been used both to facilitate social control on the part of the Catholic Church and to boost national prestige. Their latter claim is congruent with Carroll's (1983, 1986) claim that even when countries have similar frequencies of reports of Marian apparitions, such as Spain and Italy, social and political factors have led to differential legitimatization of the apparitions by central Church authorities.

More relevant to the empirical psychology of religion is the fact that Carroll's theoretical orientation is largely classical Freudian theory, in which it is assumed that repressed sexual desires largely account for hallucinations and fantasies. Thus Carroll treats all apparitions of the Virgin Mary as hallucinations, differentially legitimated by central Church authorities. His empirical efforts focus upon predicting characteristics of Marian apparitions from history in terms of classical Freudian theory. His thesis can be readily summarized in three major claims.

First, the Catholic doctrine of the Virgin Mary incorporates three beliefs: Mary is virginal conceived, her maidenhead (hymen) was never ruptured (*in partu* virginity); and Mary remained a lifelong virgin. Thus Mary is unique in religious mythology in that she is a perpetual virgin, totally devoid of sexuality. In Freudian theoretical terms, Mary symbolizes sexual denial.

Second, Carroll provides demographic and historical data to document that the cult of Mary is strongest in countries when the machismo complex is most common. The machismo complex essentially entails fierce sexual domination of women by men, often strongly culturally supported.

Third, Carroll provides anthropological and ethnographic data to show that in areas when the Mary cult and the machismo complex are strongest, males come from father-ineffective families. In Freudian terms, father-ineffective families assure strong and delayed attachment to the mother on the part of her male children. Using Freudian Oedipal theory, Carroll argues that males strongly attached to their mothers have intense erotic repressions that can effectively be expressed in attraction to the cult of the Virgin Mary. The idealized Virgin Mary represents the denial of sexual attraction to one's mother; the machismo complex displaces eroticism onto other women, who are treated primarily as sex objects; guilt is assuaged by attraction to the passion of Christ, in which the male identifies with the need for punishment. Thus sexual sublimation accounts for the appeal of the cult of the Virgin Mary.

Carroll's provocative thesis is rare in the psychology of religion, as it incorporates historical, anthropological, ethnographic, and social-historical facts into a single, coherent theoretical framework. It has also led to several empirical studies. For instance, Carroll utilized Walsh's (1906) extensive identification of Marian apparitions associated with the Catholic Church that included those officially recognized by the church, as well as those not legitimated. All apparitions from the years 1100 to 1896 for which three empirical criteria could be documented resulted in a sample of 50 (see Carroll, 1986, pp. 225–226, for a list of these). The three empirical criteria were as follows: (1) The seer was in a waking state; (2) the seer both heard and saw Mary; and (3) the image of Mary was not provided by a identifiable physical stimulus. Assuming sexual sublimation to foster susceptibility to Marian hallucinations (apparitions), Carroll predicted that the seer should be unmarried (and hence likely to be celibate). Table 9.5 presents the results of Carroll's study for 45 of the 50 separate appari-

TABLE 9.5. Assumed Celibacy Status of Seers at Time of Their First Apparition of the Virgin Mary

Status	n	%
Assumed celibate		
Cleric	18	40
Unmarried		
Child	8	18
Adolescent	9	20
Adult	8	18
Assumed not celibate		
Married	2	4

Note. Adapted from Carroll (1983, p. 210). Copyright 1983 by the Society for the Scientific Study of Religion. Adapted by permission.

tions for which the celibacy status of the seer could be assumed. Inspection of this table shows that 94% of the seers could be assumed to be celibate; this supports the sublimation thesis. Of course, one cannot be assured that every unmarried seer was celibate, but the available data do suggest that married and assuredly noncelibate seers were unlikely to report apparitions for the years studied (1100 to 1896).

What of women seers? Freudian theory suggest that sexual sublimation applies to females as well as males. In the female case, identification with Mary on the part of females permits expression of repressed sexuality, since a daughter obtains the father by identifying with her mother. Although Freudian Oedipal theory is controversial (Shafranske, 1995), Carroll's use of this theory does lead to specific, empirically testable predictions. In this case, Carroll predicted that the gender of the seer would relate to whether or not apparitions of Mary would contain additional male figures (such as Jesus or adult male saints). He based this prediction upon the fact that males desire exclusive possession of the mother and do not want father figures present. Since females identify with the mother in order to obtain access to the father, they should want father figures present. Classifying the same 50 apparitions noted above, this time for gender of the seer, permitted Carroll to cross-tabulate this with whether or not male figures were present in the report Mary apparition. These results are presented in Table 9.6 for the 47 of the 50 seers for whom the gender and adulthood of male figures appearing with Mary could be clearly identified. Inspection of this table indicates that most apparitions studied did not have adult males in them. However, a gender effect was clearly identified for males; that is, males were unlikely to report a male present in their Marian apparitions. For females, a male was as likely to be present as not to be present. Most importantly for Carroll's thesis, females were much more likely to report apparitions with males present than were males, whose Marian apparitions seldom included other adult male figures (Carroll, 1986).

If we assume Marian apparitions to be hallucinations (non-sensory-based imagery), than Carroll's theory argues that psychological factors predispose individuals to experience hallucinations that may be compatible with religious traditions legitimating such imagery in the form of apparitions. Thus religious tradition and psychological dispositions may interact to allow a powerful experience for some, which, when formally sanctioned by the authorities of the tradition, become powerful vicarious experiences for others within that tradition as well. They can believe through faith what the original seers have experienced firsthand. A

TABLE 9.6. Relationship between Sex of Seer and Likelihood of at Least One Adult Male in a Marian Apparition

| | Male in Marian apparition? | | | |
| | Yes | | No | |
Sex of seer	n	%	n	%
Male	2	7	25	93
Female	10	50	10	50

Note. Although these data are significant according to Fisher's exact test (one-tailed), phi = .35, $p < .05$, the cases were probably not independent, since earlier apparitions probably influenced later ones. Data from Carroll (1986, p. 145).

test of Carroll's thesis, using a sample of Protestant males and preference for images of Mary and Christ, is presented in Research Box 9.7.

Studies of hallucinations or apparitions of the Virgin Mary have important conceptual relevance for the empirical study of religion. What is crucial is the fact that the meaningful status of imagery varies with the context within which it is interpreted and with the nature of the ontological status the image is given (Bettelheim, 1976; Klinger, 1971; Singer, 1966; Watkins, 1976). Anthropological studies of apparitions have rightly cautioned against ignor-

---

Research Box 9.7. An Empirical Test of Carroll's Psychoanalytic Theory of Apparitions (Hood, Morris, & Watson, 1991)

Carroll's thesis that sexual sublimation is involved in the male attraction to the cult of the Virgin Mary in Roman Catholicism was tested by Hood et al. in a sample of non-Catholic, Christian males. Independent samples of raters were used to identify (1) crucifixes ranked according to the degree of Christ's suffering they represented, and (2) artistic renderings of the Virgin Mary rated ranked and rated for (a) eroticism and (b) nurturing quality. Four crucifixes reliably varying in degree of suffering expressed (and one plain cross, as a control) were used as stimuli. Five pictures of the Virgin Mary, reliably varying in erotic and nurturing quality (with one identified as *equally* nurturing and erotic, as a control) were also used. These stimuli were then rated for personal preference by 71 non-Catholic males, all of whom either agreed or strongly agreed on a 5-point Likert scale that "My whole approach to life is based upon my religion." These males had also taken a measure developed by Parker (1983; Parker, Tupling, & Brown, 1979) to measure self-recalled maternal bonding. This was used as a measure of strong attachment (ambivalently erotic and nurturing) to one's mother.

Participants were taken one at a time into a room in which the crucifixes and the cross were mounted on one wall and the pictures of the Virgin Mary were mounted on another wall. They were first seated in front of the wall on which the crucifixes and cross were randomly numbered and hung, and were asked to take a moment to contemplate them. They then answered the question "Which cross or crucifix best expresses what Christ means to you?" followed by "Which cross or crucifix next best expresses what Christ means to you?" This was continued until one remained, and participants were asked, "Why did you not choose this cross/crucifix?" A similar procedure was then followed as participants were seated in front of the wall with the five pictures of the Virgin Mary.

Consistent with the theory of the role of sexual sublimation in reports of Marian apparitions, Hood et al. predicted that males strongly but ambivalently attached to their mothers would have a preference for (1) a suffering Christ and (2) the ambivalently erotic/ nurturing Virgin Mary representation. Results supported these predictions. The more males recalled ambivalent and strong attachments to their mothers as measured by the bonding scales, the more likely they were to prefer a suffering Christ figure and the ambivalent Virgin Mary figure. In terms of Freudian theory, the ambivalent attraction to one's mother also involves the unconscious sense of guilt and the identification with a Christ who suffers painfully. Freudian theory is often controversial and susceptible to varying interpretations. It is best viewed as one interpretation on any set of data—even those proposed as a test of Freudian theory, as in this study of Carroll's speculative theory.

ing the cultural context of apparitions. Apolito (1998, p. 24) warns against Carroll's "relentless psychological reductionism" and states that visionary realities are complex constructions that are more than mere "hallucinations." Yet Carroll's work remains a provocative frame within which psychological factors can be shown to operate as at least one part of a complex phenomenon sanctioned with the Catholic tradition.

Visions of Christ

If Marian apparitions are largely restricted to the Catholic tradition, visions of Jesus Christ occur within both Catholicism and Protestantism. Wiebe (1997, 2000) has made an extensive study of such visions reported by 30 living visionaries. Like much of the other research on visions, his sample is largely unrepresentative and certainly not an adequate scientific sample from a specified population, Yet, as with Hardy's and Hufford's work (described earlier in this chapter), the value of Wiebe's work is in his effort to provide extensive detailed descriptions of visions from the perspective of the visionaries. Although a social scientist is likely to be reluctant to claim any non-natural basis for religious imagery, it is interesting that careful phenomenological descriptions of imagery experiences—whether they are called hallucinations, apparitions, or visions—reveal that psychologists have yet to explain them fully. Wiebe discusses efforts to explain visions of Christ in three broad areas (supernaturalistic, mentalistic, and neurophysiological). However, as Hufford (1982) concludes in regard to the Old Hag phenomenon, Wiebe (2000) concludes that "These visions elude adequate naturalistic explanation . . . and continue to provide a profound sense that a reality that does not belong to our world has been manifested" (p. 139). Thus, as in popular studies of both Marian apparitions (Garvey, 1998) and encounters with Jesus Christ (Sparrow, 1995), the belief that a reality has been encountered—that a figure has actually been seen that cannot be dismissed as merely a hallucination—is an essential part of the experience. Rodney Stark (1999) has proposed a general theory of revelations, which places the often limited psychological study of visions or hallucinations within a broader social context. His model, which is empirically testable, is presented in Table 9.7.

TABLE 9.7. Stark's General Model of Revelations

1. Revelations will tend to occur in cultures that support communication with the divine.
2. A wide variety of mental phenomena can be interpreted as communication with the divine.
3. Most revelations are confirmatory (i.e., they support existing beliefs within the tradition).
4. There are individual differences in the ability to receive revelations.
5. Novel revelations are likely to come from devout believers who perceive shortcomings within their tradition.
6. Social crises increases the probability of perceiving shortcomings within one's tradition.
7. During periods of social crises, the number of persons both receiving and accepting revelations is maximized.
8. Confidence that one has received a revelation is increased to the extent that others accept the revelation.
9. Revelations are more likely to be accepted from members of intense primary groups.
10. Further revelations are likely if the recipient is reinforced.
11. Increased revelations and reinforcement increase the probability of novel or heretical revelations.
12. As religious movements become successful, they attempt to curtail novel revelations.

Note. Data from Stark (1999, p. 308).

The Facilitation of Religious Imagery

Religious imagery plays a role in many religious traditions and is of immense relevance to any empirical psychology of religion. Much of the more clinical and conceptual literature in the psychology of religion—for instance, the literature associated with Jungian, object relations, and transpersonal theory—explores images in depth (Beit-Hallahmi, 1995; Greenwood, 1995; Halligan, 1995). Experimental study of imagery has also been of interest in the long tradition of studies of "sensory deprivation" or isolation. As we shall see, restricting external perception enhances the probability of imagery. Not surprisingly, psychologists have sought ways to enhance both solitude and isolation to facilitate the occurrence of imagery.

Few contemporary psychologists would dispute Pylyshyn's (1973, p. 2) claim that "imagery is a pervasive form of human experience and is of utmost important to humans." Indeed, as both Shephard (1978) and Lilly (1977) have noted, situations of isolation, solitude, and focused concentration often elicit unanticipated and undesired imagery that can disrupt ongoing activities. Examples of such situations include focusing upon a radar scope, attending to concerns during space travel, and surviving during prolonged periods of isolation. Thus it is not surprising that early experimental studies of isolation, using isolation tanks, often documented imagery that was disruptive and disturbing to research participants (Lilly, 1977; Zubeck, 1969). The very phrase "sensory deprivation" emphasizes the negative. However, within many religious traditions, withdrawing from "worldly" perceptions and "turning within" have long had a valuable and privileged status. For instance, some forms of both prayer and meditation involve withdrawal from external sensory attention, which may produce imagery that is religiously meaningful. LaBarre (1972a, p. 265; emphasis in original) has gone so far as to claim:

> Every religion in historic fact, began in one man's "revelation"—his dream or fugue or ecstatic trance. Indeed, the crisis cult is *characteristically* dereistic, autistic, and dreamlike precisely *because* it had its origins in the dream, trance, "spirit" possession, epileptic "seizure," REM sleep, sensory deprivation, or other visionary state of the shaman–originator. All religions are necessarily "revealed" in this sense, inasmuch as they are certainly not revealed consensually in secular experience.

Although LaBarre's position may be extreme, it does emphasize the obvious relevance of imagery to religious traditions. It is thus curious that sensory isolation research has neither focused upon the elicitation of imagery with religious samples nor concerned itself with the specific elicitation of religious imagery among samples, whether religious or not.

The exclusion of external sources of stimulation in isolation studies led early investigations to coin the term "sensory deprivation." Many assumed that the images present in such studies must be hallucinations. However, early isolation ("deprivation") studies produced exaggerated results that are now readily identifiable largely as artifacts of the experimental setting (Zubeck, 1969). In particular, the use of isolation tanks provided the means to control external sources of stimulation. A typical isolation tank is an enclosed, soundproofed, and lightproofed container filled with magnesium salt solutions, heated to external body temperature (34.1°C), and adjusted for specific gravity so that a person simply floats partly submerged. The uniqueness of the isolation tank situation, combined with excessive experimental forewarnings and precautions, elicited panic and bizarre reactions in some participants. However, as studies progressed, it was discovered that if participants were knowledgeable (i.e., were initiated into the experiences likely to be facilitated by the isolation tank), negative reactions became exceedingly uncommon. Instead, participants explored the variety of experiences common to altered-states research in an almost universally positive fashion (Lilly, 1956, 1977; Lilly & Lilly, 1976; Suedfeld, 1975). Most importantly for our interests is the imagery elicited in isolation tank experiences—imagery that is seldom appropriately identified as merely hallucinatory (Suedfeld & Vernon, 1964).

Imagery is readily elicited in isolation tanks if participants are relaxed and unfearful, and if they are given specific instructions to attend to internal states, contents, and processes. Unstructured phenomena such as focused or diffuse white light, as well as various geometric forms and colors, are common and rapidly explainable by the psychology of perception. For instance, spontaneous neural firing in the retina, a common phenomenon, is attended to in isolation studies and hence becomes a part of conscious awareness. Some of these phenomena are common in meditation and prayer, as discussed above.

More detailed instructions and time in the isolation tank can lead to more meaningful images—some similar to hypnogogic imagery, and other similar to meaningful figures not unlike those found in dreams. Both the report and content of imagery are heavily influenced by set and setting (Jackson & Kelly, 1962; Rossi, Sturrock, & Solomon, 1963). As in psychedelic research, hallucinations are rare in isolation tanks. Persons do not see images they mistakenly expect to exist in time and space, as they would see objects of everyday perception. However, with appropriate set and setting, participants do experience imagery that has ontological significance. The imagery is not simply dismissed as "subjective." In this sense, isolation tanks can facilitate genuine religious experiences. Research Box 9.8 reports one study in which set and setting were used to facilitate religious experiences under isolation tank conditions.

Other researchers have begun to explore ways to experimentally induce imagery and other forms of religious experience. Masters and Houston (1973), noted for their pioneering work on the varieties of psychedelic experience, have developed a mechanical device to induce altered states of consciousness. Essentially a suspended platform that responds to the slightest movement, the device is claimed to induce a trance state rapidly in most subjects. With proper set and setting, individuals report imagery and similar experiences. Once again, the relevant point is that when investigators take a serious interest in the elicitation of experiences, participants, especially when selected for their interest and sensitivities, may report significant religious experiences.

ᐋ

Research Box 9.8. Sensory Isolation and the Elicitation of Imagery
(Hood & Morris, 1981b)

Hood and Morris utilized an isolation tank to provide a setting in which the elicitation of imagery could be facilitated. The isolation tank was 7.5 feet long, 4 feet high, and 4 feet wide. The tank contained a hydrated magnesium sulfate solution with a density of 1.30 grams/cc with a depth of 10 inches, and a temperature of 34.1°C (approximate external body temperature). Participants were totally enclosed in the tank, which was also soundproofed and lightproofed. The tank itself was in a small soundproofed room. Participants were nude in the tank and floated there for 1 hour.

continued

Research Box 9.8. *continued*

A person can expect a variety of imagery phenomena under isolation conditions, including geometric forms, light, and images of meaningful figures. As part of the appropriate ethical concerns in doing such research, participants were forewarned to anticipate such experiences. However, participants were also instructed to try to control their images.

In a double-blind procedure, half the participants were instructed to try to imagine religious figures, situations, and settings, while the other half were instructed to try to imagine cartoon figures, situations, and settings. Thus the researchers attempted to encourage specific imagery among religious types, for whom such imagery should be relevant. Furthermore, it was predicted that intrinsically religious persons would report more religious imagery, based upon the assumption that their participation in religion is more devoutly experientially based than that of extrinsically religious persons. Twenty intrinsically and 20 extrinsically religious participants had been selected for their extreme scores on either the Intrinsic or Extrinsic religious orientation scale.[a] Results of this study are presented in the table below.

Reported imagery	Set condition	Religious type			
		Intrinsic		Extrinsic	
		Mean	SD	Mean	SD
Religious figures	Cartoon	2.10	0.86	1.10	0.32
	Religious	3.10	0.74	1.90	0.74
Cartoon figures	Cartoon	2.30	0.95	2.50	1.27
	Religious	1.30	0.68	1.50	0.71
Meaningful figures	Cartoon	2.30	0.95	2.30	1.06
	Religious	2.00	1.16	2.50	0.97
Geometric forms	Cartoon	2.40	1.08	1.60	0.70
	Religious	2.00	1.05	2.30	0.82
Light	Cartoon	2.30	1.16	2.10	0.88
	Religious	2.10	0.74	2.90	0.57

Note. From Hood and Morris (1981b, p. 267). Copyright 1981 by the Society to the Scientific Study of Religion. Reprinted by permission.

Statistical analyses of these data revealed that there was no overall tendency for either religious group to report more imagery when the images were those well documented to occur under isolation conditions (e.g., geometric forms, meaningful figures, light). However, under the set conditions, intrinsically religious persons reported more cued religious imagery than extrinsically religious persons did, while the groups did not differ in cartoon imagery. Thus the report of more religious imagery under cued conditions was not a function of the intrinsic participants' greater tendency to report imagery. Indeed, the intrinsic participants even reported more religious imagery under the cartoon cue than extrinsic participants reported religious imagery under the religious cue. That these results were are not simply functions of demand characteristics (with intrinsic participants more sensitive to reporting more religious imagery when cued) is supported by additional work in which intrinsic participants did not report more religiously relevant imagery than extrinsic participants when asked to give religious responses to Rorschach cards.

[a]The intrinsic participant group had an Intrinsic scale mean of 38.9 (*SD* = 4.01) and an Extrinsic scale mean of 26.4 (*SD* = 5.12). The extrinsic participant group had an Extrinsic scale mean of 35.4 (*SD* = 3.93) and an Intrinsic scale mean of 20.9 (*SD* = 4.22). The Allport and Ross (1967) scales were used.

In a similar vein, Goodman (1990) claims to have discovered 30 specific body postures that can reliably elicit altered states of consciousness. These postures are derived from ancient cave drawings as well as from anthropological research. Unique in Goodman's research is her claim that these specific body postures elicit states of consciousness in which perceptions of an expanded reality are accessible. Although her thesis is controversial, it is clearly empirically testable. Again, the issue is that sympathetic researchers are taking seriously not simply the induction of altered states of consciousness, but the ontological reality of what is revealed in the experience. In this sense, the psychology of religion is forced to confront spiritual claims as it explores the reports of individuals whose experience may have evidential force.

Prayer and Religious Imagery

One of the earliest topics in psychology, and one that continues to occupy the interests of psychologists of religion, is the efficacy of prayer. However, it is only recently that psychologists have become interested in empirical (much less experimental) studies of prayer, which Heiler (1932) argued to be central to religion. Since there are few firm data on which to base a theory of prayer, it is not surprising for Janssen, de Hart, and den Draakk (1990) to note that "no convincing psychological theory [of prayer] exists."

Part of the problem is that instead of focusing upon the content and phenomenology of prayer, researchers have focused upon its correlates. Galton (1869), one of the earliest measurement psychologists, argued persuasively on the basis of statistical analysis that prayer has no demonstrable objective benefits However, he argued just as persuasively for the beneficial effects of prayer on subjective well-being. The shift to a focus upon subjective well-being in prayer research has been helpful for the study of religious experience in two senses. First, subjective well-being involves experience—how one feels or reacts to situations as a function of prayer. Second, few religionists or scientists would find a test derived from a subject's own wishes to be very meaningful, and thus there has been a shift away from study of the mere efficacy of prayer in objective terms. The scientists find such studies deficient because people obviously cannot wish the world to conform to their desires in any efficacious sense, and few researchers would bother to think futher empirical tests of such hypotheses worthwhile. The religionists find such theorizing inadequate because mature faith in virtually every tradition is likely to be seen as shifting from requesting that a person's own will be done to asking that the divine will be done. In the latter case, apparently unanswered prayers (outcomes not corresponding to those requested) can be successfully interpreted as meaningful in terms of a more mature reflection upon the nature of faith, as emphasized by Godin (1968, 1985).

Poloma and her colleagues have made significant contributions to the contemporary empirical study of prayer (Poloma & Gallup, 1991; Poloma & Pendleton, 1989). Not only have they reliably measured several types of prayer (colloquial, meditative, petitionary, and ritualistic), but they have focused upon the more psychologically meaningful measures of (1) experiences during prayer and (2) subjective consequences of prayer. Thus much of Poloma et al.'s work is in the quality-of-life tradition, which meaningfully assesses the subjective aspects of human experience (Poloma & Pendleton, 1991).

"Quality of life" is a multidimensional construct that includes existential well-being, happiness, life satisfaction, religious satisfaction, and negative affect (reverse-scored). Prayer is also multidimensional, with various types of prayer differentially relating to experienced quality of life. For instance, meditative prayer is most closely related to religious satisfaction and existential well-being. On the other hand, only colloquial prayer predicts the absence of negative affect, whereas ritual prayer alone predicts negative affect (Poloma & Pendleton, 1989). Thus not simply frequency of prayer, but the nature and type of prayer, determine the experiential consequences of prayer.

Another contribution of Poloma and her colleagues is to focus upon the measurement of actual experiences during prayer. Poloma's prayer index is presented in Table 9.8. This index consistently correlates with quality of life, regardless of the objective status of those who pray. Thus in the specific case of variables used in religion, assessing objective outcomes may be less relevant than assessing subjective ones, as others have noted (Brown, 1966, 1994). Specifically, in research on prayer, Brown (1966, 1968) has noted that the belief in the objective efficacy of even petitionary prayer decreases with age and spiritual maturity.

This turn away from attempting to document the physical consequences of prayer makes work such as Loehr's (1959) on the efficacy of prayer on plant growth less worthy of critical methodological commentary than irrelevant. It is simply the wrong kind of issue to address. If the focus is upon the change in intentionality, consciousness, or affect of those who pray, then the focus of prayer is rightly on its subjective quality.

In this regard, both Poloma and her colleagues, and Hood and his, have derived remarkably similar factors in their multidimensional approach to the measurement of prayer. Table 9.9 presents their similar factor structures, which are remarkable for their independent derivation—one by a team of sociologists, the other by a team of psychologists. Furthermore, the high reliability of all scales suggests the robust nature of the multidimensional criteria of prayer that Poloma's and Hood's groups have both identified.

Both Poloma's and Hood's groups have noted that "contemplative" (Hood's term) or "meditative" (Poloma's term) praying—a nonpetitionary attempt merely to become aware of God—leads to unique experiences. For instance, Poloma and Pendleton (1989, p. 43) note that with the exception of life satisfaction, each of their quality-of-life measures relates to only one type of prayer. Consistent with our focus on subjective experience, meditative prayer relates most closely to an existential quality of life. Similarly, Hood and his colleagues found that contemplative (Poloma's meditative) prayer related most strongly to measures of mystical awareness (a feeling of unity), religiously interpreted for intrinsically religious individuals who prayed (Hood, Morris, & Watson, 1989). On the other hand, extrinsically religious individuals who prayed had disruptions of both religious and nonreligious imagery during

---

TABLE 9.8. Poloma's Index of Prayer Experience

1. How often during the past year have you felt divinely inspired or "led by God" to perform something specific as a result of prayer?
2. How often have you received what you believed to be a deeper insight into a spiritual or Biblical truth?
3. How often have you received what you regarded as a definitive answer to a specific prayer request?
4. How often have you felt a strong sense of God during prayer?
5. How often have you experienced a deep sense of peace and well-being during prayer?.

Answer options: ____once or twice, ____monthly, ____weekly, ____daily.

Note. Adapted from Poloma and Pendleton (1989, p. 53). Copyright 1989 by the Religious Research Association. Adapted by permission.

TABLE 9.9. Poloma's and Hood's Prayer Factors Compared

Poloma's four factors[a]	Hood's four factors[b]
Meditative (alpha = .81)	Contemplative (alpha = .82)
How often do you spend time just "feeling" or being in the presence of God?	When you pray or meditate, how often do you seek to be one with God or ultimate reality?
How often do you spend time worshipping or adoring God?	When you pray or meditate, how often do you seek a perfect harmony?
Ritualistic (alpha = .59)	Liturgical (alpha = .81)
How often do you read from a book of prayers?	When you pray or meditate, how often do you recite sacred phrases or words?
How often do you recite prayers that you have memorized?	When you pray or meditate, how often do you read from sacred texts?
Petitionary (alpha = .78)	Petitionary (alpha = .90)
How often do you ask God for material things you might need?	When you pray or meditate, how often do you seek blessings for others?
How often do you ask God for material things your friends or relatives may need?	When you pray or meditate, how often do you seek forgiveness for yourself?
Colloquial (alpha = .85)	Material (alpha = .65)
How often do you ask God to provide guidance in making decisions?	When you pray or meditate, how often do you seek material things for yourself?
How often do you talk with God in your own words?	When you pray or meditate, how often do you seek material things for others?

[a]Adapted from Poloma and Pendleton (1989, p. 48). Copyright 1989 by the Religious Research Association. Adapted by permission.

[b]Adapted from Hood, Morris, and Harvey (1993). Adapted by permission of the authors.

contemplative prayer—suggesting the inability to quiet the mind and eliminate images. Furthermore, they did not experience a sense of unity, as intrinsic participants did. Thus it may be that different interpretations of experience reflect actual differences during experience, as well as differences in the types of prayer intrinsically and extrinsically religious persons engage in.

Although more research is clearly needed, it is readily apparent that the shift away from the study of the efficacy of petitionary prayer is a step in the right direction. Brown (1994, pp. 45–46) has argued that if one restricts prayer to the narrow view of merely "asking for things," than prayer is perhaps more characteristic of unbelievers. Faber (2002) argues that a naturalistic understanding of prayer links it to magical behavior as understood in contemporary anthropology. Measurement-based research has clearly established the multidimensionality of prayer, and future research will undoubtedly contribute to a deeper understanding of the subjective experience of prayer. Although the empirical study of prayer is an established part of the psychology of religion (Francis & Astley, 2001), no generally agreed-upon theory of prayer has emerged. In this sense, theories such as Sundén's role theory will become more relevant, as knowledge of traditions and texts is required to illuminate the meaningfulness of prayer within the communities of those who pray. Research Box 9.9 reports one of the few empirical studies of the needs stated for prayer, the content of prayer, and its effects.

ENTHEOGENS AND RELIGIOUS EXPERIENCE

It has long been recognized that many religions have employed various naturally occurring and synthetic substances in their religious rituals. However, until the discovery of psychedelic drugs, it was rather arrogantly assumed that concern with the facilitation of experience by drugs was the domain of anthropology and sister disciplines concerned with less "advanced" religions. In a new and controversial discipline with the cumbersome name "archeopsychopharmacology," researchers combine ancient texts and artifacts with contem-

---

Research Box 9.9. A Content Analysis of the Praying Practices of Dutch Youths (Janssen, de Hart, & den Draak, 1990)

In 1985, a sample of 192 Dutch high school students was asked to respond to three openended questions regarding prayer: (1) "What is praying to you?", (2) "At what moments do you feel the need to pray?", and (3) "How do you pray?" Using a computer technique to analyze the content of the response to these three questions, Janssen and colleagues were able to summarize prayer structure according to the following sentence: "Because of some reason, I address myself to someone in a particular way, at a particular place, at a particular time, to achieve something." They diagrammed this sentence as follows:

	2. Action (predicate)	
	3. Direction (indirect object)	
	4. Time (adverbial adjunct 1)	
1. Need (conditional adjunct)	5. Place (adverbial adjunct 2)	7. Effect (direct object)
	6. Method (adverbial adjunct 3)	

The percentages of content references to each structural category for the four most frequent citations within that category were as follows[a]:

1. *Need (83%)*: personal problems (60%); sickness (23%); happiness (20%); death (16%).
2. *Action (83%)*: talk/monologue (38%); talk/dialogue (36%); ask/wish (33%); meditate (22%).
3. *Direction (60%)*: God/Lord (80%); Spirit/Power (13%); Someone (11%); Mary/Jesus (2%).
4. *Time (20%)*: evening/night (90%); day (8%); dinner (8%); anytime (5%).
5. *Place (34%)*: bed (86%); home (11%); church (11%); outside (9%).
6. *Method (55%)*: alone (55%); prayer, formal (17%); low voice (19%); aloud (4%).
7. *Effect (37%)*: help/support (38%); favor (34%); remission (13%); rest (10%).

[a]Percentages for the seven structural aspects are based upon $n = 192$. Percentages for content within each structure are based upon the number of participants who reported that structural aspect. See the Janssen et al. paper, p. 102, Table 1.

porary cross-cultural studies of the use of naturally occurring psychedelic substances to speculate on the origins of religions. For example, Allegro (1971) contends that the origin of the Judeo-Christian tradition may have been heavily influenced by altered states facilitated by the use of naturally occurring psychedelic substances, such as the mushroom *Amanita muscaria*. So influenced, too, Wasson (1969) argues, was the sacred *Soma* of the ancient Indian text *Rig Vedat* by the use of a mushroom with psychedelic properties, the fly agaric. Indeed, Kramrisch, Otto, Ruck, and Wasson (1986) argue that all religions originated from the use of psychedelic mushrooms. Finally, Wasson, Hofmann, and Ruck (1978) have argued that an ergot similar to LSD was integral to the Eleusinian mystery cults of ancient Greece, and from there influenced Western philosophy. Although the widely speculative theories of archeopsychopharmacology cannot be empirically confirmed, they have raised a crucial question at the center of the social-scientific study of religion and the more general study of psychedelic drugs: Can psychedelic drugs facilitate or produce religious experiences? Those who argue the case most persuasively prefer the term "entheogens" to describe plants or chemical substances that facilitate primary religious experiences (Forte, 1997). It is the term we currently prefer, especially as we focus upon the facilitation of religious experience by means of chemical substances.

The literature on the psychology of entheogens is immense, easily running to several thousand studies. Much of the U.S. research has been stopped by legislation against these drugs, so that Rätsch (1990, p. 2) has concluded: "Since the beginning of the 1970s, there has been little new research into psychedelic substances." While Rätsch's claim must be qualified—given both the significant current research by anthropologists and ethnobotanists with naturally occurring plants around the world, and the study of entheogens in European countries (where laws are more flexible)—the measurement-based empirical study of entheogens has clearly been drastically curtailed by U.S. drug laws. However, there nevertheless remains an extensive body of research on psychedelic drugs (Lukoff, Zanger, & Lu, 1990). Selective reviews are readily available, including the general overall review by Aarson and Osmond (1970), Dobkin de Rios's (1984) cross-cultural survey, and Barber's (1970) methodological review. Masters and Houston's (1966) review focuses upon the varieties of psychedelic experience, while Lukoff et al. (1990) focus upon religious and transpersonal states facilitated by psychedelic drugs. Finally, Roberts and Hruby (1995) have produced a useful bibliographic guide to entheogens.

Curiously, very few studies to date have used religious variables for directly assessing the religious importance of entheogens, despite a vast, often contentious conceptual literature on chemical substances and religion. Although the archeopsychopharmacological speculations of Wasson and his colleagues may be extreme, their basic assumption has been common within both psychological and religious studies. It has long been noted that there is an obvious similarity between various religious experiences and drug-induced experiences. Before the turn of the 20th century, in fact, Leuba (1896) argued that religious experiences in advanced traditions must be invalidated, because of their similarity to drug-induced states in less advanced traditions. The essentials of Leuba's argument have been more recently advanced by Zaehner (1972), who argues that because an experience is drug-induced, it cannot be genuinely religious. These largely conceptually based debates do little to advance a scientific understanding of the possible religious importance of entheogens. One can no more invalidate an experience because its physiology is known than one can invalidate physiology because its biochemistry has been identified. As Weil (1986) has emphasized, the similarity of psychedelic substances found within plants, animals, and the human brain suggest that any simple distinction between natural and artificially induced states is arbitrary.

Our concern is with the religious significance of chemical substances. In particular, we focus upon the question of whether or not some chemicals can induce or be used to facilitate a religious experience. We include as "entheogens" such drugs as LSD, mescaline, and psilocybin, since in both scientific studies and street use, reports indicate similar psychological experiences from these drugs (Aarson & Osmond, 1970; Stevens, 1987; Wells & Triplett, 1992). However, as Brown (1972) cautions, drugs that produce similar psychological effects need not have identical biochemical properties.

The term "psychedelic," the most common precusor to "entheogen," has a controversial history (Stevens, 1987). Debates over the common name for the class of drugs we are discussing have produced a range from "hallucinogenic" to "psychotomimetic" to "psychedelic" to "entheogen." "Hallucinogenic" is the most inadequate term, since hallucination is one of the *least* common response to psychedelic drugs (Barber, 1970). Although these drugs do produce various visual and imagery effects, whether users' eyes are open or closed, they do not produce perceptions that have no external stimulus (hallucinations). "Psychotomimetic" was the term favored by early researchers who thought that this class of drugs produces psychoses or psychotic-like states. Given the cultural evaluation of psychoses, the negative connotations of "psychotomimetic" are obvious; however, it is well established that the ability of psychedelics to elicit sudden psychoses in otherwise normal persons is highly exaggerated (Barr, Langs, Holt, Goldberger & Klein, 1972). "Psychedelic" was the term most favored by those who favored the "mind-manifesting" aspect of these drugs. It is the most common term today, despite its positive connotations among participants in the 1960s deviant drug culture and its still-current association with the illicit street drug culture (Stevens, 1987). As noted above, those who prefer to focus upon the religious significance of these plants and chemical substances prefer the term "entheogens."

For well-established physiological reasons, entheogens can be expected to produce reliable alterations in visual and other imagery, which to informed and stable participants are likely to be interesting objects of conscious exploration (Durr, 1970; Strassman, 2001). Meaningful images that occur under the influence of these substances, with the user's eyes closed, are not typically attributed to the object expected to exist in the world (in the sense that if the user were to open his or her eyes, the object would be in physical reality). Likewise, when the user's eyes are open, alterations in perception of objects are noted as perceptual alterations of existing objects, not changes in the actual physical objects or the perception of objects that in fact are not real. However, the user's ability to interpret perceptions in terms of a meaningful frame can transform his or her perception of the world. In Sundén's theory, a religious frame should enhance the power of entheogens to facilitate religious experiences. With an appropriate religious set and setting, entheogens can facilitate religious experiences, insofar as one under the influence of these substances may for the first time see the world in terms appropriate to a particular system of meaning. In this sense, the "other-worldly" property of entheogens is well established and provides their obvious link to religion. Religious beliefs often assert realities and possibilities of experience that are quite foreign to everyday secular experience. In addition, as noted in Chapter 12, religions often encourage such experiences in believers (or, at a minimum, urge believers to respect these experiences in others).

Masters and Houston (1966) found that under the influence of entheogens, religious imagery was quite common, even when many participants did not identify themselves as having a "religious" drug experience. For instance, religious architecture was one of the most common images reported, but Masters and Houston (1966) claim that this was more a sense of aesthetic appreciation than a genuine religious interest. Still, the commonality of religious imagery in their sample of 206 subjects is impressive. These data are presented in Table 9.10.

The frequent report of religious imagery is likely to be a function of set and setting, long known to be major determinants of the content of imagery elicited by entheogens (Barr et al., 1972; Barber, 1970). In light of Sundén's role theory, we would expect that if given the appropriate familiarity with religious frames, many substance-facilitated experiences would be experienced as religious. It would be naive to claim that religious experiences are substance-specific effects. Rather, the power of entheogens to facilitate religious experience lies in the extent to which states of consciousness, altered by chemical substances, are seen as relevant in religious terms. Within U.S. culture, the ironic fact is that mainstream religions sends mixed signals relative to religious experience—often encouraging and validating experiences when interpreted as originating in God, but discouraging and invalidating experiences that are known to be chemically facilitated. The fact that many participants in studies using entheogens experience religious imagery and use religious language to describe otherwise secular imagery (e.g., cosmological events) is difficult to assess. Masters and Houston (1966) noted that the use of sacramental or religious metaphors was a common practice for their participants, even though genuine religious experiences may have been rare. Here the problem is how to judge the genuineness of any experience; obviously verbal reports of religious imagery and religious language are, even in Sundén's theory, necessary but not sufficient criteria for religious experience.

Grof (1980) has argued that the therapeutic use of entheogens often provides a set and setting that encourage the report of religious and transpersonal experiences. Many of these experiences are interpreted in terms of Jungian theory, which is particularly favorable to describing religious imagery. Thus would expect religious imagery in LSD psychotherapy sessions to be common and to increase if the set and setting are made even more explicitly religious—for instance, by having religious symbols in the therapeutic room. Leary (1964)

TABLE 9.10. Spontaneous Religious Imagery Elicited by Entheogens

Imagery	%
Overall religious imagery of some kind (*n* = 206)	96
Specific religious imagery	
Architecture, such as temples, churches	91
Sculpture, paintings, stained-glass windows	43
Symbols, such as cross, yin and yang, Star of David	34
Mandalas	26
Persons, such as Christ, Buddha, and saints	58
Devils and demons	49
Angels	7
Abstract imagery interpreted religiously	
Numinous visions, such as pillars of light, God in the whirlwind	60
Cosmological imagery, such as heavily bodies, galaxies	14
Religious rituals	
Christian, Jewish, and Muslim rites	8
Oriental rites	10
Ancient rites (such as Greek, Egyptian, Mesopotamian)	67
Primitive rites	31

Note. Adapted from Masters and Houston (1966, p. 265). Copyright 1966 by Robert Masters and Jean Houston Masters. Adapted by permission.

compared the reported LSD experiences of clients of two different therapists—one who used an explicitly religious context for therapy, and one who did not. These data are presented in Table 9.11. Inspection of this table indicates that the evaluation of the LSD experience as the greatest personal experience was a function of religious context; in addition, whether an experience was interpreted as religious or not was clearly affected by the religious context of the therapy. Although these results confound possible differences in therapists with set/setting differences, if we assume that therapists in religious contexts are global contextual factors, having a religious context clearly facilities a religious experience. Research Box 9.10 presents a study in which autobiographical accounts of various experiences, including hallucinogenic drug experiences, were shown to differ reliably in the way they were described.

Although the hostility of mainstream religion to the use of entheogens is well documented, the irony is that entheogens have relevance to the range of experiences typically called "religious." It is a mistake not to acknowledge the possibility that chemically facilitated states of consciousness may have ontological validity. Indeed, identifying them as religious both contextualizes them and gives them such validity. However, the mere elicitation of a single experience, however "religious," probably lacks sustained life-transforming power if it is not contextualized within some tradition. Roszack (1975, p. 50; emphasis in original) has argued that the focus upon specific behaviors or experiences elicited as "religious" can be distorting:

> The temptation, then, is to believe that the behavior which has thus been objectively verified is what religious experience is *really* all about, and—further—that it can be appropriated as an end in itself, plucked like a rare flower from the soil that feeds it. The result is a narrow emphasis on special effects and sensations: "peak experiences," "highs," "flashes" and such. Yet even if one wishes to regard ecstasy as the "peak" of religious experience, that summit does not float in midair. It rests upon tradition and a way of life; one ascends such heights and appreciates their grandeur by a process of initiation that demands learning, commitment, devotion, service, sacrifice. To approach it in any hasty way is like "scaling" Mount Everest by being landed on its top from a helicopter.

Stevens (1987) has documented the history of the original "psychedelic movement" and its failure to have mind-altering substances accepted for sacramental use within a religious frame. In this sense, the "psychedelic movement" must be judged in terms of the cultic and sectarian movements discussed in Chapter 12. However, exceptions include some Native

TABLE 9.11. LSD Therapy Experience as a Function of Religious Set/Setting

	Percentage of clients saying yes	
	Therapist A, using no religious context ($n = 74$)	Therapist B, using religious context ($n = 96$)
Felt LSD was greatest personal experience	49	85
Felt LSD was a religious experience	32	83
Felt a greater awareness of God, higher power, or ultimate reality	40	90

Note. Data from Leary (1964, p. 327).

❧

Research Box 9.10. The Language of Altered States
(Oxman, Rosenberg, Schnurr, Tucker, & Gala, 1988)

Oxman and his colleagues collected 94 autobiographical accounts of personal experiences. The texts were divided into four categories: schizophrenic experiences; drug-induced hallucinogenic experiences; mystical/ecstatic experiences; and autobiographical controls (identified as personally important experiences). The texts were coded into 83 lexical categories by means of standardized computer programs.[a] The four groups were significantly different in word frequencies in 49 of the 83 lexical categories. Using lexical content to classify the three altered states of consciousness and the control experiences indicated that the altered states of consciousness were more different from one another than similar. Schizophrenic experiences were characterized by an abnormal illness experience associated with a negative self-evaluation. Drug-induced hallucinogenic experiences were characterized by positively aesthetically experienced visual and auditory phenomena. Mystical/ecstatic experiences were characterized by life-altering encounters with God, associated with a sense of power and certitude. When discriminant functional analysis was employed, 84% of the experiences could be correctly identified by their word frequencies. The authors assumed that the actual experiences were different, given that different words were used to describe the experiences.

[a]These were the General Inquirer Computer Content Analysis Program and the Harvard-111 Psychosociological Dictionary (see Stone, Dunphy, Smith, & Ogilvie, 1966).

American religions, whose long history of sacramental use of peyote demonstrates that entheogens can be incorporated into religious frameworks and used to facilitate experiences whose meaning is truly religious (Bergman, 1971; LaBarre, 1969).

The cultural bias against entheogens has not only affected serious study of these chemicals, but has made it difficult to take a balanced view of the range of their effects (Forte, 1997; Walsh, 1982). Furthermore, several reviewers have argued that typical double-blind studies are particularly inappropriate ways to investigate entheogens, especially since participants who are assigned to the control conditions are likely to be immediately aware of this fact (Bakalar & Grinspoon, 1989; Yensen, 1990). Many researchers have supported the view that ingestion of psychedelic substances on the part of researchers is a valid (and, some claim, necessary) method of study. Such self-involvement has plagued the history of the "psychedelic movement" in the United States and promises to fuel future controversies in which research on entheogens and religion takes on many of the characteristics of religious movements, as discussed in Chapter 12.

OVERVIEW

Religious experience is as varied as the interpretations individuals can bring to their lives. It is less relevant to seek the common elements of religious experiences than to find higher-order abstractions for identifying a class of varied phenomena. The James–Boisen formula that religious experience is a successful resolution of discontent is basic to most faith traditions. However, few studies have placed religious experience within a context to determine its functionality over time. The particulars of discontents and resolutions are provided by Sundén's role theory, which not only allows tradition, text, and practice to model appropriate perceptions and interpretations that facilitate religious experiences within a faith tradition, but permits longitudinal studies needed for true tests of the James–Boisen formula.

Common religious practices, such as prayer and meditation, have been studied in terms of the physiological correlates and subjective contents of these experiences. Speculations as to the neurophysiology of dramatic religious experiences, such as glossolalia and hallucinations, demand additional empirical investigation. Dynamic theories illuminating processes involved in determining the content of hallucinations have been tested and promise to foster both controversy and additional research.

Imagery has returned as a focus of study, with new psychological orientations offering interpretations of imagery that are sympathetic to faith traditions concerned with their reality. Entheogens remain of interest, despite legal impediments in the United States to research. The fact that religious imagery can be facilitated by entheogens, in the appropriate set and setting, assures the continued relevance for the psychology of religion of techniques to alter states of consciousness.

Chapter 10

MYSTICISM

In Hinduism, in Neoplatonism, in Sufism, in Christian mysticism, in Whitmanism, we find the same recurring note, so that there is about mystical utterances an eternal unanimity which ought to make a critic stop and think and which brings it about that the mystical classics have, as has been said, neither birthday nor native land.

How can an individual human claim union with God without compromising divine transcendence and elevating the creature beyond its proper status? Are not claims to union inherently blasphemous?

According to our yogic traditions, *samadhi* means complete awareness of God, or to put it in less religious terms, *samadhi* means that your mind and the mind of the universe are, for a time, merged in an absolute ecstatic union.

The fascination of the subject of mysticism is not, I suggest, simply a fascination with some intense psychological experiences for their own sake, but rather because the answers to each of these questions are also ways of defining or delimiting authority.

The breadth and intensity of the interest in mysticism during the last half of the twentieth century have given rise to many different interpretations of mysticism and many conflicting theories about it.

This problem of the secularized interpretation of amorphous mystical experiences has been raised repeatedly since the Enlightenment.[1]

The focus upon mysticism in this chapter highlights the central role that mystical experience has occupied in conceptual discussions of religion for the last century. The claims of mystics dominate contemporary discussions concerned with the evidential value of religious experience. "Evidential force" and "evidential value" are the phrases most linked to debates as to whether or not religious experiences such as mysticism provide sufficient grounds for asserting the truth of various religious beliefs (Clark, 1984; Davis, 1989; Swinburne, 1981). For some, mystical experience cannot support a belief that one has united with God or experienced ultimate reality. For others, mysticism is an experience that provides sufficient warrant for belief in God or ultimate reality; for these latter individuals, mystical experience has evidential force. As Katz (1977) notes, those who assert the evidential force of mystical

---

1. These quotations came, respectively, from the following sources: James (1902/1985, p. 324); McGinn (1989, p. vii); Lenz (1995, p. 215); Jantzen (1995, p. 1); Ruffing (2001, p. 1); and Scholem (1969, p. 16).

experience provide an ecumenical umbrella under which diverse religious claims can be sheltered as simply different expressions of one fundamental truth. This avoids the embarrassing particulars of religious experiences, which, like the particulars of religious belief expressed in dogmatic terms, tend to separate one faith from another (Schuon, 1975). Although as social scientists we need not address theological or philosophical debates directly, our methods and analyses cannot avoid philosophical and religious implications. As Jones (1994) has noted, science and religion are not identical, but neither can they be categorically separated or viewed as mutually exclusive orientations. Our confrontation with the conceptual issues debated by both philosophers and theologians will give us a framework to organize and guide our review of the empirical research. It will also (we hope) overcome the lack of conversation among the various disciplines that study mysticism, which, in McGinn's (1991, p. 343) words, have been "equally at fault in this unrealized conversation."

CONCEPTUAL ISSUES IN THE STUDY OF MYSTICISM

The theological and philosophical literature on mysticism is extensive (see McGinn, 1991). Our concern as social scientists is restricted to the aspects of these literatures that have direct relevance for empirical research. Of immediate concern is the clarification of the nature of mystical experience, as well as of its relationships to other forms of religious experience.

Thorner (1966), following the work of the philosopher Kaufmann (1958), contrasts mystical and prophetic experiences. Thorner first notes that persons having any religious experience believe three things: (1) Their experience is different from everyday, normal experience; (2) the experience is more important than everyday experiences; and (3) the perceptual referents are not simply to be found in the discrete aspects of the empirical world. These claims are consistent with our analysis of the wide variety of religious experiences discussed in Chapter 9. However, the third point raises serious problems. How are social scientists to respond to a claim that refuses to locate the perceptual referents of experience in discrete aspects of the empirical world? Within the conceptual literature on religion, scholars have focused upon numinous and mystical experiences as the most likely candidates for revealing a transcendent dimension to human experience. Social scientists have concurred, noting that the numinous and the mystical are empirically the most common claims of those who assert they have experienced a transcendent reality, however conceived. Social scientists differ widely in their own claims to have identified the true perceptual referents in such experiences. However, most also share the belief that the true perceptual referents need not include reference to God or an ultimate reality, and hence they attempt to explain the transcendent in purely scientific terms. Religionists tend to perceive such explanations as reductionistic.

Accordinig to Thorner (1966), what mystics claim is that the perceptual referent in religious experience is a unity within the world. This unity is not linked to any one perceptual object; instead, all objects are unified into a perception of totality or oneness. However, the mystical experience of a unity within the world emphasized by Thorner is only one form of mysticism. Following Stace (1960), we refer to this as "extrovertive mysticism." We contrast extrovertive mysticism with another form of mysticism, "introvertive mysticism." This is an experience of unity devoid of perceptual objects; it is literally an experience of "no-thing-ness." Perceptual objects disappear, and a pure consciousness devoid of content is reported. Forman (1990a) has referred to this as "pure conscious experience." What is important for now is that only extrovertive mysticism has as its perceptual referent a unity that transcends individual, discrete objects of perception. There are discrete objects of perception, but they are all seen unified in their particularity as nevertheless one. The unity in extrovertive mysticism is with the totality of objects of perception; the unity in introvertive mysticism is with a pure consciousness, devoid of objects of perception. Stace (1960, p. 131) has suggested that extrovertive mysticism is a less developed form, perhaps preparatory to introvertive mysticism. Forman (1990) argues that extrovertive mysticism is a higher form of mysticism to which introvertive mysticism is only preparatory. Hood (1989) has argued that extrovertive mysticism is likely to follow upon introvertive mystical experience, but he does not claim it to be a "higher" experience. The conceptual arguments as to whether these are two separate mysticisms has important consequences for empirical research. As we shall see, if introvertive and extrovertive mysticism can be measured, the relationship between the two can be studied as an empirical issue. Yet, whether the experience of unity is introvertive or extrovertive, it is this experience that by scholarly consensus uniquely characterizes mysticism (Hood, 1985).

Many scholars have contrasted "prophetic" or "numinous" experience with "mystical" experience. A numinous experience is an awareness of a "holy other" beyond nature, with which one is felt to be in communion. More typically, this experience is identified with the classic work of Otto (1917/1958), whose phenomenological analysis illuminates the human response to the transcendent. For Otto, the essential fact of religious experience includes a nonrational component that is psychologically characterized by a numinous consciousness. The term "numinous" is based upon the Latin term *numen*, denoting a power implicit in a sacred object. It is the object that elicits a response from the subject. Thus religion, as Hick (1989) has also argued, is a response to the transcendent. Social scientists can study this response, noting that from the believer's perspective it is a response to a transcendent object experienced as real. Numinous experiences identify a personal transcendent object, often referred to as God or Allah or Yahweh. Obviously, religious traditions assert the reality of this object, refusing to identify it merely with empirical realities described by the scientist.

Hood (1995a) refers to the transcendent object as the "foundational reality" of a faith tradition. The numinous consciousness is compelled both to seek out and explore this transcendent object (*mysterium fascinans*), and to be repelled in the face of the majesty and awfulness of this object in whose presence one's "creatureness" is accentuated (*mysterium tremendum*). Efforts to rationally confront the feelings of *tremendum* are articulated in personal conceptualizations of a holy other, such as God or Allah or Yahweh. The *fascinans* is explicated in rational concepts such as grace, in which the inadequacy of personal analogies to conceptualize the holy other are revealed. The *fascinans* thus has a mystical element, insofar as the personal analogue revealed in the *tremendum* is found to be inadequate and an impersonal language is sought to describe it. Not surprisingly, Stace's categories of "introvertive mysticism" and "extrovertive mysticism" are derived from Otto's (1932) "mysticism of introspection" and "unifying vision," respectively. Thus, although it is possible to separate the numinous and the mystical as two poles of religious experience, they are ultimately united. Mystical experiences of unity (variously expressed) can be numinous as well, eliciting the *mysterium fascinans* when the object is experienced in impersonal terms and the *mysterium tremendum* when the object is experienced in personal terms. Hick (1989) has articulated this duality as the *personae* and *impersonae* of "the Real." Hood (1995c) has emphasized that William James accepted both impersonal (the absolute) and personal (God) interpretations as compatible with the facts of mystical experience. As we shall see, empirical studies use measurements that tend to emphasize experiences of either a sense of presence (favoring numinous experiences) or a sense of unity (favoring mystical experiences).

The focus upon the numinous and the mystical as two poles of religion is important, in that it links the empirical studies of mysticism to current theological and philosophical considerations of mysticism. Much as modern physics employs both wave and particle conceptualizations of light, Hick (1989) argues that what he simply refers to as "the Real" can be either personal or impersonal. Similarly, Smart (1964) has argued that although the numinous and the mystical must be carefully conceptually distinguished, they are incorporated into a single unifying doctrine in some religious traditions. Elsewhere, Smart (1978) has noted that "nature mysticism," the extrovertive experience of unity in nature, is in fact a numinous experience. This parallels Stace's (1960) view that extrovertive mystical experiences incorporate an awareness of an inner subjectivity to all that is perceived. Likewise, Stace has emphasized that the category of the holy applies to both introvertive and extrovertive mystical experiences and most probably accounts for their religious quality. Thus we can separate the numinous and the mystical for conceptual purposes, depending upon whether the personal or impersonal aspects of foundational reality are emphasized. Mysticism tends toward the impersonal; the numinous tends toward the personal. As we shall shortly note, measurement studies can identify both numinous and mystical experiences, based upon whether one experiences a sense of presence (numinous experience) or a sense of unity (mystical experience).

For the purposes of this chapter, we refer to mystical experiences as either "mystical experiences proper" when experiences of unity are emphasized, or as "numinous experiences" when a sense of an other's presence are emphasized. That both components are properly mystical has been briefly noted above and extensively argued by Hood (1995a). Their importance is that from a social-psychological perspective, they are part of what religions defend as the experience of the sacred. Empirically, reports of transcendent experiences include the belief in the reality of transcendent objects. It may also be true that the belief in their reality is necessary for the experience to occur. Thus, although social scientists cannot confirm any transcendent realities, they can construct theories compatible with claims to the existence of such realities. Hodges (1974) has argued that the scientific taboo against the supernatural can be broken, as long as hypotheses about the supernatural can be shown to have empirical consequences. In Garrett's (1974) phrase, "troublesome transcendence" must be confronted by social scientists as much as by theologians and philosophers.

There is no reason why scientists cannot include specific hypotheses derived from views about the nature of transcendent reality in empirical studies of religious experience, as long as specific empirical predictions can be made. The source of the predictions may reference even the unobservable and the intangible. All that is required is that there be identifiable empirical consequences. As Jones (1986) has stated the case,

> Invoking Occam's Razor [i.e., the philosophical principle that the best explanation of an event is the simplest one] to disallow reference to factors other than sensory observable ones is question begging in favor of one metaphysics building up an ontology with material objects as basic. (p. 225)

Jones echoes the classic claim of William James that mystics base their experience upon the same sort of processes that all empiricists do—direct experience. James would restrict the authoritative value of mystical experience to the person who had the experience, but value it as a hypothesis for the social scientist to investigate (Hood, 1992a, 1995c). However, mystics are united in the belief that such experiences are real, and many non mystics are convinced of the reality of the experience even if they personally have not had it. Thus, as Swinburne (1981) argues, mystical experience is also authoritative for others:

> . . . if it seems to me I have a glimpse of Nirvana, or a vision of God, that is good grounds for me to suppose that I do. And, more generally, the occurrence of religious experience is prima facie reason for all to believe in that of which the experience was purportedly an experience. (p. 190)

What makes numinous and mystical experiences so important to study is that they are the strongest claims to experience foundational realities. Social scientists are often too quick to boast that their own limited empirical data undermine ontological claims. Whether we use Hick's term "the Real" or Hood's phrase "foundational reality," the point is that religious traditions cannot be adequately understood without the assumption that transcendent objects of experience are believed to be real to those who experience them. It is also possible that not only are they believed to be real, but that they are in fact real as well. Furthermore, their reality may be revealed in experience. Carmody and Carmody (1996, p. 10) define "mysticism" as "a direct experience of ultimate reality." This definition remains a hypothesis capable of empirical investigation. To presuppose otherwise is less persuasive than once thought. Bowker (1973), after critically reviewing social-scientific theories of the sense of God, has noted that it is an empirical option to conclude that at least part of the sense of God might come from God. In our terms, religious views of the nature of the Real suggest ways in which it can be expressed in human experience. This can work in two directions, both deductively and inductively. Deductively, one can note that if the Real is conceived in a particular way, then certain experiences of the real can be expected to follow. Thus we anticipate that expectations play a significant role in religious experience, often confirming the foundational realities of one's faith tradition. Inductively, we can infer that if particular experiences occur, than the possibility that the Real exists is a reasonable inference—a position forcefully argued by Berger (1979). Thus we can anticipate that experiences, some unanticipated, may lead some to seek religions for their illumination. O'Brien (1965) has gone so far as to include in his criteria for a mystical experience that it be unexpected. Religious traditions adopt both options in confronting mystical and numinous experiences.

Not surprisingly, then, these experiences have long been the focus of empirical research and provocative theorizing among both sociologists and psychologists. We first explore classic efforts to confront these experiences. These classic views are of more than historical interest, as they set the range of conceptual issues that continue to plague the contemporary empirical study of mysticism. Our focus upon classic views is not exhaustive; we focus upon representatives of three major social-scientific views regarding mystical experience. These are as follows:

1. *Mysticism as erroneous attribution.* Mystics attribute to transcendence objects and processes that can in fact be explained in social-scientific terms. These processes have been variously identified as physiological, psychological, or sociological. The mistaken attribution is to assume that something more is involved in such experiences. Most commonly the "more" is believed to be something transcendent, including, in cases of personal mysticism, God, Allah, or Yahweh.

2. *Mysticism as heightened awareness.* Mysticism is an awareness of ultimate reality that occurs with heightened or altered awareness. This awareness may be cultivated or occur spon-

taneously. The awareness may be variously interpreted, or the interpretations may reflect different reality claims. Although social-scientific and physiological processes can be identified that permit the experience of transcendence to occur, they need not deny genuine ontological status to the object of transcendence. In simple terms, both the mystical experience and its object are real in the terms of which they are experienced.

3. *Mysticism as evolved consciousness.* Mysticism is an evolved form of consciousness. It is variously interpreted to be a capacity potentially common to all humans (only some of whom actualize it), or to be a capacity that only some humans now possess. Typically, this form of consciousness is interpreted in purely natural-scientific terms. The transcendent is merely a naturally evolved form of consciousness.

REPRESENTATIVE CLASSICAL VIEWS OF MYSTICISM

Mysticism as Erroneous Attribution

Preus (1987) has emphasized that the classical social-scientific theorists of religion, with only a few exceptions, had little doubt that they could provide genuine reductive explanations of religion. Such explanations purported to replace religious attributions with purely secular claims to processes involved in mystical experience as illuminated by science. Furthermore, it was commonly assumed that once the social sciences illuminated the true nature of religious experience, then religious claims based upon such experiences would lose much of their persuasive force.

The early psychologists of religion could not help confronting mysticism in light of this assumption. The mystical claim to have experienced God could not be uncritically accepted by psychologists. Much of the scientific validity of psychology was seen to rest upon its ability to provide scientific explanations for spiritual and religious claims. Thus, despite the fact that in the popular mind psychology was seen as a spiritual discipline, most psychologists saw the public interest in spiritual matters as a way to help develop the science of psychology, if psychology could explain the spiritual in natural-scientific terms (Coon, 1992; Taves, 1999). In *The Psychology of Religious Mysticism*, Leuba (1925) provided one of the earliest physiological theories of mysticism. Considerably less sympathetic to religion than William James was, Leuba insisted that mystical experience could be explained in physiological terms. He also insisted that no transcendental object is necessary for mystical or numinous experience, and that only physiological processes and a natural-scientific framework can illuminate these experiences. He was one of the first psychologists to argue forcefully that mystical experience provides no evidential force for religious beliefs. Mystics do not encounter God in their experience, Leuba claimed; rather, mystics use their beliefs to interpret their experience, ultimately erroneously. His now-classic study of mysticism was echoed in the general French tradition of the emerging discipline of psychiatry, in which mental states—including many religious ones interpreted by those who experienced them—were understood in terms of their origins in physiological and psychological processes that were often deemed pathological. Charcot, who was part of this French tradition, heavily influenced Freud, whose attitude toward religion was complex but ultimately unsympathetic.

In *The Future of an Illusion* (1927/1961), Freud argued that religious *beliefs* are illusory—the products of wishes, rather than responses to the reality of the world. Later, he responded to a criticism of the Nobel laureate Romain Rolland that he had focused only upon religious belief and had underestimated the value of religious *experience*. Rolland found the essence of religion in what he termed the "oceanic feeling," was a state of unity with the world (mysticism); Rolland claimed validity for this feeling, independent of Freud's devastating challenge to religious beliefs. Freud's response in *Civilization and Its Discontents* (1930/1961) was that this feeling is not originally religious, but only later becomes attached to religious beliefs. The actual "oceanic feeling" is only a recollection of an infantile state, perhaps of unity with the mother. Mysticism is thus a regression to an earlier infantile state. Thus mystical experience does not provide evidence for unity with the world or even with God; it is simply a feeling attached to religious beliefs that God exists and can be experienced. The religious beliefs themselves are not simply illusional, but delusional as well. Religion is thus a double error: an erroneous belief in the existence of a God, and the erroneous interpretation of regressive experiences as evidence of union with God. Thus Freud was one of the first theorists to argue that there is no essential relationship between mystical experience and religious beliefs. Current criticism of Freud's view of mysticism, especially based upon claims that he misunderstood the oceanic feeling of Rolland (Parsons, 1999) and that mystical experience is not inherently regressive (Hood, 1976a), allow for nonpathological views of mysticism even within classical Freudian theory (Hood, 1992b; Parsons, 1999).

Leuba and Freud represent examples of genuine explanations of mysticism, if one assumes that the experience is capable of being reductively explained by either physiological processes (Leuba) or psychological processes (Freud). Basic to both views is that persons who believe they have confronted or merged with transcendent objects are wrong. Similar arguments have been made by sociologists. For instance, Durkheim (1915) argued for mystical experience as the apprehension of individuals' dependence upon a transcendent object; however, that object is society, not a divine being or reality. The genuine experience of being part of a larger unity is correct, but a misattribution applies this to God instead of its real origin, society. Thus any theory that claims to explain experiences of union with the Real by processes that can be identified as purely physiological, psychological, or social must claim to interpret mysticism by misattribution. A corollary is that when individuals realize the true source of their experience of union, the religious quality (in terms of transcendent claims) will disappear.

These classical theories set the tone for modern studies of mysticism. Inherent in their views is that mystical experiences offer no ontological proof for religious belief, and assuredly no proof that one has experienced union with God. Although they may be acted upon as authoritative by those who have them, insofar as they are misattributions, the individual who so acts risks being defined as delusional or pathological (if not simply naïve). The authoritative basis of these experiences for an individual who has them may be susceptible to destructive analyses by experts, in which the experience itself is demonstrated to be due to processes more appropriately identified by social scientists, whether they are physiologists, psychologists, or sociologists.

Mysticism as Heightened Awareness

Although most early social scientists reveled in the apparent power of psychology to explain religion in general and mystical experiences in particular, William James best represented the paradoxical position of the emerging science of psychology. Hood (1992a, 1995c) has traced the efforts of James to avoid religious concepts, such as the soul, in developing psychology as a natural science. In the *The Principles of Psychology* (1890/1950), James saw no need for the concept of a soul or for any transcendent dimension to human consciousness; however, in *The Varieties of Religious Experience* (1902/1985), James noted that the facts of mystical experience require a wider dimension to human consciousness. He favored Myers's (1903/1961) notion of a subconscious, in which James argued that a wider self may emerge. Furthermore, he argued that this natural process may be one in which the human self merges with God. Thus, although the empirical facts cannot prove the existence of a God, mystical experience provides the basic experiential fact from which God as a genuine "overbelief" to explain the process is a viable hypothesis. Mystical experiences thus have reasonable evidential force, in James's view (Hood, 2000a, 2002a).

James's views created much controversy among early psychologists, who were anxious to separate psychology from religious views associated with the science in the popular mind. But James's insistence that mystical experiences are valid forms of human experience—incapable of being reductionistically explained by either physiological or psychological processes—provided a counter to the emerging natural-scientific and psychoanalytic psychologies, which denied the possibility that religious experiences may have a truly transcendent dimension (Hood, 2002a; Taves, 1999). James's view was simply that one may encounter God in numinous and mystical experiences, regardless of the processes identified by the scientists that are operating during the experience. In terms used previously, science cannot rule out that a mystical or numinous experience is an experience of the Real or of a foundational reality that may be necessary for the experience to occur. At a minimum, the *belief* in the reality must be there. As James stated in his notes for his lectures on mysticism in *The Varieties*, "Remember, the whole point lies in really believing that through a certain point or part in you you coalesce and are identical with the Eternal" (quoted in Perry, 1935, Vol. 2, p. 331).

Mysticism as Evolved Consciousness

Evolutionary theory has been a continuous influence on psychology since its inception. Mysticism has been proposed by some as a form of consciousness that is evolving, much as consciousness has evolved from the nonreflective consciousness that characterizes animals to the reflective consciousness that characterizes people. Not only are persons aware, but they are aware that they are aware; that is, they can reflect upon their awareness. Bucke (1901/1961) is most closely identified with the theory that following upon reflexive awareness in the evolution of consciousness is a cosmic consciousness or mystical state of awareness of unity with the world. He documented the increased presence of individuals over time whom he saw as examples of persons who express this cosmic consciousness. Basic to his theory is the notion that cosmic consciousness is evolving in the human species, becoming more frequent (even though by citing as exemplars of mystics such persons as Buddha and Christ, Bucke made the absolute frequency of mystical experience quite rare in any population). Nevertheless, as opposed to theorists who described mysticism as pathological or as a union with a religiously defined transcendent object, Bucke saw cosmic consciousness as the natural, advanced form of consciousness toward which the human species is evolving. As consciousness evolves, it evolves into a mystical consciousness. The philosopher Bergson gave the major impetus to evolutionary theories of mysticism by identifying mystical experience with the direct awareness of the evolutionary process itself (*élan vital*), which he saw as the basis of all life. Kolakowski (1985) has argued that sociological studies of mysticism both support and are compatible with Bergson's linking of mystical experience and his *élan vital*.

Alister Hardy (1965, 1966) proposed a similar theory of evolution, in which a cosmic consciousness is gradually emerging within the human species as a whole and provides a thoroughly naturalistic basis for mystical experiences that were previously interpreted in religious terms.

Unlike Bucke, Hardy assumed that mystical states are common. Late in his life, after his retirement from a career in zoology, he began soliciting reports of religious experiences and intiated efforts to provide a classification system of them. We have mentioned his empirical work in Chapter 9, and we discuss it further in the section on survey research below.

Perhaps the most mystical of the dynamic theorists, Jung, offered a different twist to evolutionary theories of mysticism. Indeed, many have claimed that Jung's entire psychology is inherently mystical. For our purposes, it is sufficient to note that in terms of evolution, Jung's theory assumes that archetypes are evolutionarily based tendencies to experience the world in particular ways. When imagined, experience is archetypal and has a numinous sense (Jung, 1954/1968). The archetypes are collectively shared as profound religious symbols, inherent in the human psyche. Thus one who follows Jung expects numinous experiences to occur in everyone, whether or not they are expressed in religious language. In Catholicism, the symbols are objectively protected and identified; in Protestantism, the symbols are allowed to emerge outside of institutional controls (Jung, 1938). Yet even when these experiences occur in dreams outside of religious interpretations, as normal processes inherent in the human psyche, only the absence of their report is problematic. Jung had carved in the arch to his home: *Vocatus atque non vocatus deus aderit.* The phrase has been variously translated, but a good English rendering is "Whether called or not, God will be present."

From our brief consideration of the conceptual issues involved in the study of mysticism, as well as the three major classical theories of mysticism, four key issues can be identified that have significant empirical consequences:

1. How is mysticism to be operationalized and measured? Clearly, how mysticism is measured brings with it the conceptual consequences that have been well discussed in the scholarly literature on this topic. It is unlikely that any empirical measure can avoid serious conceptual criticism, given the controversies that dominate this literature.

2. What empirical relationships exists between mystical experience and its interpretation? How does language affect experience? The conceptual literature ranges from the claim that mystical experiences are identical despite different interpretations (the "unity thesis") to the claim that differences in descriptions of experience constitute different experiences (the "plurality thesis").

3. What kind of persons report mystical experiences? Do such experiences occur across the developmental spectrum? Are they characteristic of healthy or of disturbed persons? Do they occur only among religiously committed persons?

4. What triggers such experiences? Can they be facilitated or do they occur only spontaneously? Is an experience affected by how it is produced? For instance, are experiences reported under the influence of entheogens (see Chapter 9) possibly the same as those reported during prayer?

These four issues are central to the conceptual literature on mysticism and have generated extensive discussion. Much of this discussion is quite philosophically and theologically sophisticated. However, our task in the remainder of this chapter is to focus on the empirical literature. As we shall see, many of the issues raised in the conceptual literature are paralleled in the empirical literature. By interrelating these two, we hope to contribute to what McGinn (1991, p. 343) has termed the "unrealized conversation" between social-scientific investigators and those involved in the history and theory of mystical traditions.

THE EMPIRICAL STUDY OF MYSTICISM

Central to any empirical study of mysticism is measurement based upon operationalized terms. There are almost as many definitions of "mysticism" as there are theorists. Over 100 years ago, Inge (1899) evaluated at least 26 definitions of it and concluded that no word in the English language had been employed more loosely. Not surprisingly, much of the current conceptual literature on mysticism debates various definitions and classifications of mysticism—often, obviously, on the basis of prior theological or religious commitments. For instance, Zaehner (1957) has argued for a clear distinction between "theistic mysticism" and other forms of mysticism, primarily on theological grounds. Likewise, in an often-cited example, the renowned Jewish scholar of mysticism Buber (1965) referred to his own experience of an "undivided unity," which he had thought to be union with God, but later felt to be an inappropriate interpretation. In a similar vein, James (1902/1985) refused to give serious consideration the considerably refined classification systems of mystical states associated with the Catholic mystical tradition, believing them to be primarily driven by theological considerations unrelated to actual experience. The Protestant theologian Ritschl claimed that neo-Platonism had so influenced the history of mysticism that it had become the theoretical norm for mystical experience, and that the universal being viewed as God by mystics is a "cheat" (quoted in McGinn, 1991, pp. 267–268). Finally, feminist theorists have accused both authorities within mysticism and scholars who study mysticism of falsely universalizing perspectives that, when deconstructed, can be seen as efforts to silence women—including accepting "ineffability" as a criterion of mysticism precisely so that women can say nothing of their experience (Jantzen, 1995).

From this sampling of views, it is clear that any definition of mysticism is likely to encounter conceptual criticism. However, at the empirical level it is clear that the distinction between experience and its interpretation and/or evaluation carries some weight. Thus, even in the case of Buber cited above, an experience of unity can be identified, regardless of how it is interpreted. The measurement of mysticism is possible once some operational indicator is identified. A considerable consensus exists that an experience of unity is central to mystical experience. Indeed, debates on mysticism often center on precisely how this unity is to be interpreted. Accordingly, measurements of mysticism identifying an experience of unity that is variously interpreted are quite congruent with the conceptual literature. They can also provide empirical tests of some of the issues central to that literature.

Whereas unity characterizes mysticism proper, we have noted above that numinous experiences focus more upon a fascinating and awe-inspiring sense of presence. Again, theological traditions determine how this presence is identified. In social-psychological terms, expectations determine interpretations of an experience (and, as we shall see, perhaps the nature of the experience itself). The measurement of a sense of presence is another indicator of mystical states, one that has been operationalized in a measure derived from the work of William James—the Religious Experience Episodes Measure, or REEM (Hood, 1970). We discuss this measure later in this chapter. However, more sociologically oriented social psychologists utilize survey data; this approach necessitates limited numbers of questions, which can be answered via phone surveys or interviews. Thus, on the sociological side, both numinous and mystical experiences have been measured by a limited number of questions that have been repeatedly used across a variety of survey studies. These too must be noted. Finally, several investigators have simply asked respondents to reply to a single item they believe to tap mystical experiences.

In summary, we can anticipate three major ways in which mysticism has been operationalized and measured in empirical research:

1. Open-ended responses to specific questions intuitively assumed to tap mystical or numinous experiences. These responses may then be variously coded or categorized.
2. Questions devised for use in survey research. Of necessity, these questions are brief, limited in number, and worded in language easily understandable for use in surveys of the general population. However, they are relevant as indicators of both a numinous sense of presence and an experience of unity.
3. Specific scales to measure mysticism.

As we shall see, how mysticism is operationalized and measured is related to the kinds of data provided to answer the various key issues in mysticism noted above. Accordingly, we discuss empirical studies in terms of the predominant operational and measurement strategies employed.

Studies Using Open-Ended Responses to Assess Mystical Experiences

Laski's Research

One of the more curious mainstream references in the empirical study of mysticism is Laski's (1961) research on ecstasy—curious, because of its severe methodological inadequacies. Laski, a novelist untrained in the social sciences, became interested in whether or not the experience of ecstasy she had written about in a novel was experienced in modern life. Initially using a convenience sample of friends and acquaintance sampled over a period of 3 years, she essentially asked persons to respond in an interview to the primary question: "Do you know a sensation of transcendent ecstasy?" (Laski, 1961, p. 9). If she was asked to explain what was meant by transcendent ecstasy, she told her respondents to "Take it to mean what you think it means" (Laski, 1961, p. 9). It only took 63 persons to produce 60 affirmative responses, perhaps because of the highly educated and literary nature of Laski's friends (20 of the 63 identified themselves as writers). Laski's own belief was that the transcendent ecstasy is most likely to be related to a family of terms that includes "mysticism," "oceanic feeling," and "cosmic consciousness" (1961, p. 5). However, an attempt to replicate her interview results with a sample distributed through mailboxes to 100 homes in a working-class area of London resulted in only 11 returns, with only 1 of these responses answering affirmatively the reworded question: "Have you ever had a feeling of unearthly ecstasy?" (Laski, 1961, pp. 526–533). We need only note here that different methods with different samples radically alter the nature of the data one may collect!

Thus Laski's 1961 text primarily analyzed responses obtained from her 60 interviews and from comparisons to 27 literary and 24 religious excerpts from published texts (selected for their intuitive demonstration of ecstatic experiences similar to those reported by the interview group). Her work is an extensive discussion of various means of classifying and identifying the nature of these experiences, primarily in terms of the language used to describe them. Laski's own limited data-analyzing skills were balanced by her perceptive analysis of language. The citations of the primary texts and interviews make it easy for the reader to judge the value of Laski's own analyses. Her conclusions raise several issues that have been the focus of more rigorous studies, to be discussed below.

Among Laski's conclusions is that transcendent ecstasy is a subset of mystical experience, defined and demarcated by the language used to describe it. It can be of three subtypes: experience of (1) knowledge, (2) union, or (3) purification and renewal. It is transient, and is triggered or elicited by a wide variety of circumstances and contexts. Generally, it is pleasurable and have beneficial consequences. However, it need not have unique religious value or provide evidential force for the validity of religious beliefs. Laski's own preference was to interpret transcendent ecstasy as a purely human capacity to experience joy in one's own creativity. She concluded that in both the past and the present, those who believe that they have experienced God are indeed mistaken; they have made a misattribution (Laski, 1961, pp. 369–374).

Social scientists continue to cite Laski's work, less for its methodological rigor than for its powerful description and analysis of instances of mystical experience. The assumption of many that mysticism is a rare phenomenon, characteristic of only a few, is belied by Laski's work. Her examples ring true to many persons' experiences, as we shall see. Furthermore, her interview procedures and her willingness to use the participants' own terms and language to analyze experiences have parallels in modern phenomenological research (Wulff, 1995).

Pafford's Research

One of Laski's contributions was to identify mystical experiences among adolescents. In her interview sample, there were two girls aged 14 and 16, and one male aged 10. This unwittingly opened the door to a series of studies identifying mystical experiences among children and youths. Especially among those influenced by literary works, the poet Wordsworth has given an implicit model of mystical experience relevant to children and adolescents. Laski (1961, p. 399) used two excerpts from Wordsworth's poetry in the literary texts she analyzed. In his autobiography, *Surprised by Joy*, C. S. Lewis (1956) extensively analyzed three boyhood experiences central to his religious development, noting that such descriptions had also been furnished by such poets as Wordsworth and could be "suffocatingly subjective" (p. viii). However, they gained ontological validity as they pointed to something "outer" and "other" (Lewis, 1956, p. 238). Pafford (1973) later titled a book that was partly based upon questionnaire responses from both grammar and university students *Inglorious Wordsworths*. Implicit in all these observations is a model purporting that children have an intense longing for transcendent experiences, which often are realized. Much of adult life is assumed to involve a longing for such experiences once again. Such a model can be contrasted with psychoanalytic and object relations theories, which assume mystical experiences to be regressive in a pathological sense. "Inglorious Wordsworths" have transcendent experiences that are valuable and healthy, and are capable of being recovered in adulthood.

As part of a questionnaire study, Pafford had both university and grammar school students respond to a literary description of an experience typical of Wordsworth's poetry—an experience that was specified as occurring in childhood, and one that involved consciousness of something more than a mere child's delight in nature (Pafford, 1973, p. 251). The actual text was from W. H. Hudson's (1939) autobiography *Far Away and Long Ago*. Participants were to describe in writing any experience of their own that they felt was is in any way similar to the one described in the passage. Pafford analyzed responses from 400 participants, half each from the university and grammar school samples; there were equal numbers of males and females in each sample. He found that 40% of the grammar school boys and 61% of the grammar schools girls had had such experiences. In the university sample, the percentages were 56% for the men and 65% for the women (Pafford, 1973, p. 91).

Although Pafford's samples can be classified and analyzed in as many intuitive ways as Laski's, he did at least attempt some crude quantitative and statistical analyses. One quantitative effort was to have respondents check off, on a list of 15 words, those that applied to their experience. These results are presented in Table 10.1. It is interesting to note that whereas Pafford claimed, partly from his own transcendental experiences, that such experiences are part of the essence of what he termed "real" religion, his own respondents checked the two most religion-related words ("holy" and "sacred") quite infrequently. It is unlikely that the most frequently checked word ("awesome") was interpreted by the respondents in a religious sense.

Pafford found that transcendental experiences were most typical in the middle teens, under conditions of solitude. The experiences were positive, and most respondents wished to have such experiences again. However they were less frequent in adulthood. One of the most common outcomes of the experience was some effort at creativity, although Pafford (influenced by Laski) specifically asked about creative acts following the experience, perhaps setting an expectation among respondents to list such activities.

Other Research on Children and Adolescents

Both Laski and Pafford found most mystical-type experiences to be uncommon in childhood—Laski because she sampled so few children, and Pafford because his samples reported most such experiences in middle adolescence, even though the literary example he cited stated 8 years of age as the beginning of such experiences. Since in Pafford's sample sixth-form grammar school students would have tended to be 18 and university students 19 or above, it may be that his respondents simply reported their most recent experience, hence minimizing reports of possible experiences in childhood. Some have argued that the commonalty of religious experience reported in adolescence reflects a North American Protestant bias, linked to the early focus on conversion experiences discussed in Chapter 11.

TABLE 10.1. Endorsement of Words Characterizing Transcendental Experiences

	Frequency of endorsement	Percentage of subjects endorsing
Awesome	119	54
Serene	87	39
Lonely	81	37
Frightening	77	35
Mysterious	65	29
Exciting	64	29
Ecstatic	47	21
Melancholy	45	20
Sacred	39	18
Sad	33	15
Holy	28	13
Sensual	21	10
Irritating	7	3
Erotic	5	2

Note. Number of respondents = 222. Adapted from Pafford (1973, p. 262). Copyright 1973 by Hodder and Stoughton. Adapted by permission.

One such critic, Klingberg (1959), sought to focus upon the study of religious experience in children, sampling only the age ranges from 9 to 13. Klingberg's study was done in Sweden in the mid-1940s, but was not published in English until 1959. Two sets of data were collected, intended to be "mutually supplementary" (Klingberg, 1959, p. 212); one of these consisted of adults' religious memories from childhood. Our concern is with compositions collected from 630 children (273 boys and 357 girls) in Sweden from 1944 to 1945. Most were 10 to 12 years of age. All children responded in writing to the statement "Once when I thought about God. . . ." Of the 630 compositions received, 566 contained accounts of personal religious experiences (244 from boys and 322 from girls). An unspecified number of compositions contained accounts of more than one experience. Assessing the experiences for depth indicated "phenomena which call to mind the experiences of the mystic" (Klingberg, 1959, p. 213). These primarily included both apparitions of objects of religious faith, such as Jesus, God, and angels; more importantly for our interests, however, they also included a felt sense of an invisible presence. Although Klingberg recognized the facilitating role of a religious culture, school, and home in encouraging such reports among children, he claimed that the value of the study is that it shows that mystical experiences *can* take place during childhood. Klingberg argued that maturational mechanism cannot eliminate mystical experiences in children, and suggested their universality. Fahs (1950) has persuasively argued for the awakening of mystical awareness in children by avoiding narrow religious indoctrination, which might preclude a sense of wonder, curiosity, and awe.

David and Sally Elkind (1970) studied the compositions of 149 ninth-grade U.S. students who were asked to respond to the questions "When do you feel closest to God?" and "Have you ever had a particular experience of feeling especially close to God?" (p. 104). The former question was assumed to tap recurrent religious experiences, and the latter acute religious experiences. The researchers concluded that the majority of respondents regarded personal religious experiences as a significant part of their lives, even though many resisted formal religious activities and participation. Across all respondents, 92% wrote compositions indicating recurrent experiences, and 76% wrote compositions indicating acute experiences (Elkind & Elkind, 1970, p. 104). Again, asking people in friendly or institutional contexts to write or talk about religious and mystical experiences readily yields responses from most participants.

Hood's Research

Open-ended responses to specific questions such as the ones we have been discussing can yield massive material, difficult to summarize. Statistical rigor and classification often yield to a rich descriptive presentation. However, such studies can be used to test empirical hypotheses as well. Hood (1973b) selected two extreme groups from a sample of 123 college students who responded to Allport's Intrinsic and Extrinsic religious orientation scales. The 25 highest-scoring subjects on each scale (Intrinsic mean = 41.8, *SD* = 2.9; Extrinsic mean = 49.2, *SD* = 3.7) were invited to participate in interviews regarding their "most significant personal experience." The 41 ubjects who participated (20 "intrinsic subjects" and 21 "extrinsic subjects") described a wide variety of experiences, few of which were explicitly identified as religious. However, coding experiences for their mystical quality on five criteria revealed that, as predicted, intrinsic subjects' most significant personal experiences were reliably coded as mystical more frequently than were extrinsic subjects' most significant personal experiences (see Table 10.2). This held not only for the total, global assessment of mysticism,

TABLE 10.2. Most Significant Personal Experiences Coded for Mystical Criteria in Intrinsic and Extrinsic Persons

Mystical criteria	Intrinsic ($n = 20$)	Extrinsic ($n = 21$)	Chi-square	Contingency coefficient[a]
Total				
Mystical	15	3		
Nonmystical	5	18	13.0***	.49
Loss of self				
Yes	14	3		
No	6	18	10.9***	.46
Noetic				
Yes	17	3		
No	3	13	7.6**	.39
Ineffable				
Yes	19	4		
No	1	17	21.0**	.58
Positive				
Yes	19	12		
No	1	9	6.0*	.36
Sacred				
Yes	18	6		
No	2	15	13.8***	.56

Note. Adapted from Hood (1973b, p. 446). Copyright 1973 by the Society for the Scientific Study of Religion. Adapted by permission.

[a]Upper limit of contingency coefficient = .71.

*$p < .02$. **$p < .01$. ***$p < .001$.

but for each of the five criteria used to identify mysticism. Despite the wide diversity of actual experiences (from childbirth to drug experiences), these could be coded as mystical more often for the intrinsic subjects than for the extrinsic subjects. It is important to note that few participants spontaneously described any experience as mystical; coders using theory-derived criteria categorized experiences as mystical or not. The role of language in defining experience from both first- and third-person perspectives is complex and is a topic of intense conceptual debate (Jantzen, 1995; Katz, 1992; Scharfstein, 1993). Yet at the purely empirical level, Hood's study indicates that experiences can be reliably coded as mystical by independent raters using theory-based criteria, even if the respondents themselves do not spontaneously define their experiences as either "religious" or "mystical."

Research by Thomas and Cooper, and by the Hardy Centre

However, if individuals affirmatively respond to an item measuring mysticism, does it mean that their experience was mystical as judged by others? Thomas and Cooper suggest that it may not be so. In two studies (Thomas & Cooper, 1978, 1980), they had persons from colleges, religious groups, and civic organizations respond to one of the items most frequently used in survey research (to be discussed below) to assess mystical experience. The item was "Have you ever had the feeling of being close to a powerful spiritual force that seemed to lift you out of yourself?" (Thomas & Cooper, 1978, p. 434). Research Box 10.1 describes these two studies in greater detail.

Research Box 10.1. Measurement and Incidence of Mystical Experiences (Thomas & Cooper, 1978 [Study 1], 1980 [Study 2])

In Thomas and Cooper's first study, only young adults aged 17–29 were used (44 males, 258 females). In the second study, 305 persons representing three different age groups— 17–29 years ($n = 120$), 30–59 years ($n = 110$), and 60 years and older ($n = 75$)—responded to the same survey question. In each study, those who answered "yes" went on to describe their experience in open-ended fashion, and raters coded the responses to place them in one of the categories described below. The percentage who answered "yes" was identical in both studies and is typical for survey research (34%). However, when the open-ended descriptions were analyzed for frequency and type of experience reported, all experiences were reliably placed into one of four response categories derived from a portion of the initial sample.

The frequencies and types of experiences reported, based upon open-ended descriptions to "yes" responses to the question "Have you ever had the feeling of being close to a powerful spiritual force that seemed to lift you out of yourself?", were as follows. (Note that these percentages are based on n's of 302 for Study 1 and 304 for Study 2; coder agreement was 94% overall for both studies.)

Type 0: No experience (Study 1, 66%; Study 2, 66%). Respondents answered "no" to question.

Type I: Uncodable (Study 1, 8%; Study 2, 10%). Respondents answered "yes," but responses were irrelevant or could not be reliably coded.

Type 1: Mystical (Study 1, 2%; Study 2, 1%). Responses included expressions of such things as awesome emotions; a sense of the ineffable; or a feeling of oneness with God, nature, or the universe.

Type 3: Psychic (Study 1, 12%; Study 2, 8%). Responses included expressions of extraordinary or supernatural phenomena, including extrasensory perception, telepathy, out-of-body experience, or contact with spiritual beings.

Type 4: Faith and consolation (Study 1, 2%; Study 2, 16%). Responses included religious or spiritual phenomena, but without indications of either extraordinary or supernatural elements.

Depite minor variations in frequencies of experience categories between these two studies (perhaps because of the larger age range in Study 2), there is remarkable agreement not only in the identical percentage of affirmative responses in both studies, but also in the fact that the *least* frequent content category for the open-ended responses was mystical.

The importance of these two studies is that if affirmative responses in a single-item survey question are accepted at face value, many diverse experiences may be clustered together. In terms of our specific concern with mystical experiences, no more than 2% of the 34% who responded to the survey question presumed to be a measure of mysticism actually described mystical experiences in open-ended descriptions. The criteria for mysticism compatible with those typically cited in the conceptual literature—such as an ineffable sense of union with God (personal) or the universe (impersonal)—were not evident. Thus survey items to assess mysticism may do so poorly according to more rigorous criteria, and may overestimate the actual incidence of reported mystical experience in samples.

The findings of Thomas and Cooper are supported by classifications of the religious experiences solicited from and sent in to the Alister Hardy Religious Experience Research Centre, as described in Chapter 9. Much as Alister Hardy collected and classified samples of plankton during his career as a zoologist, numerous samplings from over 5,000 reports of religious experience at the Hardy Centre have been collected and variously classified. The most extensive classification is based upon the initial 3,000 cases Hardy collected. Variations occurred in the wording of the appeal for reports of such experiences, depending on the source of publication. In some cases, brief descriptions from literature were given to illustrate the type of experience in which the researchers were interested (Hardy, 1979, p. 18). Most common was this one in a pamphlet widely circulated in the United Kingdom:

> All those who feel they have been conscious of, and perhaps influenced by, some Power, whether called God or not, which may either appear to be beyond their individual selves or partly, or even entirely, within their being, are asked to write a simple account of their feelings and their effects. (Hardy, 1979, p. 20)

Not surprisingly, Hardy and his colleagues found that the reports of the materials submitted defied easy classification: "So many of them were a mixture of widely different items" (Hardy, 1979, p. 23). Hardy's own elaborate classification system, composed of 12 major categories (most with numerous subclassifications), yielded a total of 92 classifications. Some of these referred to the development and consequences of the experience, and did not describe the experience proper. Each experience was rated for the presence or absence of any classification category. Most relevant to our concerns in this chapter are those experiences that were coded in terms of mystical or numinous criteria. Few were: The most specific mystical category, "Feeling of unity with surroundings and/or with people," characterized only 168 of the initial 3,000 experiences coded, or 5.6% (Hardy, 1979, p. 26). The most numinous classification, "Sense of presence (not human)," characterized 369 or 12.3% of these 3,000 reports (Hardy, 1979, p. 27). Thus, despite the fact that Hardy felt his appeal would yield reports of evidential value, akin to spiritual reports in the Bible and accounts by mystics, only a small minority of the experiences were either mystical or numinous when coded for relevant criteria by independent raters.

However, a cautionary note must be sounded regarding materials from the Hardy Centre. Access to these materials by various scholars has led to numerous classification systems, few of which have been rigorously established by methodological or statistical means. Hence widely varying reports of the content of these materials persist. For instance, Hay (1994) has identified six major types of religious experiences in the Hardy archives, one of which is "an awareness of the presence of God"and the other "experiencing in an extraordinary way that all things are One" (Hay, 1994, pp. 21–22). These correspond to numinous and mystical experiences, respectively, but Hay's results differ dramatically from Hardy's own analysis as described above.

Hay's Research

Hay and Morisy (1985, p. 14) asked a random sample of 266 residents of Nottingham, England, a version of the Hardy appeal: "Have you ever been aware or influenced by a presence or power, whether you call it God or not, which is different from your everyday self?" Of the 172 who consented to be interviewed, 72% (124) answered "yes." Eliminating 17 of these (who apparently misunderstood the question or who could not describe the experience) left 107 persons who were able to describe in detail the experience (or the most important experience, if they had more than one). Using the respondents' own language, the researchers classified the experiences into one of seven categories as follows: presence of or help from God (28%), assistance via prayer (9%), intervention by presence not identified as God (135), presence or help from deceased (22%), premonitions (10%), meaningful patterning of events (10%), and miscellaneous (8%) (Hay & Morisy, 1985, p. 217). Although these categories were purely provisional, once again it is evident that persons who were responding to particular questions were in fact reporting a wide range and type of experiences. This was true even though the specific wording of the Hardy appeal used in this study was field-tested and assumed to draw out both the mystical and numinous qualities of religious experience. Yet no mystical experiences could be coded (except perhaps if included under "miscellaneous"), and only 28% were explicitly numinous in terms of a sense of presence identified with the holy (God).

In a similar study, Hay (1979, p. 165) found a high (65%) affirmative response rate to whether an individual could ever remember "being aware of or influenced by a presence or a power, whether you call it God or not, which is different from your everyday self." Respondents were 100 randomly selected students in a postgraduate teacher certificate course at Nottingham University, England. Despite the fact that the question was worded to cover mystical or numinous experiences—by focusing upon whether the experience was of a personal ("presence") or impersonal ("power") nature—classification of extended interviews in which affirmative respondents described their experience yielded only 32 of 109 (29.4%) experiences that were clearly either mystical or numinous. These were 10 (9.2%) experiences of unity (mystical experience), and 22 (20.2%) experiences of an awareness of God (numinous experience).

Summary of Studies Using Open-Ended Responses

Overall, we can conclude that open-ended responses to specific questions presumed to elicit reports of either mystical or numinous experiences reveal little of scientific value, beyond the fact that individuals (from children through senior citizens) readily report such experiences. The richness of their reports varies with their linguistic capacities. They cannot be taken as uncritical evidential value for the realities they describe, and they may be highly influenced by personal concerns of those making such reports. Finally, depending on investigators' own classification interests, such reports can be almost interminably classified and cross-referenced. This means that first-person descriptions of experience are unlikely to correspond closely to third-person classifications of these same experiences. Perhaps the very richness of these descriptions means that they are best approached by techniques of literary criticism. However, this research tradition does remind us that responses to such questions, even if reliably quantified, mask a rich subjective variation of immense importance to those whose experiences are studied.

Survey Research

Emerging simultaneously with, and influenced by, open-ended reports of mystical and numinous experience are survey studies. As noted earlier, such studies use a few specific questions, often answered simply "yes" or "no." What survey studies lose in terms of the range and depth of description of experiences, they gain in terms of identifying the frequency and reporting of such experiences in the general population. Their results are also easily quantified and allow correlations with a wide variety of demographic and other variables to provide a distinctive empirical base that complements merely conceptual discussions of these experiences. We focus here on the body of survey research that has asked questions intended by the researchers to be direct measures of mystical and numinous experiences. Fortunately, several surveys have used identical questions over several years and even within different cultures, so some comparisons over time and cultures can also be made, at least at the descriptive level.

One caution must be noted before we begin. Intercorrelations among different items to measure mystical experiences across different surveys are not available. Although we can anticipate positive correlations, it is not clear that this will always be the case, nor can we be certain of the magnitude of such correlations. Hence each item must be judged in itself as an operational measure of the experience in question. Four major questions have dominated the majority of surveys covering since 1960. Accordingly, we summarize these data in terms of the survey questions used, each identified by the name most closely associated with the formulation of the initial question. Therefore we have the Stark, Bourque, Greeley, and Hardy questions.

The Stark Question

As part of an early multidimensional model of religion, Glock and Stark (1965) proposed five dimensions to religion, one of which is the experiential dimension. This dimension includes religious emotions, as well as claims to direct experiential awareness of ultimate reality. The survey question used in their initial sampling of churches in the greater San Francisco area in 1963 was this: "Have you ever as an adult had the feeling that you were somehow in the presence of God?" (Glock & Stark, 1965, p. 157, Table 8-1). With a sample size just under 3,000 respondents (2,871), 72% answered "yes." Although we might expect the various dimensions of the Glock and Stark model of religion (ritual, belief, consequences, experience, belief) to intercorrelate simply because they are all religious items, the model attempts to assess experience independently; hence the question refers to a *feeling* of God's presence, which is presumed to tap religious experience rather than belief. Not surprisingly, the majority of religiously committed, institutionally involved persons answered "yes." Only 20% of all Protestants sampled ($n = 2,326$) and 25% of all Catholics sampled ($n = 545$) answered "no."

Vernon (1968) isolated a small sample of 85 persons who indicated "none" when asked religious commitment. In this sample of "religious nones," 25% nevertheless answered the Stark question affirmatively. Thus, even among those with no institutional religious commitment, a significant minority of adults reported experiencing a sense of God's presence.

More recently, Tamminen (1991) used the five religious dimensions of Glock and Stark (1965) to organize his longitudinal study of religious development in Scandinavian youths. Modifying the Stark question slightly by omitting the phrase "as an adult," Tamminen asked, "Have you at times felt that God is particularly close to you?" Percentages of responses by grade level for the 1974 sampling are presented in Table 10.3. The steady decline in the percentage of students reporting experiences of nearness to God by grade level (and hence age) is obvious. This decline is further evident in Table 10.4, which contains responses to the same question in 1986 from this longitudinal study. Tamminen's study is thus the only major longitudinal study to document the steady decline in the report of religious experience from

TABLE 10.3. Scandinavian Students' Reports of Experiencing Nearness to God (1974)

Response	Percentage responding by grade level					
	I	III	V	VII	IX	XI
Yes	84	—	—	—	—	—
Very often	—	42	17	10	10	8
A few times	—	30	40	33	31	27
Maybe once	—	18	12	15	14	13
No	16	10	31	43	44	53

Note. $n = 1,336$. Level I answered only "yes" or "no." Adapted from Tamminen (1991, p. 42). Copyright 1991 by Soumalainen Tiedeaktemia. Adapted by permission.

childhood through adolescence. It suggests that such experiences (or their report) are quite common in childhood, supporting the claims of Pafford and others discussed above.

The Bourque Question

In a series of surveys, Bourque and her colleagues utilized the following question to assess religious experience: "Would you say that you have ever had a 'religious or mystical experience'—that is, a moment of sudden religious awakening or insight?" (Back & Bourque, 1970, p. 489). They also cited results from three Associated Press surveys using this question; these surveys were conducted in 1962, 1966, and 1967 in the United States. Over time, the percentage of persons answering "yes" increased from 21% in 1962 ($n = 3,232$) to 32% in 1966 ($n = 3,518$) to 41% in 1967 ($n = 3,168$). Bourque (1969) administered this question, along with the Stark question above and another question, to a sample of 3,168 and found that 32% answered "yes." Gallup (1978) used this item in a U.S. national survey in 1976 and found that 31% answered affirmatively in a sample of 1,500. More recently, Yamane and Polzer (1994) reported the results of two Gallup surveys in 1990—one in June and one in September, each using a sample of 1,236—and found a stable affirmative response frequency of 53%.

Thus, over a period exceeding a quarter of a century, representative samples of persons in the United States reported having a religious or mystical experience, defined as a moment of sudden religious awakening or insight. The range of affirmative responses was large (from 21% to 53%), but lower than the typical affirmative response to the Stark question, which

TABLE 10.4. Scandinavian Students' Reports of Experiencing Nearness to God (1986)

Response	Percentage responding by grade level						
	III	IV	V	VI	VII	VIII	IX
Very often	19	19	13	10	5	1	4
A few times	31	33	44	29	20	13	15
Maybe once	18	20	19	27	24	18	22
No	32	28	24	34	52	68	59

Note. $n = 971$. Adapted from Tamminen (1991, p. 43). Copyright 1991 by Soumalainen Tiedeaktemia. Adapted by permission.

asks active, institutionally affiliated religious persons whether they have ever had a sense of God's presence.

The Greeley Question

Another question widely used in survey research and accepted as an operational measure of reported mystical question is associated with the work of Greeley (1974). The question most typically used is "Have your ever felt as though you were close to a powerful spiritual force that seemed to lift you out of yourself?" It has been administered as part of the General Social Survey (GSS) of the National Opinion Research Center. The GSS is a series of independent cross-sectional probability samples of persons in the continental United States, living in noninstitutional homes, who are 18 years of age and English-speaking. It was found that overall, in a GSS sample of 1,468, 35% of the respondents answered "yes" to this question (Davis & Smith, 1994).

Hay and Morisy (1978) administered a similar question to a sample of 1,865 in Great Britain and found that 36% answered in the affirmative. In the two studies by Thomas and Cooper (1978, 1980) discussed above, the 34% affirmative responses revealed few responses that were truly mystical when independently coded for criteria of mysticism. On the other hand, Greeley (1975, p. 65) found that a very high percentage (29%) of those who positively answered his question agreed with "a sense of unity and my own part in it" as a descriptor of their experience. Thus most of the 34% answering "yes" to the Greeley question also appeared to accept a mystical description of unity as applying to the experience. It may be that, methodologically, checking descriptors of experience increases the positive rate of mystical experiences over spontaneous descriptions of the experiences in open-ended interviews.

In a survey of 339, McClenon (1984) found the lowest affirmative response rate to the Greeley question (20%). More recently, Yamane and Polzer (1994) analyzed all affirmative responses from the GSS to the Greeley question in the years 1983, 1984, 1988, and 1989. A total of 5,420 individuals were included in their review. Using an ordinal scale where respondents who answered affirmatively could select from three options—"once or twice," "several times," or "often"—yielded a range from 0 (negative response) to 3 (often). Using this 4-point range across all individuals who responded to the Greeley question yielded a mean score of 0.79 ($SD = 0.89$). Converting these to a percentage of "yes" as a nominal category, regardless of frequency, yielded 2,183 affirmative responses, or an overall affirmative response rate of 40% of the total sample who reported ever having had the experience. Independent assessment of affirmative responses for each year suggested a slight but steady decline. The figures were 39% for 1983–1984 combined ($n = 3,072$), 31% for 1988 ($n = 1,481$), and 31% for 1989 ($n = 936$).

Bourque and Back (1971) created an index of religious experience composed of three questions—the Stark and Bourque questions already noted, plus a third: "Have you ever had a feeling of being saved in Christ?" In a sample of 3,168, a total of 990 (31%) answered affirmatively to all three questions; 794 (25%) to any two; and 566 (18%) to at least one (Back & Bourque, 1971, p. 10).

The Hardy Question

As noted above, Alister Hardy's interest in religious experience focused methodologically on soliciting open-ended responses from persons to both literary examples and descriptions of religious experiences. The most common description used by Hardy (noted above) was slightly modified by Hay and Morisy and used in several survey studies.

The precise wording of the Hay and Morisy question was "Have you ever been aware of or influenced by a presence or power, whether you call it God or not, which is different from your everyday self?" (1978, p. 207). Their survey was conducted in Great Britain. Respondents were chosen from a two-stage stratified sample: names randomly drawn from the electoral register, supplemented with names drawn at random of nonelectors from the households of the selected electors. In their sample of 1,865, 36% answered affirmatively to the question. In the more restricted sample of 172 homes in an industrial area of England (described earlier), Hay and Morisy (1985) found the high affirmative response rate of 72%. The high rates were probably a function of face-to-face interviews, which have been shown to increase the number of affirmative responses to survey questions dealing with religious experience. However, Hay (1994) also found a 65% affirmative response rate to his version of the Hardy question in a random sample of postgraduate students at Nottingham University, England. He extensively interviewed respondents regarding their experiences, but the actual affirmation of the experiences occurred before the interview. It may be that anticipating a discussion of reports of religious experience increases their rate of report. Hay (1994, p. 8, Table 3) also cites a study by Lewis, in which a high affirmative response rate to the Hardy question was obtained in a British sample of 108 nurses from two different hospitals in Leeds. Again, face-to-face interviews may have been a factor increasing response rates.

In a Gallup sample of 985 British citizens, Hay and Heald (1987) found a rate more typical of other general surveys using the Hardy question: 48% of their sample responded affirmatively to the question. This closely matches the 44% rate found in previously unpublished data based upon an Australian sample of 1,228 by Morgan Research (the Australian affiliate of the Gallup Poll organization) and cited by Hay (1994, p. 7). A survey in the United States of 3,000 sampled produced a 31% affirmative response rate, closely matching the 35% response rate produced in a sample of 3,062 from the Princeton Research Center (1978) a few years earlier. Hay (1994, p. 7, Table 1) also cites two unpublished Gallup Polls commissioned by the Hardy Centre in 1985, indicating a 33% affirmative response to the Hardy question in a sample of 1,030 in Britain, and a 10% higher rate (43%) for a similar sample of 1,525 in the United States. Finally, Back and Bourque (1970) reported three different Gallup surveys done in the United States, with affirmative response rates to the Hardy question of 21% in 1962 ($n = 3,232$), 32% in 1966 ($n = 3,518$), and 41% in 1967 ($n = 3,168$).

Thus surveys from 1962 through 1987 in the United States, Britain, and Australia suggest a fairly wide range (21–72%) of affirmative responses to the Hardy question. However, when the higher rates obtained from anticipated in-depth interviews are ignored, the affirmative response rates average in the 35–40% range for the Hardy question—paralleling fairly closely those for the Greeley and Bourque questions, and for the Stark question when the respondents are not restricted to church or synagogue members. Thus, overall, it appears that 35% of persons sampled affirm some intense spiritual experience, felt by the researchers to measure mystical and/or numinous experience. At a minimum, then, the reports of such experiences have been clearly and conclusively established by survey studies to be statistically quite common among normal samples. What are we to make of these reports?

Most survey studies have included additional questions and demographic characteristics that can be correlated with the reports of religious experience. No simply pattern has emerged from the studies mentioned above, and unfortunately each study must be considered in terms of its sampling and the statistical models used. The range of data analysis is large, from naïve to state-of-the-art sophistication. The major consistent findings are easily summarized: Women report more such experiences than men; the experiences tend to be age-related, increasing with age; they are characteristic of educated and affluent people; and they are more likely to be associated with indices of psychological health and well-being than with those of pathology or social dysfunction. Thus Scharfstein's (1973) "everyday mysticism" is supported by survey research in affirming the commonalty of mysticism among both institutionally and noninstitutionally committed religious persons within the United States, the United Kingdom, and Australia.

Several studies have focused upon the communication patterns of persons who have such experiences, noting that these persons do *not* talk about their experiences with others. Even Tamminen (1991, p. 62) noted this among his Scandinavian sample; the failure to communicate such experiences starts in childhood. This may well account for the persistence of the belief that such experiences are uncommon. The irony is that at least one-third of the population claims to have such experience, but few people talk about them publicly. This hidden dimension of religious experience is well documented and can be clarified by other studies, to be discussed below. However, before we discuss these studies, one cautionary note is needed—one that confronts the issue of the language and experience central to much of the conceptual and empirical literature on mysticism.

A CAUTIONARY NOTE:
MYSTICISM AND THE PARANORMAL

Since its inception, North American psychology has been linked in the popular mind with psychic phenomena. As Coon (1992) has documented, many founding North American psychologists fought hard to separate the emerging science of psychology from "spiritualism" and "psychic," to which it was connected in the popular mind. Few psychologists, then or now, believe in the reality of parapsychological phenomena. Hood (1994, 2000a) has identified religion and parapsychology as perhaps the most controversial research area in the psychology of religion.

Yet within research on mysticism, several empirical facts emerge that are problematic. Several of the key theoreticians and empirical researchers have explicitly linked mysticism to parapsychology, with varying degrees of sympathy to both. These include such major figures as Greeley (1975), Hardy (1965, 1966), and Hood (1989). Historians have also documented the relationship of paranormal phenomena to the history of religious experience in North American Protestantism (Coon, 1992; Taves, 1999). Second, in classifications of open-ended responses to single-item questions to measure mysticism, one of the most common code categories is "paranormal." Thus many persons who affirm what the researcher assumes to be a mystical or numinous item are in fact reporting paranormal experiences, such as telepathy, clairvoyance, or contact with the dead. Third, survey studies of mysticism commonly include items to assess paranormal experiences. For instance, paranormal experiences are included in the 1984, 1988, and 1989 GSS data. In virtually every survey, paranormal and mystical experiences are positively correlated: Persons who report paranormal experiences often report mystical experiences as well, and vice versa. Seldom is only one type of experience reported. Further support for this claim is that factor analysis of survey items including mysticism and paranormal experience indicate that extrasensory perception, clairvoyance, contact with the dead, and mysticism form a single factor; this means that these are empirically measuring one thing in the popular mind. Thalbourne and his colleagues propose the term "transliminality" to account for the common factor underlying all these experiences (Thalbourne, Bartemucci, Delin, Fox, & Nofi, 1997; Thalbourne & Delin, 1999). If we exclude *déjà vu* experiences, which are also included in survey studies but neither conceptually nor empirically linked to paranormal experiences, the pattern of affirmative responses is as high as or higher than the range of affirmative responses to religious items. As an example, Table 10.5 compares the distribution of affirmative responses to three items assessing paranormal experiences with the distribution of such responses to the Greeley question about mysticism.

Clearly, Table 10.5 reveals that reports of parapsychologcial experiences are at least as common as those of mystical experiences. This fact, combined with the strong intercorrelation among parapsychological and religious items that in a general sample often yield a single factor, suggest that what is being tapped in these surveys is some assertion of experiencing a reality different from that postulated by mainstream science (Targ, Schlitz, & Irwin, 2000; Thalbourne et al., 1997; Thalbourne & Delin, 1999). However, the nature of that reality is open to serious question. We have seen that open-ended responses to survey questions yield a wide range of experiences. It is likely that some respondents simply want to affirm experiences that offer evidential support not only for alternative beliefs, but also for their own self-importance. Furthermore, it is likely that to tease out separate reports of such experiences as mystical and numinous experiences would require studies of sophisticated populations for whom such distinctions can be made, in terms of both conceptualizations and actual experience. However, it would seem that sampling from religiously committed persons would best allow distinctions between the religious and parapsychological experiences often associated with religion but perhaps best independently identified. For instance, the conceptual literature on mysticism clearly separates paranormal experiences from mystical ones. Measurement studies that find a common factor such as the one noted above may need more

TABLE 10.5. Comparison of Affirmative Responses to Four Questions about Mystical or Paranormal Experiences in Three Years of the GSS

Year	Extrasensory perception	Clairvoyance	Contact with the dead	Mysticism
1984	$n = 1,439$	$n = 1,434$	$n = 1,445$	$n = 1,442$
	67%	30%	42%	41%
1988	$n = 1,456$	$n = 1,440$	$n = 1,459$	$n = 1,451$
	64%	28%	40%	32%
1989	$n = 922$	$n = 983$	$n = 991$	$n = 988$
	58%	23%	35%	30%

Note. The four questions asked were as follows:

Mysticism: Have you ever felt as though you were close to a powerful spiritual force that seemed to lift you out of yourself?

Extrasensory perception: Have you ever felt as though you were in touch with someone when they were far away from you?

Clairvoyance: Have you ever seen events that were happening at a great distance as they were happening?

Contact with the dead: Have you ever felt as though you were in touch with someone who had died?

Adapted from Fox (1992, p. 422). Copyright 1992 by the Association for the Sociology of Religion. Adapted by permission.

sophisticated samples to separate responses to parapsychological and mystical items. Moreover, many religious traditions carefully dissociate themselves from what they would term "occult" practices.

Some empirical evidence for this view is that when samples are carefully selected for their religious identification, paranormal experiences are infrequently cited (if at all) as instances of religious experiences. For instance, Margolis and Elifson (1979) carefully solicited a sample of persons who were willing to affirm that they had had a religious experience that the researchers accepted as indicating some personal relationship to ultimate reality. Forty-five respondents were then carefully interviewed about their experiences; to avoid interviewer bias, a structured format was employed. The 69 experiences described were content-analyzed, yielding 20 themes. These were then factor-analyzed, yielding four factors—the major one of which was a mystical factor, "very similar to the classical mystical experience described by Stace and others" (Margolis & Elifson, 1979, p. 62). Two of the other three factors (a life change experience factor and a visionary factor) were clearly religious experiences. One factor, vertigo experience, was a loss of control experienced negatively, often triggered by drugs or music. No paranormal experiences were reported. Thus it is likely that survey questions worded to avoid religious language probably elicit a variety of experiences, including paranormal ones, that otherwise would not be identified as religious by the respondents.

However, in a survey study in the San Francisco Bay area, Wuthnow (1978) found not only that the majority of all respondents claimed to have experienced paranormal phenomena, but that those affirming that they had "ever been in close contact with the sacred or holy" were the most likely to report paranormal experiences. The conceptual literature on mysticism is replete with discussion of traditions that warn against confounding paranormal and mystical experiences, even though they are often related both empirically and historically (Coon, 1992; Hood, 2000a; Taves, 1999; Zollschan, Schumaker, & Walsh, 1995). It is unlikely that members of the general population make such distinctions, because they usually lack either the experiential base or the conceptual sophistication to make such distinctions. As Yamane and Polzer (1994) have argued, religiously committed persons may be quite adept at distinguishing religious experiences from other types of intense or anomalous experiences. Of course, some people outside mainstream religious traditions may define paranormal experiences as "religious," or more likely by the more general term "spiritual." It is likely that the specific presence or absence of the term "God" in survey items produces different results, in that persons committed to a mainstream religion are most likely to respond to religious language and to make distinctions among various experiences based upon religious knowledge.

Clearly, avoiding religious language in survey questions encourages the reporting of a wider range of experiences. Teasing out reports of experiences from a whole host of complex factors affecting their reporting requires more complex techniques than the methodology of survey research permits. Some of these issues have been explored in more measurement-based studies, many of which are correctional. However, there are also more laboratory-based and quasi-experimental studies. These permit even more precise identification of determinants of the reports of mystical experience.

Measurement Studies

Academic psychology of religion is heavily committed to what Gorsuch (1984) has called the "measurement paradigm." One goal of measurement is to create reliable scales from clearly operationalized concepts. Many have thought that religious experiences, particularly the numinous and mystical varieties, cannot be reliably measured. However, two approaches to their measurement have been reasonably successful and used in several studies.

The Religious Experience Episodes Measure: The Influence of James

One approach to measurement of mystical and numinous experiences has been to operationalize and quantify what might be called the "literary exemplar approach" of many of the more open-ended studies discussed above. Laski, Pafford, and Hardy gave particular examples of experiences and asked respondents whether they had ever had an experience like the one described. Hood (1970) essentially systematized this procedure in constructing the Religious Experience Episodes Measure (REEM). He selected 15 experiences from James's *The Varieties of Religious Experience*, presented them in booklet form, and had respondents rate on a 5-point scale the degree to which they had ever had an experience like each of these. Hood's approach standardized the experiences presented to research subjects, and allowed a quantification of the report of religious experience by summing the degree of similarity of one's own experiences to those described in the REEM. Rosegrant (1976) modified the REEM by rephrasing "the elegant 19th century English" (p. 306) and reducing the number of items from 15 to 10. Examples of REEM items as modified by Rosegrant are presented in Table 10.6.

Both Hood's initial version and Rosegrant's modified version of the REEM have high internal consistencies, suggesting that the experiences described cluster together. Unpolished factor analysis of the REEM also yields a single factor. Overall, the mixture of more numinous and mystical items with explicit or implicit religious language suggests that the REEM is best used with religiously committed samples. It also reflects religious experience perhaps most

---

TABLE 10.6. Items from the Modified REEM

<u>To what extent have you ever had an experience like this?</u>

God is more real to me than any thought or person. I feel his presence, and I feel it more as I live in closer harmony with his laws. I feel him in the sunshine, or rain, and my feelings are best described as awe mixed with delirious restfulness.

<u>Or like this?</u>

I would suddenly feel the mood coming when I was at church, or with people reading, but only when my muscles were relaxed. It would irresistibly take over my mind and will, last what seemed like forever, and disappear in a way that resembled waking from anesthesia. One reason I think that I dislike this kind of trance was that I could not describe it to myself; even now I can't find the right words. It involved the disappearance of space, time, feeling, and the things I call my self. As ordinary consciousness disappeared, the sense of underlying essential consciousness grew stronger. At last nothing remained but a pure, abstract, self.

<u>Or like this?</u>

Once, a few weeks after I came to the woods, I though perhaps it was necessary to be near other people for a happy and healthy life. To be alone was somewhat unpleasant. But during a gentle rain, while I had these thoughts, I was suddenly aware of such good society in nature, in the pattern of drops and every sight and sound around my house, that the fancy advantages of being near people seemed insignificant, and I haven't thought about them since. Every little pine needle expanded with sympathy and befriended me. I was so definitely aware of something akin to me that I thought no place could ever be strange.

Note. From Rosegrant (1976) as adapted from Hood (1970). (Also see Hill & Hood, 1999a, pp. 222–224.) Copyright 1976 by the Society for the Scientific Study of Religion. Reprinted by permission.

common in North American Protestant experience—a common criticism leveled against James's classic text, from which items for the REEM were selected. Holm (1982) found it difficult to make a meaningful translation of the REEM into Swedish, and had to create a version of the REEM appropriate to Swedish culture by selecting Nordic tales.

Hood (1970) initially created the REEM to test the hypothesis that intrinsically religious persons would score higher on the REEM than extrinsically religious persons. In a sample of college students this hypothesis was supported, with intrinsic persons scoring significantly higher on the REEM than extrinsic persons. These findings are compatible with the survey research noted above, in which religiously committed persons are often identified to have high rates of reported mystical experiences. It further suggests, however, that among religiously committed individuals, intrinsic persons have higher scores (and hence perhaps report more experiences) than extrinsic persons. Using Allport's Intrinsic and Extrinsic scales to create a fourfold typology, based upon median splits on the Intrinsic and Extrinsic scales, indicated that "indiscriminately pro" (IP) persons (with high Extrinsic/high Intrinsic scores) could not be distinguished from intrinsic persons based upon their REEM scores. Likewise, "indiscriminately anti" (IA) persons (with low Extrinsic/low Intrinsic scores) could not be distinguished from extrinsic persons based upon their REEM scores. Survey researchers have often worried about "false positives" and "false negatives" in their surveys. How do we know that persons who report experiences are telling the truth? Some might not have had the experiences they report (false positives). On the other hand, how to we know that persons denying these experiences are telling the truth? Some may refuse to admit experiences they have had (false negatives).

In this study, Hood (1970) linked the methodological problem of distinguishing between intrinsic and IP persons and between extrinsic and IA persons with the possibility that IP persons often represent false positives and IA persons represent false negatives with respect to reports of mystical experience. The basis for this hypothesis is that Allport believed the indiscriminate types to be motivated by conflicting stances with respect to religion: IA persons may deny religious impulses they may in fact feel, while IP persons may feign religious impulses they may not actually experience. It is this sort of dynamic and conflictual process that Allport and Ross (1967, p. 442) felt made the indiscriminate categories potentially of significant research interest and of "central significance" for Allport's theory.

In a second study, Hood (1978b) replicated the relationship between Allport's fourfold typology and REEM scores. This time, using Rosegrant's modification of the REEM and categorizing persons according to their religious type produced similar high REEM scores for intrinsic and IP persons and similar low scores for extrinsic and IA persons, as indicated in Table 10.7.

In order to directly test the possibility that the indiscriminate categories might represent false positives (in the case of IP persons) and false negatives (in the case of IA persons), Hood had interviewers in a double-blind condition conduct a bogus interview that included nearly 40 personal and religious questions. These served as baseline data and also served to mask the key final question, which was prefaced by the comment that many of the preceding questions were designed to tap whether or not one had ever had a mystical experience. Persons were then asked whether they had in fact ever had such an experience. The answer to this key question, whether "yes" or "no," was then analyzed with a "Stress Analyzer," a device that measures stress by means of detecting small voice tremors. Each subject's stress level was measured by comparing the affirmation or denial of mystical experience to the baseline levels of stress in response to the bogus inventory. The numbers of persons affirm-

TABLE 10.7. REEM Scores According to Religious Type

Religious type	Score
Intrinsic ($n = 31$)	Mean = 48.81, $SD = 12.21$
IP ($n = 46$)	Mean = 50.89, $SD = 14.79$
Extrinsic ($n = 39$)	Mean = 39.51, $SD = 17.07$
IA ($n = 31$)	Mean = 39.13, $SD = 18.8$

Note. $F (1, 143) = 15.69$, $p < .05$; post hoc comparisons grouped according to significant differences *between* clustered categories, at least $p < .05$. Categories *within* parentheses did not differ: (IP, I); (IA, E). Adapted from Hood (1978b, p. 426). Copyright 1978 by the Society for the Scientific Study of Religion. Adapted by permission.

ing and denying mystical experiences, and the numbers showing stress when responding, are reported in Table 10.8 according to religious type.

As predicted, the proportions of persons affirming mystical experiences were similar in the intrinsic and IP groups, as were the proportions denying mystical experiences in the extrinsic and IA groups. However, intrinsic persons as a group expressed little stress when affirming mystical experiences, while IP persons showed much stress. The case was less clear for extrinsic persons. Still, more than half the IA persons exhibited stress, and while many did so when reporting mystical experiences, it may be that indiscriminate persons (whether pro or not) indicate stress when talking about their religion (or lack of it), due to their conflictual stance with respect to religion. In any case, the large number of IP persons affirming mystical experiences with great stress is consistent with the possibility that they are "false positives," attempting to appear religious by reporting experiences they believe they should experience but perhaps have not.

However, it is also possible that as Rosegrant (1976, p. 307) found, stress is often associated with the report of mystical experience; this was indicated by a .29 ($p < .05$) correlation between REEM scores and a measure of stress in a nature setting with 51 students. Although Rosegrant did not measure religious orientation in his study, it may be that the *lack* of correlation between mysticism and a measure of meaningfulness used in his study indicates that mystical experiences are experienced as stressful only when subjects are asked for a meaningful religious framework for interpretation. Consistent with this claim is that mys-

TABLE 10.8. Affirmation and Denial of Mystical Experience and Associated Stress by Religious Type

Religious type	Mystical experience		Stress level	
	Affirming	Denying	High	Low
Intrinsic ($n = 46$)	28	3	3	28
IP ($n = 31$)	40	6	31	15
Extrinsic ($n = 39$)	3	36	8	31
IA ($n = 31$)	12	19	18	13

Note. There was an error in the original article: The numbers for mystical experience for the extrinsic group were reversed. All differences were significant at least at $p < .05$ for all groups except the IA group for both mystical experience and stress. Adapted from Hood (1978b, p. 427). Copyright 1978 by the Society for the Scientific Study of Religion. Adapted by permission.

tical experience as measured by the REEM is not only higher among intrinsically oriented persons, but also among religious denominations with strong norms for eliciting and interpreting mystical experiences.

Rosegrant's finding that mystical experiences as measured by the REEM were associated with stress experiences in a solitary nature setting may be misleading. It is unlikely that stress per se should serve to elicit mystical experience. Rather, the incongruity between anticipatory stress and setting stress is postulated to be a likely trigger of mysticism. In a study to test this hypothesis specifically in a nature setting, Hood (1978a) administered Rosegrant's modification of the REEM to 93 males who, as part of the requirements for graduation from a private high school, participated in a week-long outdoors program. One portion of this program entailed having students "solo." Each student was taken alone by Hood into a wilderness area; was issued minimal equipment (a tarp, water, and a mixture of nuts and candy for food); and was then left to spend the night in solitude. Various students were taken out over a five-night period, regardless of weather conditions. As some indication of the power of this experience, 29 of the 93 participants "broke solo," meaning that they returned to camp before dawn. Before each outing, anticipatory stress was measured by having the students fill out a measure of subjective stress. In addition, setting stress was fortuitously varied by the fact that some students soloed on nights when there were strong rain and thunderstorms. Table 10.9 presents the means on the REEM for participants in this exercise, according to anticipatory stress and setting stress conditions. Appropriate statistical tests indicated not only that set–setting incongruity elicited higher REEM scores, but that it made no difference whether the incongruity was between high anticipatory stress and low setting stress or low anticipatory stress and high setting stress. Either incongruity would work.

Subcultural differences in the emphasis upon and support of intense religious experiences should also be reflected in REEM scores. Hood and Hall (1977) had anthropologists select five REEM items deemed "culturally fair" in order to compare four samples. All participants were Catholics and were matched for education, gender, age, and socioeconomic status. The four groups were Native American, acculturated Mexican Americans (spoke English 100% of the time), Mexican Americans (spoke Spanish at least 25% of the time), and European Americans. As hypothesized, the two groups whose subcultures encourage intense experiences (Native Americans, Mexican Americans) had higher REEM scores than either European Americans or acculturated Mexican Americans. The matching on relevant vari-

TABLE 10.9. Mean REEM Scores for Participants under High- and Low-Stress Nature Solo Conditions, According to Anticipatory Stress Levels

Anticipatory stress	Setting stress	
	High	Low
High	32.44 ($SD = 12.75$) ($n = 16$)	52.83 ($SD = 14.72$) ($n = 12$)
Low	51.43 ($SD = 9.37$) ($n = 21$)	42.07 ($SD = 4.95$) ($n = 15$)

Note. Adapted from Hood (1978a, p. 283). Copyright 1978 by the Society for the Scientific Study of Religion. Adapted by permission.

ables suggests that differences in the REEM scores reflect genuine subcultural differences in either the experiences themselves or the reporting of such experiences.

Several investigators have postulated that mystical and other intense religious experiences are related to and perhaps often elicited by hypnotic trance states. For instance, Gibbons and Jarnette (1972) suggest that at least some religious experiences may be trance states induced by stimuli outside awareness. Both historians (Taves, 1999) and anthropologists (Lewis, 1971) have long argued for the similarity between hypnotic and religious ecstatic states. Hood (1973a) found a correlation between the original form of the REEM and the Harvard Group Scale of Hypnotic Susceptibility (Shor & Orne, 1962) of .36 ($p < .01$) in a sample of 81 fundamentalist Protestants willing to be hypnotized. This is consistent with the finding that fundamentalist Protestants who report significant conversion experiences are also hypnotically suggestible (Gibbons & Jarnette, 1962), and with the historical linkage of hypnosis with Protestant conversion experiences in North America (Taves, 1999). Perhaps the loss of sense of self reported in mystical experience parallels the loss of self in hypnotic states. However, we must be careful *not* to equate mysticism and hypnosis on the basis of similar processes that might operate in both.

It is also worth hypothesizing that the wide diversity of triggers or conditions facilitating mystical experiences (as noted in survey and other studies) may have in common the fact that an individual fascinated by any given trigger experiences a momentary loss of sense of self, being "absorbed" or "fascinated" by his or her object of perception. Tellegen and Atkinson (1974) have proposed "absorption," or openness to absorbing and self-altering states, to be a trait related to hypnosis. The only empirical study using both their measure of absorption and a measure of mysticism is a study by Mathes (1982) relating mysticism, absorption, and romantic love. Unfortunately, Mathes did not report the correlation between mysticism and absorption. However, in his study a measure of romantic love (Rubin, 1970) was correlated with mysticism for both males and females. This is consistent with being fascinated or "absorbed" by the object of interest in both experiences. It is also consistent with the fact that both love and sexuality are frequently cited as triggers of mysticism in open-ended questionnaire and survey studies.

The relationship between mysticism and hypnosis has been negatively interpreted, particularly by psychodynamically oriented investigators. Both hypnotic susceptibility and intense religious experiences, especially mystical ones, are interpreted either as regressions to early states of ego development or as signs of weak adult ego development (Allison, 1961; Owens, 1972). Both Hood (1985) and Parsons (1999) have noted that claims to a relationship between weak ego development and religious experience are derived from primarily a priori theoretical commitments of dynamic theorists that not only are conceptually unwarranted, but lack empirical support. In the only direct empirical test of a relationship between weak ego development and intense religious experience, both the conceptual and empirical inadequacies of this hypothesized relationship were demonstrated.

Hood (1974) administered the most psychometrically sophisticated measure of ego strength (Barron's [1953] ego strength scale) to a sample of 82 college students who also took the initial 15-item version of the REEM. Overall, there was a significant negative correlation ($r = -.31$) between the REEM and Barron's scale, appearing to support the claim that intense experience is related to weak ego strength. However, part of the problem is conceptual, in that Barron's scale contains several religiously worded items; these religiously worded items are scored so that agreement indicates weak ego strength. This suggests a conceptual bias against religious experience, so that one can simply assume that many religious beliefs reflect poor ego development and then use them as a measure of weak ego strength. Hood separated Barron's scale into two parts: the religiously worded items and the residual, nonreligiously worded items. Correlating these with the REEM yield markedly different results, as noted in Table 10.10.

Inspection of this table is instructive in two senses. First, negative correlations, supposedly indicating weak ego strength among persons reporting mystical experiences, were found with religiously worded items scored to indicate weak ego strength! This link reveals the conceptual basis of these items, and confounds many supposedly empirical findings. Removing the religious items removed any significant relationship between weak ego strength and religious experience. Furthermore, using a nondynamically oriented measure developed for use in survey research revealed that among a sample of 114 college students, those with higher adequacy in psychological functioning as measured by this index had significantly higher REEM scores than those with lower adequacy as measured by this index.

Thus, not only is there little conceptual or empirical support for the claim that weak ego strength must characterize persons who have intense religious experiences; such persons may be *more* psychologically adequate than those who do not report such experiences. This latter claim is consistent with the normality of the report of mystical and numinous experiences noted in survey studies, and also with theories that are more sympathetic to religion. For instance, Maslow's (1964) popular theory of self actualization postulates that more actualized persons are most likely to have and report "peak experiences" (Maslow's term for mystical and other related experiences). Although his theory has generated little rigorous empirical research to support this claim. it serves as a useful conceptual counter to dynamic theories that postulate a relationship between regression and religious experience, for which there is also little rigorous empirical support.

The Mysticism Scale (M Scale): The Influence of Stace

James was the source for the range of experiences, both numinous and mystical, selected for the REEM. One criticism of the REEM is that while it does contain both numinous and mystical experiences according to the criteria discussed earlier, it is not particularly theory-driven. However, this is not the case with the Mysticism Scale (M Scale). It was developed as a specific operationalization of Stace's (1960) phenomenological work, in which he iden-

TABLE 10.10. Correlations between the REEM and Barron's Total Ego Strength Scale, Religiously Worded Items, and Residual Items

	Nonreligiously worded items	Religiously worded items	REEM
Total ego strength scale	.47*	.93*	−.31*
Religiously worded items		−.46*	−.55*
Nonreligiously worded items			−.16

Note. Adapted from Hood (1974, p. 66). Copyright 1974 by the Society for the Scientific Study of Religion. Adapted by permission.

*p < .01.

tified both introvertive and extrovertive mysticism and their common core. It is commonly employed as the most widely used empirical measure of mysticism (Lukoff & Lu, 1988).

Prior to the development of the M Scale, Stace's criteria of mysticism had influenced assessments in psychedelic research seeking to document the ontological validity of experiences elicited under drugs. Stace's criteria were developed under the assumption of causal indifference. That is, the examples used by Stace were accepted as mystical, whether elicited under drug conditions or not (Stace, 1960, pp. 29–31). Research Box 10.2 presents a summary of, and follow-up data from, what is perhaps the most famous study in the psychology of religion—Pahnke's Good Friday experiment.

Pahnke's original study and Doblin's long-term follow-up are important in demonstrating the effect of set and setting on drug-facilitated mystical experiences, using Stace's explicit criteria. The general discussion of entheogens and religious experience in Chapter 9 obviously applies to this experiment. Yet in terms of this chapter, Pahnke was the first investigator to attempt explicitly to operationalize Stace's criteria of mysticism. His original questionnaire has been variously modified through the years, with many additional, nonmystical items added. However, basic items relating to Stace's core criteria of mystical experience have remained virtually unchanged. The most recent, expanded versions of Pahnke's questionnaire include items relevant to peak experiences. It is clear that the concept of "peak experience" has been broadened to include a wide variety of experiences, only some of which are mystical in Stace's sense of the term. The M scale is explicitly designed to measure Stace's criteria of mysticism—distinct from a wide range of other experiences, including peak experiences.

Common-Core Theorists versus Diversity Theorists.   Given that the M Scale is based upon Stace's demarcation of the phenomenological properties of mysticism, it is also of necessity driven by some of Stace's theoretical concerns. Most central is the fact that Stace has become the central figure in the debate between what we call the "common-core theorists" and the "diversity theorists." Common-core theorists assume that people can differentiate experience from interpretation, such that different interpretations may be applied to otherwise identical experiences. This theory is often characterized by its opponents as if it claims that there is an absolute, unmediated experience. In fact, Stace (1960) and other common-core theorists simply distinguish between degrees of interpretation, arguing that at some level different descriptions can mask quite similar if not identical experiences.

Diversity theorists—led by Katz (1977), who edited an entire volume in response to Stace's work—argue that no unmediated experience is possible, and that in the extreme, language is not simply used to interpret experience but in fact constitutes experience. Proudfoot (1985) is among the contemporary theorists (heavily influenced by psychology) who argue for the role of language in the constitution of, and not simply in the interpretation of, experience.

Just as Katz marshaled a series of scholars in opposition to Stace's common-core thesis, Forman has recently marshaled others in opposition to the diversity position of Katz. In two edited works (Forman, 1990b, 1998), scholars associated with Forman argue that at least with respect to introvertive mystiicsm, the diversity thesis fails. The basic argument is that since introvertive mysticism is an experience devoid of content, it cannot be qualified by various descriptors, nor can language play a role in its construction. Hence introvertive experience (identified as "pure conscious experience" by Forman, 1990a) may be variously interpreted after the fact, but as experience it lacks content. It thus is legitimately as Stace conceptualized it—a common core to mysticism independent of both culture and person—

Research Box 10.2. Drugs and Mysticism: Pahnke's "Good Friday" Experiment (Pahnke, 1966; Doblin, 1991)

In the psychology of religion's most famous and controversial study, Pahnke, as part of his doctoral dissertation, administered the drug psilocybin or a placebo in a double-blind study of 20 volunteers, all graduate students at Andover–Newton Theological Seminary. The subjects met to hear a broadcast of a Good Friday service after they had been given either psilocybin (experimental group) or nicotinic acid (placebo group). Participants met in groups of four, each consisting of two experimental subjects and two controls matched for compatibility. Each group had two leaders assigned, one of whom had been given psilocybin. Immediately after the service and then 6 months later, participants were administered a questionnaire, part of which consisted of Stace's specific common-core criteria of mysticism.

Nearly a quarter of a century later, from November 1986 to October 1989, Doblin contacted the original participants in the experiment. By either phone or personal contact, he was able to interview nine of the control participants and seven of the experimental participants from the original study. In addition, he was able to administer Pahnke's questionnaire to them. Thus we have the responses on Stace's criteria of mysticism immediately after the service, then 6 months later, and finally nearly 25 years later. Assigning each score as the percentage of the possible maximum for that criteria, according to Pahnke's original procedure, yields the following results.

	Original Pahnke study				Doblin follow-up study (nearly 25 years later)	
	Immediate		6 months later			
Stace category	Exptls. ($n = 10$)	Controls ($n = 10$)	Exptls. ($n = 10$)	Controls ($n = 10$)	Exptls. ($n = 7$)	Controls ($n = 9$)
1. Unity:						
a. Internal	70%	8%	60%	5%	77%	5%
b. External	38%	2%	39%	1%	51%	6%
2. Transcendence of space/time	84%	6%	78%	7%	73%	9%
3. Positive affect	57%	23%	54%	23%	56%	21%
4. Sacredness	53%	28%	58%	25%	68%	29%
5. Noetic quality	63%	18%	71%	18%	82%	24%
6. Paradoxicality	61%	13%	34%	3%	48%	4%
7. Ineffability	66%	18%	77%	15%	71%	3%
8. Transience	79%	8%	76%	9%	75%	9%

Note. Our table has been constructed to allow direct comparison between Doblin's percentages and Pahnke's. Terms have been altered to correspond more closely to M Scale terminology where relevant. Some of Pahnke's criteria were not employed by Stace (e.g., transience) and some of Stace's criteria were not employed by Pahnke (e.g., inner subjectivity). Paradoxicality is not assessed by the M Scale. Smith (2000, pp. 99–105) has revealed that in the original study, one experimental subject had a psychological disruptive experience that had to be handled by administration of thorazine—a fact unfortunately not reported in the original description of the study. Exptls., experimental participants.

and has become the basis for constructing what Forman (1998) refers to as a "perennial psychology." Recently, Parsons (1999) has also championed this phrase.

Although we cannot further engage this rich conceptual literature here, we can note that three fundamental assumptions implicit in Stace's work and in that of the common-core or perennialist psychologists should be emphasized. First, the mystical experience is itself a universal experience that is essentially identical in phenomenological terms, despite wide variations in ideological interpretation of the experience (the common-core assumption). Second, the core categories of mystical experience are not all definitionally essential to any particular mystical experience, since there are always borderline cases, based upon fulfillment of only some of the criteria. Third, the introvertive and extrovertive forms of mysticism are most conceptually distinct: The former is an experience of unity devoid of content (pure consciousness), and the latter is an experience of unity in diversity, one with content. The psychometric properties of the M Scale should reflect these assumptions, and insofar as they do, they are adequate operationalizations of Stace's criteria. The question for now is this: Does empirical research support a common-core/perennialist conceptualization of mysticism and its interpretation?

Factor-Analytic Tests of the Common-Core/Perennialist Claim.   The M Scale consists of 32 items (16 positively worded and 16 negatively worded items), covering all but one (paradoxicality) of the original common-core criteria of mysticism proposed by Stace. Independent investigators (Caird, 1988; Reinert & Stifler, 1993) have supported Hood's original work indicating that the M Scale contains two factors. For our purposes, it is important to note that Factor I consists of items assessing an experience of unity (introvertive or extrovertive), while Factor II consists of items referring both to religious and knowledge claims. This is compatible with Stace's claim that a common experience (mystical experience of unity) may be variously interpreted. The factor analysis by Caird (1988) supported the original two-factor solution to the M Scale. Reinert and Stifler (1993) also supported a two-factor solution, but suggested the possibility that religious items and knowledge items might emerge as separate factors. This would split the interpretative factor into religious and other modes of interpretation, which would not be inconsistent with Stace's theory. This would allow for an even greater range of interpretation of experience—a claim to knowledge that can be either religiously or nonreligiously based. This is consistent with the distinction between spirituality and religion, to be discussed later in this chapter. However, the factor-analytic studies cited above were from definitive; notably, they suffered from adequate subject-to-items ratios. Overall, however, they consistently demonstrated two stable factors— one an experience factor associated with minimal interpretation; the other an interpretative factor, probably heavily religiously influenced.

Hood and his colleagues proposed a three-factor solution to the M Scale, based upon a more adequate sample size (Hood, Morris, & Watson, 1993). This three-factor solution fitted Stace's phenomenology of mysticism quite nicely, in that both introvertive and extrovertive mysticism emerged as separate factors, along with a third interpretative factor. Hood and his colleagues then undertook to directly test Stace's common-core theory of mysticism with both exploratory and confirmatory factor-analytic procedures.

A persistent problem with the M Scale is that it attempts to be neutral with respect to religious language. For instance, the scale refers to experience with ultimate reality, not to experience of union with God. However, the language of neutrality is perplexing, as emphasized by the diversity theorists: How do we know that union with God is the same experience as union with ultimate reality? Two issue are empirically relevant.

First, no language is neutral. Hence, to attempt to speak of union with "God" or "Christ" in language that references only "ultimate reality" suggests to some conservative religionists a "New Age" connotation. Likewise, to reference "God" or "Christ" is itself problematic for secularists. Although the distinction between experience and interpretation acknowledges that language is an important interpretative issue, it also forces us to focus upon the experiential basis from which genuine differences in interpretation can arise. Like texts, measurement scales use particular language and thus confound the distinction between interpretation and experience. However, empirical methods are available to suggest how this confound can be clarified. One method is to show similar factor structures despite different language.

Second, individuals demand that profound experiences be interpreted. In Barnard's (1997) extended treatment of James's theory of mysticism, a mystical experience is defined as one that is necessarily "transformative" with respect to contact with some transpersonal reality. Although we do not accept this definition of mysticism as properly Jamesian, it does indicate that intense transformative experiences will be acknowledged in some language that identifies, defines, and expresses what the experienced transpersonal reality is. In Jamesian terms, this language is less constructionist of the experience than descriptive of it. Therefore, those who have experienced "ultimate reality" may not wish to claim it as "God." Even more, Christians may want that reality to be identified as "Christ"—something that non-Christian mystics may eschew. Thus the claim of what is experienced is important as part of the "social construction" of the expression of experience. However, differently expressed experiences may have similar structures if we can avoid confounds with language issues.

Hood and Williamson (2000) created two additional version of the M Scale. Each paralleled the original M Scale, but, where appropriate, made reference either to God or to Christ. Both the original M Scale and either the God-language version or the Christ-language version were given to relevant Christian-committed samples. The scales were then factor-analyzed to see whether similar structures would emerge. Basically, whether the M Scale items were phrased in terms of God, Christ, or more "neutral" words, the structures were identical.

The structures for all three versions matched Stace's phenomenologically derived model quite well. For all versions of the scale, clear introvertive, extrovertive, and interpretative factors emerged. The exception was that, as Hood and Williamson (2000) anticipated, ineffability emerged as part of the introvertive factor in all samples, and not as part of the interpretative factor (as suggested by Stace). However, as Hood and Williamson note, an experience devoid of content is inherently "ineffable," as there is no content to describe.

In additional research, Hood and his colleagues translated the M Scale into Persian and administered this scale to a sample of Iranian Muslims (Hood, Ghorbani, et al., 2001). The scale in its original English version was also administered to a U.S. sample. Confirmatory factor analysis was then used to directly compare Hood's model of mysticism in both samples (with ineffability as part of introvertive mysticism) to other possible models, including Stace's (where ineffability is part of the interpretative factor). The overall results showed that both Stace's and Hood's models were better than any other models, and that Hood's model of mysticism was better than Stace's. Thus, empirically, there is strong support to claim that as operationalized from Stace's criteria, mystical experience is identical as measured across diverse samples, whether expressed in "neutral language" or with either "God" or "Christ" references. Both Stace's and Hood's versions of the basic structure of mysticism emerging from this research are presented in Table 10.11.

Three-factor solutions to the M Scale clearly provide most adequate overall measures of mysticism in terms of compatibility with Stace's theory. Furthermore, Hood's three-

TABLE 10.11. Conceptual (Stace's) and Empirical (Hood's) Models of
Mystical Experience: The Perennialist View

The Stace model of mystical experience—phenomenologically derived

Introvertive Mysticism	*Extrovertive Mysticism*
a. Contentless Unity	a. Unity in Diversity
b. Timeless/Spaceless	b. Inner Subjectivity

Interpretation

a. Noetic
b. Religious
c. Positive Affect
d. Paradoxicality (not measured in M Scale)
e. Ineffability (alleged)

The Hood model of mystical experience—empirically derived

Introvertive Mysticism (12 items)	*Extrovertive Mysticism (8 items)*
a. Contentless Unity items	a. Unity in Diversity items
b. Time/Space items	b. Inner Subjectivity items
c. Ineffability items	

Interpretation (12 items)

a. Noetic items
b. Religious items
c. Positive Affect items

---

factor solution with ineffability as part of introvertive mysticism is clearly the most psycho-metrically adequate. It is preferred for future research. However, for now it seems fair to con-clude that the perennialist view has strong empirical support, insofar as regardless of the lan-guage used in the M Scale, the basic structure of the experience remains constant across diverse samples and cultures. This is a way of stating the perennialist thesis in measurement-based terms.

Correlational and Empirical Research with the M Scale and Other Measures

Most empirical research with the M Scale to date has used the two-factor solution initially reported by Hood, in which introvertive and extrovertive mysticism are not independently measured, forming as they do part of the minimal phenomenological factor (Factor I). Thus the majority of studies of mysticism to date using two-factor solutions do not separately iden-tify differential predictions for introvertive and extrovertive mysticism, but rather merge these two as a single factor expressing experiences of unity (see Hood, 2002b).

The initial publication of the M Scale related it to several other measures. The M Scale might be anticipated to correlate with the REEM, since the latter contains a mixture of items relating to numinous and mystical experiences. However, given the overall religious language (explicit or implicit) in the REEM, it was anticipated that the interpretative factor would cor-relate more strongly with the REEM than the phenomenological factor would. This was the case in a sample of 52 students enrolled at a Protestant religious college in the South: Factor I correlated .34 with the REEM, while Factor II correlated .56 with the REEM (Hood, 1975). It was also found in another sample of 83 college students that Factor I of the M Scale correlated

(−.75) more strongly with a measure of ego permissiveness (Taft, 1970) than did Factor II (−.43) (Hood, 1975). Insofar as Taft's ego permissiveness measure is related to openness to a wide rang of anomalous experiences, including ecstatic emotions, intrinsic arousal, and peak experiences, it is not surprising that Factor I correlated more strongly with this measure than Factor II. The differential correlation of Factors I and II in the two studies is congruent with Stace's theory that experience can be separated from interpretation in varying degrees. Factor I correlates more strongly with measures of experience minimally interpreted, and Factor II with measures of experience more extensively interpreted in religious language.

In Hood's (1975) original report, the M Scale factors correlated with a measure of intrinsic religion in roughly the same magnitude in a sample of 65 fundamentalist college students enrolled in a religious college in the South (I = .68, II = .58), supporting the research noted above linking the REEM and intrinsic religion. Furthermore, if in light of the assumption that intrinsically religious persons are likely to be frequent church attendees, Hood's (1976b) finding that both frequent attendees and nonattendees had similar high scores on Factor I of the M Scale, but only frequent church attendees had high Factor II scores, makes sense in terms of Stace's distinction between experience and interpretation. Both frequent attendees and nonattendees reported mystical experiences in terms of their minimal phenomenological properties of an experience of union, but only frequent church attendees were likely to interpret these experiences in religious terms. The nonattendees did not use traditional religious language to describe their experiences.

Holm (1982) prepared a Swedish translation of the M Scale and administered it to a sample of 122 Swedish informants. Unlike the REEM, the M Scale could be meaningfully translated into Swedish and could be studied similarly to the way it was investigated in North America. Holm not only confirmed a two-factor solution closely paralleling Hood's initial mysticism and interpretation factors, but also found that in correlating the M Scale with ratings of a person's most significant personal experiences, Factor I correlated best with experiences reported by individuals without a Christian profile, while Factor II best related to more traditional Christian experiences. The revised Swedish version of the REEM, using Nordic accounts of intense experiences appropriate to Finnish–Swedish culture, also showed similar patterns to Hood's research with the REEM in North America. Holm (1982) stated.

> We also discovered one factor which could be called a general mysticism factor and another where the experience was interpreted on a religious/Christian basis. The "religious interpretation factor" had strong correspondences with religious quality in the interviews and with the background variables of prayer frequency, Bible study, church attendance and attitude towards Christianity. This factor thus covered experiences with an expressly Christian profile. It showed high correlations with the intrinsic scale, with the expressively Christian narratives on the REEM and with the religious quality on the interviews. Thus, overall, in a Finnish–Swedish culture the M Scale and REEM functioned very closely to how they function in American culture. (p. 273)

Interestingly, Holm also noted that the distinction between a general mysticism factor (or impersonal mysticism) and a religious factor (or personal mysticism) has parallels with early research on mysticism in Sweden by Solderblom, who identified these as "infinity mysticism" and "personality mysticism," respectively (see Holm, 1982, pp. 275–276). This parallels our earlier discussion of the distinction between impersonal and personal aspects of mystical experience, as noted by several investigators.

Although the relationship between the religious factor of the M Scale and the more explicitly religiously worded REEM items is reasonable, the question of more general personality factors related to mysticism is of interest. M Scale scores have been correlated with scores on standardized personality measures in two studies. In one, Hood (1975) found that most scales of the Minnesota Multiphasic Personality Inventory (MMPI), a widely used measure to assess pathology, failed to correlate with the M Scale. Furthermore, differential patterns of significant correlations between Factors I and II were compatible with a nonpathological interpretation of mysticism. For instance, Factor II (but not Factor I) significantly correlated with the Lie (L) scale of the MMPI. This scale presumably measures the tendency to lie or present oneself in a favorable social light. However, insofar as Factor II represents a traditional religious stance, Hood suggested that high L scores for Factor II may represent the fact that traditionally religious individuals are less likely to engage in deviant social behaviors as measured by the L scale. Factor I did significantly correlate with two scales on the MMPI concerned with bodily processes (Hypochondriasis) and intense experiential states (Hysteria), which in nonpathological terms are likely to be compatible with mystical experience.

Possible relationships between absorption or hypnosis, discussed above in connection with the REEM as a measure of religious experience are consistent with the work of Spanos and Moretti (1988). They directly correlated the M Scale with the Tellegen and Atkinson (1974) Absorption scale and with three measures of hypnosis. Overall, the M Scale correlated positively with all these measures. When mysticism was used as the criterion variable, regression analyses using the four hypnosis measures, absorption, and two other variables (neuroticism and psychosomatic symptoms) indicated that absorption was the single best predictor, accounting for 29% of the variance; hypnotic depth was second best, adding a further 5%. None of the other hypnosis scales, or the neuroticism or psychosomatic symptom scales, added predictive power. Spanos and Moretti concluded that although mystical experience can occur among distraught and troubled individuals, it is as frequent among psychologically untroubled people.

A study of the M Scale along with other indices of mysticism is relevant to this issue. Hood and Morris (1981a) took virtually all items used in previous empirical assessments of mysticism and factor-analyzed them into scales, all with adequate reliability. These were then administered to a sample of respondents who rated the items for their applicability to defining mysticism as they understood it. Next, they rated each item as to whether or not they had ever had experienced it. The respondents did not differ in knowledge about mysticism, including whether or not they personally identified themselves as having had a mystical experience. However, persons denying having a mystical experience did not mark items they knew to define mysticism as experiences they had had, whereas those affirming mystical experience did. Thus persons who were equally knowledgeable about mystical experiences differed in whether nor not they marked an item as being experienced as a function of having a mystical experience. This suggests that persons can know what mysticism is and yet not have an experience of it. This further suggests, despite the possibility that both demand characteristics and the abstract nature of many items assessing mysticism may contribute to "false positives" in studies of mysticism (Wulff, 2000), that respondents can be knowledgeable about mysticism and still deny that they have had the experience. Perhaps Scharfstein (1973) is correct in warning that mysticism may be more common than social scientists have heretofore thought. Certainly his claim to an "everyday mysticism" is supported by survey research and by measurement-based studies. It may be that the true fulfillment of mysticism, like love, may be rare, but few also are those who have no experience of it at all.

The report of mystical experience is thus firmly established as a normal phenomenon among healthy individuals—who, if lacking a religious commitment, are unlikely to use traditional religious language to describe the experience, or only reluctantly use it as the only available language to express their experience. However, the fact that mystical experience is a normal phenomenon reported among healthy individuals does not mean that others cannot also report such experience. The only empirical study to date of the M Scale with both disturbed and nondisturbed populations supports this view. Stifler, Greer, Sneck, and Dovenmuehle (1993) administered the M Scale along with other measures to three relevant samples (n = 30 each): psychiatric inpatients meeting formal diagnostic criteria for psychotic disorders; senior members of various contemplative/mystical groups; and hospital staff members (as "normal" controls). Using total M Scale scores, Stifler et al. found that the psychotic and contemplative groups could not be distinguished from one another, but that both differed from the hospital staff controls. Thus both psychotic and contemplative individuals report mystical experiences more often than controls. Although these data are correlational, it is reasonable to assume that mysticism neither causes nor is produced by psychoses. Rather, psychotic individuals, like contemplative persons, can have or report such experiences.

Consistent with research affirming that mysticism is unlikely to be pathological is work on temporal lobe epilepsy, commonly assumed to be associated with reports of mystical and other religious experiences (see Chapter 3). For instance, Persinger (1987) has argued that what he terms the "God experience" is an artifact of changes in temporal lobe activity. However, in a study of 46 outpatients in the Maudsley Epilepsy Clinic, Sensky (1983) found that patients with this type of epilepsy did not have a higher rate of mystical experiences (or general religious experiences) than a control population. By contrast, a study by Persinger and Makarec (1987) found positive correlations between scores on their measure of complex epileptic signs and the report of paranormal and mystical experiences in a sample of 414 university students. Although neither of these studies used the M Scale to measure mystical experience, their findings overall suggest that even if mystical experience is commonly associated with temporal lobe activity, it is no more common in actual patients with such epilepsy than in control populations with normal temporal lobe activity. Hence there is no firm empirical basis from which to assume neurophysiological deficiencies in those reporting mystical experiences. On the contrary, as noted in Chapter 3, the biological basis of religious experience in general and mysticism in particular suggests that, if anything, such experiences are normal. It is also worth emphasizing that despite the identification of neurophysiological processes that facilitate mystical experiences, the neurophysiology does not rule out that such experiences have a basis in reality (d'Aquili & Newberg, 1993, 1999). As Deikman (1966) has said, the unity revealed in mysticism may be the unity of reality.

Triggers of Mystical Experience

Accepting that mystical experience is normal has led some to search for personal and cultural factors that affect what might be appropriate triggers for mystical experiences. Survey research has long established that a variety of triggers can elicit mystical experiences. Although some triggers are consistently reported—prayer; church attendance; significant life events, such as births and deaths; and experiences associated with music, sex, and entheogens—one seeks in vain for a common characteristic shared by such diverse triggers. Empirically, it is more useful to focus upon what triggers function to elicit mystical experience in different persons. Research Box 10.3 presents the results of a study in which the evaluation of experi-

◆

Research Box 10.3. Differential Evaluation of Experiences and Triggers by High- and Low-Dogmatism Persons (Hood, 1980)

Hood was interested in how the evaluation of intense experiences would vary as a function of the identification of triggers among open- and closed-minded persons. From published sources, he selected one true report each of an aesthetic, a mystical, and a religious experience, independently operationalized for equal intensity. These unlabeled experiences were then presented in a booklet along with Rokeach's Dogmatism scale, claimed to be a measure of "open-mindedness." Three versions of the booklet were constructed, so that the experiences described could be described as a result of drugs, prayer, or unspecified factors. The experiences were rated on an evaluative semantic differential scale, with higher scores indicating a more positive evaluation. This part of the study clearly showed that the more normative the experience, the more positively it was viewed, so that religious experiences were evaluated more positively overall. Aesthetic and mystical experiences were evaluated less positively overall than religious ones, but did not differ from each other in valence of evaluation. In addition, as predicted, the more normative the trigger, the more positively it affected the evaluation of the experience. Experiences triggered by prayer were more positively evaluated than those with unspecified triggers. Drug triggers lowered the evaluation of all experiences. These effects were most pronounced for the high-dogmatism persons. The actual mean evaluations for each experience coded by trigger for high- and low-dogmatism groups were as follows. (This table is based upon 93 low- and 93 high-dogmatism subjects; 31 subjects in each group rated the three experiences as triggered by drugs, 31 as triggered by prayer, and 31 as triggered by unspecified factors [none].)

Subjects		Aesthetic experience triggered by			Religious experience triggered by			Mystical experience triggered by		
		Drugs	Prayer	None	Drugs	Prayer	None	Drugs	Prayer	None
High-dogmatism	Mean	53.16	62.65	59.94	55.97	66.68	60.03	47.87	59.87	54.00
	SD	9.4	4.1	8.3	9.6	8.9	9.3	12.3	9.5	10.7
Low-dogmatism	Mean	51.988	61.32	57.86	54.50	62.10	59.61	48.02	57.45	53.65
	SD	9.9	7.3	9.0	8.7	8.1	8.6	11.4	9.7	10.7

Note. From Hood (1980). Copyright 1980 by the Religious Research Association. Adapted by permission.

ence was shown to be a function (1) of the normative legitimacy of the trigger, (2) of the experience, and (3) of the alleged open-mindedness of respondents.

Sex and eroticism are often cited as triggers of mystical experience. Consistent with the vast conceptual literature relating mysticism and eroticism (Kripal, 2001), Hood and Hall (1980) hypothesized that individuals would use similar gender-based descriptions to describe both mystical and erotic experiences. Open-ended descriptions of mystical and erotic experiences by both males and females were coded for the use of active, agentive language or receptive language. As predicted, females used receptive terms to describe both their erotic and mystical experiences. However, while males used agentive language to describe their sexual experiences, they did not describe their mystical experiences in such terms. Rating their mystical and erotic experiences on words independently established to be either agentive or receptive also showed that females described both erotic and mystical experiences in receptive terms, but that males described only their sexual experiences in agentive terms. The researchers have suggested that the compatibility of erotic and mystical experiences for females is aided by the masculine imagery common in the Christian tradition, which facilities congruent expression of eroticism and mysticism for females but inhibits it for males. Consistent with this claim is a study by Mercer and Durham (1999), who found scores on the M Scale to be significantly correlated with scores on a measure of gender orientation; specifically, persons with female and androgynous orientations had higher M Scale scores than persons with masculine orientations. Mercer and Durham suggest that persons scoring high on the M Scale are those who have developed a feminine self-schema (cognitive structure), through which they process data in a way that facilitates the unity of reality and facilitation of mystical experiences. Similar arguments have been made within the conceptual literature on mysticism (Kripal, 2001).

Rather than focusing upon particular concrete triggers, Hood has argued that more abstract conceptualization may permit a more empirically adequate investigation of conditions and circumstances that trigger mystical experience. In particular, theological and philosophical interest in the concept of "limits" is useful (Grossman, 1975). At the conceptual level, the idea of limits entails transcendence; in fact, awareness of limits makes the experience of transcendence possible. Perhaps the sudden contrast that occurs when a limit is suddenly transcended yields a contrast effect similar to a figure–ground reversal, in which what was previously unnoticed is thrown into stark relief. Hood (1977) has noted that such sudden contrasts are common in nature settings, particularly those in which stress is involved. The fact that nature is a common trigger of mystical experiences is well documented in survey studies, and often such experiences are associated with stress, which is itself sometimes cited as a trigger. In one study described earlier, the set–setting incongruity hypothesis was supported when the REEM was used as a measure. It has also been supported in research using the M Scale.

Hood (1977) took advantage of a week-long outdoors program at a private all-male high school. In a week-long program, graduating seniors took a trip in which they engaged in a variety of outdoor activities varying in degree of stress. Three particularly stressful activities were examined: rock climbing and rappelling (for the first time, for many students); whitewater rafting (down a river rated as difficult); and the experience (described earlier in this chapter) of staying alone in the woods at night with minimal equipment). A nonstressful activity (canoeing a calm river) was selected as a control. Just prior to participating in each activity, participants were administered a measure of subjective, anticipatory stress for that activity. Immediately after each activity, the participants completed the M Scale, to assess mystical experience. The comparisons between set and setting stress for each high-stress activity supported the hypothesis that the interaction between these two types of stress elicits reports of mystical experience. It is important to note that anticipatory stress varied across situations, such that whether or not a particular person anticipated a given situation as stressful was not simply a function of its independently assessed situation stress. Second, in stressful situations, those anticipating low stress scored higher on mysticism than those anticipating high stress. Thus set–setting stress incongruity elicited reports of mystical experience—not simply stress per se, either anticipatory or situational. Additional support for this hypothesis was found by using the canoe activity as a control; no student anticipated this activity to be stressful. Given the congruity between anticipated stress and setting stress (both low), low M Scale scores resulted, as predicted. However, in high-stress activities anticipated as high in stress, low M Scale scores were also hypothesized and obtained. Only the incongruity between setting and anticipatory stress produced high M Scale scores. Furthermore, with only one exception, these results held for both Factor I and Factor II scores; this suggested not only that the minimal phenomenological properties of mysticism were elicited, but also that they were seen as religiously relevant in the broad sense of this term. This replicates the findings discussed above with solo experiences in a nature setting when the REEM was used as a measure. Thus it would appear that anticipatory and setting stress incongruities can elicit both mystical experiences of unity (M Scale) and more numinous religious experiences (REEM) in nature.

The fact that both nature and prayer settings reliably elicit reports of mystical experience in traditionally religious persons has led some to suggest that prayer should be correlated with the report of mystical experience, particularly if the prayer is contemplative in nature. Hood and his colleagues have documented such a correlation in two separate studies, using a modified form of the M Scale (Hood, Morris, & Watson, 1987, 1989). They found that among persons who prayed or meditated regularly, intrinsically religious persons had higher M Scale scores than extrinsically religious persons, in terms of both the minimal phenomenological properties of mysticism and its religious interpretation. This finding is consistent with survey research by Poloma and Gallup (1991), in which meditative prayer was related to experiences of closeness to God. Thus several studies suggest that meditative prayer, as opposed to petitionary or other forms of prayer, relates to both mystical (unity) and numinous (nearness) experiences of God. Finney and Malony (1985c) have developed a theoretical model in which contemplative prayer should be a useful adjunct in psychotherapy when spiritual development is a treatment goal, and therapeutic progress should be associated with greater mystical awareness. However, they failed to find empirical support for their theory when mysticism as measured by the M Scale did not increase during successful therapy aimed at spiritual development, even though time spent in contemplative prayer did increase (Finney & Malony, 1985b).

Mystical experiences are common in nature and meditative prayer, both often solitary conditions. Hence factors that meaningfully enhance solitude may facilitate the report of mystical experience. Experimentally, it is possible to enhance solitude through the use of an isolation tank. If a religious set is given in an isolation tank, would the combination of set and enhanced isolation facilitate the report of mystical experience? Research Box 10.4 reports a study in which Hood and his colleagues explored this question.

Overall, then, studies (mostly employing the M Scale) have been successful in correlating mysticism with predicted variables of theoretical significance. Quasi-experimental studies involving efforts to elicit mystical experience have also produced useful results. It is simply not true that mystical experiences cannot be elicited under experimental or quasi-experimental conditions. Of course, we make no claim that investigators have caused such experiences—only that they have produced conditions under which such experiences are likely to occur.

TOWARD A THEORY OF MYSTICISM: RELIGIOUS AND SPIRITUAL

The rather substantial body of conceptual and empirical literature on mysticism has not yielded any coherent theory that has been accepted by more than a few investigators. Perhaps consistent with Chapter 3 are neurophysiological theories of mysticism. As Wulff (2000) concludes, his own survey of research on mysticism suggests that some fundamental internal mechanism is operating. Yet Wulff also notes the methodological issue raised by the fact

---   ❧   ---

Research Box 10.4. The Differential Elicitation of Mystical Experience in an Isolation Tank (Hood, Morris, & Watson, 1990)

Solitude is often cited as one trigger of religious and mystical experiences. Hood and his colleagues placed individuals in a sensory isolation tank to maximize solitude. The tank was approximately 7.5 feet in diameter and 4 feet high. It contained a hydrated magnesium sulfate solution with a density of 1.30 grams/cc, a constant temperature of 34.1°C, and a depth of 10 inches. The tank was totally enclosed, lightproof, and soundproof. It was equipped with an intercom system so that a participant could communicate with an experimenter in another room.

Each participant in the study was placed in the isolation tank after being told about the typical images likely to occur under these conditions. In addition, participants were given a specific religious set (in boldface) or nonreligious control set (italics) as follows:

> I am now going to invite you to keep silent for a period of ten minutes. First you will try to attain silence, as total silence as possible of heart and mind. Having attained it, you will expose yourself to whatever (**religious revelation**/*insight*) it brings.[a]

Participants had previously taken the Allport religious orientation scales and could be classified as intrinsic, extrinsic, and "indiscriminately pro" (IP) individuals. A modified version of the M Scale was used that allowed a simple "yes" or "no " response to each item, so that the participants could respond over the intercom while still in the isolation tank. Results were as predicted: Under the religious set, both intrinsic and IP participants reported more religious interpretation of their experiences (higher Factor II scores) than extrinsic participants. However, the IP participants reported less minimal phenomenological properties of mysticism (lower Factor I scores) than either the intrinsic or the extrinsic participants. This suggests that IP participants wished to "appear" religious by affirming religious experiences they did not actually have. Extrinsic participants had these experiences, as indicated by their Factor I scores, but did not describe them in religious language. Intrinsic participants both had the experiences and described them in religious language.

Further support for these views was evident in the control conditions. When participants were not presented with a religious set, none of the groups differed in the minimal phenomenological properties of mysticism (Factor I). However, intrinsic persons still interpreted their experiences in religious terms (Factor II), whereas neither extrinsic nor IP persons described their experiences in religious language in the control condition. Thus the isolation tank elicited similar experiences in subjects of all religious types. The difference in Factor II under set conditions for the types suggests that intrinsic persons consistently interpreted their tank experiences as religious; extrinsic persons consistently interpreted their tank experiences as less religious; and IP persons only interpreted their tank experiences as religious when given an explicit religious set.

[a]These instructions were adapted from those used by de Mello (1984) in his study of prayer.

that it is not uncommon for investigators who were originally neutral about mysticism to become convinced of its reality as other than a merely subjective state, and to seek out explanations compatible with the ontological assertions of the experience. William James followed this path (Hood, 2000, 2002b), and insofar as mystical experiences are noetic, perhaps so should we. Thus we end this chapter with a theory of mysticism that is not linked to proposed internal mechanisms, but to Deikman's (1966) claim noted previously that the unity of the mystical experience may in fact be a unity that is objectively real. However, our theory, rooted in the pioneering but neglected work of Troeltsch's (1931) description of two types of mysticism, remains neutral with respect to theological or cosmological claims to the reality experienced as unity. Nevertheless, it is rooted in historical processes that facilitated the emergence of mystics as independent types, and is consistent with the empirical data on mysticism, religion, and spirituality.

Mysticism within and outside Religious Traditions: The Emergence of "Mystics"

Both Bouyer (1980) and Smith (1977) note that the word "mysticism" comes from the Greek and derives its meaning from the verb "to close." Applied initially to the very specific Greek mystery rites whose rituals were secret or "closed" to outsiders, the term gradually evolved to refer simply to any knowledge that is enigmatic (Bouyer, 1980, p. 44). The term has a distinct history within Christianity, emerging in three distinct transformative stages. Bouyer identifies these stages as "Biblical," "liturgical," and "spiritual."

Only later in its history has the term come to mean a particular experience—what Bouyer has described as an "ineffable mode of experimental knowledge of divine things" (1980, p. 51). It is important to note that "mystical experience" was formerly not thought to be psychologically illuminated by a mere subjectivity, but was viewed as an experience grounded in what is ontologically "real" in terms of the objective description of Biblical truth that also inspired all Christian liturgy. Smith (1977) suggests that the derivation from the pagan rites came to mean the closing of the mind to all external things (i.e., all things not of divine illumination). The crucial point for our empirical concerns is that whatever the focus upon mystical experience may have been, it was contextually dependent upon claims for it as the objective realization of a truth less ineffable than that contained in sacred texts and expressed in sacred liturgy. Thus, as Katz (1983) has argued, mysticism is often conservative—expressing itself with a tradition, not standing outside and opposed to it. Furthermore, empirical studies suggest that mystical experiences interpreted within a tradition have the most meaning and transformative power (Deikman, 1966; Ruffing, 2001; Wittberg, 1996).

As McGinn (1991) has noted, self-identified "mystics" are a more recent historical phenomenon. It thus behooves social scientists to develop a theory of how mysticism became divorced from specific faith traditions. The separation, while never complete, suggests a tension that mystics in the third ("spiritual") sense of Bouyer's classification have always faced within their traditions. It also serves as an umbrella under which the contemporary debate over religion and spirituality can be meaningfully covered.

The Religion–Spirituality Debate in Relation to Mysticism

Recently, as we have discussed in Chapters 1 and 2, this tension has been best captured in the social science literature by the comparison and contrast between two terms—"religion" and "spirituality" (Pargament, 1999). For some, "religion" has become a term that identifies institutional aspects of a faith tradition. This includes beliefs and rituals adhered to and practiced, but seen by some people as devoid of an "inner, experiential dimension." For these people, the preferred term is "spirituality." Wulff (1997) claims that the "new spirituality" employs an emergent model of a journey or quest whose goal is the realization of some innate capacity, variously conceived. He rightly notes that this model has deep roots in historical faith traditions. He states with reference to the Christian tradition, "Indeed, the classic Christian mystics would find every element in the model familiar" (Wulff, 1997, p. 7). He further notes that the shift from "religious" to "spiritual" is simply the focus upon inner processes emphasized by the latter rather than the former term. He goes on to assert that what is "conspicuously new" in contemporary spirituality is the lack of an explicit transcendent object outside the self (Wulff, 1997, p. 7). Here, of course, are serious ontological issues not to be avoided (Deikmann, 1966; Hood, 2002b; Parsons, 1999). However, our focus here is upon a theory to account for the emergence of spirituality within the framework of a larger theory of mysticism.

Pargament (1999, p. 7) has argued that discussions and studies of spirituality lack theoretical grounding—something that is desperately needed. Although there are some interesting efforts underway to develop theoretically grounded views of spirituality (Helminiak, 1998), our intent is to develop a theory that is grounded in historical facts and can frame the empirical data.

Troeltsch's Model: Church, Sect, and Two Types of Mysticism

Troeltsch's theory, as developed in *The Social Teaching of the Christian Churches* (1931), is explored in Chapter 12 in terms of the distinction between church and sect. However, Troeltsch was clearly using an expanded typology derived from Weber, in which besides church and sect as forms of religious organization, he identified a third type—mysticism. Ironically, Troeltsch was popularized among North American scholars by H. R. Niebuhr, especially in his *The Social Sources of Denominationalism* (first published in 1929 and thus antedating the English translation of Troeltsch's text by 2 years). Niebuhr dropped Troeltsch's third type, mysticism, so that subsequent theorizing and empirical research on church–sect theory has largely ignored mysticism. The reasons for this are in dispute, but it is clear that neither Niebuhr nor Troeltsch thought fondly of mysticism and that neither saw it as characteristic of the North American religious landscape (Garrett, 1975; Steeman, 1975). Whatever the reason, as Garrett (1975, p. 205) has noted, mysticism has experienced "wholehearted neglect" at the hands of sociological investigators. Among psychologists, the wholehearted neglect is of a historically grounded theory. Thus, if sociologists have a relevant theory, psychologists have the relevant data—many of which have been presented above. In the remainder of this chapter, we develop a general theory of mysticism that incorporates two mysticisms—that of the church and of what Parsons (1999, p. 141) has called "unchurched mysticism."

According to both Bouyer (1980) and Troeltsch (1931), one form of mysticism is an inherent tendency to seek personal piety and an emotional realization of a faith within the individual; it serves simply to intensify commitment to a tradition. Only when mysticism emerges as an independent religious principle—as a reaction to the church and the sect form—does it become a new social force and seek an independent philosophical (today, psychological!) justification. These two forms of mysticism must be clearly distinguished—something social scientists have failed to do even when acknowledging Troeltsch's mysticism. Garrett (1975, pp. 214–215) simply identifies these two forms as M_1 and M_2.

In the widest sense, mysticism is simply a demand for an inward appropriation of a direct inward and present religious experience (Troeltsch, 1931, p. 730). It takes the objective characteristics of its tradition for granted, and either supplements them with a profound inwardness or reacts against them as it demands to bring them back "into the living process" (Troeltsch, 1931, p. 731). This is Garrett's M_1 or Troeltsch's "wider mysticism. " We identify this as "religious mysticism" for two reasons. It is a mysticism that, according to both Troeltsch (1931, p. 732) and Bouyer (1980, p. 51), is found within all religious systems as a universal phenomenon. Thus, as an empirical fact, it entered Christianity partly from *within* (insofar as Christianity entails the same logical form as all traditions relative to this type) and partly from *without* (from other sources that were "eagerly accepted" by Christianity) (Troeltsch, 1931). Concentrating among the purely interior and emotional side of religious experience, it creates a "spiritual" interpretation of every objective side of religion, so that mystics typically stay within their tradition (Katz, 1983).

However, Troeltsch also identifies a "narrower, technically concentrated sense" of mysticism (1931, p. 734). This is Garrett's M_2. It is a mysticism that has become independent in principle from, and is contrasted with, religion. It gives rise to "spiritual religion." It claims to be the true inner principle of all religious faith. This we refer to as "spiritual mysticism," but the term "spiritual" is redundant. This type of mysticism breaks away from religion, which it disdains. It accepts no constraint or community other than ones that are self-selected and self-realized. It is a "spiritual religion," with the term "religion" as redundant here as "spiritual" is above. It is the basis of what Forman (1998) and Parsons (1999) identify as a "perennial psychology" rooted in mysticism that now allows one to be identified as a mystic, rather than as a Buddhist, Catholic, or Jew. It is what many today profess to be "spirituality" as opposed to "religion."

Research on Distinctions between Religiousness and Spirituality

Kenneth Pargament and his students have taken the lead in descriptive and correlational work identifying distinctions between religious and spiritual self-identification (Zinnbauer et al., 1997). One motivation for Zinnbauer et al.'s study, to paraphrase part of the title of the article in which these data are presented, was to "unfuzzy the fuzzy" (a phrase first coined by Spilka). In an essentially forced-choice procedure, participants were asked to endorse one of the following five options:

1. Religiousness and spirituality overlap, but they are not the same concept.
2. Spirituality is a broader concept than religiousness, and includes religiousness.
3. Religiousness is a broader concept than spirituality and includes spirituality.
4. Religiousness and spirituality are the same concept and overlap completely.
5. Religiousness and spirituality are different and do not overlap.

In addition, participants rated themselves on spirituality and religion on a 5-point scale. Participants also identified themselves as either "religious," "spiritual," "both," or "neither," again in a forced-choice context. Finally, a content analysis was performed on each participant's personal definitions of religiousness and spirituality.

Data were solicited from 11 different small convenience samples, ranging from "conservative Christian college students" to "New Age groups. " Most of the 364 participants were either college students or members of some religious group. Exceptions included a small sample of residents of a nursing home ($n = 20$) and of mental health workers ($n = 27$). Over-all, 78% of participants identified themselves as "religious," while 93% identified themselves as "spiritual." It is worth noting that in both Roof's (1993, 1999) research on "baby boomers" (see Research Box 10.5, below) and the Zinnbauer et al. (1997) study, most religious persons considered themselves to be spiritual (74% in the latter study). Overall, few of Zinnbauer et al.'s participants thought religiousness and spirituality to be identical concepts (2.6%) or entirely nonoverlapping concepts (6.7%). Thus, for most, religiousness and spirituality were somehow and variously intertwined. Nearly identical percentages identified themselves as religious but not spiritual (4%) or as neither (3%); all we need note is that very few people considered themselves religious but not spiritual. Hence, for most participants, religion was inherently involved with spirituality.

Zinnbauer et al.'s content analysis for personal definitions of spirituality and religiousness revealed a fact consistent with our discussion of the interview data above: Namely, the most common categories for spirituality were experiential, while those for religion were belief-based. This is consistent with Day's (1994) distinction, found in his interview with Sandy and with other Sierra Project participants (see Research Box 10.6, below). It was also found that for *all* groups, self-rated spirituality equaled or exceeded self-rated religiousness. Not surprisingly, the greatest differences between self-ratings were found among participants who were members of religious groups distant from traditional expressions of faith, such as "New Age groups" and Unitarians. Although members of more traditional faiths might differ in levels of self-rated religiousness and spirituality, within specific groups such as Roman Catholics there was no significant difference, whereas among "New Age groups" self-rated spirituality greatly exceeded self-rated religiousness. Furthermore, consistent with Roof's (1993, 1999) perceptive observation, more conservative religious groups made less distinction between spirituality and religiousness (Zinnbauer et al., 1997).

These data are congruent with previous empirical work. In particular, the finding that mental health workers are more "spiritual" than "religious" replicates previous work on mental health professionals. Shafranske (1996) has reviewed the empirical research on the religious beliefs, associations, and practices of such professionals. Focusing primarily on samples of clinical and counseling psychologists who are members of the American Psychological Association, Shafranske notes that psychologists are less likely to believe in a personal God, or to affiliate with religious groups, than other professionals or the general population. In addition, while the *majority* of psychologists report that spirituality is important to them, a *minority* report that religion is important to them (Shafranske, 1996, p. 153). Shafranske summarizes his own data and the work of others to emphasize that psychologists are more like the general population than was previously assumed. However, Shafranske (1996, p. 154) lumps together various indices as the "religious dimension," and this is very misleading. In fact, psychologists neither believe, practice, nor associate with the institutional aspects of faith ("religion") as much as they endorse what Shafranske properly notes are "noninstitutional forms of spirituality" (1996, p. 154). One could predict that in forced-choice contexts they would be most likely to be "spiritual" but not "religious." Empirically, three facts about religious and spiritual self-identification ought to be kept quite clear.

First, most persons identify themselves as *both* religious and spiritual. These are largely persons sampled from within faith traditions, for whom it is reasonable to assume that spirituality is at least one expression of and motivation for their religion (e.g., institutional participation). Hence many measures of spirituality simply operate like measures of religion (Gorsuch & Miller, 1999).

Second, a significant minority of individuals use spirituality as a means of at least partly refuting or even ridiculing religion. This is particularly obvious in qualitative studies, where individuals identify their spirituality in defiant opposition to religion. They actually oppose various aspects of institutional religion, such as its authority, its more specific ("closed") articulation of beliefs ("dogma"), and its practices ("ritual"); they seek to move away from religion in order to become "more developed" spiritually. The move is from belief to experience, as Day (1994) perceptively notes.

Third, religiousness and spirituality overlap considerably, at least in North American populations. The majority of the U.S. population in particular is religious *and* spiritual, in terms of both self-identification and self-representations. Exceptions are easy to identify, but one ought not to lose sight of the fact that they are *exceptions.* Significantly, they include not only scientists in general, but psychologists in particular (Beit-Hallahmi. 1977; Shafranske, 1996). Among these people, a hostility to religion as thwarting or even falsifying spirituality is evident. This hostility is readily revealed in qualitative studies in which there is some degree of rapport between interviewer and respondents. One sociological study—Roof's research on baby boomers, which has already been discussed to some extent in Chapter 6—is presented in Research Box 10.5.

Research Box 10.5. Qualitative Sociological Study of Religion versus Spirituality (Roof, 1993, 1999)

Roof (1993) has characterized the 76 million U.S. adults born in the two decades after World War II as a "generation of seekers" who are either "loyalists" (those who have stayed with their religious tradition), "returnees" (those who experimented with options before returning to their religious tradition), or "dropouts" (those who have left their tradition). Roof (1993) noted that a distinguishing feature among the "highly active seekers" he interviewed was a preference to identify themselves as "spiritual" rather than "religious." Twenty-four percent of these had no religious affiliation. Such highly active seekers were but a minority (9%) of all Roof's participants, but they seem to have captured the interest of researchers in what we might identify as the "spiritual turn" in the scientific study of religion. Roof's (1999) follow-up text reveals similar findings regarding self-identification. Asking, "Do your consider yourself religious?" and "Do you consider yourself spiritual?" in nonconsecutive places in open-ended interviews (but always in that order) revealed an overall weak association between the two identifications (gamma = .291). However, among "strong believers" the association was higher (gamma = .439) than among "highly active seekers" (gamma = .196). Other data, including the question "Which is best: to follow the teachings of a church, synagogue or temple, or to think for oneself in matters of religion and trust more one's own experience?" (Roof, 1999, pp. 320–321), suggested that those identified as seekers were least likely to rely upon institutional authority or to think that such authority should overrule their own conscience. An Asian American participant who was no longer active in the Methodist Church captured what we are suggesting well: "You can be spiritual without being religious. I think religious . . . would be more specific. The faith is more specific, certain doctrines. Spiritual would be general, wider. I think that's how you can be spiritual without being religious. Maybe even religious without being spiritual. Show up for church and go through the motions" (Roof, 1993, p. 78).

The emergence of the discussion of spirituality among psychologists of religion parallels sociological concern with a vocal minority of highly active seekers whose spirituality is most typically identified as mystical (Bellah, Marsden, Sullivan, Swidler, & Tipton, 1996; Roof, 1993, 1999). A qualitative psychological study is presented in Research Box 10.6.

Empirical support for qualitative studies that have identified a minority of persons intensely opposed to religion while identifying themselves as spiritual is readily available. For instance, Zinnbauer et al. (1997, p. 553) used a modified form of Hood's M Scale (unity items only) and found that in their overall sample, self-rated religiousness did not correlate with mystical experience ($r = -.04$), but self-rated spirituality did ($r = .27, p < .001$). Furthermore, there was a significant difference between the mean mysticism scores for the "equally spiritual and religious" group and the "spiritual but not religious" group, with the latter scoring significantly higher. The percentages of self-identification into groups ("neither religious nor spiritual,") "religious but not spiritual," "spiritual but not religious," and "equally religious and spiritual" in Hood's data reasonably parallel Zinnbauer et al.'s (1997) data for mainstream college students. The scores on the M Scale, as well as the group comparisons, are also consistent with Zinnbauer et al.'s data. However, use of the complete M Scale provides

---

ॐ

Research Box 10.6. A Qualitative Psychological Study of Religion versus Spirituality (Day, 1994)

The Sierra Project, which was specifically designed to advance students' stages of moral development, began with the 1979 class at the University of California–Irvine. A crucial aspect of this study (and its continuation since 1987 by researchers associated with Boston University) is the use of both traditional empirical and narrative-based qualitative methodologies (see Day, 1991, 1994; Whiteley & Loxley, 1980). Day (1994) reported the results of in-depth interviews with three Sierra participants chosen by the Boston research team after listening to hundreds of hours of audiotaped interviews. Day wrote up the results of an interview with one participant, "Sandy," in an idiographic presentation rare in psychology.

The interview probed Sandy's views on both religion and spirituality—a tactic based upon researchers' belated recognition that earlier Sierra participants might have purposefully avoided discussion of religion, especially religious beliefs (Day, 1994, p. 160). Thus questions on religion and spirituality were strategically placed within the schedule on subsequent interviews.

Sandy took great care to distinguish religion from spirituality. In her words, "Religion is organized, dogmatic, and social. Spiritual is individual, intimate, personal. Religion tells you what is good or true and tells you who is favored and who is not. It operates in fixed categories. Spirituality is developed. You have to work hard at it and to be conscious about it and take time for it. Sometimes, in order to grow spiritually, you have to go beyond or even against religious doctrine" (Day, 1994, p. 163). Sandy's concern with doctrine was important. Day noted that she would probably protest if identified as a "believer." She neither identified herself nor wanted others to label her as "religious" (Day, 1994, p. 165).

further clarification. As with Zinnbauer et al.'s data, the means for the two experiential factors were greater for the "spiritual but not religious" group than for the "equally spiritual and religious" group. However, the difference was not significant for the introvertive factor (one that is quite compatible with classical Christianity), but it was significant the extrovertive factor (an experience less traditional within Christianity) (see Hood, 1985). The truly significant difference lay between the "spiritual but not religious" and "equally spiritual and religious" groups on the one hand, and the "religious but not spiritual" and "neither" groups on the other. A crucial point, consistent with previous research, was that both "spiritual-only" and "equally religious and spiritual" persons reported mystical experience more often than "religious-only" or "nonreligious" persons. Also important was that on the interpretative factor, the "equally religious and spiritual" group scored higher than the "spiritual but not religious" group; again, however, the real difference was between these two groups and the "religious but not spiritual" and the "neither" groups.

Thus we can summarize these data by stating that mystical experience ("spirituality") is commonly reported by individuals who identify themselves as spiritual rather than religious, and by those who identify themselves as equally religious and spiritual. In other words, there is a mysticism ("spirituality") both within and outside of religious traditions. This ought not to surprise us. As noted earlier, Katz (1983) reminds us that most mystics, even when struggling against their faith tradition, stay within it. Religious mysticism is inherently conservative in this limited sense. For most religious people, belief serves to adequately express their mystical experiences, and their religious rituals facilitate them (Hood, 1995a). But for some "independent" mystics, spirituality is only constrained and choked by belief. These independent mystics are those who consider themselves spiritual but not religious.

Hood (2003) has reviewed several empirical studies using various indices of mysticism. Overall, a clear pattern emerges: Spirituality is more closely identified with mystical experience, whereas religion is more closely identified with a specific religious interpretation of this experience. Thus the current debate on religiousness and spirituality is really neither new nor theoretically unexpected. It has been more than three decades since Vernon (1968) noted that those who answered "none" to questions of religious preference were ignored in the scientific study of religion. He argued that perhaps a parallel could be drawn to those in political surveys who identify themselves as "independents." Such person, he noted, are not without political convictions (1968, p. 223). "Spiritual but not religious" persons, or "nones," are perhaps religious independents, paralleling political independents. In response to the question "Have you ever had a feeling that you were somehow in the presence of God?", Vernon found that those who rejected membership in formal religious groups (the "nones") answered either "sure" (5.9%) or "I think so" (20%). Thus 26% of the "nones" nevertheless thought or were sure they had had an experience of God. This percentage closely matches survey reports of mystical experience across a wide range of populations, religious and otherwise, as discussed above. They are also congruent with psychological research indicating that "nones" often score higher on measures of the minimal phenomenological properties of the experience than on the religious interpretation of the experience (Morris & Hood, 1980). Vernon also noted the problem that his religious "nones" had with using religious language to describe mystical experiences. So there is not simply the finding of spirituality emerging in opposition to religion, but the persistent failure by social scientists of religion to study the experiences of those who do not primarily identify themselves as religious. If these people are more willing to identify themselves as "spiritual" than as "religious," it has been a social-scientific oversight to think that they have nothing to do with "religion."

OVERVIEW

Clearly, mystical experience remains a central concern for those who would link the conceptual and empirical literatures on religious experience. The mystical and the numinous remain contenders for the unique in religion. They also provide an experiential basis that may require serious attention to the ontological claims of those who have such experiences. McClenon (1990) has argued that the uniformity in the reporting of a wide range of anomalous experiences suggests that cultural determination of these interpretations may account for less variance than many suppose. We have discussed many examples of such experiences in Chapter 9. Similar arguments apply to numinous and mystical experiences. Although social scientists may not offer "proofs" for such claims, neither can they without hubris deny the possibility that religion contains truths. Indeed, such truths may be as necessary for the experience as the more restricted claim that the *belief* in such truths is necessary. Few persons have such experiences without believing in their possibility in advance or becoming converted to their truth after the fact.

Research on mystical experiences is best approached in terms of what each methodology can contribute. The descriptive material of open-ended and qualitative studies enhances the narrowness and precision of survey research. Yet both methods have revealed similar triggers and consequences of these experiences, and both methods have confirmed the normality of their occurrence. Survey research provides correlations and patterns suggestive for laboratory and quasi-experimental studies, which in turn have shown that mystical experience can be facilitated and follows patterns compatible with the results from open-ended and survey research. All these are then given various conceptual alternatives by the theological and philosophical and historical literature.

If there is any picture to be suggested at this point, it must be sketched in broad lines. Yet even this picture is helpful. Mysticism is a normal phenomenon, reported by healthy and functioning persons who struggle to find a meaningful framework within which to live out this experience as foundational—as at least what is real for them, if not in some sense as the ultimate "Real." Mysticism, real or Real, has proven itself susceptible to empirical investigation. Clearly, much remains to be done. Future progress will surely be interdisciplinary. Even if McGinn (1991, p. 343) is correct in his fear that an empirical reading of mystical texts from a psychological perspective has only an "ambiguous contribution" to make, he is correct in noting that psychological investigators and those involved in studying the history and theory of mysticism must cooperate in what to date is an "unrealized conversation."

Chapter 11

CONVERSION

Riding home with a friend that evening in the back seat of a car, I
listened incredulously as my companions spoke glowingly about the
message that they had just received. In fact, they were so moved by
the guru's words that they made tentative plans to return the next
day to pay homage to him by kissing his feet. I was flabergasted,
stunned. How could anybody have thought this guy was a spiritual
master?

There are two lives, the natural and the spiritual, and we must lose
the one before we can participate in the other.

He was down and out, the Catholics took him in and before he
knew it, he had faith. So it was gratitude that decided the issue most
likely.

But the Muslim believes that the propositional tenets of his faith are
self-evident if they are properly presented and understood, and the
focus of his proselytization is the proclamation of these tenets rather
than the experiences of human beings.

All conversions (even Saul's on the road to Damascus) are mediated
through people, institutions, communities, and groups.

And Priests in black gowns were walking their rounds,
And binding with briars my joys & desires.[1]

In the early months of 1881, G. Stanley Hall delivered a series of public lectures at Harvard
University. His topic was religious conversion, and much of the material he covered was later
incorporated into his classic two-volume study of adolescence (Hall, 1904). The young science of psychology was courageous enough to tackle some of the most profound and meaningful religious phenomena of the times. Because the emerging psychology was linked in the
popular mind with religious and parapsychological phenomena (Coon, 1992), some of the
first North American psychologists divided along lines claiming to debunk or support such
phenomena (Hood, 1994). Hall eventually went on to write a two-volume treatise with the
title *Jesus, the Christ, in Light of Psychology* (1917). The title reveals the Christian bias of the
emerging science of psychology: When they said "religion," most psychologists meant Christianity. Furthermore, when they said "Christianity," most psychologists meant Protestant-

---

1. These quotations come, respectively, from the following sources: Kent (2001, p. xvi); James (1902/1985,
p. 139); Kundera (1983, p. 308); Poston (1992, p. 158); Rambo (1993, p. 1); and Blake (1789/1967, Plate 44).

ism. Thus, not surprisingly, the North American psychology of religion emerged as a psychology of North American Protestant Christianity—a bias that dominates the field to this day (Gorsuch, 1988).

At the turn of the 20th century, religious revivals were common in North America, especially in evangelical Protestantism (Gaustad, 1966; Taves, 1999). Evangelicals focused upon the "born-again" experience. In his Gifford Lectures, James distinguished between those "once-born," who are cultivated within their faith and gradually socialized to accept it unproblematically, and those "twice-born," with a more melancholy temperament, who are literally compelled through crises to accept or realize their faith within an instant (James, 1902/1985, Lectures VI through VIII). Not surprisingly, North American psychologists were fascinated by this predominantly Protestant phenomenon, and conversion became the earliest major focus of the psychology of religion.

Sociologists were also concerned with conversion. Jackson (1908) chose conversion as his topic when he gave the Cole Lectures at Vanderbilt University. James (1902/1985) devoted two of his Gifford Lectures in Edinburgh to the specific topic of conversion (Lectures IX and X). James's lectures relied heavily upon the research of his contemporaries, especially Edwin Starbuck and James H. Leuba. Both had been students of Hall's at Clark University. Leuba (1896) published the first psychological journal article on conversion; this was rapidly followed by Starbuck's (1897) article on conversion and by his first book-length treatment of the topic (Starbuck, 1899). Not surprisingly, Leuba's and Starbuck's research methods paralleled Hall's, including the use of questionnaires and personal documents. Despite James's aversion to questionnaire studies, he utilized material supplied by Starbuck from his questionnaire studies of religious converts. Another early investigator, Coe (1916), added quasi-experimental techniques to the investigation of religious converts.

Whereas these early investigators tended to focus upon dramatic cases of sudden conversion, others argued against the selection of such extreme cases as the basis for developing a general model of conversion. For instance, Pratt (1920), a student of James's at Harvard, focused upon gradual converts, whose experiences were less dramatic, required intellectual seeking, and were hypothesized to be more genuinely characteristic of conversion within both Christianity and other religious traditions. As we shall soon see, from the beginning of the study of conversion, fundamental issues were identified and debated that continue to characterize the contemporary study of the subject. Yet as the psychology of religion waned in North America, conversion was ignored by psychologists. By the late 1950s, W. H. Clark bemoaned the fact that psychology had all but abandoned the study of conversion:

> For students of religion and religious psychology there is no subject that has held more fascination than the phenomenon called conversion. Yet of recent years a kind of shamefacedness becomes apparent among those scholars who mention it. . . . among the more conventional psychologists of the present day, who infrequently concern themselves with the study of religion and practically never with the subject of conversion. It is quite obvious that the latter is regarded as a kind of psychological slum to be avoided by any respectable scholar. (Clark, 1958, p. 188)

Even now, critical reviews of the literature on conversion reveal that there are no systematic programs of methodologically sophisticated research on conversion. The necessary longitudinal studies are nearly nonexistent. As Paloutzian, Richardson, and Rambo (1999, p. 1048) note, "most of the research is retrospective and cross-sectional, and no systematic program of research has ever been sustained."

It is primarily social psychologists who produce the majority of the empirical measurement-based research in the psychology of religion. Social psychology is divided into sociological social psychology and psychological social psychology (Stephan & Stephan, 1985). Although contemporary research on conversion is rapidly increasing in volume, the clear tendency is for sociological social psychology to dominate the field. Much of this can be attributed to the sociological interest in new religious movements, discussed in Chapter 12. For instance, a major bibliography on new religious movements by Beckford and Richardson (1983) contained at least 145 references pertinent to conversion, only 5% of which appeared prior to 1973. An earlier bibliography specifically on conversion literature prepared by Rambo (1982) listed 252 references, only 38% of which were published prior to 1973. Despite the claim of Beit-Hallahmi and Argyle (1997, p. 115; emphasis in original) that conversion has been "*the* classical topic in the psychology of religion," we see a reemergence of studies of conversion as a major focus for the contemporary social psychology of religion, but with a distinctive sociological rather than psychological emphasis.

Quite naturally, we can focus upon two major approaches to conversion, roughly identified with what we term the "classic" and the "contemporary" periods in the social-psychological study of conversion. The classic approach, influenced primarily by psychological social psychology, has been dominated by a concern with North American Protestantism. Many different of techniques and methods characterize this research, but the focus is primarily upon intraindividual processes. The contemporary approach is influenced primarily by sociological social-psychological studies of conversion. The research is focused upon new religious movements, or varieties of communal Christian groups; it is less likely to be strongly measurement-based, and the focus is upon interpsychological processes. These major distinctions are not exclusive and overlap in significant ways, but as we shall see, they provide differing (and to some extent even contradictory) views of conversion. The extent to which the differences between the classic and contemporary approaches are confounded by claims about the nature of conversion processes is an open question.

THE CLASSIC RESEARCH PARADIGM: PSYCHOLOGICAL DOMINANCE

What we have chosen to call the classic research approach to conversion is not merely of historical interest. The early psychologists utilized a variety of methods to study conversion. They also accepted as raw data for analysis various types of material; these included personal documents such as private letters and confessions, as well as autobiographical and biographical materials. Questionnaires, interviews, and public confessions were also employed. Although contemporary psychology tends to minimize the use of many of these sources, especially personal documents, their value can be immense (Capps, 1994; Capps & Dittes, 1990). They cannot be used to identify the causal processes in conversion, but they are essential and valid as rich descriptions of the process of conversion as a human experience.

Classic Conceptualizations of Conversion

Snow and Machalek (1984) have appropriately noted that any effort to understand the causes of conversion presupposes the ability to identify converts. However, they have also noted that few investigators have bothered to give clear conceptualizations of conversion. Most psychologists define "conversion" as a radical transformation of self; these definitions emphasize intrapersonal processes. Furthermore, early psychologists such as Cutten (1908) and Pratt (1920) emphasized that such definitions rely heavily upon a Protestant understanding of Saul's (Paul's) conversion on the road to Damascus as typical of all conversion (Richardson, 1985b).

The use of Paul's conversion as prototypical so dominates the classic paradigm of conversion research that Richardson (1985b) refers to the "Pauline experience" as the exemplar for conversion research in an article contrasting the classic paradigm with an emerging contemporary paradigm. Ironically, contemporary views echo Pratt, who argued that the fascination of psychologists with Paul's conversion as a model for all crisis-precipitated sudden conversion accounted for its overrepresentation in textbooks on psychology of religion. In Pratt's own words, "I venture to estimate that at least nine out of every ten 'conversion cases' reported in recent questionnaires would have no violent or depressing experience to report had not the individual in question been brought up in a church or community which taught them to look for it if not to cultivate it" (1920, p. 153).

As was the case with psychology at the beginning of the 20th century, much of the contemporary psychology of religion is really a study of Christianity, particularly Protestantism (Gorsuch, 1988; Taves, 1999). Gorsuch (1988, p. 202) has appropriately cautioned against extending the psychology of Christianity to other religions. However, social psychologists have not been appropriately cautious in this respect: They have generalized from Paul's conversion not only to all conversion within Christianity, but even to conversion experiences in other religions as well.

Defining conversion as a radical transformation of self is probably itself heavily influenced by the conversion of Paul. Even sociologically oriented investigators tend to define conversion in terms that imply radical change in self, even if these terms are deemphasized or if conversion is empirically assessed by other indicators as well. For instance, in an often-cited definition, Travisano (1970, p. 594) refers to conversion as "a radical reorganization of identity, meaning, life." Heirich (1977, p. 674) refers to conversion as the process of changing one's sense of "root reality," or of one's sense of "ultimate grounding." After critical analysis of definitions of conversion as radical personal change, Snow and Machalek (1984) define conversion in terms of a shift in the universe of discourse, which carries with it a corresponding shift in consciousness. However, as Coe (1916, p. 54) long ago noted, if self-transformation is used to define conversion, "Conversion is by no means co-extensive with religion." Indeed, most psychologists are likely to focus upon changing the self outside religious contexts (Brinthaupt & Lipka, 1994). What then makes conversion, contextualized as a radical transformation of self, distinctively religious?

It does little good to define conversion in distinctively religious terms, by imputing causal power to a deity to distinguish religious from nonreligious conversions. For instance, Rambo (1993, p. xiii) admits his own predilection to define as genuine only conversions as transformation of the person by the power of God, though he recognizes that this is not a useful definition for empirical psychology. However, whether or not one makes attributions to the self-transforming power of God is capable of being empirically investigated. The use of religious attributions or a religious universe of discourse is what makes conversion *religious* conversion (Snow & Machalek, 1984). After conversion, religious attributions defining and identifying the new self become "master attributions," replacing secular attributions or religious attributions that were peripheral prior to conversion (Snow & Machalek, 1984). In this sense, early clarifications of conversion mesh nicely with contemporary considerations. Coe (1916, p. 152) spoke of "self realization within a social medium" as defining conversion. James (1902/1985, p. 162) noted that "To say a man is 'converted' means . . . that religious ideas, peripheral in his consciousness, now take a central place, and that religious aims form the habitual center of his energy."

Most empirical studies of conversion implicitly, if not explicitly, utilize criteria that correspond to Coe's analysis of conversion. First, conversion is a profound change in self. Second, the change is not simply a matter of maturation, but is typically identified with a process (sudden or gradual) by which the transformed self is achieved. Third, this change in the self is radical in its consequences—indicated by such things as a new centering of concern, interest, and action. Fourth, this new sense of self is perceived as "higher" or as an emancipation from a previous dilemma or predicament. Thus conversion is self-realization or self-transformation, in that one adopts or finds a new self. The process also occurs within a social medium or context. Specifically, in religious conversion this entails a religious framework within which the transformed self is described, acts, and is recognized by others. The fact that conversion may result in new habitual modes of action links any purely *intrapsychological* processes of conversion to the *interpsychological* processes that maintain them. Long ago, Strickland (1924) argued against James's distinction between once-born and twice-born believers, on the grounds that anyone who consciously adopts a religious view (whether gradually or suddenly), is twice-born: "And if action from new ideals and changed habits of life do *not* follow, there has been no conversion" (p. 123; emphasis in original).

Although admittedly some change must occur in conversion, the nature of that change must be carefully delineated. Psychologists frequently focus upon personality change. Paloutzian et al. (1999) argue that the two distinct literatures on conversion and personality change ought to be related. Adopting contemporary views of personality that recognize levels or domains to personality (Emmons, 1995) suggests that one can organize the empirical literature on conversion by the extent to which it produces changes in particular domains or levels of personality. For instance, research at the basic personality level, using such indicators as the "five-factor model of personality" (McCrae, 1992), has produced little if any evidence that conversion changes basic personality. However, at other levels of personality functioning, changes resulting from conversion can clearly be identified. Research Box 11.1 summarizes the conversion literature with respect to the changes conversion produces in various levels of personality functioning.

Contemporary Distinctions Refining the Classic View

Numerous investigators have recognized that self-transformation within a religious context is a useful definition of conversion, capable of a variety of operational indicators. Unfortunately, no studies exist empirically assessing the interrelationship among various operational measures of conversion. The study of conversion requires additional conceptual refinements so that variations in closely related phenomena can be distinguished. Five common phenomena closely related to conversion are apostasy, deconversion, intensification, switching, and cycling.

1. "Apostasy" refers to the abandonment of one's religious commitment in favor of the adoption of a nonreligious framework.

2. "Deconversion" refers to the process by which previous converts leave. Deconversion does not necessarily imply apostasy.

ह&

Research Box 11.1. What about the Personality Changes in Conversion? (Paloutzian, Richardson, & Rambo, 1999)

The empirical study of conversion interfaces two bodies of literature in psychology: the literature on conversion, a perennial topic in the psychology of religion, and that on personality change, a topic of renewed interest in personality theory. Paloutzian, Richardson, and Rambo have reviewed and organized these two literatures according to levels of personality. Identifying three levels or domains of personality and the accompanying empirical literature of the effects of conversion reveals a fairly consistent picture. The magnitude of the effects of conversion across these three levels or domains of personality is consistent, whether conversion is sudden or gradual, or whether it is active or passive. They also appear to hold regardless of whether conversion is to a Western or Eastern faith tradition. We can summarize these findings as follows:

Personality level or domain	Effects of conversion
Level I: Basic functioning	No or minimal change
Level II: Midlevel functions (attitudes, feelings, behavior)	Significant change[a]
Level III: Self-defining personality functions (purpose in life, meaning, identity)	Profound change[a]

[a]Change may not be permanent if continual conversions occur (this is common among active seekers).

---

3. "Intensification" refers to a revitalized commitment to the religion in which one was raised or of which one has been only a nominal member (Rambo, 1993, p. 183). It is distinguished from conversion proper, as one does not adopt an entirely new faith commitment or change one's religion. Many religious traditions have routine procedures whereby intensification experiences are to be anticipated by the faithful. For instance, among many evangelicals, there is a moment when one is "born again."

4. "Switching" refers to a change of religious membership without radical change in one's self. Typically, changing from one denomination to another closely related denomination entails no radical self-transformation and hence is merely switching. We discuss denominational switching in Chapter 12.

5. "Cycling" refers to patterns of religious participation that vary across the lifespan. Participation is episodic; many drop out of religious anticipation, only to return at various points in their lives. We also discuss religious cycling in Chapter 12.

It is unreasonable to expect a single model of conversion to account both for conversion and for these five related but distinguishable phenomena.

Age and Conversion

Investigators have persistently studied the relationship between age and conversion. Although conversion can conceivably occur at any age, a reasonable hypothesis is that it is most likely to occur in adolescence. Adolescence is a time in which individuals challenge and test normative systems, eventually selecting and identifying with those within which they forge their identity or sense of self (Erikson, 1968). It is also a time when secondary socialization provides a variety of options in a world that is largely recognized to be socially constructed (Berger & Luckmann, 1967). Religions exist as one type of meaning system within which individuals can orient themselves and can understand, interpret, and direct their lives. Adolescence is a likely time in which the very existence of a variety of religions testifies to the necessity of choice, even if only to affirm one's already existing religious faith (Berger, 1979). As Starbuck (1899, p. 224) noted, "Theology takes the adolescent tendencies and builds upon them; it seems that the essential thing in adolescent growth is to bring the person out of childhood into the new life of mature and personal insight."

In a review of five major studies of conversion that had a total sample size exceeding 15,000 persons, Johnson (1959) found the average age of conversion to be 15.2 years, with the range from 12.7 to 15.6 years. Roberts (1965) found adolescence to be the typical time of conversion in Britain; the typical age at conversion was 15. Gillespie (1991) found 16 to be the typical age of conversion in samples he reviewed. These data correspond to critical summaries of the literature fixing adolescence as the customary time of conversion (Argyle & Beit-Hallahmi, 1975; Beit-Hallahmi & Argyle, 1997). Thus, in general, the empirical literature on age of conversion is consistent and has been for over 40 years, although admittedly based upon a biased sampling range that seldom extends beyond youth (Silverstein, 1988).

There is a fairly narrow age range for conversion, centering around middle to late adolescence. If sex differences are considered, females convert from 1 to 2 years earlier than males. However, this is true only for conversion in Western countries—primarily in the United States and Canada, and to a lesser extent in the United Kingdom and some parts of Europe. It also may be most characteristic of conversion within specifically Christian traditions; for instance, Köse (1996a, 1996b) found that the average age of conversion of 70 native British converts to Islam was approximately 30 years. Furthermore, in most cases studied, the phenomena reported as conversion are mixed with intensification experiences, in which adolescents consciously come to adopt the faith within which they were raised or switch to a similar faith commitment. Few investigators linking age to conversion have adequately empirically assessed the possibility of radical self-transformation by sophisticated psychometric procedures. Most rely upon either verbal reports of conversion or of reported church participation. Finally, anticipating a bit, we might note here that conversion to new religious movements appears to be age-related. Most typically, such conversion is likely to occur in late adolescence, and early youth. Unfortunately, few investigators directly survey age and participation in new religious movements, other than to report the mean ages of their samples. Typically these are college-age students, who are readily available to be sampled but are perhaps not truly representative of the age of conversion to new religious movements in general.

Age and Apostasy

The "secularization thesis" discussed in Chapter 12 is relevant to contemporary studies of conversion, in that apostasy has increasingly become a topic of social-scientific interest. Secularization provides the context within which the complete rejection of religion is possible and perhaps increasingly frequent. However, it remains true that most North Americans identify with religion, insofar as they at least affirm some religious identification. When asked in surveys for their religious identification, only a minority mark "none" (Vernon, 1968; Welch, 1978). Hadaway (1989) notes that from 1972 to 1988, 93% of U.S. residents identified themselves as either some variety of Protestant, Catholic, or Jew, based upon National Opinion Research Center surveys; only 7% identified themselves as having no religion. Brinkerhoff and Burke (1980) note that religious disidentification is an extreme form of apostasy only when persons both sever ties with religious institutions and disavow religious self-identification. However, the most typical operational indicator of apostasy is refusing to indicate a religious identity in questionnaire or phone survey studies. These are religious "nones." Often it is simply assumed that these "nones" were raised within a religion and hence are apostates. Furthermore, Hadaway and Roof (1988) note that U.S. apostates have dropped a religious identity within a culture in which religion remains a dominant value. They report that the rate of apostasy increased by 2% from 1972 to 1987, remaining fairly constant (ranging between 7.2% and 7.8%) for the most recent years surveyed.

Studies using this operational indicator have found that, like conversion, apostasy is age-related. Apostates tend to be late adolescents or very young adults (Roof & Hadaway, 1979; Roof & McKinney, 1987; see also Chapter 5). Thus both apostasy and conversion are primarily phenomena of youth. However, one must not lose sight of the fact that typical ages of conversion and apostasy reported are often confounded by limiting sampling to adolescents and young adults, typically in high school or college. It does not mean that these phenomena do not occur across the lifespan, from early adolescence through old age. In Chapter 12, apostasy and cycling are explored across a broader spectrum of the lifespan.

Efforts to Explain Conversion

The process of conversion can be gradual or sudden. It is the speed of this process that has led to the most intense theoretically guided discussions purporting to provide explanations of it.

Sudden Conversion

Early investigators did not fail to classify conversion types into simple dichotomies. The most obvious was derived from a continuum of duration. Some persons convert quickly, appearing suddenly to adopt a faith perspective previously unknown (conversion) or to make a faith that was previously of peripheral concern suddenly central (intensification). Other people seem to mature and blossom gradually within a faith perspective that in some sense has always been theirs. We have already noted the dispute surrounding James's once-born and twice-born types. James (1902/1985) acknowledged the possibility of gradual conversion, but focused upon sudden conversion, probably precipitated by crises. Many of James's examples of crisis-precipitated conversion are what Rambo (1993) identifies as intensification experiences.

In his fascination with sudden conversion, James was not alone. Starbuck (1899) focused upon "conversions of self-surrender" and "voluntary conversions." The former were thought to be elicited by a sense of sin, suddenly overcome; the latter by a gradual pursuit of a religious ideal. Ames (1910) favored restricting the term "conversion" to sudden instances of religious change associated with intense emotionality. Coe (1916) noted at least six senses of conversion, but likewise favored limiting the term to intense, sudden religious change.

Johnson (1959, p. 117) later echoed these views succinctly when he stated, "A genuine religious conversion is the outcome of a crisis."

So influential were the early psychologists in focusing conversion upon sudden, intense experiences of religious self-transformation that Richardson (1985b, p. 164) summarizes their implicit conceptualization as the "old conversion paradigm." The prototype is the conversion of Paul in the Christian tradition. It suggests what Miller and C'deBaca (1994) refer to as "quantum change." Its major characteristics can be summarized as follows (see Richardson, 1985b, pp. 164–166):

1. The prototype is Paul's conversion.
2. The process is more emotional than rational.
3. The convert is a passive agent acted upon by external forces.
4. The conversion entails a dramatic transformation of self.
5. Behavior change follows from belief change.
6. Conversion occurs once and is permanent.
7. It typically occurs in adolescence.
8. It typically occurs suddenly.

Richardson emphasizes that what we have called the classical model implies a passive subject transformed by forces that may be differentially identified. However, whether these forces are identified as "God" or "the unconscious" makes little difference. The convert is not seen as an active agent; instead, emotion dominates the irrational transformation of self that suddenly changes belief, and subsequent behavior change follows.

Richardson's model has similarities to Strickland's (1924) summary of the success of sudden conversions common among evangelical and fundamentalist Protestant groups in North America, including those that occurred during revivalist meetings. Strickland also emphasized the institutionalization of Paul's conversion as the valued form of entering the Christian faith, with the emphasis upon sin and guilt as eliciting conditions joyously relieved in the emotionality of a sudden conversion. Strickland's perspective thus adds a more dynamic understanding to Richardson's assertion that the classical conversion paradigm is facilitated by emotional factors that are likely to erupt suddenly in late adolescence.

Not surprisingly, several empirical studies have related emotional states to sudden conversions. For instance, in a classic study by Clark (1929), 2,174 cases of adolescent conversions were classified as either sudden or gradual. Approximately one-third were sudden and were precipitated by either emotion or crisis; they also tended to be linked with a stern theology. Starbuck (1899) studied adolescent conversions and found that two-thirds were at least partially triggered by a deep sense of sin or guilt. However, he found that in later adolescence, conversion was likely to be more gradual. Pratt (1920) went so far as to identify the view that prior to their conversions, twice-born individuals wallow in extreme feelings of unworthiness, self-doubt, and depreciation that are released or overcome via conversion, as in the James–Starbuck thesis. The James–Starbuck thesis recognizes conversion as a functional solution to the burdens of guilt and sin, which are found to be unbearable prior to conversion. Research Box 11.2 presents a more detailed analysis of Clark's (1929) classic study of conversion, which supports the James–Starbuck thesis.

In light of the James–Starbuck thesis, one must be cautious not to interpret negative emotions such as guilt, sin, and shame as necessarily psychologically unhealthy Watson and his colleagues have provided a series of studies relevant to this thesis (Watson, 1993; Watson,

---

Research Box 11.2. The Psychology
of Religious Awakening (Clark, 1929)

In this classic study, E. T. Clark classified 2,174 conversions as to whether they were sudden or gradual. Sudden conversions (32.9%) were subdivided into two types: (1) "definite crisis awakening," in which a personal crisis was suddenly followed by a religious transformation (6.7%, majority males); and (2) "emotional stimulus awakening," in which gradual religious growth was interrupted by an emotional event that was suddenly followed by religious transformation (27.2%, equal proportions of males and females). Gradual conversions were described as "gradual awakening," a steady, progressive, slow growth resulting in gradual religious transformation (66.1%, slightly more females). A stern theology was associated with sudden conversions, equally distributed between crises and emotional awakenings. This was as would have been predicted from the James–Starbuck thesis. Almost all gradual conversions were associated with compassionate theologies that emphasized love and forgiveness.

Clark suggested that sudden conversions were associated with fear and anxiety. In addition, 41% of these conversions occurred during revivals, which were likely to be highly emotional settings. The dominant emotional states reported were joyful reactions, assumed by Clark to result from the alleviation of negative feelings that occurred prior to conversion, which were elicited by stern theologies emphasizing sin and guilt. This study suggests that negative emotional states can precipitate experiences within a religious setting, and that conversion then provides positive relief of these negative feelings.

Morris, & Hood, 1993). Watson argues that negative emotions such as shame and guilt can function positively when interpreted within an "ideological surround" that provides a context for both their meaningfulness and their resolution. Clearly, one individual's personal religious reactions may be another's madness. Just as many people refuse to experience the necessity of salvation from sin insisted upon by some fundamentalist groups, so may others perceive fundamentalists to be encased in a rigid, outmoded religious framework. Nevertheless, the functionality of sin, shame, and guilt within fundamentalism is hard to dispute (Gordon, 1984; Hood, 1992c). As Hood (1983) has documented, the empirical issues involved in studying fundamentalist religious groups are clouded by differences, often value-based, between investigators and those who are investigated.

That sudden conversion is often correlated with emotionality seems well established. However, such correlations do little to provide meaningful causal claims, such as that emotional feelings trigger conversions or that guilt and sin are resolved by such conversions. Nevertheless, essentially correlational studies can be suggestive. A classic study by Coe (1916) compared 17 persons who anticipated striking conversions that actually occurred with 12 persons anticipating striking conversions that did not occur. Emotional factors were dominant in the group for which striking conversions occurred; cognitive factors were dominant in the group for whom striking conversions did not occur. In addition, the actual converts were more suggestible than the other group. Although Coe's research suggests that emotional factors may be causally involved in sudden conversions, no true experimental studies or longitudinal studies documenting this claim exist. However, recent research in cognitive psychology suggests a reason to link emotionality and sudden dramatic conversions. McCallister

(1995) has noted that emotional situations such as dramatic conversions may restrict the encoding of knowledge about experience, leading dramatic converts to utilize narrative formats to reconstruct their experience.

Still, in many studies it may be that emotionality and sudden conversions are merely correlated phenomena. For instance, Spellman, Baskett, and Byrne (1971) divided persons in a small Protestant town into sudden or gradual converts and compared them to non-converts. They found sudden converts to score higher on an objective measure of anxiety than gradual converts or nonconverts. Yet this difference found was *after* conversion; there was no evidence that greater emotionality differentiated the groups prior to their conversion, as postulated by the James–Starbuck thesis. Furthermore, as Poston (1992) has noted, emotional and crisis-triggered conversions are uncommon in many non-Christian religions—they do not, for instance, characterize conversion to Islam. Woodberry (1992) notes that traditional Islamic thought does not even have a term for "conversion." Finally, the specific case of sudden conversion associated with claims to mind control and "brainwashing" is discussed in Chapter 12. It is a recent and case of emotion-induced sudden conversion associated with analyses of new religious movements, primarily sects and cults.

Gradual Conversion

Like sudden religious conversions, gradual conversions result in a transformation of self within a religious context. Yet gradual conversions occur almost imperceptibly; they are usually distinguished empirically by not being identified with a single event. Some investigators have argued that gradual conversions need not result in radical shifts in personality, self, or even religious beliefs. These researchers have essentially redefined conversion or have accepted as empirical criteria such things as merely joining a new religious group. Scobie (1973, 1975) even argues for "unconscious conversion," referring to persons who cannot recall *not* having been religious. Clearly, characteristics associated with joining a new religious group need not precisely parallel those defining conversion in the classic sense. Neither do continual faith commitments without an intensification experience. We must note in each case the empirical criteria used to assess conversion, and must keep these in mind when comparing individual empirical studies.

Strickland (1924) contrasted gradual and sudden conversions. In gradual conversions, the emphasis is upon a conscious striving toward a goal. The convert is not likely to experience a single decisive point at which conversion is either initiated or completed. There is an absence of emotional crises and of feelings of guilt and sin. The process is cognitive rather than emotional.

THE CONTEMPORARY RESEARCH PARADIGM: SOCIOLOGICAL DOMINANCE

Strickland's distinction between gradual and sudden conversion laid the foundation for the emergence of what we term the contemporary paradigm of conversion. The focus upon an active agent, seeking self-transformation, has become the target of extensive research among more sociologically oriented investigators. No single theory dominates the research literature, but most theories share enough common assumptions to contrast them with the classic psychological paradigm.

Five characteristics of the contemporary paradigm are notable. First, the research is done primarily by sociologists or sociologically oriented social psychologists, rather than by psychologists or psychologically oriented social psychologists. Second, the research focuses upon new religious movements, many of non-Western origin or influence (or, if Christian, often fundamentalist groups of a sectarian nature). Third, the research is often participatory in nature, with single groups studied over a period of time. Investigators are less likely to take a single set of measurements on a group, as is typical of classic research by psychologists on conversion. Both structured and unstructured interviews with religious converts are common. Fourth, almost by definition, the research focuses upon gradual conversion rather than sudden conversion. Finally, the process of deconversion is investigated, in which individuals who have converted and then left new religious movements are studied. (We cover deconversion in greater detail later in this chapter.)

Major Differences between the Classic and the Contemporary Paradigms

Richardson (1985b) has been the most articulate theorist arguing that the old paradigm, based upon the "Pauline experience," is being abandoned in favor of an emerging paradigm. Some have debated the claim that there is a new emerging paradigm; they argue instead that perhaps the nature of conversion itself has changed over time (Lofland & Skonovd, 1981). It is difficult to compare the classic and contemporary paradigms empirically, given differences in research methods and the nature of religious groups studied. It is also unwise to think that both paradigms cannot operate, with some conversions being sudden and others gradual. The empirical issue seems to be under what conditions do each type of conversions occur.

What undoubtedly characterizes the contemporary paradigm is the use of typologies, often based upon assumed contrasts widely acknowledged in the classic paradigm. In the classic paradigm, sudden change was contrasted with gradual transformation, and associated with this distinction were other contrasts (such as passive vs. active and emotional vs. intellectual). The classic and contemporary paradigms are contrasted in Table 11.1. It is noteworthy that all these contrasts were noted by early investigators (Starbuck, 1899), as well as emphasized by contemporary investigators (Richardson, 1985b).

TABLE 11.1. The Classic and Contemporary Conversion Paradigms Compared

Classic paradigm	Contemporary paradigm
Conversion is sudden	Conversion is gradual
Middle adolescence to late adolescence	Late adolescence to early adulthood
Emotional, suggestive	Intellectual, rational
Stern theology	Compassionate theology
Passive	Active
Release from sin and guilt	Search for meaning and purpose
Emphasizes intraindividual psychological processes	Emphasizes interpsychological processes

The classic paradigm acknowledged a series of contrasts between sudden and gradual conversion, although empirical research was focused upon the more dramatic case of sudden religious conversion. Perhaps it was this narrowed focus in the empirical literature that allowed the contemporary paradigm to emerge. In addition, the emergence of new religious movements and their obvious appeal to converts altered that typical pattern of research, almost by definition. Thus intensification experiences within traditions that focused upon intrapsychological processes (studied by psychologists) gave way to conversion to new religious movements focused upon interpersonal processes (studied by sociologists and social psychologists).

Below, we summarize the characteristics of the emerging paradigm in conversion research as described by Richardson (1985b, pp. 166–172):

1. Conversion occurs gradually.
2. It is rational rather than emotional.
3. The convert is an active, seeking agent.
4. There is self-realization within humanistic tradition.
5. Belief change follows from behavior change.
6. Conversion is not permanent; it may occur several times.
7. It typically occurs in early adulthood.
8. No one experience is prototypical.

It is readily apparent, however, that Richardson's claim to an emerging paradigm ironically meshes quite closely with earlier psychological research on gradual conversion. Perhaps appropriate is the fact that the Lofland and Stark (1965) model, seen by Richardson (1985b) as transitional between the old and new paradigms, is still useful insofar as it permits identification of both predisposing psychological factors (typically studied in sudden conversions) and situational and contextual factors (typically studied in gradual conversions). This model is based upon Lofland's (1977) provocative research in what was then only a minor new religion. He was one of the earliest investigators to study the Unification Church (popularly known as the "Moonies") at a time when it was a minor cult, and had not yet emerged to prominence on the world scene. As discussed in Chapter 12, research on the Unification Church, like research on many religious cults, is often dichotomized into psychological and sociological studies. In the former, sudden conversion is associated with denigrating popular metaphors, such as "brainwashing" and "mind control." Yet more sociologically oriented studies of the gradual and voluntary process of conversion to the Unification Church are consistent with empirical findings concerning a variety of new religious movements, and are not compatible with denigrating models of conversion as pathological (Barker, 1984).

Long and Hadden (1983) have argued for a "dual-reality" approach, in which conversion may involve either sudden, emotional processes (associated with intrapsychological processes, which can be denigrated in terms of a "brainwashing" metaphor) or more gradual processes (associated with interpsychological processes). However, we need not assume conversion to be an either–or process, based upon dichotomies such as sudden–gradual or passive–active. The distinction primarily reflects differing psychological and sociological interests. Investigators would best profit from studying actual processes of conversion in particular cases, and the degree to which characteristics typically assumed to operate in what we have termed the classical and contemporary paradigms can be empirically identified. One may assume, as Rambo (1992) does, that there are no fundamental differences among the processes of conversion to various religions. However, we must be careful to identify the various factors that actually do operate in conversion before we can take such an assumption as proven.

Conversion Motifs

Among those studying conversion to new religious movements, the emphasis upon gradual processes has suggested a variety of empirical phenomena operating in conversion, viewed as a process occurring over time. Several investigators have attempted more diversified classifications of conversion types, identifying various possible "conversion careers" (Richardson, 1978b). It is undoubtedly true that personal accounts of conversions often reflect biases elicited by investigators who rely upon interviews and observation after the fact to assess factors operating in conversion, as Beckford (1978) has noted. Classifications of conversion that rely upon psychological dispositions and intrapsychological processes ought not to be simply opposed to those that rely upon social contexts and interpsychological process. The union of both is needed.

One classification system admirably linking the classic and contemporary models, the psychological and the sociological, is that of Lofland and Skonovd (1981). These scholars have coined the concept "conversion motif" to take account of the "phenomenological validity" of "holistic subjective conversion experience." (p. 374). They have postulated six conversion motifs, and five major dimensions that apply to each motif. These are presented in Table 11.2.

The Lofland and Skonovd typology allows for variations in conversion without forcing arbitrary dichotomies. It permits a distinction among basic objective phenomena, identified along the five dimensions; it also respects the subjective account of conversion by the convert. Thus their six conversion motifs provide "phenomenological validity" to the objective factors (dimensions) postulated to be operative in conversion (Lofland & Skonovd, 1981, p. 379). Their motifs are capable of operationalization and empirical study. They also cut across the psychological and sociological concerns that mediate between the classic and contemporary paradigms of conversion discussed above. For instance, their mystical motif fits the classical Pauline prototype of conversion, emphasizing intrapsychic factors; by contrast,

TABLE 11.2. The Lofland and Skonovd Conversion Motifs

	Intellectual	Mystical	Experimental	Affectional	Revivalist	Coercive
Degree of social pressure	None or low	None or low	Low	Medium	High	High
Temporal duration	Medium	Short	Long	Long	Short	Short
Level of affective arousal	Medium	High	Low	Medium	High	Low
Affective content	Insight	Awe or love	Curiosity	Affection	Love and fear	Fear and love
Belief–behavior sequence of change	Belief first	Belief first	Behavior first	Behavior first	Behavior first	Behavior first

Note. Adapted from Lofland and Skonovd (1981, p. 375). Copyright 1981 by the Society for the Scientific Study of Religion. Adapted by permission.

the experimental motif focuses upon the processes by which "seekers" creatively transform themselves, often by interacting with others who model proper converted behavior, as in the contemporary paradigm (Straus, 1976).

Embedded in the conversion motif typology is the assumption that there are three levels of reality to consider. The first is what Lofland and Skonovd (1981, p. 379) call "raw reality," or the actual truth of conversion, which is only imperfectly available to the social scientist. The second level is the convert's experience and interpretation. The third is the analytic interpretation provided by the social scientist. The change in conversion motifs over time may reflect a change in any one or all of these levels of reality. Obvious examples are the clearly historical contingency of coercive motifs (discussed in detail in Chapter 12) and the revivalist motif (now less common among nonevangelical forms of Protestantism).

The processes of conversion within each motif need to be empirically researched. Once again, psychological and sociological social psychologists actually parallel one another in their analyses. For instance, whereas sociological social psychologists tend to focus on accounts (Beckford, 1978; Snow & Machalek, 1983), a parallel literature exists among psychological social psychologists in terms of attributions (Spilka & McIntosh, 1995; Spilka, Shaver, & Kirkpatrick, 1985). To a large extent, various conversion motifs exist because of the linguistic frameworks within which conversion is understood. These include biographical reconstructions, the adaptation of master attribution schemes, and various rhetorical indications that one has indeed been converted. Mafra (2000) has even argued that conversion can be treated as a narrative genre in its own right.

Active Conversion

Much of the sociological literature on the process of conversion emphasizes how people behave in such a way that they essentially "convert themselves." Whereas classic conversion research focused upon what happens to passive converts, the contemporary research focuses upon what converts actively do to produce their conversions. For instance, Balch (1980) has emphasized how individuals must learn to act like converts by performing particular role-prescribed behaviors expected of people who have been converted. Thus behavior change occurs before an individual internalizes beliefs and perceptions characteristic of a convert. Perhaps actual perceptual changes require a reconditioning of habitual patterns of perception, aptly captured by Deikman's (1966) notion of "deautomatization." However, it is only after participating in activities associated with new religious groups that such alterations in perceptions can occur. Thus behavior change precedes belief change. Several investigators have documented this via participation research with new religious groups. For instance, Wilson (1982) has demonstrated such a process with converts to a yoga ashram, and Preston (1981, 1982) has demonstrated this same tendency among converts becoming Zen practitioners.

In terms of empirical assessment, it is important to note that the use of either behavior change or belief change as an indicator of conversion will determine at what point conversion occurs (if at all). The two types of change need not occur at the same time. In addition, the temporal duration of conversion may be different for belief change and behavior change, even within a single conversion process. An individual may gradually be socialized into a new religious group and at some point suddenly experience a deautomatization, resulting in new perceptions congruent with the group's world view. This is apparently particularly true of some Eastern traditions that emphasize practice over belief, such as Zen and yoga (Preston, 1981, 1982; Wilson, 1982; Volinn, 1985). In this sense, a person may not be able to actively pursue deautomatization as a goal; it is a product of successful socialization into religious groups, and becomes possible once proper techniques and practices are mastered (Balch, 1980; Deikman, 1966). Much of the research literature has reintroduced classic cognitive dissonance theory to provide theoretical justification for a sequence of behavior change–belief change. The focus has been upon maintenance of conversion within groups when prophecy appears to fail.

Maintenance of Conversion When Prophecy Appears to Fail

One theory that has had considerable influence in the study of conversion is the theory of cognitive dissonance, first proposed by Festinger (1957). Basic to his theory is the notion that cognitions more or less map reality. Hence there is pressure for individual beliefs to be congruent with reality—whether physical, psychological, or sociological (Festinger, 1957, pp. 10–11). This has led some researchers to puzzle over how it is that individuals can maintain membership in religious groups when prophecy fails. The classic study by Festinger and his colleagues was titled *When Prophecy Fails* (Festinger, Riecken, & Schachter, 1956). This participant observation study of a group that believed in flying saucers and predicted the end of the world began a series of participant observation studies of religious groups whose success in maintaining converts is paradoxically linked to failed prophecies. Part of the appeal of Festinger's theory is undoubtedly due to its counterintuitive claim—that prophecies proven to be incorrect result both in maintenance of conversion and in efforts to convert others. How is this possible?

Central to Festinger's theory is that cognitions can be dissonant. Dissonance exists if the obverse of one belief follows from the other. When this is the case, the believer is motivated to reduce this dissonance. However, since the dissonance of two cognitions is defined by psychological as well as logical means, Festinger's theory has undergone a series of modifications as investigators have continued to study religious groups and what perhaps are only apparent prophetic failures. As in much of the literature on conversion, the more psychologically oriented and the more sociologically oriented social-psychological studies yield different results.

Psychologically Oriented Social-Psychological Studies of Failed Prophecy

Festinger et al. (1956) infiltrated a religious group in which a housewife began experiencing automatic writing that revealed to her the coming end of the world. Included in this prophetic claim was that superior beings would come in flying saucers and save those who, like this housewife, believed in them. Festinger and his colleagues infiltrated this group and, as participant observers, sought to test their own prophecy—namely, that when this group's prophecy of the world's destruction failed, the group would both continue in its beliefs and attempt even greater proselytization. Simply put, in Festinger's theory of cognitive dissonance, proselytization increases when prophecy fails. Why?

Festinger's theory requires five basic conditions: First, the belief must be sincere and held with one's "whole heart"; second, and closely related, the person must be committed to this belief; third, he or she must actually take "irrevocable action" based upon it; fourth, the individual must be presented with "unequivocal and undeniable" evidence that the belief is wrong; and, finally, there must be social support subsequent to disconfirmation (Festinger et al., 1956).

Festinger's theory seems straightforward enough and is uniquely relevant to religious groups for two basic reasons. First, religious groups do seem to make predictions and assert beliefs that from other perspectives seem disconfirmed. This is especially the case when clear prophecies are made that do not come true. Second, Festinger sidetracked the issue of pathology by noting that the beliefs are shared among individuals—there is social support. In Festinger et al.'s (1956) classic study, the predicted date came and passed, apparently falsifying the prophecy. Nevertheless, Festinger and colleagues claimed that the group did not disband because of the failed prophecy, but continued—renewed in its faith commitment, and passionate in its efforts to convince others of the truth of its beliefs. Although this has been widely reported by psychologists as a positive test of Festinger's theory, we shall shortly note that more sociologically oriented social psychologists have criticized this claim.

Festinger's claim to have identified the consequences of failed prophecy has been applied to many historical examples of failed prophecy, such as the Montanists, the Millerites, and even Christianity itself. For instance, it is claimed that the 2nd-century failure of Montanus to predict the return of Jesus led to renewed commitment and the success of the Montanists (Hughes, 1954). Similarly, William Miller's mid-19th-century prediction of the end of the world never materialized, and yet the Millerites prospered as a consequence (so we are led to believe) of their failed prophecy (Sears, 1924). Perhaps most dramatic is the interpretation that Christianity itself succeeded largely because of the failed prediction of Christ's second coming (Wernik, 1975). Although Festinger and his colleagues were careful only to suggest that historical examples of failed prophecy can be explained by cognitive dissonance, specific historical studies of the prophetic traditions of the Bible have considerably modified their claims—particularly their claim to have objectively identified actual failed prophecies (Carroll, 1979). However, psychologically oriented social psychologists continue to interpret dissonant beliefs objectively, offering even quasi-experimental support for Festinger's basic theory (see, e.g., Batson, Schoenrade, & Ventis, 1993, pp. 210–216). Thus psychologically oriented social psychologists have tended to see in Festinger's theory a classic model of theory construction that has allowed specific empirical tests, which are viewed as largely supportive of the theory. However, sociologically oriented social psychologists have argued quite the opposite.

Sociologically Oriented Social-Psychological Studies of Failed Prophecy

Sociologically oriented social psychologists have found major flaws in cognitive-dissonance-based interpretations of failed prophecy. First, Festinger et al.'s (1956) classic study has been faulted on methodological grounds. Bainbridge (1997) noted that often almost one-third of the members were participant observers, and that the group members were continually badgered by the press to account for their commitment. Thus the increased proselytizing and affirmations of faith may have been influenced by media pressure. Others have noted that Festinger's interpretation of historical cases in the light of dissonance theory is flawed. For instance, Melton (1985) has argued that the Millerites were not simply focused upon prophecy and did not disband in the manner Festinger claimed in order to provide support for his theory. Melton (1985, p. 20) further notes that "within religious groups prophecy seldom fails." Likewsie, Van Fossen (1988) has noted that the continual citation of Festinger et al.'s (1956) classic study provides a deficient guide to the study of prophetic groups. Bader (1999, p. 120), after critically reviewing his own and Festinger et al.'s study, concludes that "Nevertheless no study of a failed prophecy, the current research included, has provided support for the cognitive dissonance hypothesis."

How can psychologically and sociologically oriented social psychologists have such different evaluations of dissonance theory? The answer is largely methodological. Psychologically oriented social psychologists tend to take an outsider perspective—as if they could identify dissonant beliefs by more objective criteria, or identify "unequivocal and undeniable disconfirmation of a prophecy" (Festinger et al., 1956, p. 3). Yet as Coyle (2001, p. 150) notes, the term "religious gap" has become common with reference to the difference between mental health professionals and the general population in regard to religious beliefs. Table 11.3 shows the nature of this gap.

The religious gap hypothesis is relevant when it is recognized that researchers tend to describe for themselves when beliefs are dissonant or when prophecy has failed. This is crucial, since Festinger's theory requires that beliefs must be *proven* false—in his group's own words, that the disconfirmation must be "unequivocal and undeniable." However, as Carroll (1979) noted when applying cognitive dissonance theory to Biblical prophecy, there are no simple objective criteria by which one can identify failed prophecy. What outsiders (especially researchers!) see as failed prophecy is seldom seen that way by insiders. Tumminia (1998, p. 165) notes that "what appears to be seemingly irrefutable evidence of irreconcilable contradictions to outsiders, like Festinger, can instead be evidence of the truth of prophecy to insiders." Carroll (1979) observes that among the faithful, there is a transcendental dimension to prophecy, securing it from failure. Sociologically oriented social psychologists have noted this as well, recognizing that failed prophecy entails hermeneutical considerations that make claims to "unequivocal and undeniable" falsification problematic.

Sociologically oriented social psychologists have tended to take an insider's perspective and to focus upon interpersonal processes that maintain a socially constructed reality incapable of any simply falsification. "Failed prophecy" is thus a negotiated term and depends upon negotiated claims to reality (Berger & Luckmann, 1967; Carroll, 1979; Pollner, 1987). Furthermore, among prophetic groups, prophecy is less central than outsiders assume. The exclusive focus upon prophecy leads outsiders to assume that the major concern of the group is prophecy; it ignores the complex cosmology that serves to integrate the group (Melton, 1985). Participant observation studies of prophetic groups have begun to show how rare

TABLE 11.3. Religious Gap between Mental Health Professionals and the General Population

Group	Religious	Nonreligious
General population	72%	9%
Family therapists	62%	15%
Social workers	46%	9%
Psychiatrists	39%	24%
Psychologists	33%	31%

Note. Religious respondents endorsed the statement "My whole approach to life is based upon my religion." Nonreligious respondents identified themselves as atheist, agnostic, humanistic, or otherwise nonreligious. Data from Coyle (2001, p. 150).

increased proselytization is as a reaction to what is only apparently failed prophecy (Stone, 2000). Zygmunt (1972, p. 245) defines "prophecy" as a prediction that a "drastic transformation of the existing social order will occur in the proximate future through the intervention of some supernatural agency." The recognition of the transformation is socially constructed, and hence it cannot be unequivocally or undeniably disconfirmed. Thus, from the insider's perspective, prophecy cannot fail.

The denial of failure of prophecy is the most common response from within prophetic groups as members struggle to stay within the group and to seek a proper interpretation of what must be only an apparent failure (Carroll, 1979; Dein, 1997, 2001; Melton, 1985; Tumminia, 1998). Increased proselytization is actually an uncommon response to failed prophecy (Stone, 2000). As Dein (2001) notes, dissonance theory is utilized too often to persuade others that those who stay within prophetic groups are irrational and driven by forces they do not understand. Such claims are possible only when researchers assume an objectivist stance and can claim that in fact prophecy has failed. However, researchers who adopt the perspective of the insider avoid committing what James (1890/1950) identified as the "psychological fallacy"—assuming that others must experience the world as psychologists do. The task is to understand how believers confront a more spiritual understanding of prophecy, rather than a simple literal understanding of its "failure" (Carroll, 1979; Dein, 2001). For instance, Dawson (1999) notes that increased proselytization is only one way to decrease dissonance, and that it is not at all a common way in the face of failed prophecy. More common than increased proselytization is the denial of failed prophecy (Zygmunt, 1972). This can take the form of "spiritualization"—a reinterpretation of the prophecy so that it has been fullfilled. For instance, Bainbridge (1997) notes that when Charles Taze Russell of the Jehovah's Witnesses apparently failed to predict Christ's return in 1874, he argued that Christ had indeed returned invisibly. Likewise, Tumminia (1998) studied the Unarius Academy of Science in El Cajon, California, over a period of 5 years (1988–1993). Failed prophecies were reinterpreted in terms of past lives and reincarnation, thus allowing denial of the failure of prophecy in terms of experiencing its fulfilment in a more spiritual sense. Both historical and contemporary participant observation studies of diverse prophetic groups—such as the Baha'i sect (Balch, Farnsworth, & Wilkins (1983), a Mormon sect called the Morrisites (Halford, Anderson, & Clark, 1981), and the contemporary Lubavitcher Hasidic movement (Dein, 2001)—reveal that members continue to struggle with their beliefs and membership within groups, sometimes become disillusioned, and occasionally leave groups. However, they always rationally struggle with the meaning of prophecies that become not simply false, but problematic.

One common interpretation is that failed prophecies are a test of faith (Hardyck & Braden, 1962; Tumminia, 1998). Again, however, the struggle is always rational and meaningful from an insider's perspective. As Dein (2001, p. 399) notes, individuals within a prophetic religious group "are not a group of fanatics who follow doctrine without question. They are sane people trying to reason their way through facts and doctrine in the pursuit of understanding." Finally, as Bader (1999) has noted, the theoretical task is to propose testable hypotheses that not only clarify under what conditions failed prophecy will have specific effects, but also specify which members will leave a group if they perceive prophecy to have failed. Research Box 11.3 presents the results of a contemporary study of a religious group, Lubavitcher Hasidism, in which the complexities of apparently failed prophecy are explored in the tradition of Festinger's classic study.

Research Box 11.3. What Really Happens When Prophecy Fails?
(Dein, 2001)

Simon Dein, a nonreligious Jew, lived in the Stamford Hill Lubavitcher Hasidic community in England over a 3-year period (1992–1995). While working part-time as a physician, he studied the ways in which Lubavitchers dealt with illness. Beginning in 1993, intense messianic fervor emerged in the community. Dein interviewed 30 Lubavitchers (24 were males, and the majority of these were rabbis).

The Lubavitcher movement is a worldwide movement of Hasidic Jews who emphasize feelings over intellect and emphasize that one's thoughts should be continually upon God. They believe that their spiritual leader (*zaddik* or *rebbe*) is a perfectly righteous man. In accordance with traditional Jewish teachings, Lubavitchers believe that in each generation there is a potential messiah (*moshiach*). However, although each *zaddik* is a potential messiah, the *zaddik* himself may not realize this potential because the generation is unworthy of him.

Rebbe Menachem Mendel Schneerson became the leader of Lubavitcher Hasidism in 1951. He has been described by Lubavitchers as the "most phenomenal Jewish personality of our time" (quoted in Dein, 2001, p. 390). He became an intense focus of the Lubavitchers, many of whom suggested that he was the messiah. Rebbe Schneerson (or simply "the Rebbe," as he was called) did little to diminish this expectation. For instance, in April 1991 he stated, "Moshiach's coming is no longer a dream of a distant future, but an imminent reality which will very shortly become manifest" (quoted in Dein, 2001, p. 391).

The Rebbe's statements had profound effect on the Stamford Hill Lubavitchers. A "Moshiach Awareness" caravan was held that toured Britain; public discussions were held on messianic issues; and, while never publicly identifying the Rebbe as the messiah, many Lubvatchers privately acknowledged that he was. Others expressed doubt. As one Lubavitcher told Dein, "The Rebbe may be Moshiach, but I am unsure. I hope he is" (p. 393). The Rebbe died on June 12, 1994, having been comatose from a stroke and on a respirator since March 1994. His death was widely reported in the news media. After his death, several themes arose among the Lubavitchers. Many believed that he would be resurrected. Others emphasized his continual spiritual presence in the world. All continued to hope and pray for the messianic arrival. Lubavitchers began to visit the Rebbe's tomb, and miracle stories continue about people who have visited his grave. Some Lubavitchers noted that although the Rebbe was a potential messiah, the generation did not possess enough merit to warrant his coming. Others simply admitted that they had been wrong—that only God knows when the messiah will come. Dein notes that the Lubavitchers have adapted an apparently failed prophecy in complex ways that have not only preserved, but enhanced, their commitment to messianic prophecy.

CONVERSION PROCESSES

Contemporary research has been guided by a focus upon gradual conversion to new religious movements. In addition to typologies, numerous investigators have presented models of the process of conversion. Some are formal in scope and propositional in nature (Gartrell & Shannon, 1985). The majority are qualitative models that have been inductively arrived at and used to organize the empirical literature (Lofland & Stark, 1965; Rambo, 1993); it is not clear that such models can be easily submitted to empirical tests capable of falsifying them (Kilbourne & Richardson, 1989; Kuhn, 1962; Masterman, 1970; Richardson, 1985b). Most models share a recognition that conversion is a complex process in which a variety of factors must be considered. In general terms, we can identify these factors under four headings: context; precipitating events; supporting activities; and finally participation/commitment.

Context

Conversion always takes place within a context. The term "context" is broad and vague enough to incorporate historical, social, cultural, and interpersonal situations that make conversion possible. For instance, Wallace (1956) noted that historical figures such as Jesus, Mohammed, and Buddha have become foci of revitalization movements. Within varieties of North American Protestantism, we have already seen how Paul's conversion has served as a prototype for a model of transformation that permits the expected "born-again" experience associated with conversion or intensification experiences. Yet the cautionary note that this is only one model of transformation is now well substantiated by empirical research. Research Box 11.4 presents a study of conversion within Islam, in which emotional, Pauline-type experiences are neither modeled by the religion nor typically reported by converts. Clearly, the context of Islamic culture does not facilitate such experience.

Included among the contextual factors facilitating religious conversion are purely social and cultural phenomena that alter the probability of conversion. For instance, Bulliet (1979) has argued from a historical perspective that conversion to new religions follows the typical S-curve established to characterize diffusion of innovation in cultures. Psychologists will readily recognize the S-curve as a summated normal "bell curve." What is important for

---

Research Box 11.4. An Empirical Study of Conversion to Islam (Poston, 1992)

Poston attempted to obtain questionnaire responses from 20 Muslim organizations. Only 8 of these 20 responded at all, and from these 8, only 12 completed questionnaires were obtained. Poston notes that this is typical of Muslims (at least in North America), who are suspicious of research into their beliefs and practices. By contrast, Christians and members of many new religious movements in North America readily cooperate in completing questionnaires on reports of their conversion experiences.

Reverting to reports of conversion experience in Islamic publications, Poston was able to obtain 72 testimonies of conversion, 69% of which were from males. Classifying these testimonies, Poston found that most converts (57%) had been raised as Christians. Only 3 of the 72 converts reported an emotional, Pauline-type conversion in which supernatural factors were perceived to account for the conversion. All but one of the converts were seekers who sought out a variety of religious options before becoming converted to Islam, with 21% stating the reasonableness of the faith as the motive for conversion, and 19% giving the universal brotherhood of all as the reason.

studies of conversion is Bulliet's classification of those who converted at various points in history along the curve. Using the history of Islam as his example, he described the first 16% who converted as the "innovators" (2.5%) and "early adopters" (13.5%). Then came the 34% constituting the "early majority," followed by the next 34%, the "late majority." Finally, the remaining 16% who converted were described as the "laggards" (Bulliet, 1979, pp. 31–32). Figure 11.1 illustrates Bulliet's classification curve.

Bulliet's theory has been operationalized and tested for the historical dominance of Islam in various cultures, but this model could be empirically tested within other historical contexts as well. What is important is the fact that the social-psychological processes of conversion may vary, depending upon the historical moment at which one converts to a religion and its dominance at that time in the culture. The kinds of persons and the processes by which they convert to new religious movements may vary as such movements gain ascendancy within the culture. Bulliet's historical perspective can be linked to other models of conversion, particularly those sensitive to the varieties of conversion motifs. Research Box 11.5 presents a study of British converts to Islam, interpreted in terms of the conversion motifs of Lofland and Skonovd (1981).

Precipitating Events

The effort to dichotomize theories of conversion often focuses upon whether or not precipitating events can be identified, and if so, within what time frame they operate. We have seen how proponents of sudden conversions often cite crises or emotional events as the turning point. Yet as Rambo (1993) has noted, crises can vary in length, scope, and duration. Proponents of gradual conversion emphasize interpersonal processes and the active seeking of meaning and purpose over a longer time interval as key factors in conversion (Gerlach & Hine, 1970).

The use of the conversion motifs discussed earlier allows for many variations, compatible with the existing empirical literature. There are many pathways to conversion, varying in length, scope, and nature (Heirich, 1977). For instance, crisis-precipitated conversions,

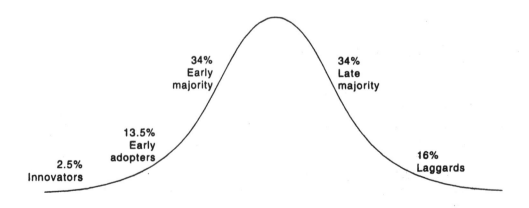

FIGURE 11.1. A bell curve model of conversion types, based upon time of conversion relative to percentage of population converted. Data from Bulliet (1979, pp. 31–32).

⅋⬥

Research Box 11.5. Conversion Motifs among British Converts to Islam
(Köse & Loewenthal, 2000).

Köse and Loewenthal (2000) studied 70 contemporary British converts to Islam. Köse, a male Muslim, interviewed each convert; both he and a female psychologist then independently rated the interviews in terms of the six conversion motifs of Lofland and Skonovd (1981). There results are summarized in the following table.

Motif[a]	Males	Females	Factors significantly associated with conversion motif
Intellectual	38	12	Cognitive concerns before conversion
Mystical	9	1	Sufism; new religious movements
Experimental	28	14	None
Affectional	28	18	Sufism; marriage; being female
Revivalist	0	0	(Not applicable)
Coercive	3	0	None

[a]Motifs are not mutually exclusive; actual numbers, not percentages, are reported in this table.
These investigators note that the conversion motifs of Lofland and Skonovd (1981) allow for a shorthand representation of complex religious autobiographies that permits them to be linked to normative features of conversion. They also note that the antecedents of conversion vary with conversion motifs. It is also noteworthy that revivalist conversion, which is associated with the classical paradigm largely derived from Christianity, does not apply at all to converts to Islam.

---

including the affective and coercive motifs, vary widely among themselves in terms of duration, intensity, and scope (Straus, 1979). Furthermore, a crisis may be intrapsychic or interpsychic; the former often refers to some variety of personal stress, the latter to some variety of social strain (Seggar & Kunz, 1972). Likewise, actively seeking meaning and purpose (as in the experimental and intellectual motifs) varies in the range and nature of meaning sought, as well as in the motivation for seeking such meanings (Rambo, 1993). It may be, as Gerlach and Hine (1970) have shown, that some converts gradually employ new systems of rhetoric that allow them to see themselves and the world transformed. Similarly, in a study that employed a comparison group to look at differences among Catholic Pentecostals, Heirich (1977) found that converts were most likely to be persons introduced to the group by friends or spiritual advisors who facilitated the gradual use of new religious attributions in the process of conversion. Nonconverts were not introduced to the group by friends or spiritual advisors and failed to acquire the appropriate language (attributions or rhetoric) of conversion. Thus mundane factors can precipitate conversion. Straus (1979) has documented how several converts to Scientology managed to seek and find beliefs, and to enter groups that allowed them to convert themselves by "creative bumbling."

Thus no one process of conversion applies to all conversion motifs. Generalizations concerning the conversion process are highly suspect if proffered as other than hypotheses for empirical investigation. Furthermore, it is not clear how the nature of the religious group to which a person has converted interacts with whatever general conversion processes have been empirically proposed. For instance, Seggar and Kunz (1972) found that one widely cited process model of religious conversion accounted for only 1 of the 77 cases of conversion to Mormonism in their study. Likewise, compensatory models of religious conversion must be tempered by the empirical assessment of the consequences of conversion, which are typically positive (Richardson, 1995). This is the case even when the conversion is to religious groups that remain marginal to the larger culture. Research Box 11.6 reports a study evaluating the legitimacy of conversion based upon the factors that precipitated conversion.

Ullman (1982) made empirical comparisons of conversion processes across different religious groups. Emotional factors, rather than cognitive factors, differentiated converts to all four religious groups from nonconverts. This was not a direct test of the relative contribution of cognitive and emotional factors in conversion, given that all converts were selected according to criteria that included actual changes in religious identity but excluded such changes when they were made for interpersonal reasons, such as marrying a spouse in the new faith. We have already noted the role of interpersonal factors in some conversion motifs, especially those unlikely to be precipitated by crises or emotional factors. In addition, all four of Ullman's groups cultivated intense, emotional experiences, perhaps biasing the sample toward an affective conversion motif. Still, Ullman's study is one of the few empirical studies that have used appropriate measurement procedures to compare converts to a variety of religious groups with matched controls. Some highlights of this research are presented in Research Box 11.7.

Research Box 11.6. Evaluating the Legitimacy of Conversion Based upon the Five Signs in Mark 16:17–18 (Hood, Williamson, & Morris, 1999)

Judgments regarding the legitimacy of conversion experiences can be expected to be based either upon prejudice or upon reasoned, rational rejection of certain practices. The serpent-handling sects of Appalachia practice all five signs specified in Mark 16:17–18—casting out demons, laying hands upon the sick, speaking in tongues, handing serpents, and drinking poison. A sample of 453 undergraduate psychology students were asked to evaluate the legitimacy of individuals' hypothetical conversion experiences, in terms of each of the five signs. As anticipated, results indicated that both prejudiced and rational rejection of conversion was associated with the two most extreme signs—serpent handling and drinking poison. Prejudiced rejection included stereotyping, negative affect, and specific behavioral intentions to avoid associating with converts.

However, when the effects of rational rejection were controlled for, there remained a strong relationship between prejudice and the evaluation of the legitimacy of conversion, including stereotyping. Conversion based upon serpent handling and drinking poison was still less accepted than conversion based upon casting out of demons, speaking in tongues or the laying of hands upon the sick. The relevance of separating prejudice from rational rejection is important, given the legal repercussions for serpent-handling sects in many states. It may be the case that even reasoned disagreement with serpent-handling sects masks an underlying prejudice, especially since knowledge of this tradition is largely available only from stereotyped presentations of these sects in the mass media.

હ

Research Box 11.7. Emotional versus Cognitive Factors in Precipitating Conversion (Ullman, 1982)

Ullman studied 40 white, middle-class individuals raised as Jews and Christians, who had converted from 1 to 10 months previous to the study. Half the converts were male and half female. They were compared on the basis of both objective measures and in-depth interviews to each other and to 30 controls (nonconverted subjects). All converts actually changed religious denomination. The four converted groups consisted of 10 subjects each, who were now Orthodox Jews, Roman Catholic, Hare Krishnas, and Baha'i adherents. The major differences between converted and nonconverted groups were on emotional, not cognitive, indices. Among the major significant differences between all converts and the control group were a greater frequency of both childhood and adolescent stress, as well as a greater frequency of prior drug use and psychiatric problems, among the converted subjects. Converts recalled childhoods that were less happy and filled with more anguish than those of nonconverts. The emotions recalled for adolescence followed the childhood patterns, with the addition of significant anger and fear in adolescence for the converts but not the nonconverts. Converts also differed from nonconverts in having less love and admiration for their fathers, and more indifference and anger toward them. Differences among the converted groups were less relevant than the consistency across all converted groups, suggesting that similar processes operated regardless of the faith to which a subject converted.

Supporting Activities

The classification of conversion motifs is helpful in directing research into factors in the conversion process that have long been ignored. Among these are interpersonal relationships between a potential convert and what Rambo (1993) refers to as the "advocate."

The advocate is often a friend who initiates and sustains the potential convert in the group. Sometimes simple factors (such as marriage) convert one partner. Much of the literature has documented the importance of social networks in facilitating conversion, especially among noncommunal religions. For instance, Snow and Machalek (1984, p. 182) found that the vast majority (from 59% to 82%) of Pentecostals, evangelicals, and Nichiren Shoshu Buddhists that they studied were recruited through social networks.

Much of the research has focused upon how social networks may facilitate gradual emotional conversions by the mere fact that intensive interaction among group members increases the likelihood of affective bonding among the members (Galanter, 1980; Snow, Zurcher, & Ekland-Olson, 1980, 1983; Stark & Bainbridge, 1980a; Straus, 1979). Jacobs (1987, 1989) has reintroduced the analogy of conversion and falling in love into the contemporary literature on conversion to groups with charismatic leaders. William James (1902/1985) used the same analogy, as did Pratt (1920), who went so far as to state that "In many cases getting converted means falling in love with Jesus" (p. 160). Cartwright and Kent (1992) have noted that new religious movements provide alternative pathways to intimacy and love within a familial perspective.

More psychologically oriented social psychologists have also focused on affective bonding, operationalized more rigorously in terms of attachment theory (discussed in Chapter 4). Individuals with the less secure types of attachment may exhibit higher rates of sudden conversions in adolescence or adulthood, regardless of the religiosity of their parents (Kirkpatrick, 1992, 1995; Kirkpatrick & Shaver, 1990). Kirkpatrick (1997) has provided one of the few longitudinal studies of this issue, in which he demonstrated that women readers of a Midwest newspaper surveyed approximately 4 years apart were more likely to report a changed relationship to God at the second assessment if they had insecure rather than secure attachment styles. Insecure-anxious women were most likely to report a conversion experience within this 4-year period. Granqvist (2002a) has suggested that the attachment literature can clarify some of the relationships between gradual conversion (or the contemporary paradigm) and sudden conversion (or the classical paradigm). Secure attachment leads to the gradual acceptance of the religiosity or nonreligiosity of parents. When there are religious changes, they are likely to be gradual and associated with loving and intimate God images. However, among the insecure attachment types, the influence of parental religiosity is minimal. Religious changes are likely to be sudden and associated with a distant and unloving image of God. In these types, the image of God serves as a compensatory attachment figure. Thus much of the attachment literature parallels the sociological literature of relationships. Once again, the literatures of sociological and psychological social psychology have focused upon similar concerns, although unfortunately these are not often cross-referenced. In addition, Beit-Hallahmi and Argyle (1997, p. 120) have noted how the attachment literature "seems to lend clear support to the psychodynamic view of religious conversion."

Thus various theories converge to suggest that religious conversion can be compensatory for psychological deficiencies linked to childhood experiences. For instance, Oksanen's (1994) meta-analysis of 25 studies sampling a total of over 4,500 converts found considerable support for the view that, however interpreted, conversion can be seen as serving a compensatory function for difficulties in interpersonal relationships with significant others (in either adulthood or childhood). However, as the data reviewed earlier suggest, by no means are all conversion experiences compensatory. Furthermore, qualitative studies often suggest correctives to exclusively quantitative research. For instance, Streib (2001b) has used qualitative/biographical research to study both converts and deconverts to new fundamentalist religious movements. He has found "no typical sect biography and no typical set of motivational factors" (p. 235). Furthermore, although childhood trauma and anxiety were identified in fundamentalist biographies, they were found in nonfundamentalist biographies as well (Streib, 2001b). Likewise, Zinnbauer and Pargament (1998) found that persons reporting spiritual conversions were similar to nonconverts who had become more religious. The only difference between the two groups were that spiritual converts reported more postconversion life transformation. Thus psychologists ought to be sensitive to the extent to which qualitative studies may add depth and clarification to purely measurement-based approaches (Streib, 2001a; Zinnbauer & Pargament, 1998). What is clear is that various theoretical and methodological orientations are beginning to converge and to clarify how individual differences in interpersonal styles (whether attachment-based, psychodynamically based, or sociologically based) may affect the conditions under which conversion may be sudden or gradual, and compensatory or not.

Social networks may also function to facilitate more cognitively motivated conversions, by providing interpersonal support for world views associated with what amount to cognitive reformulations of converts' sense of themselves and others. Religious converts not only use more religious attributions, but use those associated with their new group. For instance, Beckford (1978) has demonstrated the process by which Jehovah's Witnesses converts gradually come to cognitively assess the world in light of a master attribution scheme consistent with Jehovah's Witnesses' theology. One rhetorical indicator that conversion is occurring is the utilization of such a master attribution scheme, which both defines and produces conversion. Interacting within a given social network supports the scheme and serves to differentiate the newly emerging convert. It is the new religious attribution scheme that permits a biographical reconstruction of the transformed self. Often such reconstructions are solidified by participation in appropriate rituals confirming one's conversion (Boyer, 1994; Morinis, 1985).

The more sociologically oriented research on rhetorical indicators of conversion meshes nicely with psychologically oriented measurement-based research on cognitive change among converts. For instance, Paloutzian and colleagues have demonstrated an increase in scores on a measure of purpose in life for converts, as compared to nonconverted controls or controls who were unsure they were converted (Paloutzian, 1981; Paloutzian, Jackson, & Crandell, 1978).

Participation/Commitment

It is not likely that conversion as a process can be identified in temporal terms as having been completed once and for all. After conversion, commitment and participation can be expected to vary. It is not uncommon for converts to new religious movements to follow "conversion careers," joining and leaving a variety of religious groups over time (Richardson, 1978b). Bird and Remier (1982) note that only a small percentage of converts to new religious movements remain members of one movement. Furthermore, participation in religious groups is not necessarily higher among converted individuals than among those born and socialized into the groups (Barker & Currie, 1985).

DECONVERSION AND RELATED PHENOMENA

The concept of conversion careers makes it clear that for some converts, a variety of conversion experiences can be expected. This especially characterizes converts to new religious movements, the majority of whom can be expected to leave within a few years. "Deconversion" is the term most typically used to identify this process. Compared to the massive research literature on conversion, few studies of deconversion exist, and the few existing studies are of fairly recent origin. For instance, Wright (1987) could document only three studies of deconversion published prior to 1980.

Not surprisingly, the literature on deconversion parallels that for conversion. With the exception of the special case of "brainwashing" discussed in Chapter 12, most studies of deconversion have been done by sociologists using participant observation or descriptive research strategies. Assessment is often carried out via interviews, either structured or open-ended, with former members. Most studies of deconversion have focused upon defectors from new religious movements, paralleling the tremendous literature on new religious movements and conversion discussed above. Unlike the literature on apostasy, the deconversion literature focuses upon the processes involved in leaving religious groups, not simply correlates and predictors of leaving.

Deconversion within New Religious Movements

Skonovd (1983) studied former members of fundamentalist Christian groups, as well as of Scientology, the Unification Church, the People's Temple, and various Eastern groups. He identified a process of deconversion consisting of a precipitating crisis, followed by review and reflection, disaffection, withdrawal, and a transition to cognitive reorganization. His model, however, does not distinguish between voluntary and involuntary leaving—an issue of concern, given the debate on deprogramming discussed in Chapter 12.

Wright (1986) studied matched samples of those remaining and those voluntarily defecting from the Unification Church, Hare Krishna, and a fundamentalist Christian group. He focused upon precipitating factors that initiated the process of deconversion. Among those identified were breakdown of insulation from the outside world, development of unregulated interpersonal relationships, perceived lack of success in achieving social change, and disillusionment. Wright's research parallels conversion research, in that both emotional and cognitive factors can trigger the process of deconversion, and the process itself can be sudden or gradual. Furthermore, he identified different modes of departure, based upon the length of time people were committed to a group. Most of those who were members for 1 year or less (92%) left by quiet, covert means. Those who were members for more than a year left by either overt means or direct confrontations, often emotional and dramatic in nature ("declarative" means).

Downton (1980) has documented the gradual process of deconversion from the Divine Light Mission (the sect associated with Guru Maharaj Ji). Intellectual and social disillusionment predominated. The breaking of bonds within the group occurred only as new bonds were established outside the group. Galanter, Rabkin, Rabkin, and Deutsch (1979) found that converts to the Unification Church who had not completely severed nonsanctioned emotional attachments within the group were likely to deconvert even when they believed in the doctrine of the group.

Jacobs (1989) studied 40 religious devotees, most of whom where involved in either charismatic Christian, Hindu-based, or Buddhist groups. All groups had charismatic leaders, were patriarchal in orientation, and had structured hierarchies with rigid disciplines of behavior and devotion. The 21 male and 19 female participants were predominantly middle-class, white, and well educated. Among the 40 deconverters, both social disillusionment and disillusionment with the charismatic leader were major reasons cited for discontent leading to deconversion, as noted in Table 11.4. Jacobs (1989) notes that the total process of deconversion for these individuals required severing ties both with the group and with the charismatic leader. The total process of deconversion included a period of initial separation, often accompanied by an experience of isolation and loneliness; this was followed by a period of emotional strain and readjustment, culminating in the reestablishment of identity outside the group.

Descriptive studies of deconversion, like those on conversion, run the risk of confounding the natural history of groups with causal processes assumed to operate in them (Snow & Machalek, 1984). Furthermore, investigators tend to avoid measurement in favor of utilizing subjective accounts of deconversion, placed within descriptive systems proposed by the investigators as explanatory. Few tests of these models have been undertaken. Longitudinal research is virtually absent. Finally, no studies have compared subjects who have deconverted from several religious groups to see whether the same process of deconversion occurs each time.

TABLE 11.4. Sources of Disillusionment among 40 Deconverters

Source	%
Disillusionment with a charismatic leader and his actions	
Physical abuse	31
Psychological abuse	60
Emotional rejection	45
Spiritual betrayal	33
Social disillusionment	
Social life	75
Spiritual life	50
Status/position	35
Prescribed sex roles	45

Note. Adapted from Jacobs (1989, pp. 43, 92). Copyright 1989 by Indiana University Press. Adapted by permission.

Disengagement within Mainstream Religious Groups

Although most of the research on deconversion has focused upon new religious movements that are sectarian or cult-like in nature, most religious participation in North America is within denominational religious groups. Such established groups have long been noted to have transitional memberships. As a general pattern, participation in religious groups waxes and wanes. Probably 80% of denominational members withdraw at some point in their lives, only to return at some later point (Roozen, 1980). Thus only a minority of persons socialized into religious groups in North America ever truly reject religious identity or participation. As we have noted, the percentage of apostates in the United States has remained fairly constant at about 7%. This means that well over 90% of the U.S. population belonging to a religious group engages in some form of religious participation, whether this takes place at a church, mosque, or synagogue. However, the frequency of this participation fluctuates. For instance, Albrecht, Cornwall, and Cunningham (1988) mailed questionnaires to a stratified random sample of 32 active and 45 inactive families in each of 27 different Mormon wards (similar to congregations). Seventy-four percent of the active families and 44% of the inactive families responded. Phone follow-ups to the inactive families raised their participation rate to 64%. Two measure of disengagement were used: (1) behavioral (a period of 1 month or more of no church attendance), and (2) belief (a period of at least 1 year when the Mormon church was not an important part of a family's life). Summarizing the results for every 100 families revealed that 74 became disengaged, either in terms of behavior (55) or belief (19). Only 4 families remained engaged nonbelievers; only 22 remained engaged believers. Of the 55 families that were disengaged nonbelievers, 31 returned to church participation (Albrecht et al., 1988; see also Albrecht & Cornwall, 1989). These data are consistent with studies of disengagement and reengagement among Catholics (Hoge, with McGuire & Stratman, 1981). They are also consistent with the studies of denominational switching and the cycling of religious participation discussed in Chapter 12. However, in light of the historical context within which new religious movements have emerged, it appears that many disengaged from mainstream religion have explored new religious movements as one form of reengagement.

Baby Boomers and Disengagement/Reengagement

As noted in earlier chapters, several investigators have been concerned with what has been called the "baby boomer" generation. Although not precisely defined, this generation includes those raised in the 1960s in North America during a period of intense social upheaval (Roszak, 1968). Associated with this upheaval was the emergence of new religious movements, competing with and often congruent with a variety of countercultural movements (Tipton, 1982). Participants in these countercultural movements were largely youths reared in mainstream religious traditions. For instance, Roof (1993) found that two-thirds of all baby boomers reared in mainstream religious traditions dropped out or disengaged from mainstream religious participation in their late adolescence or early youth. The average ages of disengagement for different birth cohorts are presented in Table 11.5.

Roof used a commercial firm to conduct focused group interviews with subjects from randomly digit-dialed samples. Households in four states (California, Massachusetts, North Carolina, and Ohio) were sampled. A 60% participation rate was obtained from an initial sample of 2,620 households. Baby boomers were defined as those born between 1946 and 1962 ($n = 1,599$; 61% of sample). The sample was further divided into older boomers (1946–1954; $n = 802$) and younger boomers (1955–1962; $n = 797$). Follow-up interviews were conducted with older boomers, and eventually 64 in-depth, face-to-face interviews and 14 group dialogues were conducted with these participants (Roof, 1993).

As discussed in Chapter 5, religious disengagement tends to follow a pattern that includes religious socialization and participation, followed by youthful rebellion and departure, and subsequently by return. Thus high rates of disengagement among boomers would not be surprising, nor would a return of most of most of these to mainstream religious participation. Indeed, Roof found that a return to mainstream religion occurred as expected for many of those who were disengaged. Furthermore, categorizing participants by the extent to which they were part of the mainstream culture (in terms of having settled into a community, married, and had children) indicated that the more normalized a subject's current lifestyle was in terms of the dominant culture, the more likely the subject was to have returned to religious involvement, as noted in Table 11.6.

The fact that those who disengage from religion tend to return as they participate more fully in the dominant culture is readily understandable in terms of life cycle theories of socialization. As noted earlier in this chapter, youth is a time for exploration and rebellion—or, in more psychological terms, a time in which one searches for identity (Erikson, 1968). However, it is also the case that theories of social change suggest the relevance of youthful participation in radical social movements aimed at altering society (Keniston, 1968, 1971; Roszak, 1968). Kent (2001) has marshaled considerable empirical evidence to support the thesis that the youthful

TABLE 11.5. Average Age of Disengagement by Birth Cohort

Birth cohort	Average age at disengagement
1926–1935	29.4 years
1936–1945	25.1 years
1946–1954 (older baby boomers)	21.1 years
1955–1962 (younger baby boomers)	18.2 years

Note. Adapted from Roof (1993, pp. 154–155). Copyright 1993 by HarperCollins Publishers. Adapted by permission.

TABLE 11.6. Baby Boomers' Reengagement in Mainstream Religion

Normative criteria	% reengaged
Single, no children, not settled	14 ($n = 51$)
Married, no children, not settled	16 ($n = 50$)
Married, children, not settled	52 ($n = 71$)
Married, children, settled	54 ($n = 124$)

Note. Adapted from Roof (1993, p. 165). Copyright 1993 by HarperCollins Publishers. Adapted by permission.

political protest to mystical religions.[2] Whereas religions denominations tend to be at ease with the dominant culture, religious sects and cults are at tension with at least some aspects of this culture, as discussed in Chapter 12. New religious movements are likely to appeal to individuals not committed to the dominant culture, and thus may recruit members whose initial protest was expressed in political terms (Kent, 2001). Montgomery (1991) has argued that the spread of new religions is facilitated when the new religions either are a threat to society or come from a source other than the society; they provide sources of identity and resistance for those alienated from the dominant culture. Although Montgomery's theory applies to the emergence of new religions within a historical context and focuses upon macrosocial relations, it also applies to the emergence of new religions within a culture where a dominant culture opposes a subculture—a phenomenon characteristic of the 1960s in North America (Tipton, 1982). The subculture is likely to accept new religious movements that promulgate behaviors and beliefs at odds with the dominant culture, as sects and cults do.

One empirical prediction that is congruent with these macrosocial assumptions is that exposure to countercultural values should make a person more susceptible to new religious movements and to disengagement from mainstream religion. Roof's research provides data relevant to this claim. Using an index of exposure to the 1960s counterculture, Roof found that the preference for sticking to a mainstream cultural expressions of faith varied as a function of such exposure, as did willingness to explore other teachings and religions. These results are summarized in Table 11.7.

The high rate of former drug use among members converted to new religious movements is well documented. In some new religious movements, the rate of former drug use is reported to be almost 100%. For instance, Volinn (1985) used in-depth interviews and extensive participatory observation to study 52 members of an ashram in New England. Forty-seven of these admitted to smoking marijuana, and 46 had used it 50 times or more. Likewise, all but 8 admitted to using LSD, but only 6 had used this more than 50 times, and 14 had used it only "once or twice" (Volinn, 1985, p. 152). Other investigators have documented former drug use among converts to new religious movements. Among new religious movements Judah (1974) has documented abandonment of drug use among converts to Hare Krishna; Galanter and Buckley (1978) have obtained similar results for converts to the Divine Light Mission; Anthony and Robbins (1974) have documented abandonment of drug use

---

2. However, the conversion to religious frames may have been only temporary. For instance, Whalen and Flacks (1989) studied 17 political activists convicted for a Bank of America bombing in 1970. The majority did turn temporarily to countercultural religions, but eventually resumed political activities, although in a less extreme form.

TABLE 11.7. Responses to the Question "Is It Good to
Explore the Many Differing Religious Teachings, or Should
One Stick to a Particular Faith?" as a Function of Exposure
to the 1960s

Exposure to 1960s index[a]	Explore many teachings	Stick to faith
0	49%	39%
1	60%	32%
2	63%	23%
3	80%	14%

Note. Adapted from Roof (1993, p. 124). Copyright 1993 by HarperCollins
Publishers. Adapted by permission.

[a]Exposure to 1960s index: "Did you ever: 1. Attend a rock concert? [67% yes];
2. Smoke marijuana? [50% yes]; 3. Take part in any demonstrations,
marches, or rallies? [20% yes]." For each positive response, 1 point was scored.

among converts to Meher Baba; and Nordquist (1978) also found such outcomes for converts to Ananda, a "New Age" community in Sweden.

The low rates of illicit drug use among members of mainstream religions have long been
established (Gorsuch, 1976), and both mainstream religions and new religious movements
discourage the use of illicit drugs. However, it appears that prior drug experience varies according to whether one is a member of a mainstream denomination or a new religious movement,
whether sect or cult. In denominational religion, norms and beliefs serve to decrease the probability of illicit drug use among participants. However, among those who use illicit drugs, spiritual seeking can result in conversion to new religious movements that then discourage illicit
drug use. Several investigators have described new religious movements as providing an alternative to drug experiences. Some argue that conversion can even be a new form of addiction
(Simmonds, 1977a); new religious converts may simply substitute one addiction for another.
Others, such as Volinn (1985), have focused upon the spiritual experiences of converts to new
religious movements as meaningful alternatives to illicit drug "highs."

It would appear that with few exceptions, institutional forms of religion—whether denominations, sects, or cults—tend to discourage drug use. An interesting exception is the Native American use of peyote (LaBarre, 1969). Yet many who utilize drugs outside of religion
define themselves as spiritual seekers. Roof (1993) noted that among his baby boomers, those
most exposed to the counterculture of the 1960s were least likely to be conventionally religious,
but most likely to define themselves as spiritual. Eighty-one percent of those scoring highest
on his index of exposure to the 1960s defined themselves as spiritual, whereas 92% of those
who scored zero on his index defined themselves as religious. Not surprisingly, 84% of those
scoring highest on the exposure-to-the-1960s index were religious dropouts (Roof, 1993).

THE COMPLEXITY OF CONVERSION

It has been over half a century since Allport (1950, p. 37) claimed that "no subject within
the psychology of religion has been more extensively studied than conversion." However,
despite the massive empirical literature—first from psychologically oriented and more recently from sociologically oriented social psychologists—no simple conclusion can be reached

that has any degree of empirical validity. Clearly, conversion can entail significant changes in persons, even if changes in basic personality functions are unlikely. The questions of precisely how and why these changes occur demand systematic programs of research (Paloutzian et al., 1999, p. 1048). Such programs are unlikely to be useful if they are not guided by theories or models as complex as the empirical realities they hope to illuminate.

With this in mind, Rambo (1993) has proposed an integrative model that utilizes insights from anthropologists (Berkhofer, 1963), missiologists (Tippett, 1977) and sociologists (Lofland & Stark, 1965). It is not simply developmental, although it does propose stages or sequences that can serve as a heuristic model. Unlike many purely psychological approaches, the stages or sequences are neither unidirectional nor invariant. Finally, the stages are interrelated in complex dialectical ways that allow them to be interactive, so that not only can early stages influence later stages, but these in turn can influence earlier ones (Paloutzian et al., 1999). The model is summarized in Table 11.8.

OVERVIEW

Conversion has occupied the interest of social scientists since the beginning of the 20th century. The early research was dominated by psychologists, who focused upon adolescence and sudden emotional conversions. The classic paradigm for conversion was fashioned after Paul's experience. Gradual conversion were recognized to occur, and were linked to an active search for meaning and purpose, but were seldom studied except to be contrasted with sudden conversions.

In the early 1960s, sociologically oriented social psychologists began to study conversion as a phenomena linked to new religious movements. They have focused upon gradual conversions, postulating models of the conversion process most typically derived from participant observation or interview studies of converts.

TABLE 11.8. An Integrative Model for Conversion

Stages or facets of the conversion process	Factors that must be assessed in this stage
Stage 1: Context	Factors that facilitate or hinder conversion. These include cultural, historical, personal, sociological, and theological factors.
Stage 2: Crisis	May be personal, social or both.
Stage 3: Quest	Intentional activity on part of potential convert.
Stage 4: Encounter	Recognition of alternative spiritual or religious option. May be facilitated by individual ("advocate") or institution (missionary activity).
Stage 5: Interaction	Extended engagement at many levels with new religious/spiritual option.
Stage 6: Commitment	Identification with new spiritual or religious reality.
Stage 7: Consequences	Transformations as a result of new commitment, including beliefs, behaviors, and identity.

Note. See Rambo (1993) and Paloutzian, Richardson, and Rambo (1999).

Studies employing cognitive dissonance theory have shifted the focus from research-ers' and outsiders' claims about failed prophecy to insiders' perspective on how such prophecy becomes interpreted in ways to maintain group commitment and cohesion. Studies are be-ginning to look at the conditions under which different individuals may leave prophetic groups to which they have converted.

Apostasy and deconversion have been studied as phenomena closely linked to conver-sion. Like conversion, apostasy has been linked to adolescence or young adulthood. Rela-tively few individuals remain apostates; most return at some point in the life cycle. This typi-cally occurs when they are married, have children, and settle in an established community. However, spiritual seekers may remain outside religion altogether. Deconversion from a new religious movement is likely to be a gradual process of disillusionment, both with the reli-gious group and with its leader.

Chapter 12

THE SOCIAL PSYCHOLOGY
OF RELIGIOUS ORGANIZATIONS

The people of Jonestown could not have had a compelling reason for what they did, for the integrity of our own social existence would thereby be placed in doubt. Giving credence to Jones' account would require concluding the unthinkable: that the people of Jonestown were "justified" in taking the action of terminating the lives of an entire community.

Between you and God there stands the church.

Amish values, Amish limits, and the Amish definition of success cannot be grafted onto American culture. It would be pointless to imitate their use of bonnets, buggies, and kerosene lamps. The value of the Amish lies, rather, in making clear limits of some kind and in their insistence in defining for themselves the limits within which they will live.

Muslim traditionalists are not fantasizing when they identify divorce, abortion, more open sexual experimentation, sexually transmitted diseases, and women's demands for equality in the workplace and in decision-making as threats to traditional values.

When a society would turn its eyes away from the deepest questions of responsibility, brainwashing becomes an explanation that avoids the responsibility of looking inward.[1]

The process of becoming religious continues to intrigue social scientists and to foster both theoretical and empirical debate. The simple fact that persons are not born religious means that they must become religious if they are to be religious. The process of becoming religious entails numerous possibilities. Persons may be born into a family with a particular faith commitment and simply be socialized to adopt that faith as their own. These individuals are those whom William James (1902/1985) dubbed the "once-born." On the other hand, persons may be born into one faith tradition and later change to another. Those born outside any faith tradition may later choose to commit to one. Those previously committed may fall away. Persons may have a series of different faith commitments throughout their lives. Some may simply engage in an interminable quest, in which spiritual issues

---

1. These quotations come, respectively, from the following sources: Hall (1989, p. xiii); statement attributed to the bishop presiding at the trial of Joan of Arc, quoted in Stobart (1971, p. 157); Olshan (1994, p. 239); Awn (1994, p. 76); and Scheflin and Opton (1978, p. 50).

absorb their interest but never find a resolution. Much of this flux is the subject matter of religious conversion; converts are James's (1902/1985) "twice-born," discussed in Chapter 11.

Yet this individual religious change does not take place in a vacuum. The maintenance of faith, as well as conversion, is not an individual affair. Those with faith tend to seek companions in a social context within which their faith may be both shared and practiced. In this flux of individual religious change also lie the rise and fall of churches and the growth and decline of denominations. In addition, the emergence of novel religious forms from within established groups creates the sects and from without the cults. James (1902/1985) typifies the psychologist's propensity to emphasizes religious experience in individual terms, as we have discussed in Chapter 9. The renowned philosopher Whitehead (1926) even went so far as to define religion in terms of what individuals do with their solitude. There is a rich conceptual literature linking spirituality and solitude (Koch, 1994; Storr, 1988). As we have seen in Chapter 10, there are also many empirical data supporting a spirituality that is more closely linked to solitude than to tradition. Yet is remains true that religion has an inherently social dimension. Even solitude is a retreat from the social and takes with it the very language shared by others within which private thoughts are possible (Berger & Luckmann, 1967).

Thus the social characteristics of the groups within which persons are socialized, to which individuals convert, or from which individuals withdraw are of obvious relevance to understanding how persons become religious. Our task in this chapter is to present theory and data on the social psychology of religious organizations. In so doing, we confront issues that have long been of concern to social scientists and that have recently emerged into public debate and controversy. Both the rise and fall of religious collectivities and the commitments and disaffections of religious individuals cannot be discussed for long without controversy (Richardson, 1999b).

THE CLASSIFICATION OF RELIGIOUS ORGANIZATIONS

Although it may be true that psychologists are particularly prone to define religious commitments in terms of individuals, it remains abundantly clear that these are shared and under varying degrees of organizational control. Whitehead's (1926) focus on the great solitary images of religious imagination—Mohammed brooding in the desert, Buddha resting under the Bodhi tree, and Christ crying out from the cross—is balanced by the fact that such solitary religious figures maintain their importance within great traditions maintained by generations of the faithful, organized into "churches" or "denominations" and "sects." Furthermore, novel forms of religious commitment centered upon newly identified charismatic figures are likely themselves quickly to take an organizational form, however unstructured, if they are to survive. These are the religious "cults." Hence, to be either traditionally or innovatively religious is to be related in some fashion to a religious group. The solitary religious figure is a myth reconstructed and abstracted from the organizational forms that both define this figure and give her or him meaning. The classification of these religious forms has been of much interest to the more sociologically oriented psychologists of religion. Of the various classification schemes proposed, the most influential has been "church–sect theory."

CHURCH–SECT THEORY

Church–sect theory was never intended as a theory of origins, and hence it is a bit surprising that it has so dominated the empirical literature on both established and new religious movements. Furthermore, as Dittes (1971c) has noted, the careers of Troeltsch's church–sect theory and of Allport's theory and measures of Intrinsic versus Extrinsic religion (discussed in Chapter 2) have numerous parallels. Both theories have dominated their conceptual and empirical literatures; both have numerous critics; and both have, in Dittes's phrasing, "some considerable promise of surviving their obituaries" (1971c, p. 382).

A common criticism shared by these two theories is the confounding of evaluation with description. This often entails implicit claims to "good" and "bad" religion—whether in terms of organizational structure, as in Troeltsch's theory, or in terms of religious motivation, as in Allport's theory (Dittes, 1971c; Kirkpatrick & Hood, 1990). As we note later in this chapter, religious cults have to a large extent shared the burden of various pejorative connotations. They are typically perceived as "bad" religion. As social psychologists, we must explore the empirical reasons for such connotations. To do so requires an empirical grounding of the relationship between forms of religious organizations and their dominant or host cultures. In this section, we draw upon the roots of church–sect theory and attempt to show how these have influenced the sociologically oriented social-psychological literature. Only a few would argue against the importance of church–sect theory (Robertson, 1975; Snook, 1974). We hope that our discussion of this theory's roots in the work of Troeltsch will demonstrate both its relevance and its usefulness in organizing contemporary empirical studies on the social psychology of religious organizations.

Origins of Church–Sect Theory

The main source of church/sect theory in modern social psychology has been Reinhold Niebuhr's (1929) work on the social sources of denominationalism. Denominations are what many persons think of as "churches"—groups commonly accepted as legitimate religious organizations within their host cultures. Most people identify themselves by reporting their denominational membership when asked for their religious identification. Thus, as Wimberley and Christenson (1981) have noted, individual religious identity is largely synonymous with group religious membership.

Niebuhr's work is a modification and popularization of church, sect, and mysticism—three types of religious organizations articulated in Troeltsch's (1931) classic work *The Social Teachings of the Christian Churches*. Niebuhr's popularization significantly altered Troeltsch's conceptualizations. As discussed in Chapter 10, Niebuhr ignored Troeltsch's three-part typology (church–sect–mysticism) in favor of a two-part typology (church–sect). Furthermore, Niebuhr added a dynamic tendency to the theory: He suggested that persons who are dissatisfied with the commonness and permissiveness of churches as they successfully appeal to the masses seek more demanding criteria for membership. This exclusiveness creates a sectarian movement. Although Niebuhr thought that sects would be unable to gain control from elites within churches, and hence that the direction of change would be from church to sect, but not from sect to church, others argued against this. Johnson (1963, p. 543) argued that a shift from sect to church was theoretically "conceivable." Eister (1973) argued more forcefully for what he referred to as the "paradox of religious organizations":

Dynamic processes produce sects from churches, but sects then tend to become like the churches they once criticized.

Niebuhr's modification of Troeltsch's typology is further confounded when it is recognized that Troeltsch's three-part typology was derived from two independent dichotomies elaborated by Max Weber (Gerth & Mills, 1946; Weber, 1922/1963). As Swatos (1976) has emphasized, Weber had two typologies: church–sect and mysticism–asceticism. Troeltsch's single typology of church–sect–mysticism was itself a modification intended both to simplify and to clarify his friend Weber's dual typologies. The extent to which Troeltsch's single typology is compatible with Weber's dual typologies is a matter of dispute among scholars. Steeman (1975) argues that Troeltsch's treatment of church–sect–mysticism at least approximates Weber's intent with his dual typology. On the other hand, Garrett (1975) argues that a significant disjuncture separates Weber and Troeltsch's typologies, especially when consideration is given to mysticism.

For our purposes, it is important to emphasize that the Weber and Troeltsch theories share a crucial defining criterion that differentiates churches (denominations) from sects: Churches are inclusive, while sects are exclusive. By focusing upon the single criterion of degree of exclusiveness, church–sect theory can contribute to organizing the empirical literature in value-neutral terms. The criterion of exclusiveness is easily operationalized, and it permits us as social scientists to sidestep issues of evaluating "good" and "bad" religion.

A further clarification of the origins of Troeltsch's theory will aid us greatly in organizing the empirical literature, as well as in suggesting how a focus upon the original intent of Weber's and Troeltsch's typologies makes them less evaluative than subsequent theorists' development of these concepts.

Troeltsch and Church–Sect Theory

Troeltsch's theory has been critiqued or modified by numerous theorists, most of whom ignore Troeltsch's own analytical use of this typology within a limited historical context. Furthermore, Troeltsch's typology was intended only for Christianity. Contemporary theorists apply church–sect theory to a variety of new religious movements, many of which are non-Christian. However, despite these serious limitations, Troeltsch's theory remains viable as it focuses upon two assumptions likely to have universal validity. First, church, sect, and mysticism are logical tendencies within Christianity. Such tendencies are likely to be inherent not only in Christianity, but in any faith tradition centered upon a charismatic figure, regardless of particular histories or contexts (Troeltsch, 1931, Vol. 2, pp. 993–994). The second assumption is that contingent historical factors often structure the emergence of the types as actual empirical embodiments of these logical tendencies (Troeltsch, 1931, Vol. 2, pp. 994–1004). Troeltsch saw the logical tendencies of church, sect, and mysticism exhausted in their empirical forms insofar as Christianity was concerned. He argued that the church form was most purely expressed in medieval Catholicism, the sect form in Calvinism, and mysticism form in Quakerism. However, mysticism needs little formal organization. Instead, it enshrines radical subjectivity and individuality either within or outside faith traditions as forms of spirituality claiming direct access to the transcendent. Hence mysticism is of little relevance to religious organizations. As Steeman (1975) has succinctly noted, the mysticism type is more or less the end of the road in Troeltsch's historical scheme. Thus we do not further discuss mysticism in this chapter. (It has been separately treated in Chapter 10 of this text.)

The Troeltsch legacy for the modern study of religion is the "free church." Here, as new denominations of Christianity emerge, each a free expression of a fellowship of faith. These denominations exhibit dynamic tendencies, competing for universality (an expression of the church type) while also demanding ascetic purity (an expression of the sect type). Denominations are expressions of religious tolerance in a host culture that accepts and demands religious diversity. The historical exhausted realities of Troeltsch's forms of Christianity remain as logical tendencies within denominations, with their propensity for universalization (church) and personal purity (sect). These tendencies are expressed in much of the contemporary empirical literature.

The Empirical Tradition Influenced by Church–Sect Theory

Not surprisingly, contemporary social scientists have divided into two camps regarding church–sect theory. One camp continues the classical tradition of modifying church–sect theory and of debating its validity and value, mainly at the conceptual level (Eister, 1973; Johnson, 1963, 1971; Wilson, 1970). Most of the resulting classification systems are qualitatively derived, relying upon appeals to face validity. Few in this camp seek empirical verification of predictive consequences for their typologies. In the rare instances when these classifications have been empirically assessed, they have been found to be less than adequate. As Welch (1977, p. 127) has noted, "Few existing set classification schemes—both unidimensional and multidimensional varieties—are able to offer true discriminatory power when put to the empirical test."

Members of the other camp have opted for more precise operationalization of their typologies, often employing quantitative procedures to construct their typologies (Eister, 1973; Finke & Stark, 2001; Johnson, 1963, 1971; Stark & Bainbridge, 1987; Wilson, 1970), and seeking systematic testing of hypotheses derived from these classifications. One of the most systematic efforts has been made by Stark (1985a), whose model has moved the debate beyond mere conceptual criticisms to the testing of empirical hypotheses based upon operational measures.

Stark owes much to a now-classic paper by Johnson (1963), who first operationalized the essential difference between church and sect that he felt both Weber and Troeltsch set forth with varying degrees of explicitness. Churches are inclusive (e.g., accepting infant baptism) and are widely accommodating to their host cultures, seldom being at significant odds with their major values. On the other hand, sects are exclusive (e.g., often demanding adult baptism), and seek a religious purity that often puts them at odds with their culture. The universalizing tendency of the church type accommodates to the host culture, accepting many persons who meet only minimal criteria for membership. The perfectionist tendency of the sect type sets rigorous criteria for membership; as such, it is less accommodating to the host culture as it limits membership. Johnson (1963) operationalized these tendencies as follows: "*A church is a religious group that accepts the social environment in which it exists. A sect is a religious group that rejects the social environment in which it exists*" (p. 542; emphasis in original). Johnson further restricted church and sect to religious groups, stopping by definitional fiat the efforts to extend church–sect typologies to other groups (such as political ones) that some theorists have found useful (Robertson, 1975).

Stark and Bainbridge (1979, 1985, 1987) have refined Johnson's definition by further operationalizing acceptance and rejection according to degree of difference, antagonism, and separation between a religious group and its host culture. In our view, the most fruitful operational indicator is the degree of difference, indicated by beliefs and behavioral norms, between sects and the dominant host culture. Salient differences are likely to lead to mutual rejection, but whether or not they do is an independent empirical question. Furthermore, antagonism is largely a corollary of different beliefs and behavioral norms. Difference itself can be operationally equated with subcultural deviance when the beliefs produce tension between religious groups and their host culture. Low-tension beliefs are congruent with being part of mainstream culture and characteristic of denominations (churches).

Given this operationalization of church and sect along a continuum of tension, embedded within a more general theory of religion, numerous novel hypotheses have been generated and empirically tested (Stark & Bainbridge, 1980b). Perhaps the most hotly disputed among these is the concept of a general religious economy, in which religious views must compete in an open market. As such, extreme sects become more successful (gain members) by reducing their tension with the host culture. Over time, sects tend to shed their other-worldly and perfectionist tendencies as they accommodate to the culture. They may, but are unlikely to, remain isolated instances of subcultural deviance. Thus, in the Stark and Bainbridge theory, churches reemerge from sects as essentially secularized religious groups—insofar as secularization is recognized to be a process of accommodation to the dominant host culture. In other words, they become acceptable forms of denominational religious expression.

Finke and Stark (2001) have refined this theory to argue that under conditions of free competition, religious organizations can gain membership by moving to increase or decrease tension with their host culture. Their argument rests on the assumption that participation in religious organizations approximates a bell-shaped curve. Degree of tension, defined as the degree of distinctiveness, separation from, and antagonism with the host culture, ranges from very low ("ultraliberal") to very high ("ultrastrict"). Organizations at the extremes can only grow by moving toward the center; thus increasing tension facilitates growth at the more liberal end, whereas decreasing tension facilitates growth at the more sectarian end. Figure 12.1 presents the bell curve model of Finke and Stark.

As Finke and Stark (2001, p. 176) note, "To the extent people seek religion . . . the demand is highest for religions that offer close relations with the supernatural and distinctive demands for membership, without isolating individuals from the culture around them."

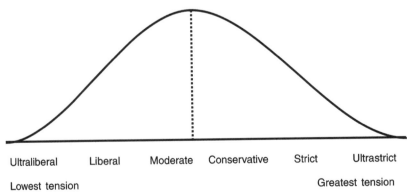

FIGURE 12.1. Hypothetical bell curve distribution of religious organizations. Data from Finke & Stark (2001, p. 177).

Thus, in North America, most religious people are members of congregations that fall somewhere between the extremes of the ultrastrict religious sects and the ultraliberal New Age and Unitarian/Universalist groups (Finke & Stark, 2001). Denominations predominate in the middle of the curve. However, this does not mean that only a "middle-of-the-road" religion can be successful.

Another novel hypothesis derived from Stark and Bainbridge's general model of religion is that in similar religious markets, novel forms of religion can be expected to thrive. As we shall soon see, if cults are defined as novel religious organizations, cults can be expected to thrive precisely where churches or denominations are weak. This follows from the hypothesis that churches have already accommodated to the mainstream culture and that sects are unlikely to maintain for long a novel stance vis-à-vis the larger host culture, to which they also must accommodate to be successful. The hypothesis that weak church environments lead to increased probabilities of cult formation has yet to be fully empirically substantiated, but it remains as viable a hypothesis as it is controversial (Bibby & Weaver, 1985; Bruce, 1999; Wallis, 1986). Still, the tendency for sects to lead to churches is inherent in any view that, almost by definition, social groups that survive have accommodated to their culture to at least the degree that their survival is assured. Garrett (1975, p. 211) has refereed to this tendency, most evident in Niebuhr, as the "Americanization of the Troeltschian typology."

It is important to emphasize that although accommodation to the host culture can be identified as a secular move, it is inherent in the nature of religious organizations that they devise objective means to permit universality at the expense of ethical perfection. For instance, churches permit membership on the basis of minimal criteria that can be objectively specified. In Troeltsch's (1931, Vol. 2, p. 993) terms, the church allows an "institutionalization of grace." Sects can maintain exclusivity by rejecting members who can be objectified as "too worldly." As such, a sect is a religious subculture by definition. Exclusivity both defines and characterizes sects as they emerge from churches. Yet they tend toward universality as they survive. Furthermore, religious subcultures, if sufficiently at odds with their host cultures and not in a process of accommodating to them, are likely to be targets of legal retaliation and control—something that has characterized the history of sects in the Western world (Johnson, 1963). It has also become a major issue with respect to the contemporary analysis of cults, as we shall shortly note. For now, it is sufficient to note that religious organizations are continually in dynamic processes of change, with individuals joining and leaving religious groups partly on the basis of their appeal to either sectarian (high-tension) or denominational (low-tension) characteristics. Research Box 12.1 presents data on this issue from a large sample of African Americans.

With church–sect theory, the useful empirical indicator is not simply a religious group's accommodation to or rejection of the host culture, but how the host culture in turn reacts to the religious group. What empirically distinguishes churches and sects is the degree to which their host cultures seek to control and minimize the influence of particular religious groups. In many Western cultures, especially North America, the generally favorable attitude toward "religion" suggests that both churches and sects are likely to do fairly well. Churches, or what we might call mainline denominations, are likely to fare better than sects, but both accommodate enough to their host cultures to be acceptable in varying degrees. As Redekop (1974) has emphasized, the useful empirical task is to identify the specific aspects of tension with the host culture that create problems of retaliation. The bell curve model illustrated above places tension along a single dimension, but tension with the host culture is clearly a multidimensional construct. We first focus upon this issue in terms of denomi-

2♣.

Research Box 12.1. Church–Sect Transitions among African Americans (Sherkat, 2001)

Sherkat hypothesized that among African Americans, preference for religious organizations should correspond to the dynamics implied by church–sect theory. Successful sects tend to lesson tension with their host culture as they become more accommodating of members' worldly behaviors and demand less of their total commitment. Sherkat hypothesized that within sects, generational differences are important factors for the transition of sects into churches and for the new formation of sectarian groups out of older churches.

Identifying birth cohorts ranging from those born before 1925 to those born between 1956 and 1980, Sherkat was able to identify a total sample of 5,075 African Americans from the 1972–1998 versions of the General Social Survey. Frequency of church attendance was reported for eight religious groups, including one group of traditionally "white liberal" churches (e.g., the Episcopal and Lutheran Churches) and another group of sects (e.g., Church of God in Christ, Pentecostal, and Holiness). For each religious group in each cohort, Sherkat identified the percentage of the cohort who were members of that group, and the percentage within each group who had switched to that group. He hypothesized that sectarian groups ought to gain membership among younger African American members but to lose membership among older church members, who should seek religious organizations that are less in tension with their host culture. Thus the sect–church–sect thesis ought to have empirically identifiable generational components. Shekart demonstrated this via cohort analysis, a procedure that samples distinct age categories from the same groups over periods of time. Using this technique Sherkat found that Methodists and Baptists accounted for 78% of the pre-1925 cohort, but 19% less (59%) of the 1956–1980 cohort. On the other hand, sects accounted for 3% more of the youngest cohort than of the oldest cohort. For all groups, the results were as follows:

	Birth cohort							
	Pre-1925 (*n* = 1,009)		1925–1943 (*n* = 1,205)		1944–1955 (*n* = 1,419)		1956–1980 (*n* = 1,442)	
Religious group	% of cohort belonging to group	% within group who switched to group	% of cohort belonging to group	% within group who switched to group	% of cohort belonging to group	% within group who switched to group	% of cohort belonging to group	% within group who switched to group
"White liberal"	2.7	30	3.7	48	3.3	34	2.4	26
Methodist	17.2	29	11.8	31	10.3	27	6.4	13
Baptist	61.2	19	60	14	53.8	12	53	9
Sects	10.4	75	10.3	70	12.1	58	13.5	40
Non-denominational	1.3	77	1.6	95	2.1	80	2	66
Catholic	4.6	48	7.1	31	8.9	22	9.6	12
Other	0.9	100	1.4	94	2.7	85	3.4	67
None	1.7	82	4.1	84	6.7	88	9.7	62

Note. Adapted from Sherkat (2001, p. 229). Copyright 2001 by the Society for the Scientific Study of Religion. Adapted by permission.

continued

Research Box 12.1. *continued*

Sherkat's study is important, in that it demonstrates that sectarian groups tend to grow by attracting religious "switchers." Forty percent of the sectarians in the youngest cohort, and 70% or more of those in the two oldest cohorts, were raised in some other religious group. However, in the traditionally "white" denominations, rates of participation were low and switchers constituted smaller percentages of the membership. Thus Sherkat notes that only high-commitment groups attract high-commitment switchers.

---

national and sectarian forms of religion. In a later section, we explore it in terms of cults—the area where it has generated the majority of recent empirical research in the face of popular controversies.

Operational Indices on the Church–Sect Continuum

Johnson's operationalization of church–sect theory in terms of degree of tension with the host culture permits Troeltsch's typology to be placed upon a continuum. Religions enforcing norms that are sharply distinct from the more generally accepted norms of the host culture are relatively sectarian; those permitting members to participate freely in all aspects of secular life of the host culture are more church-like (Johnson, 1963). They occupy the large middle range of the bell curve model of Finke and Stark (2001). Bainbridge and Stark (1980b) have provided survey data consistent with Johnson's operationalization. Their data are taken from a sample of church members in four counties of northern California; our focus is upon responses from 2,326 members of different Protestant denominations. Denominations "intuitively" identified as sects included the Church of God, the Church of Christ, the Church of the Nazarene, Assemblies of God, and Seventh-Day Adventists (Bainbridge & Stark, 1980b, p. 107).[2] Mainstream Protestant denominations were classified into those more compatible (low-tension) and those less compatible (high-tension) with their host culture. Our focus is only upon low-tension denominations contrasted with high-tension sectarian groups. We have selected from the survey data certain behaviors permitted by most of secular society but differentially forbidden by religious groups. It ought to be the case that the more sectarian groups should more frequently forbid behaviors permitted by the host culture than more church-like religious groups (denominations) should do. Table 12.1 compares results from the low-tension mainstream Protestant denominations (grouped together) and the five Protestant sects on differences in some common cultural behaviors and beliefs.

The fact that more sectarian groups hold beliefs at odds with the dominant culture simply indicates one dimension of tension. To oppose dancing or drinking within the host culture, where they are approved and considered normal, separates sect members by belief and behavior from certain cultural activities. Likewise, to oppose such beliefs as the

---

2. Certain groups (Gospel Lighthouse, Foursquare Gospel Church) classified as sects had too few respondents to be included in the statistical tables. We focus upon mainstream denominations only, contrasted with sects for which the sample size is sufficient. For additional details on the sample, the research instrument, and groups we have excluded, see Glock and Stark (1966, pp. 86–122).

TABLE 12.1. Comparison of Mainstream Protestant Denominations and Five Protestant Sects on Selected Behaviors and Beliefs

	Percentage of respondents endorsing behavior/belief					
	Mainstream Protestant (*n* = 1,032)	Church of Christ (*n* = 37)	Church of God (*n* = 44)	Church of the Nazarene (*n* = 75)	Assemblies of God (*n* = 44)	Seventh-Day Adventist (*n* = 35)
Behaviors						
Disapprove of gambling	62	100	89	92	98	97
Favor censorship	31	57	57	73	82	66
Disapprove of dancing	1	95	77	96	91	100
Beliefs						
Reject Darwin	11	78	57	80	91	94
Believe Devil exists	14	87	73	91	96	97
Believe Jesus will return	22	78	73	93	100	100

Note. Percentages must be cautiously interpreted, given the variation in sample sizes. Adapted from Bainbridge and Stark (1980b, pp. 111–112). Copyright 1980 by the Religious Research Association. Adapted by permission.

theory of evolution puts sect members at odds with normative educational forces in the culture. Even the support of more literal religious beliefs, such as the reality of the Devil or Christ's return, may put sect members at odds with other, more culturally congruent religions. In the comparisons in Table 12.1, the differences among the sectarian groups are never as large as between all sectarian groups and mainstream Protestants. This supports the contention that sects are at odds with the dominant culture and with denominations within that culture.

Additional evidence for the usefulness of operationalizing sectarian religions by belief tension with their host culture can be gleaned from Poloma's (1991) interesting study of Christian Scientists. Here a single axis of tension, appropriate medical care, is of overriding importance.

It is clearly the case that medical perspectives on physical illness dominate modern cultures; most persons seek medical treatment for illness. However, many persons use religious techniques such as prayer to facilitate healing. Several investigators have emphasized that spiritual healing is not as marginal in modern society as one might expect from the official dominance of medical perspectives. For instance, Johnson, Williams, and Bromley (1986) found that 14% of their sample of 586 adults claimed to have experienced a healing of a "serious disease or physical condition" as a result of prayer. Likewise, Poloma and Pendleton (1991) found that 72% of randomly chosen respondents from a Midwestern U. S. population believed that persons sometimes receive physical healing as a result of prayer. Nearly one-third of these (32%) claimed a personal experience of healing, and a third of this subsample (34%) claimed that the healing was of a life-threatening accident or medical problem. It is clear that spiritual healing is a widely diffused belief and practice through a broad range of the general population (Poloma, 1991; Johnson et al., 1986).

Although Poloma (1991, p. 337) is correct in her general assessment that religious healing is widely practiced, it is important to note that prayer as an adjunct to orthodox medical treatment is not a significant source of tension with the dominant culture. For instance, Trier and Shupe (1991, p. 355) have shown that among participants randomly selected from telephone numbers in the Great Lakes area, prayer was commonly used as an adjunct to traditional, mainstream medical care. They found no evidence that prayer was used in lieu of traditional medical treatments. Furthermore, frequency of prayer correlated positively with consulting a physician. Prayer is most frequently used in conjunction with and not in opposition to orthodox medical treatment (Gottschalk, 1973). As such, prayer for recovery is hardly sectarian in nature.

However, the use of prayer as an adjunct to medical treatment is a far cry from the articulation of a religious ideology that argues against both the concept of disease and the relevance of medical treatment to a cure. Christian Science is one religion that argues for healing in opposition to, not in conjunction with, orthodox medical treatment (Gottschalk, 1973). This is clearly a belief at odds with the dominant host culture, and even with mainstream Christian interpretations of spiritual healing by faith or miraculous intervention (Peel, 1987). Thus the sectarian nature of Christian Science can best be revealed when comparisons are made between the beliefs of Christian Scientists and mainstream Protestant Christians who claim to have experienced a spiritual healing.

In a follow-up study of the 1985 Akron Area Survey, Poloma and Pendleton (1991b) contacted 97 of 179 potential participants who had agreed to be interviewed for another study. These were those who reported having "experienced a healing of an illness or disease as a result of prayer" (Paloma, 1991, p. 339). They were interviewed this time on the topic of spiritual healing. The vast majority of participants were "born-again" Christians (82%) and identified themselves as charismatic, Pentecostal, or both (86%). Two were Christian Scientists, who were later used to obtain an additional sample of 42 members of the Church of Christ, Scientist (Christian Science). Comparisons between the 95 mainstream Protestants and the 44 Christian Scientists on matters on beliefs regarding spiritual healing revealed expected differences, as noted in Table 12.2.

It should be stated that these differences in beliefs in spiritual healing between Christian religious groups were found despite similarities in beliefs on other religious matters. For instance, the majority of both Christian Scientists and mainline Christians in Poloma's (1991) sample agreed that Jesus healed in order to show compassion and divinity, as well as to gain followers and to glorify God. Furthermore, in terms of actual reported medical practices, the majority of both mainline Christians and Christian Scientists practiced their beliefs—the

TABLE 12.2. Differences between Mainline Christians and Christian Scientists in Beliefs about Spiritual Healing

	Percentage of respondents endorsing belief	
Belief	Mainline Christians ($n = 44$)	Christian Scientists ($n = 95$)
God always heals if faith enough	57	85
God withholds healing for spiritual good	72	10
Healing operates with fixed laws	69	95
God punishes evil with illness	24	0
God usually heals through doctors	73	12
God usually does not use divine healing	47	3

Note. All differences were significant at $p < .01$. Adapted from Poloma (1991, p. 341). Copyright 1991 by the Religious Research Association. Adapted by permission.

former seeking and utilizing orthodox medical care, the latter much less likely to do so. Some comparisons are reported in Table 12.3.

As can be seen from Table 12.3, neither Christian Scientists nor mainstream Christians acted perfectly in conformity with their stated beliefs: 10% of Christian Scientists reported visiting a doctor within the last year, while an almost equal percentage of mainline Christians failed to visit one. Still, the Christian Scienctists' rejection of orthodox medicine was related to very high rates of nonparticipation in its practices. Clearly, rejecting orthodox medicine is a point of tension that separates Christian Scientists from other Christians and from the mainstream culture as well.

ORGANIZATIONAL DYNAMICS

The operationalization of tension with the host culture along a single continuum is useful, but it also can be misleading. Cultures are not homogeneous entities; they are not defined by a single set of norms. Cultures are heterogeneous, with conflicting and often incompatible norms existing simultaneously. In a word, cultures are pluralist. Some social scientists refer to this as "postmodernism" (Rosenau, 1992). Although little consensus exists on the meaning of this term, the fact that no single perspective dominates postmodern cultures suggests that tension with a culture must be defined in terms of opposition arising in significant power groups within the culture, which have vested interests in the support of particular norms. Deviation from norms whose enforcement is of little concern is less crucial than deviation from norms that arouses reactions from those with significant power within the host culture. More sectarian groups arouse reaction from the powerful, not simply because they harbor different beliefs, but because they harbor different beliefs on a continuum considered salient or important to the powerful within the culture (Becker, 1963).

To take an obvious example, Christian Science, in opposing modern medical science, raises concern among the powerful in a culture dominated by belief in modern medicine. Numerous instances arise when parents from belief traditions such as Christian Science or the Jehovah's Witnesses, which oppose some or all of orthodox medicine, have children in need of medical care. Here, the confrontation between orthodoxy in medicine and the opposition to these powerfully sanctioned norms within sectarian traditions illustrates a sig-

TABLE 12.3. Differences between Mainline Christians and Christian Scientists in Reasons for Seeking Medical Care and Medical Visits

	Percentage of respondents endorsing belief	
	Mainline Christians (n = 95)	Christian Scientists (n = 44)
Likely would seek help for:		
Relief of headache	100	0
Flu-like symptom	35	6
Severe chest pain	76	10
Severe injury	76	5
Visited doctor within last year	88	10

Note. All differences were significant at $p < .01$. Adapted from Poloma (1991, p. 344). Copyright 1991 by the Religious Research Association. Adapted by permission.

nificant tension. Outside of particularly specified religious alternatives, it is simply "common sense" that one treats disease by orthodox medical procedures. Yet common sense is but the culturally shared knowledge of reality defined within a tradition (Berger & Luckmann, 1967). The criteria for assessing claims to truth are often incommensurate between traditions. The very specifications of the criteria of judgment are themselves contextually bound. Thus the claim that medical treatment is "obviously" necessary for diseases does not simply affirm one reality, but rejects others, such as those articulated within Christian Science. The question of how to treat these issues empirically without imposition of value claims has long plagued the social sciences.

Before we address one possible resolution to this problem, we simply emphasize that the existence of differences between reality claims in which groups within the culture have dominant interests is not simply a source of identity, but one of conflict as well. To identify oneself as a Christian Scientist is both to belong to a group at odds with orthodox medicine and also to be at odds with the educational elite of the culture, who support and defend the perspective of orthodox medicine. It is almost axiomatic in the social sciences that strong identification of members with divergent groups increases prejudice, as measured by the social distance groups attempt to maintain from one another (Beit-Hallahmi, 1989; Tajfel & Turner, 1986). Watson (1993) has defined the social distance between groups in terms of the concept of "ideological surround."

Ideological Surround

In a series of empirical studies, Watson and his colleagues have utilized a methodological procedure that permits the identification of different meanings attributed by persons of a given tradition to various phenomena. This is consistent with the position that both ideological and methodological pluralism characterizes postmodern culture (Rosenau, 1992; Roth, 1987). Watson and colleagues utilize empirical measures corrected for their ideological content, thus producing measures acceptable to the internal definition of the group to which they are applied (Watson et al., in press). Since all descriptions are theory- and value-laden, it is of little use to attempt arguments across traditions. Furthermore, even within the physical sciences, attempting a neutral, presumably objective, context-free description of reality is neither possible nor desirable (Schlagel, 1986). It is even less so with the realities dealt with by social psychologists, which are obviously socially constructed. These constructions both define groups and provide identities for their members that can place them at odds with one another. Watson's "ideological surround" method is an empirical procedure that permits identification of different meanings for identical scale items Empirically, considerations of the ideological surround of any operational measure permits groups to communicate with one another, based upon the differing meanings any measure may have in groups identified with different ideologies.

For instance, the fact that intrinsic religiosity often correlates positively with social desirability measures is not interpreted to mean that intrinsically religious people only wish to appear socially desirable (Batson, Schoenrade, & Ventis, 1993). This interpretation of the empirical data fails to account for the meaning of social desirability items within the ideological surround of an intrinsically religious person. An alternative explanation can readily be derived from simply having individuals rate the various items on social desirability scales for their religious relevance. For instance, among intrinsically religious persons, positive endorsement of social desirability items reflects the ideological surround of their religious tradition, which defines such items as desirable social behaviors (Watson, Morris, Foster, & Hood, 1986). Thus intrinsic religiosity correlates with social desirability on measures that intrinsically religious persons see as desirable socially. In a similar vein, correcting scales to measure self-actualization for their different ideological surround reveals different meanings of the term for religiously and humanistically committed persons (Watson, Morris & Hood, 1987, 1990b). Thus whether or not people describe themselves as self-actualized is dependent upon the relevance of the meaning of any measure of self-actualization within a given tradition. The meaning of any measure is established within a given ideological surround; no measure is an Archimedean point by which all traditions can be judged. Both humanists and religionists can be self-actualized, within criteria acceptable to their beliefs. More importantly, when the ideological surround of any operational measure is understood, communication between groups is established by one's understanding of the different meaning identical operational measures may have for diverse groups.

More sociologically influenced social psychologies, especially those rooted in the work of G. H. Mead (1934), have long held that social phenomena can be predicted best when the meaning of the phenomena from the actors' perspective is taken into account. Most forcefully expressed in symbolic interactionism, this tradition argues that positivistic methods, which assume that an objective measure is equally meaningful across persons, are limited (Blumer, 1969). Persons react to meanings that in terms of religions are defined by their traditions. These meanings are often dismissed as merely subjective, or are assessed by measures assumed to be objective indices of belief, regardless of the meaning they may have for a subject. Yet, as Blumer (1969, p. 3) has noted, "To ignore the meaning of things toward which people act is seen as falsifying the behavior under study." Subjective meanings shared among persons defines an intersubjectivity that is the normative base of various groups within a culture.

Symbolic interactionists have typically used qualitative methods to study subjective meanings—a tradition often identified as the "Chicago school" (Blumer, 1969). The competing "Iowa school" of symbolic interactionism has tried to establish quantitative indices of meaning, using methods compatible with the use of reliable scales in mainstream social psychology (Kuhn & McPartland, 1954). However, these procedures ignore individual differences in meaning within groups for the same items. Watson's ideological surround permits a measurement and treatment of subjective meanings that combines the measurement considerations of the Iowa school with the sensitivity to individual subjective meanings of the Chicago school. It does not assume that meanings are identical across groups even when scales have high reliabilities. Instead, subjective meanings are determined for significant cluster of person within groups, and the scales are differentially scored for the relevance of these meanings.

The ideological surround is directly relevant to the identification of tensions that differentiate denominations from sects. Again, sects are religious groups that have significant tension with powerfully enforced norms within a host culture, based upon the different meanings those norms have for sect members and the enforcers of the dominant cultural norms. To go back to our earlier example, disease does not mean the same thing within the perspective of orthodox medicine and that of the Church of Christ, Scientist. A possible scale item such as "A good mother will take her seriously ill child to a doctor," when corrected for its ideological meaning across groups, would be scored positive for those committed to orthodox medicine and reverse-scored as negative for Christian Scientists. Thus, empirically, one has identified practices of "good mothering" that are radically different, yet each supported by a powerful tradition. Good mothers in religions compatible with the orthodox medical culture seek medical aid for their children's illness; good mothers within the Church of Christ, Scientist do not take ill children to the doctor. Here the obvious tension between sects that reject orthodox medicine and cultures that are committed to orthodox medicine is highlighted. A member of the mainstream culture is likely to wonder, "How could a mother who loves her child reject necessary medical care?" The Christian Scientist has a powerful, if clearly sectarian, response to this question.

Defining Sects versus Denominations in Terms of Change

Applying the notion of ideological surround to religious organizations helps us to grasp the dynamic nature of these groups, which might otherwise be misperceived as having a static quality. All groups are in a continual process of change, denominations no less than sects. Cultures are in a continual process of change as well. However, the issue is whether changes within religious groups are in a direction compatible with the dominant culture (denominations) or not (sects). In most cases, the issue of congruence is a function of the meanings involved. We can identify this dynamic tension as a ratio between "restorative" and "transformative" efforts to maintain a tradition or shared system of meaning. Meanings are seldom if ever merely personal or idiosyncratic; they are almost always shared by some group, and at odds with those differentially shared by other groups (Berger & Luckmann, 1967). Religions groups undergoing either restorative or transformative changes become sectarian if the dominant culture's commitments remain fairly constant or shift in a direction opposite to the religious group's concerns, respectively.

Restorative Sects

Restorative changes are attempts to maintain or restore beliefs and practices that oppose changed values in the dominant culture. These changes produce tension by supporting a particular system of meaning, with norms and behavioral expectations that the dominant culture now views as archaic. Even though the beliefs and norms may have been dominant at one time, their continuance in the face of cultural change now creates tension. If the changes are defined within a religious system of meaning, we may speak of "restorative sects."

For instance, religious fundamentalism is a modern sectarian movement within North American Protestantism directed at restoring fundamental values and commitments seen as threatened by movements within the dominant culture. It began in the early 20th century, when a series of pamphlets titled *The Fundamentals: A Testimony to the Truth* were distributed by Lyon and Milton Stewart, two California businessmen (Hood, 1983). Essentially, these pamphlets rejected the modernist techniques of textual and scientific criticism that had been applied to scripture; they asserted that historical and literary criticism was not to be utilized to undermine a literal interpretation of scripture. Scripture was avowed to be without error, and to establish authoritatively and for all time a shared system of meaning. The ideological surround of fundamentalist religion supports the meaningfulness of beliefs in such things as the divinity of Christ, the reality of the Virgin birth, and the factual truth of miracles as literally interpreted from scripture (Hood, 1983). Thus fundamentalist groups became sectarian as they refused to participate in religious denominations that accommodated their beliefs to the modernist criticisms, both scientific and literary, supported by mainstream culture.

Almost by definition, few social scientists with religious identities would identify themselves as fundamentalists, since the distance between fundamentalist ideology and that implicit in social-scientific methodologies is great. Not surprisingly, much of the empirical literature on fundamentalism finds it to be characterized by undesirable or deficient traits, such as narrow-mindedness (Altemeyer & Hunsberger, 1992; Gorsuch & Aleshire, 1974; Kirkpatrick, 1993), a lack of cognitive complexity (Kirkpatrick, Hood, & Hartz, 1991; Pancer, Jackson, Hunsberger, Pratt, & Lea, 1995), and a low level of spiritual maturity (Fowler, 1981; Richards & Davison, 1992; Streib, 2001b). However, investigators have often not appropriately noted variations within fundamentalist groups and the consequences of different operational indices used to assess fundamentalism (Ethridge & Feagin, 1979; Kellstedt & Smidt, 1991). In terms of an ideological surround, such descriptions suggest the different meanings social scientists give to phenomena that are normative and meaningful within fundamentalism. Fundamentalist groups are by definition socially functional, even when by particular psychological measures individual fundamentalists are found to be psychologically dysfunctional.

Research has demonstrated the lack of sensitivity of many social-scientific measures when applied to fundamentalist traditions. For instance, the original version of the Minnesota Multiphasic Personality Inventory (MMPI), a measure widely used to assess pathological personality, included frequency of prayer and other specific items meaningful within the ideological surround of fundamentalists. To cite but one such item, "Christ performed miracles such as changing water into wine." With the exception of an item referring to church attendance, agreement with this and all other religious items was scored to indicate pathology. To make matters even worse, many of these items were part of a subscale used in research to measure ego strength, the lack of which is often perceived as pathological (Hathaway & McKinley, 1951). Obviously, measuring pathology among religious fundamentalists by such items does not give a measure of pathology that is independent of their religious beliefs. Fortunately, the revised version of this test (MMPI-2) does not use explicitly religious items (Butcher, Dahlstrom, Graham, Tellegen, & Kaemmer, 1989). Hood (1974) demonstrated that correcting for the meaning of such items in terms of ideological surround or removing such items altogether fails to support a relationship between pathology and fundamentalism. Watson and his colleagues have shown in a systematic series of empirical studies that when measurements are made within the context of an appropriate ideological surround, empirical relationships are modified in terms of the meaning of the measures within the groups to which they apply (Watson et al., in press). Furthermore, as Stark (1971) has noted, from a purely sociological perspective ongoing groups are by definition normal, regardless of presumed pathological conditions within their membership.

Within a pluralistic society, fundamentalists maintain their sectarian nature by deliberately utilizing both religious and sectarian means to maintain the boundaries of their beliefs that are functional for their way of life. For instance, several studies have shown that fundamentalists vote as a meaningful block only when candidates take significantly different stands on issues crucial to fundamentalists' beliefs. In these instances, fundamentalists vote in a manner congruent with what has been called "boundary maintenance" (Hood, Morris, & Watson, 1985, 1986). Thus fundamentalism within Protestantism attempts to maintain a tradition in the face of broader cultural changes that threaten such beliefs, and hence it demands the restoration of these beliefs. The restorative sectarian nature of fundamentalism is widely recognized in other traditions, including Islam, despite originating as a North American phenomenon (Marty & Appleby, 1991).

Transformative Sects

Although one is often tempted to think of sectarian movements as trying to restore or maintain a tradition in the face of cultural opposition, denominations can become sectarian by attempting to maintain a tradition through transforming aspects of their beliefs or practices. For instance, within many denominations worldwide, there are efforts to alter the traditional roles of women as defined within various religions. These efforts aim to maintain the denominations' traditions through transformative modifications (Hawley, 1994a). As women's roles are radically altered within many cultures, pressure for religious groups to change increases (Hawley, 1994a). The lessening of tension with the host culture by those who would transform a religious tradition through expanding or changing the traditional roles of women within the group may operate to maintain the tradition in the face of a changed culture. Yet adapting beliefs and norms to the dominant culture on a significant axis of tension may ironically increase tension between the host culture, within which roles for women have changed, and the remaining portion of the religious tradition that would maintain the traditional norms for women.

Sectarian change is inevitable, whether it is transformative, restorative, or both. Among mainstream denominations, movements to transform traditional views of women, homosexuals, or abortion are but a few indices of the possible sources of tension. Religious groups are continually pressured to accommodate their beliefs and practices to a changing culture. They can maintain their identities by transformative moves compatible with cultural change, or can resist cultural changes in restorative sectarian efforts. In either case, change is a dynamic part of any religious group.

Placing Religious Organizations and Cultures on Axes of Change

Both restorative and transformative tendencies exist in all organizations. Within religious organizations, the crucial social dimension is whether the norms that are maintained by either of these processes are sufficiently congruent with the norms that are strongly supported by the host culture. If they are congruent, the religious group has a church (denominational) form, which assures that its members are nonproblematic to the host culture. If they are not congruent, the group has a sectarian nature, which assures that its members are problematic to the host culture. Of course, the issue is complicated by the fact that cultures are changing along with and in opposition to religious groups. Yet it is always the position of religious groups' norms relative to the cultural norm on issues of great salience that is the key to defining sects and denominations, and that probably conforms to the bell curve model presented earlier in Figure 12.1.

The Position of Sects within the Host Culture

Sects persist—but, as Bainbridge and Stark (1980b) have noted, an ongoing, functioning group that is problematic to the host culture is a deviant subculture by definition. Thus sects are best viewed as tolerable forms of religious deviance, created when religious groups differ significantly from their host culture on salient values. Sects are problematic to the dominant host culture's interests, but are of the acceptable forms of religious identity characterized by the tolerance for diversity that is common in postmodern cultures (Rosenau, 1992).

Occasionally, sectarian practices become targets of legal sanction; however, within a culture that cherishes religious freedom, efforts to constrain sectarian religious practices are likely to meet with serious obstacles. This is particularly likely to be the case where religious freedom is a strong cultural tradition and where religion is a valuable label. As Richardson (1985a) has noted, being identified as a religion in the United States has numerous benefits, not the least of which is protection from government regulations that would prohibit otherwise problematic behaviors. Benefits include tax exemptions, as well as exemptions from civil rights legislation and many laws that govern business. For instance, religions can refuse to ordain women even in the United States, where women have achieved additional legal protection from discrimination based upon gender. No Catholic woman can bring a lawsuit on discrimination because she is refused the right to be a priest, nor can a fundamentalist woman appeal on legal grounds the refusal of ordination by her church. Yet religions risk losing their religious identification if they deviate too far from cultural norms for what constitutes a "religion." As Greil and Robbins (1994) have noted, at least in the United States the law does not concern itself with claims to religious heresy; this indicates that within broad limits, religious norms, even those at odds with the dominant culture, are to be protected. However, being protected by the law does not mean that tension with the host culture is minimized. In the United States, the legal acceptance of religious diversity knows few limits. Sectarian groups are allowed to exist and even flourish as pockets of subcultural religious deviance characteristic of the religious pluralism and dynamism of postmodern culture. Among the more curious of sectarian religious practices is the handling of serpents among the Holiness sects of Appalachia, as noted in earlier chapters of this book and described in more detail in Research Box 12.2.

When tensions are extreme and reactions to religious subcultures become more intense, tolerance for diversity is likely to find its limit. In India, fundamentalist Hindus, who continue the practice of *sati* despite its illegality, support a restorative sectarian movement unlikely to find sympathy from either men or women influenced by modernity. Yet the practice of *sati* is rooted in the belief that the untimely death of a husband is due to the failure of his wife to protect him, and hence she must sacrifice herself on his funeral pyre. Cases of the reemergence of *sati* and its defense by Hindu fundamentalists have generated much social-scientific commentary and analysis (Hawley, 1994b, 1994c). Here, the tension with most cultural views is extreme, despite the long tradition of *sati* as a minority movement within Hinduism. Legal repercussions in the interest of the dominant culture suggest a retaliation and an appeal to a higher standard unlikely to be heard within the ideological surround of *sati* and its defenders.

In a similar vein, Islam has a long tradition of *jihad*, or holy war (Ruthven, 1984). Although it would be a mistake to think that Islam is inherently a violent religion, it would be equally inappropriate to fail to understand the conditions under which believers might feel justified in acting violently against those whom their tradition feels must be opposed. For instance, it is often claimed that violence in the expression of one's faith (as in Islamic fundamentalist protest movements that utilize force) is necessarily fanatical and fueled by only negative characteristics, such as paranoia and authoritarianism (Dekmejian, 1985). However, empirical studies of actual violent protesters while still alive and imprisoned fail to support such claims. A well-known study by Saad Eddin Ibrahim (1980, 1982) focused upon participants imprisoned for Islamic militancy. Ibrahim (1980, p. 427) defined Islamic militancy as "actual violent group behavior committed collectively against the state or other actors in the name of Islam." Members of two militant Islamic groups in Egypt (the Islamic Liberation Organization and Repentance of the Holy Flight) who had actually been imprisoned for Islamic militancy failed to confirm stereotypes related to any supposed personality charac-

☙

Research Box 12.2. Serpent-Handling Sects (Hood, 1998)

Early in the 20th century in the rural South, George Hensley picked up a serpent in reaction to Mark 16:17–18: "And these signs shall follow them that believe; In my name shall they cast out devils; they shall speak with new tongues; They shall take up serpents; and if they drink any deadly thing, it shall not hurt them; they shall lay hands on the sick, and they shall recover." Returning to his church, he initiated the practice of serpent handling, unique as a form of religion in the United States. For a while the practice was normative in the Church of God, where Hensley was ordained. Later rejected as a practice by the Church of God, it became normative for Holiness sects in Appalachia. Often identified as "sign-following" sects and long predicted to disappear, these sects continue to outlive their obituaries. Preachers, with their serpent boxes ever present, handle deadly snakes— either when faith alone dictates it or, for some, when they feel they have a special experience of being "anointed." Associated with serpent handling but less common is the drinking of poison, often strychnine or lye. About 80 deaths have been documented from serpent bites. Henley himself was a victim, dying of a snake bite in 1955. Serpent bites are common, and among serpent-handling sects, opinions differ on whether one ought to seek medical aid if bitten. Although many Protestant sects practice some of the signs specified in Mark 16:17–18, only the Holiness sects of Appalachia follow all five signs. For instance, many Pentecostal groups speak in tongues (glossalalia) but reject serpent handling. The tension that serpent handling presents to a modern culture is obvious. Legal sanctions have been directed against the practice in some states, such as Tennessee. In other states, such as West Virginia, the practice carries no sanction. (For a listing of laws against serpent-handling sects, see Burton, 1993.) To the outsider, this obedience to the literal Biblical imperative is the major defining characteristic of these sects.

---

teristics of religious fanaticism. The prisoners were predominantly students or recent university graduates in the sciences and medicine, with median ages in the mid-20s, and clearly had achieved greater educational success than their parents. They were motivated by Islamic ideals and felt justified in the use of force to obtain these ideals.

Similar justifications were claimed by Malcolm X in his quest for social justice as framed within the Black Muslim religion. Research Box 12.3 presents a study comparing attitudes toward Malcolm X and Martin Luther King, Jr. among lower-socioeconomic-status black and white males.

Hoffman (1995, p. 225) has presented a survey summary of Muslim fundamentalists' psychosocial profiles and concluded that the resurgence of Islamic fundamentalism often leads to the discounting of its more violent sects as "crazy," even though such claims lack empirical grounding. It is unlikely that the willingness to use force to achieve one's aims is likely to be other than a source of tension with the host culture. However, such aims and their forceful means can have meaningful religious justifications and make sense to some. Within the notion of an ideological surround, every action motivated by faith must be understood from the perspective of the actors involved, and not by some standard outside their perspective. Clearly, one major source of tension is the claim of sects to a legitimate use of violence to achieve their aims, even when this is framed within a religious perspective.

ঽ৶

**Research Box 12.3. Malcolm X and Martin Luther King, Jr. as Cultural Icons
(Hood, Morris, Hickman, & Watson, 1995)**

Malcolm X and Martin Luther King, Jr. (hereafter referred to as "Malcolm" and "Martin" both framed their protests against perceived injustice in religious terms. A major difference in the means they advocated to achieve their visions was in the justification of violence. Malcolm, taking the Black Muslim view, refused to reject violence as a means; Martin, taking the Christian view, did reject it. Hood and his colleagues reasoned that the acceptance of Martin and Malcolm would differ among culturally alienated lower-socioeconomic-status black and white males. Using a semantic differential scale to measure both evaluative assessments (i.e., approval) and potentiality assessments (i.e., estimates of power) of Malcolm and Martin, they found that black and white males did differ as predicted. The following table presents the most relevant summary of these results.

	Evaluative rating		Potentiality rating	
	Martin	Malcolm	Martin	Malcolm
Black males				
Mean	36.19	44.66	33.02	46.17
SD	9.95	6.96	9.35	5.79
White males				
Mean	32.13	24.87	30.49	47.28
SD	9.81	7.76	8.06	5.26

Analyses of these data indicated that black males evaluated Martin more highly, and Malcolm much more highly, than did white males. On potentiality, both black and white males thought Malcolm much stronger than Martin. The investigators suggested that these data are consistent with the grudging preference of Martin over Malcolm among whites, precisely because Martin's rejection of violence made him less of a threat than Malcolm's willingness to use violence if necessary. Thus the justification of violence as a means is a clear source of tension for cults within their host cultures.

CULTS

If tension with the host culture on salient values best empirically defines a church–sect continuum, what about cults? The term "cult" has such a pejorative quality, especially in the popular media, that some investigators who have profitably utilized the concept in the past have begun calling for the elimination of the term "cult" altogether (Richardson, 1993a). In one sense, it has become the sociological equivalent of psychopathology in the popular mind. Even the sociological literature on cults tends toward the dramatic and extreme, despite wide variations in the nature of cult beliefs and practices (Eister, 1979). Empirical studies of attitudes toward cults indicate that the majority of respondents have heard of Jonestown and Charlie Manson—names linked to the term "cult" in the popular media (Pfeiffer, 1992, p. 538). It is as if all sects and cults were identified with the Hindu ritual of *sati*, or as if the sensationalized press descriptions of those who advocate Islamic *jihad* as mere "terrorists" were to be taken at face value. Yet death and violence are no more essential to cults than to other social groups.

Comparing Cults and Sects

Despite the fact that the cult type was never part of the theoretical development of church–sect theory, it is probably most useful to compare cults and sects. As Stark and Bainbridge (1979, p. 125) have argued, sects tend to rise from within existing religious groups and to move toward a new religious form. Schisms create sects by what we have termed either restorative or transformative movements. Hence sects are inherently religious protest movements. On the other hand, cults lack prior ties with religious bodies and tend to emerge afresh, often under the direction of a single charismatic leader. Cults are novel forms of religion, which, not surprisingly, are likely to emerge in tension both with established religious groups (such as churches and sects) and with the host culture. As such, we can expect that sects and cults share a rejection of their host culture or at least some aspects of their host culture, and are likely to be rejected by their host culture in turn. As with sects, there are belief differences between cults and their host culture. There are also likely to be close patterns of interaction among cult members, as well as retaliatory actions on the part of the host culture toward them—all of which create an even more clearly defined religiously deviant subculture for cults than for sects. This occurs not only because cults are novel and hence lack previous religious legitimation, but also because their leader is likely to be a solitary, powerful, charismatic figure. Indeed, many characterize cults as lacking a formal organizational structure and as largely controlled in an authoritative manner by their leaders (Ellwood, 1986; Wallis, 1974). Cults are often defined and identified by the names of their leaders, at least in the popular media. Hence we have the "Manson cult," the "Jim Jones cult," and the "Moonies" (after the Reverend Sun Myung Moon). As Barnes and Becker (1938, p. 22) have noted about charismatic figures in general, "Charismatic domination is established through the extraordinary qualities (real or supposed) of the leader.... Law is not the source of authority; on the contrary, he [or she] proclaims new laws on the basis of revelation, oracular utterance, and inspiration."

Given the charismatic nature of cult leadership combined with the fact that cults (like sects) are in opposition to salient cultural values, there is often some confusion as to whether or not cults are truly "religions." The distinction between religious and secular groups has become blurred in the modern world. As Greil and Rudy (1990) have noted, many organizations are best conceived as parareligious or quasi-religious because they have mixed characteristics, some of which are sacred and some of which are secular. This applies, for example, to Alcoholics Anonymous, astrology, and many healing movements (Greil & Robbins, 1994; McGuire, 1993). In congruence with postmodern analyses, we should note that "religion" can be conceived as a category of discourse, negotiated by groups that would either desire to obtain or wish to refute the label. Although there are often benefits to the label (as noted above), there can be liabilities as well. For instance, Transcendental Meditation (TM) was successfully excluded from schools in the United States on the basis of a claim Maharishi Mahesh Yogi denied—namely, that TM was a religion (Greil & Robbins, 1994). Hence efforts to include TM as a secular activity in schools were rejected, based upon a court ruling that such practices were in fact religious in nature. Thus the category of religion must be negotiated between groups and a culture; some groups desire the label, but others do not want it (Greil, 1993).

However, as novel forms of religious identity, cults are likely to be severely challenged by mainstream culture. Pfeiffer (1992) found that the vast majority of college students in his sample (82%) described "an average cult member" only in negative terms; not a single student used positive terms. He also randomly divided his subjects into three equal groups and had them respond to one of three vignettes describing three groups. None of these three groups were identified as cults, but each was selected based upon popular notions of alleged authoritarian structures and near-total environmental control of members, who are kept isolated from the wider society. The vignettes were identical except for the groups specified— either "Marines," "Moonies," or "priests." The vignette described a typical recruit, "Bill," at the relevant group facility (with only the identification of the persons surrounding him changed across the three vignettes) as follows:

> While at the facility, Bill is not allowed very much contact with his friends or family and he notices he is seldom left alone. He also notices that he never seems to be able to talk to the other four people who signed up for the program and that he is continually surrounded by (Moonies, Marines, priests) who make him feel guilty if he questions any of their actions and beliefs. (Pfeiffer, 1992, p. 535)

Among several assessments in this study, participants were asked to select the term that best described the process Bill had undergone in order to reach the facility from among these terms: "initiation," "conversion," "brainwashing," "basic training," "resocialization," or "religious education." The most common term used to describe the process by which Bill was surrounded by Moonies was "brainwashing" (22 of 31, or 71%), whereas this term was used much less frequently to describe joining the Marines (15 of 34, or 44%) or the priesthood (10 of 34, or 29%). Still, as we shall see later in this chapter, "brainwashing" as a term to describe conversion—especially conversion to unpopular groups—has become a major issue, dividing even professional psychologists. Likewise, when participants were asked to characterize cults on the basis of the degree to which they foster "psychological growth," "community programs," "child abuse," or "brainwashing," Pfeiffer (1992) found that negative descriptive terms ("child abuse" and "brainwashing") were seen to characterize cults, whereas neither positive term was seen as characteristic of cults.

In addition, the participants rated Bill on a variety of indices on a bipolar scale, as summarized in Table 12.4.

TABLE 12.4. Mean Ratings of "Bill" Based upon Label of Group He Joined

	Marines	Moonies	Priests	
Positive process	4.41	5.22	3.97	Negative process
Happy	3.76	4.90	3.85	Unhappy
Intelligent	3.32	4.16	3.41	Unintelligent
Responsible	3.53	4.33	3.70	Irresponsible
Uncoerced	4.97	3.76	3.68	Coerced
Free to leave	6.03	6.06	5.29	Not free to leave
Treated fairly	3.55	3.55	4.71	Treated unfairly
Power to resist	4.17	5.19	4.29	Powerless to resist

Note. All ratings were made on a 7-point scale (1 = left-hand phrase, 7 = right-hand phrase). With the exception of "responsible–irresponsible," differences among the three means were significant at $p < .05$. Adapted from Pfeiffer (1992, p. 537). Copyright 1992 by V. H. Winston and Son, Inc. Adapted by permission.

Inspection of this table indicates that Bill was generally perceived as less happy and responsible if he joined the Moonies, as well as likely to have been coerced into joining them and powerless to leave. Overall, he was also perceived to have been treated unfairly by the Moonies.

Pfeiffer's study paints a negative picture of the perception of both cults and cult members that is supported by previous research. Zimbardo and Hartley (1985, p. 114) found that the most typical descriptions of cults obtained from students using a semantic differential scale tended to be those with strongly negative connotations, such as "not worthwhile" (64%) and "crazy" (60%). Consistent with the need for cults, as novel forms of religious organization, to negotiate for the validity of their label as "religious," more than one-fifth of these subjects identified cults as "nonreligious."

The problem of novel groups' negotiating to be labeled as "religious" is accentuated when these groups combine charismatic leadership with authoritarian structures that tend toward withdrawal from the dominant culture. For instance, Galanter (1989a) emphasizes the strong influence on behavior by norms supported by the attribution of divine powers to a cult leader. Richardson (1978a) emphasizes the oppositional nature of cults, which is exacerbated by the fact that they often derive their inspiration and ideology from outside the predominant religious and secular culture. Wallis (1974) has emphasized that cults need not always take their ideology from outside the dominant culture. Yet, as novel religious forms, cults clearly have an ideology at least distinct from the dominant culture. As Ellwood (1986) emphasizes, cults present a distinct alternative to dominant patterns in society, and the tension this creates is exacerbated when they are also led by charismatic persons who demand high degrees of commitment. Swatos (1981) emphasizes that the cult leader may be an imaginary figure, not a real one. Yet to focus religious novelty on a single figure, cultivating fierce commitment from members willing to withdraw from significant aspects of both religious and secular culture, is likely to create a powerful deviant subculture.

Thus models of sects as deviant religious subcultures may actually apply more forcefully to cults than to sects. As innovative deviant subcultures, cults stand in opposition to both culture and sects. Both sects and cults share the fact of tension with the dominant host culture, but cults more frequently emphasize separatist tendencies from a novel base and hence are more likely to attract intense cultural rejection in turn. As we have seen, sects tend to emerge out of religious organizations. They are likely to find some support for their aims, whether restorative or transformative, from others within the dominant culture. By contrast, cults arise as original movements within the culture and are likely to solicit opposition both from established religions and from the secular host culture.

In a postmodern culture, the acceptance of pluralism creates some added degree of tolerance—a cultic milieu somewhat favorable to both sects and cults (Kilbourne & Richardson, 1984a; Rosenau, 1992). However, tolerance has its limits. This is especially the case in light of two factors. First, as Stark (1985a) has emphasized, cults tend to appeal for recruits to members of weakened churches or to unchurched individuals. Thus in terms of the religious marketplace, denominations are either losing members to cults or failing to attract as members those individuals from the secular culture who join cults. Second, the oppositional nature of cults is directed not only against the churches' claims to appropriate accommodation to the world, but against the sects' claims to renewed efforts to maintain an exclusive religious purity. Not surprisingly, these rejections of both churches and sects as well as secular culture foster retaliation in turn. Cults are unlikely to have an easy birth or a long life. As we shall see, retaliatory efforts have created recent "anti-cult" movements, both in the United

States (Shupe & Bromley, 1985; Shupe, Bromley, & Oliver, 1984) and in Europe (Richardson & Introvigne, 2001; Robbins, 2001). Much of this movement has been aided and abetted by psychologists and psychiatrists who support the claims that cults utilize "brainwashing" to convert members against their will. We confront both of these issues, after we first give some consideration to the axis along which tension is likely to occur.

Bainbridge and Stark (1980a) have properly noted that the nature of a cult's dominant activity is likely to define its source of tension with the dominant culture. For instance, "client cults" provide personal growth and treatments for their members. Hence they are likely to be opposed by established groups that claim to provide the only legitimate avenue for these services. To give an analogy, Bergin (1980) has noted that psychiatrists and psychologists provide competing services long claimed to be the proper domain of the clergy, including the claim to be authoritative moral agents. Similarly, both London (1964) and Gross (1978) note that in secularized societies, mental health personnel often take the role previously reserved for religious healers. Likewise, Frank (1974) and Ellenberger (1970) have provided authoritative historical analyses of numerous similarities between religious and psychological systems of healing. Illich (1976) has documented the expropriation of health by orthodox medicine. Thus competition between client cults providing unorthodox treatments is likely to create significant tension with powerfully established medical and mental health groups, both of which are heavily sanctioned by the dominant culture.

Further exacerbation is readily understandable in light of the research of Kilbourne and Richardson (1984a), indicating that both established therapies and new religious movements attract persons seeking to change identities and to find new meanings in life. However, cults seek to produce more radical change than orthodox therapies, adding to tension (Kilbourne & Richardson, 1984a; Schur, 1976). In terms of an ideological surround, the very success of cults is likely to be seen as pathological by representatives of orthodox therapies. To cite but two extreme cases, who would argue for the validity of mass suicide indelibly associated with Jonestown, or the violent murders associated with the Charlie Manson "family"? Yet even in these cases, serious scholars have raised significant questions beyond the stereotype of madness and cults presented in the media. For instance, Zaehner (1974) has argued that Manson's crimes are not merely an expression of psychopathology, but have a religious significance as well: "Charlie Manson was sane: he had been *there*, where there is neither good nor evil, and he had read and reread the Book of Revelation. These two facts explain his crime" (p. 18). Likewise, Hall (1989) notes that Jim Jones, who led the mass suicide in Jonestown, is not simply to be understood in psychopathological terms:

> Ironically, Jones has become far more important for the society at large as a symbolic personification of evil than he has in any way to those who share some of the concerns that animated his movement. It is the opponents of Jim Jones who infused him with a charisma powerful enough to make him play the mythic role of scapegoat that cleanses the world of sin, even if they failed to acknowledge that the sin-offering of Jonestown had wider sources than the evil in Jones. (p. 311)

Thus we cannot ignore the religious relevance of even the most extreme of cult leaders. Feuerstein (1992) documents the relevance of madness as a category of the holy, especially for cult leaders. It is important to remember that religious extremism is also a normative part of religious history. We must be cautious not to identify all religion with cultural accommodations and compatibilities. Studies of contemporary militant movements worldwide under the broad umbrella of "fundamentalism" have shown that under appropriate conditions, militant action by religious groups is normative and cannot be attributed to the psychopathology of either leaders or followers (Marty & Appleby, 1994).

Using client cults as an example of an axis of tension identifies conflict between cults and orthodox healers that is not likely to engage massive cultural concern, except in isolated and highly publicized cases. However, an area of tension that cuts across diverse cultural groups and is perpetually a matter of intense concern is sexuality. A cult's violation of sexual norms is likely to elicit retaliatory responses from the dominant culture. We focus upon the social control of sexuality, since claims to legitimate forms of sexual expression have varied and continue to vary immensely, both within and between cultures. Yet few people have no opinion about what is appropriate.

Cults and Sexuality

Relating the control of sexuality to varieties of group formation and cohesion has a long history and firm theoretical grounding. Much of the social psychology of classical Freudian theory identifies group formation as being rooted in the control of sexuality and dyadic intimacy. As an inevitable dimension of tension with society, any form of sexuality can become problematic. The social and cultural history of sexuality is largely a religious history (Parrinder, 1980; Steinberg, 1983; Tennant, 1903/1968). Gardella (1985) has shown how Christianity, especially in North America, promoted a view of sexuality that required it to be both innocent and ecstatic. In English-speaking North America, the celibacy of Catholic priests and nuns has been challenged as abnormal, as was that of the early Shaker communities in the United States (Foster, 1984). The polygamy of early Mormons was violently criticized by a monogamous culture that was also equally opposed to what was perceived as the sexual permissiveness of the early Oneida community, which fostered free sexuality between its members (Foster, 1984).

Although monogamy has been challenged by many religious groups, retaliation is often swift, especially toward groups that put their alternative sexual beliefs into actual practice. Lewis (1989) recounts many instances of carefully constructed cultural atrocity tales directed at Catholics and Mormons, who were accused of using a wide variety of techniques of mind control to force persons to be either celibate (in the case of Catholics) or polygamous (in the case of Mormons). As we shall see, these historical instances applied to what are now mainstream religions have numerous parallels in contemporary retaliation toward cults. Lewis's discussion of atrocity tales directed at Catholics and Mormons is described in greater detail in Research Box 12.4.

Even mainstream religions have accommodated themselves to the acceptance of divorce and hence to a form of serial monogamy, seen by some as a form of polygamy. As Freud (1930/1961, p. 61) noted, there is an antithesis between sexuality and civilization, given that "sexual love is a relationship between two people, in which a third can only be superfluous or disturbing, whereas civilization is founded on relation between large groups of persons."

Not surprisingly, theorists influenced by Freud have argued for the crucial importance of sexuality in all forms of group formation, not simply religious ones (Badcock, 1980; Marcuse, 1955). Thus we should not be surprised that religious cults are likely to arouse cultural wrath if they modify established norms of sexuality. Likewise, insofar as conversion to a mainstream religious commitment is one of the best predictors of delayed loss of virginity (as noted in Chapter 7), modification of sexual norms within cults is likely to incur retaliation from mainstream churches heavily involved in the sexual socialization of adoles-

---

※

Research Box 12.4. Catholic and Mormon Atrocity Tales
(Lewis, 1989; see also Gardella, 1985)

The most popular book written in the United States before *Uncle Tom's Cabin* was a pseudoautobiography by one "Marie Monk" titled *Awful Disclosures of the Hotel Dieu Nunnery of Montreal*. With more than a quarter of a million copies sold between 1836 and the Civil War, the book told of licentious sex between priests and nuns; it also told of babies born to nuns and quickly baptized after birth, and bodily dissolved in lye. Despite being thoroughly discredited, this fraudulent text was part of an anti-Catholic genre fueled by exaggerated tales of genuine ex-nuns and of fallen priests that continues today. For instance, tales of priests forcing ladies to confess sexual sins in order to seduce them were common in English-speaking North America before the 19th century. *The Priest, the Woman, and the Confessional,* a 1984 book by C. Chiniquy, is a more recent example of this genre.

If "unnatural" celibacy fueled atrocity tales against nuns and priests, "unnatural" polygamy fueled atrocity tales against Mormons. Paralleling Marie Monk's book was another fabricated story by Marie Ward entitled *Female Life among the Mormons*. Assuming that no conscientious females would accept polygamy, the text accused Mormon males of using hypnotic techniques to force females to accept a presumably unnatural wedded life. Like ex-nuns, ex-Mormon women told elaborately embellished stories accentuating the misery of women under Mormonism. These helped to enrage the larger culture to action against Mormons, ranging from vigilante justice to government action directed against Mormon leaders and practices.

The insistence by a culture that only wedded monogamy is sanctioned by God provides a context within which advocates of other religious sexual practices, whether celibacy or polygamy, must fight to gain legitimacy for these practices.

---

cents. For example, the Unification Church has been accused by Horowitz (1983a, p. 181) of being a collectivist organization, and chided in particular for supporting arranged marriages in which persons were married who were "in some cases unfamiliar with each other up to minutes prior to the ceremony." Yet there is there firm theological justification for such marriages within the Unification Church (Barker, 1984). Moreover, Lewis (1989) has shown that dyadic intimacy is a factor in cult defection, insofar as among spouses joining cults, the best predictor is that if one partner leaves the cult the other will also leave. Not surprisingly, then, the Unification Church attempts to exert control over dyadic matching in terms of the larger group's interests, as do other religious groups such as the Hare Krishna (Judah, 1974). However, in a culture in which both free choice and romanticism are presumed to direct dyadic selection, such novel controls on sexual expression are likely to be serious sources of tension (Gardella, 1985). Similar tensions have emerged in studies of celibacy within the Catholic Church. Sipe (1990, p. 293), based upon a limited study of priests who failed to maintain their vows of celibacy, rashly concluded that the Catholic Church supports an archaic anthropological model inappropriate in light of modern understandings of human sexuality. (See Chapter 13 for a discussion of clergy sexual abuse and the recent scandals within the Catholic Church.)

When sexuality is controlled in a manner permitting multiple partners (often several partners are sexually active with a cult leader), the challenge to sexual and religious cultural norms is even more obvious. Wangerin (1993) has documented how "flirty fishing," or the use of sexual favors to gain adherents, created significant tension for the otherwise fundamentalist Children of God/Family of Love. Further confounding their otherwise fundamentalist beliefs is the confusion they have created within fundamentalist circles by supporting masturbation and a generally masculine point of view regarding sexuality (Wangerin, 1993). Chancellor (2000) has written an oral history of this movement, based upon interviews with over 700 members; he has documented the tempering of their sexual views as they continue into subsequent generations. Jacobs (1984, 1987) has documented the fact that some male cults foster romantic idealization of the cult leader by female followers. This leads to what some perceive as sexual abuse and exploitation for those who fail to carry through their attachment to the cult leader. Then, much as in a more normative love relationship, the socioemotional bonds with both the group and the leader must be broken for defection from the cult to occur (as we have seen in Chapter 11). With a charismatic male leader and a female follower, the process is accentuated, but similar processes operate in male followers as well.

THE ANTI-CULT MOVEMENT

In a partly tongue-in-cheek paper (a rarity in scientific journals), Kilbourne and Richardson (1986) described a new mental illness, "cultphobia." Although perhaps not to be taken seriously as a claim to defining a pathology, their effort was directed at "putting the shoe on the other foot" (Kilbourne & Richardson, 1986, p. 259). Richardson, a prominent sociologist and a lawyer involved in the study of new religious movements, has been a leader in arguing for researchers to abandon the term "cult" altogether, opposing his own earlier view in support of the concept (Richardson, 1978a, 1979, 1993a). Much of his concern centers upon the well-documented fact that attitudes toward new religious movements are heavily influenced by the mass media, whose presentation of cults has been largely sensationalistic and heavily slanted in a negative direction (van Driel & Richardson, 1988). Few if any distinctions are made between cults. For instance, Patrick and Dulack (1977, p. 11), activists in the anti-cult movement, have stated: "You name 'em. Hare Krishna, the Divine Light Mission, Guru Maharaj Ji, Brother Julius, Love Israel, The Children of God. Not a brown penny's worth of difference between any one of 'em."

The Empirical Study of Resistance to Cults

Empirically, the identification of resistance from groups within the culture is worthy of study. Thus we consider the pejorative connotation cults have acquired within the media an important empirical issue—one that is integral to the operationalization of cults as novel forms of subcultural religious deviance. The refusal to differentiate among cults is also worthy of empirical study. As Zimbardo and Hartley (1985) have noted, similar negative views of cults are held by adolescents, regardless of whether or not they have ever had any contact with recruiters for various cults. Yet, as Wallis (1976) has rightly noted, not all authoritatitive groups are the same. For instance, scientology has authoritarian features but most members hold down full time jobs and limit their involvement in terms compatible with their occupation and domestic responsibilities.

The empirical study of hostility toward cults is only one aspect of general tolerance for deviance, which is often examined in political science studies of civil liberties (McClosky & Brill, 1983; Stouffer, 1955; Wilcox et al., 1992). Perhaps the most consistent finding is that education and tolerance are positively correlated. Although numerous challenges and modifications of this finding have been made in specific cases, it remains as a "most durable generalization" (Sullivan, Pierson, & Marcus, 1982, p. 29).

The study of tolerance for new religious movements is almost by definition a study for tolerance of cults. Despite a relatively small literature, empirical studies are congruent with the research on support for civil liberties (Bromley & Breschel, 1992; Robbins, 2001). Within a democratic culture, retaliation against new religious movements can be expressed by attitudes in favor of legal restrictions on cults (Delgado, 1982; Galanter, 1989b; Lifton, 1985; Stander, 1987). Several studies have used this operational indicator in either general or specific cases. For instance, Richardson and van Driel (1984, p. 413) found substantial agreement with the statement that "Legislation should be passed to control the spread of new religions or cults" in a telephone survey of 400 randomly selected voters in Nevada. However, they also noted that some respondents were confused by the phrasing of the question, wanting to control cults but not new religions (Richardson & van Driel, 1984, p. 417). This confusion is consistent with the problem already discussed of negotiating a religious identity for a novel group. Cults are often refused such a label, as many do not perceive them as legitimate religions (Greil, 1993). Thus, while there is generally strong support for the right of freedom of worship for all religions, the support is strongest among educated elites rather than the mass public; it is also and tempered when the religions are seen to be too extreme, including cults, which may not be perceived as religious at all (McClosky & Brill, 1983).

When questions are more specific, the attitudes toward legal restrictions on cults are more illustrative. For instance, Bromley and Breschel (1992) utilized four specific issues to assess favorable attitudes toward cult legislation: a ban on cult recruitment of teenagers; the necessity for Federal Bureau of Investigation (FBI) surveillance of cults; the desirability of restricting solicitation by Hare Krishnas at airports; and the question of preventing the Reverend Moon from publishing a newspaper. Overall, they found that a majority of the mass public (66%), but a minority (25%) of the elites, approved of most items. Furthermore, the more religiously involved respondents were more likely to support legislation to control cults. This is consistent with the tension that cults as novel religious forms are likely to have with both secular and sacred groups within mainstream culture. In addition, it is often claimed that claims of "brainwashing" and sexual abuse (especially of children) are often used without empirical documentation, in efforts to discredit cults (Richardson, 1999a).

O'Donnell (1993) utilized a similar measure to asses attitudes toward restrictions on new religions. In addition, he added an item indicating opposition to Satan worship. Opposition to Satan worship is an important indicator of media influence on cult perception, since empirical research has failed to establish either that there is a large Satanic movement in North America or that Satan worship has any significant following or influence among adolescents (Richardson, Best, & Bromley, 1991; Swatos, 1992). O'Donnell's sample included a mass survey of 1,708 persons and an additional sample of 863 elites, selected from business, government, education, media, and religious leaders. O'Donnell used the five items as a single scale. The responses for the various groups are presented in Table 12.5. Not only did the academics within the elites have the greatest tolerance, but among the mass group, education was the best predictor of tolerance.

Thus, within the study of new religious movements, tolerance has been found to follow the similar pattern of the "most durable generalization" noted for civil liberties in gen-

TABLE 12.5. Tolerance for New Religious Movements (Cults)

Group	Overall response (1 = no, 2 = yes)
Mass public (*n* = 1,708)	1.42
Elites (*n* = 863)	
Academics (*n* = 155)	1.87
Business (*n* = 202)	1.67
Government (*n* = 106)	1.74
Media (*n* = 100)	1.79
Religious leaders (*n* = 300)	
Ministers (*n* = 101)	1.58
Priests (*n* = 100)	1.60
Rabbis (*n* = 99)	1.68

Note. The survey items were as follows:

1. There should be laws to prevent groups like Hare Krishna from asking people for money at airports.
2. Followers of the Reverend Sun Myung Moon should not be allowed to print a daily newspaper in Washington, D.C.
3. It should be against the law for unusual religious cults to try to convert teenagers.
4. The FBI should keep a close watch on new religious cults.
5. There should be laws against the practice of Satan worship.

Each item was scored on a 2-point scale (1 = yes, 2 = no). The table reports the overall mean response for the five items. Adapted from O'Donnell (1993, p. 361). Copyright 1993 by the Society for the Scientific Study of Religion. Adapted by permission.

eral. Research Box 12.5 reports an experimental study indicating that attitudes toward religious groups among educated elites can be changed by the presentation of factual material.

Still, we must confront a curious phenomenon proposed by some members of intellectual elites—one that medicalizes religious deviance and also suggests a basis for discounting much of the tolerance expressed by both elites and the educated masses toward religious cults. That phenomenon is coercive persuasion, or, in the inadequate vernacular of the popular media, "brainwashing."

The Question of Cults and Coercive Persuasion

The Medicalization of Deviant Religious Groups

The tendency for educated persons to be tolerant of new religious movements is confounded by controversies surrounding cults and the "medicalization of deviance." Although varying in precise meaning, this term generally refers to efforts to explain commitment to deviant groups in terms of dysfunctional or pathological processes (Conrad & Schnelder, 1980; Kittrie, 1971; Szasz, 1970, 1983, 1984). Thus individuals are assumed to be unable to commit freely to a new religious group. Conversion to cult beliefs and adherence to cult norms are interpreted as symptoms of illness or pathology. Not surprisingly, much of the support for this position comes from clinical psychologists and psychiatrists. For instance, in a series of papers, Clark and his colleagues (Clark, 1978, 1979; Clark, Langone, Schacter, & Daly, 1981) have claimed to clinically identify powerful mental coercion used by cults to create pathological commitments in converts. Likewise, Shapiro (1977) has claimed to have clinically identified a syndrome of "destructive cultism," which includes such phenomena as loss

---

ஓ

Research Box 12.5. Changing Views toward Serpent-Handling Sects
(Hood, Williamson, & Morris, 2000)

It is well documented that serpent handlers have been stereotyped in the popular media, which provide the basis of most persons' "knowledge" about this tradition (Brickhead, 1997). In a quasi-experimental study, college students were presented with contemporary tapes of serpent-handling services—one in which serpent handling was both demonstrated and defended, and a comparison tape in which services were shown but handling was neither defended nor demonstrated. Participants were assessed before and after viewing the tapes on a measure of prejudice that included stereotyping, negative affect, and behavioral intentions. It also included three items to assess whether one thought the practice of serpent handling to be "unfortunate," whether those who practice serpent handling are sincere, and whether one supported laws restricting the practice. Results indicated that prior to viewing the tapes, all participants held generally prejudiced attitudes toward serpent handling, thought the practice to be unfortunate, thought the handlers insincere, and favored laws against handling serpents in church. Analysis showed that viewing a videotape of serpent handling and hearing the practice explained and defended influenced attitudes. All participants in this study continued believing the practice unfortunate and holding negative affect about it, as well as not wanting to be with handlers, regardless of which tape they viewed. However, only those who actually witnessed handling and its defense decreased their stereotyping and changed their views; they now expressed beliefs that serpent handlers are sincere and that they ought to be allowed to practice their faith without legal constraint.

---

of identity, behavioral changes, estrangement from one's family, and mental control by the cult leader. Finally, Singer and her colleagues (Singer, 1978a, 1978b; Singer & West, 1980; Singer & Ofshe, 1990) have gained a considerable reputation for the clinical treatment of former cult members, whom they have described as "psychiatric casualties."

In opposition to clinical claims are the claims of most empirical researchers, who have found no evidence that cults use unique methods or techniques in order to alter normal psychological processes. Some have seen the empirical response to exaggerated clinical claims as itself overstated. As a result of all this, much of the study of new religious movements has become highly politicized. The process has forced serious debate and disclaimers among investigators as to hidden motives involved in the study of new religious movements (Barker, 1983; Friedrichs, 1973; Horowitz, 1983a, 1983b; Robbins, 1983). This has led to concerns regarding the academic integrity of research on new religious movements in general (Wilson, 1983), as well as challenges to the integrity of researchers personally committed to controversial religions such as Wicca, often simply identified as witchcraft (Scarboro, Campbell, & Stave, 1994). Segal (1985) has asked this serious question: "Have the social sciences been converted?" Others have noted that contemporary perspectives in the philosophy of science make distinctions between religious and scientific methods of knowing less distinct, blurring the boundaries of what many have tried to separate (Jones, 1994; Watson et al., in press). The debate is most heated when claims to have identified a process of coercive persuasion unique to cults is linked to the popular but scientifically unwarranted concept of "brainwashing."

A History of the Concept of Brainwashing

The term "brainwashing" has entered the popular language as a summary term for some loosely defined techniques of coercive persuasion that presumably can make persons adopt beliefs and conform to behaviors they would normally reject. Anthony and Robbins (1994) note that the term was first popularized by Hunter, a U.S. journalist who worked for the Central Intelligence Agency (CIA). This journalist claimed to have identified powerful techniques of thought reform utilized by the Chinese Communists, for which he coined the word "brainwashing" (Hunter, 1951). Research agencies of several governments—including the Nazi SS and Gestapo; the U.S. Office of Strategic Services, forerunner of the CIA; and investigators in Stalinist Russia and Communist China—had been involved in research programs to find effective procedures to obtain information from interrogation of prisoners of war, and to find ways to alter the beliefs of individuals so they would be cooperative with captor governments.

Despite widely exaggerated popular press accounts of the effects of brainwashing techniques, it was quickly recognized that no government had discovered any such techniques that were truly effective. Most efforts to alter beliefs utilized varieties of deception, often combined with the administration of drugs, or with techniques of coercion and force. Although compliance was easily produced by these crude techniques, true belief change was virtually nonexistent. "Compliance" simply means that persons conformed to demands to avoid pain and suffering within a totally controlled environment; however, their true beliefs did not change. Evidence for this was that behavioral compliance disappeared upon release from the environment. Of approximately 7,000 Korean prisoners of war subjected to harsh treatment techniques by the Chinese Communists, 30% died. Of the remainder, only 21 refused repatriation after secession of hostilities, and of these 21, 10 later changed their minds. Hence only 11 cases of over 4,500 survivors actually adopted Chinese Communist beliefs and refused ultimate repatriation (Anthony & Robbins, 1994). Not surprisingly, researchers given access to CIA material concerning all claims to brainwashing noted that no effective techniques existed, and that compliance produced by physical coercion, isolation, propaganda, peer pressure, and intense torture—in a context of total control combined with uncertainty about the future—involved no unknown social-psychological principles (Hinkle & Wolff, 1956). Indeed, the desired effects of mind change measured at repatriation indicated the complete failure of the presumed brainwashing. Thus responsible reviews of the facts indicate that no evidence exists for a technique using advanced psychological knowledge to alter a person's thoughts against his or her will.

Another phrase closely associated with brainwashing is "thought reform," a more adequate description of the Chinese Communists' intent. The term is closely linked to the research of Lifton (1961), a psychiatrist who studied Korean prisoners of war. Both thought reform and brainwashing are linked to what Schein, Schneier, and Barker (1971) have called "coercive persuasion." Although a scientifically inadequate popular literature extols the unlimited power of coercive techniques, as we shall see, the responsible scientific literature is consistent in agreeing (1) that such techniques can produce only limited attitude change and (2) that such change is highly unstable when controls on the immediate environment are lifted.

Two major varieties of coercive persuasion have been utilized in recent history, the Chinese and the European. Although the two forms overlap, as Somit (1968) has noted, their differences are evident in the extreme forms of expression. European-oriented techniques primarily emphasize the obtaining of confessions of guilt from presumably innocent persons, typically singly and in isolation. Chinese-oriented techniques focus upon efforts to change a person's total ideological orientation, typically in group situations where many are solicited as volunteers. The Chinese-oriented techniques have much in common with "totalism." Totalism seeks ultimate control of the individual through actual or threatened physical techniques of coercion and torture (see Arendt, 1979; Friedrich & Brzezinski, 1956). It is most often associated with totalitarian states. Totalism assumes the freedom of individuals to resist, and it does not postulate a unique technique or method that can make anyone (regardless of predisposing factors or strength of will) change ideological orientation. As such, it is what Anthony and Robbins (1994) refer to as a "soft determinism," quite compatible with theories of modern social science. Cults, like many other groups (both religious and secular), seek to attract persons with identifiable predispositions that can be manipulated in such a manner as to persuade the persons to become converts. Of course, such conversions remain intentional actions. They are not the process of some "hard determinant" such as brainwashing that abolishes the capacity to choose.

The popularization of a brainwashing model is compatible with neither the European nor the Chinese model of coercive persuasion, each developed independently. Although brainwashing is a thoroughly discredited concept, the broad basis of processes involved in coercive persuasion can be readily identified.

Processes of Coercive Persuasion

Since techniques of coercive persuasion have developed from pragmatic sociopolitical concerns, they have not often been linked to broader theoretical views. Overstated efforts to link a particular technique to a theory, such as Sargent's (1957) appeal to Pavlovian theory, are neither adequate to the totality of coercive persuasion nor supported by sufficient empirical evidence to be generally acceptable. Our summary of the components involved in coercive persuasion focuses only upon what is shared across several responsible efforts to reconstruct, from historical and personal accounts, the processes involved in this kind of influence (Anthony & Robbins, 1994; Bromley & Richardson, 1983; Lifton, 1961; Robbins & Anthony, 1980; Somit, 1968).

1. *Total control and isolation.* Persons are isolated (individually or in small groups), under the absolute control of authorities.

2. *Physical debilitation and exhaustion.* Persons are physically exhausted and debilitated. Causes can include constant interrogation and/or continual prodding from peers, as well as sleep and food deprivation. In extreme case, physical torture and starvation may be used.

3. *Confusion and uncertainty.* Personal belief systems and entire ideological orientations are challenged. Persons' uncertainty about their own fate is linked to uncertainty concerning their beliefs and values.

4. *Guilt and humiliation.* A sense of guilt and personal humiliation is induced by a variety of techniques. All are directed at making a potential convert feel unworthy if he or she persists in maintaining present commitments.

5. *Release and resolution.* An absolute framework provides only a single "out." Suicide is prohibited. Only by compliance or full conversion can individuals gain release from the isolation, pain, guilt, and confusion induced in them by their persuaders.

It is readily apparent that coercive techniques of persuasion are seldom of an all-or-none nature. It is best to talk about degrees of coercive persuasion, ranging from the extremes of the techniques applied to prisoners of war, to the middle-range examples of draftees into the military, and then to the minimal extremes (say, a religious summer camp to which parents may send a reluctant child). Although the degree of compliance is rather straightforwardly linked to degree of control, actual conversion or internalization of beliefs is less clearly empirically understood. What is certain is that conversion is much rarer than compliance under any system of coercive persuasion. However, as Somit (1968) has noted, compliance achieved by extreme coercive persuasion has its own limits:

> To be successful it demands a uniquely structured and controlled environmental setting and an inordinate investment in time and manpower. Despite the cost entailed, its effectiveness is limited to individual subjects or, even under the optimum conditions, to a small group of persons. (p. 142)

Coercive Persuasion/"Brainwashing" and Cults: A Contemporary Appeal to a Discredited Process

It is readily apparent that popular interest in new religious movements and cults cannot be explained by such pseudoscientific concepts as brainwashing. Nor has the term been thoroughly discredited in the contexts within which it was first applied, since no powerful psychological technique to mandate beliefs or behaviors exists. Techniques of coercive persuasion are readily identifiable and work by methods well established in the social sciences. Yet these techniques are variously associated with a variety of groups and in no sense differentially or uniquely characterize cults.

For some, the popularity of new religious movements to which close friends or relatives convert is troublesome. Yet serious issues of value and lifestyle differences are sidestepped by essentially rhetorical schemes directed at delegitimating cults. The Unification Church has been a particular target of such schemes (Robbins, 1977). For others, new religious movements can be discredited if an explanation for conversion can be offered that denies it was voluntary. Pseudoscientific terms such as "snapping" (Conway & Siegelman, 1978) and "mentacide" (Shapiro, 1977, p. 80) have been coined. Not only do such terms lack real scientific credibility; claims to a "cult syndrome" have never been substantiated, even in terms of the data provided by the most passionate champions of the claim. For instance, despite the popular appeal of one text—*Snapping: America's Epidemic of Sudden Personality Change* (Conway & Siegelman, 1978), which claims to document a "cult withdrawal syndrome"—few of the claims have withstood scientific scrutiny (Kilbourne, 1983; Kirkpatrick, 1988; Lewis & Bromley, 1987). Yet such claims are widely reported in the popular media, paralleling for new religious movements what historically occurred in terms of political ideologies (Verdier, 1977). This medicalization of the process of conversion is only part of the larger issue of the medicalization of deviance, which Robbins and Anthony (1979) have termed the "medicalization of religion." In a word, however thoroughly discredited the concept of brainwashing may be, the acceptance of brainwashing is the major way in which those who oppose conversion to cults have attempted to circumvent what would otherwise be rights of choice protected by the First Amendment to the U.S. Constitution (Anthony & Robbins, 1992).

This contemporary appeal to a discredited process follows the similar fallacious reasoning used previously to discredit political views. Applied to cults, as novel (and hence, to some, threatening) religious views, brainwashing or "snapping" implies that a person's ability to withstand such practices is severely limited. Comments offered to support a person's conversion to cult beliefs and practices are used as criteria of mental aberration, rather than as evidence of a successful search for an alternative religious view by a competent individual. When doctrines are viewed as symptoms of pathology, the process by which the individual was coerced to adopt such views is the target of concern, not the content of the beliefs or the religiously informed lifestyle the beliefs support. The right to choose even unpopular alternatives is denied to converts if the rhetorical strategies of those who would pathologize the process are successful (Robbins & Anthony, 1979).

Ironically, a largely self-fulfilling prophecy of what the rhetoricians of brainwashing fear most is realized in the anti-cult movement, portions of which support "deprogramming." Deprogrammers utilize many of the techniques of coercive persuasion to undo the presumed effects of brainwashing. The fact that cults appeal disproportionately to the young, and to others who are often in opposition to mainstream culture, fuels the anti-cult movement (Barker, 1986). Almost by definition, youths are abandoning the faiths of their parents (whether these are secular or religious) to join cults. As discussed in Chapter 5, interpersonal factors are an important factor in religious conversion. Not surprisingly, then, parent–youth conflict is both a motivating factor for conversion to cults and often a consequence of such conversion (Pilarzyk, 1978).

Parent–youth conflict plays a major role in deprogramming controversies, in which often parents must be granted legal rights to forcefully remove their children from cult groups. These legal issue are complex in their own right, and are confounded by the courts' need to evaluate scientific claims that are hotly disputed among those who defend or oppose cults as expert witnesses (Beckford, 1979; Delgado, 1977; Lemoult, 1978; Lundé & Segal, 1987; Robbins, 1985). Paradoxically, this has led to several studies of the process of deprogramming, as there are no identifiable studies on the processes of "brainwashing" presumably utilized by some of the more controversial cults (Kim, 1979). Although some have tried to sensationalize deprogramming as a new rite of exorcism (Shupe, Spielman, & Stigall, 1977) and to depict anti-cultists as themselves pathological (Kilbourne & Richardson, 1986), such rhetoric among researchers is best taken as empirical evidence the necessity of paying serious attention to issues of the ideological surround, which inevitably inform social-scientific research. The actual empirical techniques of deprogrammers are no less mysterious than are coercive persuasive techniques. The ability of deprogrammers to isolate their subjects, with extensive control over their environment, permits them to utilize established procedures to reconvert cult members. Kim (1979) has summarized this process as involving three steps: (1) motivating the persons to "unfreeze" their commitment to the cult; (2) providing information that requires the reevaluation of cult beliefs in light of the beliefs to which the persons are to be "reconverted"; and (3) obtaining a "refreezing" of the supported perspective to which the persons are now recommitted.

Cults' Actual Ability to Retain and Recruit Members

Ironically, despite controversies surrounding cult practices, the majority of cult members are not likely to stay converted. As we have noted in Chapter 11, most converts to new religious groups are "seekers" who explore a variety of beliefs and lifestyles, many associated with the new religious movements. Most cults, by their very nature, can be expected to appeal permanently only to a minority of followers. The inability of any group in a pluralist society to maintain complete social isolation, totally regulate its members' lifestyles, channel dyadic intimacy, and articulate and defend one authoritative ideology (to cite but a few examples) assures that cults will have high rates of turnover (Wright, 1987). Furthermore, most voluntary defectors from cults feel neither angry nor duped over the experience. Most feel wiser for the experience, even though they were unwilling to stay cult members. Table 12.6 indicates the results of a survey of 45 members who voluntarily left cults.

Not only do cults have significant voluntary turnover of members; their ability to recruit members through coercive techniques is severely limited, especially in a society where civil liberties are protected. For instance, in Galanter's (1989a) study of a Unification induction workshops, those who agreed to attend were followed in terms of the success of eight of these workshop to persuade attendees actually to join. Of 104 participants in the workshop, 71 dropped out within 2 days; another 29 dropped out between 2 and 9 days; and an additional 17 dropped out after 9 days. Only 9 workshop participants actually stayed over 21 days to join the Unification Church. Thus Galanter (1989a) found that even among persons self-selected to be receptive to recruitment workshops where mild degrees of coercive persuasion were used, the vast majority failed to join. Barker (1984) replicated Galanter's findings with a sample of over 1,000 workshop participants in London 1 year later. She noted that after 2 years far fewer than 1% of workshop participants were associated with the Unification Church, despite the fact that workshop participants were likely to be favorably predisposed to the Unification Church and presumably were the targets of powerful coercive techniques (Johnson, 1979). Contrary to media claims, the failure to successfully recruit large numbers of persons who voluntarily stay with deviant religious groups is typical of all cult recruitment and retention efforts.

Cults: Discussion and Summary

The research on cult recruitment suggests that the controversy surrounding new religious movements is not simply an issue of the processes employed to attract and convert members. It is more likely one of the significant tensions that mainstream religious and secular groups have with novel religions, which solicit and legitimate diverse interpretations and modes of confrontation with sacred and symbolic realities. Hence, even in the most extreme cases, we must be careful not to naively utilize and uncritically accept delegitimating modes of explanation for perspectives different from our own (Barker, 1984). The tendency to ex-

TABLE 12.6. Responses of 45 Voluntary Defectors from Three Cults

Response category	n	%
Felt angry	3	7
Felt duped/"brainwashed"	4	9
Felt wiser for experience	30	66
All other responses	8	18

Note. The three cults were the Children of God/Family of Love, Hare Krishna, and the Unification Church (*n* = 15 each). Adapted from Wright (1987, p. 87). Copyright 1987 by the Society for the Scientific Study of Religion. Adapted by permission.

plain away beliefs and practices distant from our own through labels for the processes presumed to be operating, which need not take the content of beliefs into account, is a pervasive tendency in the social sciences. Yet, as Kroll-Smith (1980) has shown, even the most private experiences of members of deviant religious groups are influenced by normal social-psychological processes. Several studies show that conversion to new religious groups helps individuals adapt to social and cultural change, of which these groups by definition are a part (Lebra, 1970; Turner, 1979; Weigert, D'Antonio, & Rubel, 1971). Even converts to deviant religious groups are often socialized by the process of conversion to accept other mainstream cultural values (Johnson, 1961). In addition, deviant religious groups socialize people into subcultures within which otherwise maladaptive behaviors are functional (Lewellen, 1979). Also, we cannot underestimate the power of such variant religious bodies to reconceptualize commonly accepted social realities, so that they both justify participation in, and legitimate the continuance of, what to mainstream culture are at best puzzling but acceptable instances of subcultural deviance (Festinger, Riecken, & Schachter, 1956; Weisner, 1974). This is particularly true of many of the practices of cult leaders, whose behaviors to an outsider appear to be no more than trickery, chicanery, or pathology (Feuerstein, 1992).

The failure of cults to be differentially associated with pathology must be emphasized. It has not yet been confirmed empirically that cults either attract or produce pathology when pathology is judged independently of the cults' own behavioral norms. For instance, Galanter (1983, 1989a) notes that deviant sects actually avoid recruiting persons who show obvious pathological characteristics. Likewise, Ungerleider and Welish (1979) have documented the absence of obvious pathology in former and current members of a variety of cults. Finally, Taslimi, Hood, and Watson (1991) failed to substantiate previous claims to pathology in a follow-up study of former members of a fundamentalist Jesus commune, Shiloh. Furthermore, the earlier claims about the presumably maladaptive characteristics of these members while in the Jesus commune failed to account appropriately for the fact that objective indices of maladaptive behavior must be judged within the particular context; behaviors that were otherwise less functional outside the commune may have been adaptive for members inside the commune (Richardson, Stewart, & Simmonds, 1979; Simmonds, 1977b). In fact, Robbins and Anthony (1982) have critically reviewed the relevant empirical literature and concluded that members of deviant religious groups are socially integrated on many criteria:

1. Likely termination of illicit drug use.
2. Renewed vocational motivation.
3. Mitigation of neurotic distress.
4. Suicide prevention.
5. Decrease in anomie/moral confusion.
6. Increase in social compassion/responsibility.
7. Decrease in psychosomatic symptoms.
8. Improved self-actualization.
9. Clarified sense of identity.
10. Generally positive problem-solving assistance.

Finally, it must be emphasized that judgments of the relative value of identities and life styles are inevitably beyond the ability of social sciences to resolve factually. Efforts to set criteria for authentic spiritual choices must be individually and collectively made, but their existential base is never simply resolved by factual descriptions or explanations of the processes by which such choices are made. Although research clearly demonstrates that identities linked to divergent social groups increase the prejudice of such groups toward one another, the ability of groups to identify superordinate goals (which can only be achieved by the cooperation of all groups) reduces conflict and prejudice (Sherif, 1953). Thus the seeking of superordinate goals that transcend religious groupings and require the collective effort of all to achieve is a worthwhile project, however ambitious it may be, if prejudices and conflicts among religious groups are to be reduced (Anthony, Ecker, & Wilbur, 1987).

SOCIAL-PSYCHOLOGICAL PROCESSES IN RELIGIOUS PARTICIPATION

Are Religion and Mainline Religious Groups Doomed to Extinction?

It has been over 30 years since two of the major researchers in the sociology of religion raised the issue of whether or not North America was entering a post-Christian era (Stark & Glock, 1968). A major factor in their questioning was survey research documenting a decline in what many perceived as core Christian beliefs—most centrally, the belief in the divinity of Christ. Stark and Glock (1968) provided a pessimistic prediction for mainline Christian denominations:

> As matters now stand we can see little long-term future for the church as we know it. A remnant church can be expected to last for a long time if only to provide the psychic comforts which are currently dispensed by orthodoxy. However, eventually substitutes for even this function are likely to emerge leaving churches of the present with no effective rationale for existing. (p. 210)

In a similar vein, the renowned anthropologist Wallace (1966) has argued that all supernatural beliefs are doomed to extinction, presumably along with the churches that rely upon such beliefs for the effectiveness of their rituals.

However, associated with predictions of the eventual extinction of churches and supernatural beliefs are two assumptions that can be seriously questioned. One is that religious beliefs and church attendance are heavily correlated, and hence that changes in the one can be used to infer changes in the other. It is assumed that people who change religious beliefs are likely to lower their rate of church attendance, or that persons who lower their rate of church attendance have probably changed beliefs. Yet belief and attendance are far from perfectly correlated, and one can be a very poor predictor of the other (Demerath, 1965). Second, the evidence (largely derived from Gallup Poll data) suggesting declines in church attendance is confounded by variations within denominational groups. For instance, Greeley (1972a) documented an increase in church attendance among Catholics, associated with a decrease in commitment to orthodox Catholic beliefs. There is no paradox in these findings when we realize that persons attend churches for a variety of reasons, many of which are only marginally related to belief issues. Furthermore, we have noted earlier that as denominational attendance falters, sectarian and cult commitments are likely to increase, so that overall levels of religious group participation may remain strong. Yet before we accept evidence for the decline in mainstream denominations, it behooves us to consider denominations that are similar to the sects and cults in terms of ideological and behavioral strictness, even though their norms are less in tension with the dominant culture than are the more extreme norms of either sects or cults.

The Kelley Thesis and Iannaccone's Modification of It:
Strictness Contingencies

While many social scientists were predicting doom for traditional Christian denominations, one investigator burst onto the scene with a book that stimulated much controversy and continues to generate empirical research. Kelley (1972) argued that overall decline in church attendance, especially among North American Protestants, masked two contradictory trends: The more liberal and ecumenical denominations were declining in membership, while the more conservative and fundamentalist denominations were increasing in membership. Ironically, then, the more a religious group was accommodating itself to mainstream culture, the less effectively it was maintaining its membership.

Kelley's thesis is more relevant to the strictness of religious groups in the enforcement of their beliefs and behavioral norms than to their strictness in the content of the beliefs they profess. However, strict groups are likely to be sectarian in nature, demanding a purity that the more lenient denominations relax as they universalize and welcome a diverse membership, which itself is accommodating to the pluralism of mainstream modern or postmodern culture. More sectarian groups demand a seriousness and strictness that are inappropriate to broader universalizing tendencies. Hence Kelley's thesis is compatible with our earlier discussion of sects as acceptable forms of subcultural deviance, and of cults as more problematic forms of religious deviance that elicit cultural retaliation. However, in Kelley's thesis it is the stricter denominations, the sects, and the cults that are increasing in membership, at the cost of the more liberal denominations. The simplicity of his thesis can be seen in his ordering of religious groups along a gradient of seriousness or strictness. Denominations that strictly enforce norms taken seriously by their membership tend toward exclusiveness; this differentiates them from mainstream denominations, which cannot (by the very nature of their beliefs and behavioral tolerance) be strong religions, according to Kelley (1972). Another way to identify this gradient is along a continuum from most exclusive (serious/strict) to most ecumenical. It is this continuum that is hypothesized to correlate with church attendance and growth. This gradient applies primarily within the Christian tradition, not across traditions, although Kelley does include Black Muslims and Orthodox Jews in his gradient for the Christian tradition. However, with these exceptions, only Christian groups are ordered; other traditions would need their own gradients (Kelley, 1972). A listing of religious organizations along Kelley's continuum is presented in Figure 12.2.

Kelley's thesis is strongly stated. Though it needs conceptual refinement, it does have the merit of identifying the postulated determinants of church growth in terms capable of empirical investigation. Several studies have tested Kelley's basic thesis in regard to particular denominations or churches, with some degree of success (Bouma, 1979; Perry & Hoge, 1981). Empirical refinements have suggested that Kelley's thesis applies not to the recruitment of new members, but to the maintenance of adult members and to the retention of children as they mature and stay as adult members of the congregation (Bibby, 1978; Bibby & Brinkerhoff, 1973). Others have argued that not all exclusive groups maintain high membership and attendance rates, and thus that Kelley's thesis is far from a general covering law (Smith, 1992).

Recently, investigators have focused upon a modification of Kelley's thesis. Unlike Kelley, Iannaccone (1994) has focused upon organizational strength rather than simply growth. He has also operationalized strictness in terms of the costs of organizational membership, and has avoided a potential tautology by using as indicators of "cost" only activities

Black Muslims   <Most exclusive
Jehovah's Witnesses
Evangelicals and Pentecostals
Orthodox Jews
Churches of Christ
Latter-Day Saints (Mormons)
Seventh-Day Adventists
Church of God
Church of Christ, Scientist
Southern Baptist Convention
Lutheran Church–Missouri Synod
American Lutheran Church
Roman Catholic Church
Russian Orthodox
Greek Orthodox
Lutheran Church in America
Southern Presbyterian Church
Reformed Church in America
Episcopal Church
American Baptist Convention
United Presbyterian Church
United Methodist Church
Ethical Culture Society
Most universal>   Unitarian–Universalists

FIGURE 12.2. Kelley's exclusive–ecumenical continuum. Adapted from Kelley (1972, p. 89). Copyright 1972 by HarperCollins Publishers. Adapted by permission.

defined as being outside normal church activities. Furthermore, Iannaccone (1996) has persuasively argued the methodological limitations of testing the Kelley thesis across denominations, arguing instead that a fair test of the thesis requires comparing strictness within groups of the same denomination. Olson and Perl (2001) found support for Iannaccone's modification of the Kelley thesis across five different denominations. Although strictness did not systematically correlate with measures of religious commitment within denominations, it did across denominations. The results are presented in Table 12.7.

Although empirical investigation is continuing, Kelley's thesis and especially Iannaccone's modification of the theory (in terms of both its conceptualization and the most appropriate statistical procedures to test the theory) suggest that strictness does indeed lead to greater religious commitment, if not simply church growth. However, growth and strictness are not unrelated. Research Box 12.6 indicates that in the Amish tradition, growth and strictness are dynamically interrelated insofar as strictness may aid in retaining children within the tradition and hence contribute to church growth. The focus upon strictness forces consideration of the problem that has been a major focus of this chapter—the dynamic processes involved in tensions between religious groups and their cultures.

TABLE 12.7. A Test of Iannaccone's Modification of the Kelley Thesis, Using Data within and across Five Denominations

Denomination (n = 125 each)	Strictness[a] Mean	Strictness[a] SD	Time commitment[b]	Receipts of congregation[c]	Mean $ donation[d]
Assemblies of God	3.04	0.92	0.19*	0.09	0.00
Southern Baptist	2.63	1.18	−0.07	−0.11	−0.19*
Catholic	0.15	0.44	−0.02	−0.02	−0.13
Lutheran	0.15	0.44	−0.02	0.00	−0.03
Presbyterian	0.31	0.67	0.28**	0.00	−0.07
All denominations combined	1.36	1.49	0.67***	0.38***	0.33***

The columns Mean, SD, Time commitment, Receipts of congregation, and Mean $ donation fall under the spanning header "Correlations of strictness with measures of religious commitment", with "Strictness[a]" spanning Mean and SD.

Note. Adapted from Olson and Perl (2001, p. 761). Copyright 2001 by the Society for the Scientific Study of Religion. Adapted by permission.

[a]Strictness was assessed with these questions: "Does your congregation teach abstinence from certain foods? Alcohol and/or tobacco? Gambling? Certain forms of entertainment? Other (specify)?" Range of scale was from 0 to 5 (most strict).
[b]Hours spent attending, planning, and leading church activities *outside* church services.
[c]Total dollars for church budget, divided by number of households in church.
[d]As self-reported in 58% response rate (n = 10,903) from 18,750 mailings (30 per congregation).
*p < .05. **p < .001. ***p < .0001.

Research Box 12.6. Four Amish Traditions (Kraybill, 1994)

The Amish are not simply a homogeneous group, and their tension with modern culture varies among the different Amish affiliations. Ninety percent of all Amish belong to one of four affiliations. Three of these emerged from the original Old Order Amish, founded in 1809. Kraybill identifies the first of these newer affiliations, the Swartzentrubers, as "legendary for their stubborn traditionalism" (1994, p. 55). For instance, indoor bathrooms are still strictly forbidden in this order of the Amish, founded in 1913. A dispute over the shunning of Andy Weaver for affiliating with a Mennonite group led to a second new Amish affiliation in 1952. In 1968, a third new affiliation emerged, whose members were more accommodating to modern culture. In Kraybill's terms, these New Order Amish developed "a more rational and individualist understanding of Christian faith" (1994, p. 57). Where reliable data are available, they support the fact that the stricter the Amish affiliation the greater the ability to retain children, as noted in the following table.

	Swartzentruber	Andy Weaver	Original Old Order	New Order
Degree of traditionalism	Extreme	High	Moderate	Low
Estimated no. in affiliation	2,500	2,750	14,400	2,750
Average no. of children	[a]	5.9	5.1	4.9
Percentage of children affiliated with Amish	90	95	86	57
Percentage of families retaining all their children	[b]	95	88	72

Note. Data from Kraybill (1994, pp. 57, 73).

[a]Not reported, but estimated to be generally larger than in the other three affiliations.
[b]Not reported but estimated to be 90–95% by local informants.

OVERVIEW

The contemporary debate over forms of religious expression is as old as religion itself. The long tradition of church–sect theory suggests that religious organizations are in a constant process of change—some adapting to cultural changes, and others trying to resist change. The temptation to postulate unique psychological processes involved in religions distant from one's own is unlikely to be fruitful. Individuals committed to cult and sect forms of religion struggle no less for significance and meaning in their lives than do those committed to more mainstream forms of religious faith. This, combined with the discussion in Chapter 10 on the emergence of forms of spirituality in opposition to religion, suggests that the empirical study of the dynamics within and between religious groups has a certain future.

Concepts such as "ideological surround" are useful in sensitizing researchers to the fact that empirical measures and assessments are unlikely to be illuminating if they cannot capture a believer's own perspective truthfully. The claim that unique psychological processes must be involved in the maintenance of religious groups in tension with their culture is as conceptually unenlightened as it is empirically ungrounded. Polemical terms such as "brainwashing" are clearly less than useful. If we maintain the concept "cult," it is because accurate descriptions of phenomena are crucial in science, and perhaps even more so in the social-scientific study of less popular forms of religion. We ought not to abandon terms whose usefulness is only threatened by popular ignorance. The fact that, in the end, evaluations must be made is all the more reason to make them only with descriptions of religious groups that are fair and accurate.

Chapter 13

RELIGION AND MORALITY

Our study leads us to believe that there are more children actually abused in the name of God than in the name of Satan.

. . . temperance was part of a new kind of effort to assert the authority of religious ideas in the public sphere, and to regroup religious forces under auspices outside the church.

NO to condom distribution in the schools, NO to taxpayer funding of abortion, NO to sex-education classes in the public schools that promote promiscuity, NO to homosexual adoptions and government-sanctioned gay marriages.

One of the clearest cultural influences on adolescent sexual behavior is religious participation. Adolescents who attend religious services frequently and who value religion as an important aspect of their lives have less permissive attitudes toward premarital sex. This finding applies equally to Catholic, Protestant, and Jewish young people. The relationship is accentuated in adolescents who describe themselves as Fundamentalist Protestant or Baptist.

. . . parents showed their deep love for children by punishing them for . . . offences such as disobedience, sloth, lying or stealing. . . . "The rod is very little hurt compared to an eternity in hell" [said the woman].[1]

DOES RELIGION DICTATE MORALITY?

Religion has a lot to say about morality. Christians, Jews, Buddhists, Muslims, and Hindus may not agree on the nature of God, or on religious rituals and teachings, but they do tend to agree about moral issues. In fact, when it comes to ethics, major world religions are amazingly consistent in their teachings about right and wrong, especially concerning murder, stealing, and adultery. In Christianity and Judaism, this distilled essence of morality is captured by the Ten Commandments. And all major world religions seem to teach some version of "Do unto others what you would have them do unto you."

Persons with a proreligious orientation would be inclined to argue that religion has tremendous potential to improve our world by teaching an ethical system that would benefit

---

1. These quotations come, respectively, from the following sources: Bottoms, Shaver, Goodman, and Qin (1995, p. 109); Schmidt (1995, p. 111); a fund-raising letter distributed in March 1995 by the Christian Coalition, quoted in Birnbaum (1995, p. 22); Newman and Newman (1995, p. 439); and the report of a former nun from a rural commune, quoted in Cox (2002, p. A7).

all of us. In fact, the theologies of such diverse religious bodies as Buddhists, Christians, and Jews have claimed that faith and morality are inseparable (Spilka, Hood, & Gorsuch, 1985). And some groups apparently want to legislate morality; for example, the conservative Christian Coalition in the United States has seemed "eager to impose what it sees as a Bible-backed morality on the American public at large" (Birnbaum, 1995, p. 22). On the other hand, some people are not convinced that religion holds the key to morality in the world, and they may argue that it can actually cause intolerance and suffering.

Religion as "Good"

We can all think of examples in which religion has apparently resulted in tolerance, helpfulness, and personal and interpersonal integrity. Mother Teresa spent her life in appalling conditions in order to help the poor, the sick, and the downtrodden in the cause of Christian charity. Martin Luther King, Jr. faced considerable danger, and was eventually assassinated, in his religiously based fight for equal rights and self-respect for black Americans. Churches also provide money, housing, and social support for refugees from other lands, and soup kitchens and halfway houses are sponsored by religious organizations. The list could go on and on.

Religion as "Bad"

On the other hand, many examples can be cited where religion has seemed to have no impact at all in encouraging positive behavior, or where it may even have contributed to dishonesty, intolerance, physical violence, and prejudice. Anti-Semitism is preached openly in some North American pulpits. The Christian-based Ku Klux Klan spreads hatred of blacks, Jews, and Catholics. Many wars and other violent conflicts in today's world are religiously based: Catholics battle Protestants in Northern Ireland; Muslims and Christians fight in the former Yugoslavia; Sikhs and Hindus die in violent conflicts in India; the Taliban in Afghanistan took away women's rights and also charged Western aid workers for being open about their Christian beliefs; extremist Palestinian Muslim groups send suicide bombers to kill Israeli civilians; and Israeli Jews respond with military violence against Palestinians. Some may well wonder whether religion does not directly contribute to violence, intolerance, and injustice.

Considering the Evidence

Clearly, it would be a mistake to oversimplify these issues and to generalize about religion's contributing to morality or immorality. Faith is complex, and there are many unique religious groups, orientations, and dimensions that may differentially relate to specific aspects of "right and wrong."

Furthermore, we should not assume that religion has an impact on ethics through the process of "moral development" in childhood and adolescence. We have pointed out in Chapter 4 that Kohlberg thought of moral development as quite distinct from its religious counterpart, and he asserted that we should not assume that religion in any way causes or even contributes to the emergence of morality. Reviews of the literature concerning the acquisition of morality typically make little or no mention of religion in this process (see, e.g., Darley & Shultz, 1990).

It has been pointed out that different religious groups may have different ways of think-ing about moral issues, possibly because of religious teachings. Cohen and Rozin (2001) found that, partly because Protestants were more likely to believe that mental states are con-trollable and likely to lead to action, they rated a target person with "inappropriate mental states" (p. 697—e.g., not honoring one's parents, or thinking about having a sexual affair) more negatively than Jewish participants did. Thus religious traditions may to some extent lead people to think about moral issues differently, and also to judge others differently, de-pending on the others' expressed thoughts about moral issues. However, recent evidence suggests that the ways in which people *reason* about religious and moral conflicts are quite similar (Cobb, Ong, & Tate, 2001).

Quite apart from formal moral development in Kohlbergian or other terms, and the ways in which people think about morality, it has been claimed that religiousness is associ-ated with being a "better person" in numerous ways. In addition to broad moral imperatives such as "love thy neighbor," many religions have specific things to say about various per-sonal issues: honesty and cheating; substance use and abuse; sexual behavior; criminal be-havior and delinquency; domestic abuse; helping others; and prejudice and discrimination. After a brief discussion of moral attitudes and religion, we explore each of these areas in turn, attempting to determine whether religion and morality are associated. In the case of help-ing behavior and prejudice, relationships with religion are especially complex and have been of considerable interest in the psychology-of-religion literature, possibly because the asso-ciations are not always what we might expect. Thus our coverage of these latter topics is more detailed; it appears in Chapter 14.

MORAL ATTITUDES

It is not surprising that religion is related to people's attitudes on a host of morality-related issues. Typically, people who are religious (as measured in many different ways) are "more conservative" in their attitudes. In general, those who are more religious show more oppo-sition to abortion (Bryan & Freed, 1993), AIDS education (Ford, Zimmerman, Anderman, & Brown-Wright, 2001), divorce (Hayes & Hornsby-Smith, 1994), pornography (Lottes, Weinberg, & Weller, 1993), contraception (Krishnan, 1993), premarital sexuality (Bibby, 2001), homosexuality (Altemeyer & Hunsberger, 1992), feminism (Wilcox & Jelen, 1991), nudity in advertising (Alexander & Judd, 1986), suicide (Domino & Miller, 1992), eutha-nasia (Shuman, Fournet, Zelhart, Roland, & Estes, 1992), amniocentesis (Seals, Ekwo, Williamson, & Hanson, 1985), heavy metal and rap music (Lynxwiler & Gay, 2000), and women going topless on beaches (Herold, Corbesi, & Collins, 1994). Highly religious indi-viduals are also more likely to support marriage (Hayes & Hornsby-Smith, 1994), capital punishment (Bibby, 1987), vengeance (Cota-McKinley, Woody, & Bell, 2001), traditional sex roles (Larsen & Long, 1988), conservative political parties (Bibby, 1987), more severe criminal sentences (Altemeyer & Hunsberger, 1992), and censorship of sex and violence in the mass media (Fisher, Cook, & Shirkey, 1994). These lists surely just scratch the surface of such relationships, but they should give the reader an idea of the many diverse links between religion and moral attitudes.

However, it is one thing to oppose premarital sex or alcohol use on the basis of religion, and quite another to act consistently with this attitude when the opportunity presents itself. Furthermore, it is possible that one's personal position on ethical issues may differ from one's public stance. For example, it has been found that people who personally oppose abortion on moral or religious grounds, may actually *favor* legal abortion (Scott, 1989). And 70% of a sample of Seventh-Day Adventist young people endorsed their church's prohibition of premarital sex, but 54% of the sample reported that they had engaged in premarital sex (Ali & Naidoo, 1999). Thus, although associations between faith and moral attitudes are informative, they do not always accurately predict how religion will relate to moral *behavior*. So we now turn to a survey of several areas of behavior with strong ethical implications, in order to assess the role of religion in people's actions. However, as we shall see, beliefs and behavior are often intertwined in the research literature; it is therefore sometimes necessary to focus on attitudes generally in order to gain insights into moral behavior, despite the problems in doing so.

MORAL BEHAVIOR

Honesty and Cheating

In light of the emphasis placed on honesty by most religions, we might expect that their adherents would be less likely to lie, cheat, or otherwise deceive others. Of course, this is a difficult issue to study. One can imagine the problems associated with simply asking people how "religious" and how "honest" they are, to see whether the two variables are correlated. For both practical and ethical reasons, it is also not easy to place people in realistic circumstances that provide an opportunity to lie and cheat, in order to observe their reactions. First, it is difficult to construct "cheating" situations that are realistic and believable to those being studied. Second, to provide an opportunity for people to lie or cheat could violate ethical standards of research, especially since it might be necessary to conceal the true purpose of such research in order to encourage "real-life" responding.

Furthermore, values such as honesty are commonly embraced in our society, and there is some evidence that such values are commonly taught in schools (Zern, 1997) as well as through religion. Therefore, it is important that we do not assume that evidence of honesty values necessarily means that these values have been taught through one's religion.

In spite of these problems, some studies have attempted to investigate these personal morality issues. And although we might expect religion to have some impact in reducing dishonesty and cheating among religious persons, the evidence in general suggests that it has little or no impact in this regard.

Early Research

Hartshorne and May (1928, 1929; Hartshorne, May, & Shuttleworth, 1930) investigated a possible link between religiousness and cheating in their massive studies involving some 11,000 school children in the 1920s. They devised ingenious tests for cheating—for example, by measuring peeking during "eyes-closed" tests, and by checking to see whether students had changed their original answers when allowed to grade their own exams. In the end, they found essentially no relationship between religion and honesty or cheating. In fact, there was even some tendency for children who attended Sunday school to be less cooperative and helpful. Other early studies, such as that by Hightower (1930), similarly found no relationship between Biblical knowledge on the one hand and lying and cheating on the other.

More Recent Studies

People who believe that honesty is an important moral or religious value would be shocked to learn how common academic dishonesty is in high school and university settings. One investigation (Goldsen, Rosenberg, Williams, & Suchman, 1960) even found that 92% of religious college students affirmed that it was morally wrong to cheat, but that 87% of them agreed with the statement "If everyone else cheats, why shouldn't I?" Consistent with this, Spilka and Loffredo (1982) reported that 72% of a group of highly religious college students admitted that they had cheated on examinations. More generally, another study (Cochran, Chamlin, Wood, & Sellers, 1999) found that 83% of college students admitted to at least one act of academic dishonesty (e.g., plagiarism on an essay, cheating on an examination). And Bruggerman and Hart (1996) noted that when given incentives to lie and cheat, their sample of both religious and secular high school students revealed "surprisingly high levels of dishonest behavior" (p. 340). Even among Mormons, a group known for a conservative and strict approach to moral issues, 70% of a sample of more than 2,000 adolescents admitted that they had cheated on tests at school (Chadwick & Top, 1993). Apparently cheating is quite widespread among high school and college students, and it does not seem to make much difference whether or not students are religious.

Other research, involving behavioral measures and diverse samples, has also confirmed that religion does not decrease cheating behavior. Guttman (1984) investigated sixth graders from religious schools in Israel and discovered that religious children indicated some resistance to temptation on a paper-and-pencil test, but were actually more inclined to cheat on a behavioral measure. Smith, Wheeler, and Diener (1975) studied undergraduate college students, categorizing them as involved in the "Jesus movement" or as being otherwise religious, nonreligious, or atheistic; no differences emerged with respect to their tendency to cheat on a class examination when the opportunity was available.

One recent study (Perrin, 2000), using a behavioral measure, did find that religious college students cheated less. Because such behavioral investigations of cheating are rare, this study is highlighted in Research Box 13.1. Unfortunately, the cheating in this research was necessarily quite mild, involving 1 point on a single weekly quiz, and just four of seven measures of religion (all single-item measures) achieved statistical significance. Therefore, the results of this study cannot be seen as representing a major shift in findings when behavioral measures are used. However, it is an important investigation, offering findings that deserve attention and follow-up research.

Some other studies have found a negative link between religiousness and cheating, but these involved self-reports rather than actual behavioral measures. For example, Grasmick and his colleagues (Grasmick, Bursik, & Cochran, 1991; Grasmick, Kinsey, & Cochran, 1991) have carried out investigations of the relationship between religion and self-reported admission of how likely respondents would be to cheat on their income taxes (and, in one study, to commit theft and to engage in littering) in the future. There was some tendency for more religious persons to indicate they were less likely to cheat on their taxes (and less likely to litter, but there was no significant relationship for theft). Similarly, a nationwide Dutch survey (ter Voert, Felling, & Peters, 1994) found that "strong Christian believers" reported holding a stricter moral code with respect to "self-interest morality" (different forms of cheating). And Storch and Storch (2001) found that higher Intrinsic religious scores were negatively related to reported rates of academic dishonesty.

ॐ

Research Box 13.1. Religiosity and Honesty (Perrin, 2000)

Perrin carried out this study in an attempt to address problems in the literature, including the paucity of studies on religion and honesty; measurement problems, such as the tendency for dependent measures to rely on self-reports rather than behavior; and inconsistencies in the results of relevant investigations.

Perrin's own study had two main components. First, students in a large lecture course at a university in the western United States completed a survey that included seven items on religiosity. These items were intended to tap frequency of church attendance, participation in religious activities (such as Bible study), frequency of prayer, belief in life after death, whether respondents considered themselves to be "born again" and to be "strong Christians," and the frequency with which they had had religious experiences (i.e., being "very close to a powerful, spiritual force that seemed to lift you out of yourself" (p. 539)). We are not told what else was on the questionnaire, or what the reliability of the seven religiosity items might be.

Second, there was a simple but effective measure of honesty. In one of the weekly quizzes in this class, the teaching assistant intentionally graded them incorrectly, so that *everyone* received 1 additional point on that quiz. Students were then informed that an error might have been made in grading. They were to regrade their own quizzes and write, at the top of an unrelated assignment that they were handing in, one of three phrases: "I owe you a point," "Quiz graded correctly," or "You owe me a point."

Results indicated that, first, honesty was hard to come by in this investigation, as had been found in previous research. Of the 130 students included in the analyses, just 32% honestly admitted receiving an extra point on the quiz. Fifty-two percent said that the quiz was graded correctly, and 16% actually tried to get another point in addition to the point they received from the teaching assistant's "mistake." More important, however, were the comparisons of honesty across the religion item responses. For all seven items, the results were in the expected direction, such that more honesty was apparent for more religious responders. However, the results achieved significance for just four of the seven items (church attendance, frequency of other religious activities, belief in life after death, and born-again status). The most dramatic difference in scores seems to have been for church attendance: 45% of weekly (or more frequent) attenders, but just 13% of those who attended once a year or less, honestly reported the 1-point error on their quiz.

Finally, the results do confirm a stark reality for "religious people." Even among the most highly religious people in this study, as defined by seven quite different items, the majority of students apparently lied about the results of their quiz. It would seem that truly high percentages of honesty are difficult to find in groups of religious or nonreligious persons.

Unfortunately, this study had a relatively small sample about which we know little (e.g., age, percentage of men and women, race/ethnicity, religious affiliation, extent of personal religiosity), as well as only a brief "home-grown" measure of religiosity. Results are reported only in percentages of some rather unique combinations of response categories, and so on. For these reasons, it would be helpful to see the results replicated, with more standard measures and more information about samples and analyses. At the same time, this study is one of very few that has attempted to use a behavioral measure of honesty, and we hope that it will stimulate additional and much-needed investigations in this area.

However, Francis and Johnson (1999) found no relationship between scores on a "lie scale" and either church attendance or personal prayer among primary school teachers (see also Francis & Katz, 1992; Gillings & Joseph, 1996; Lewis & Joseph, 1994). In other studies, religiosity has been linked with higher lie scale scores (e.g., Francis, Pearson, & Kay, 1983a; Lewis & Maltby, 1995). We must be careful with such findings, however, since they represent self-reports only; as indicated above, what people say they will do is not always consonant with their actual behavior.

Religion and Honesty: Conclusions

In summary, the available research on religion and honesty spans a considerable time period (from the 1920s to the present), and has involved many diverse samples and measures. However, there are relatively few studies in this area, at least compared to most other topics in this chapter. Also, many of the published studies in this area (but not all of them) are apparently "quick questionnaire" investigations that include one or more simple measures of religion (e.g., attendance) and a "lie scale" or comparable measure. It is then relatively simple to calculate the correlation between the two measures. These reports tend to appear in journals inclined to publish brief reports, which preclude full discussions of methodology, findings, and interpretation of results. In short, although such studies invariably come to a "conclusion" about religion–honesty relationships, the strength of their contribution to the literature may at best be difficult to assess. These concerns aside, we can offer some tentative conclusions about research findings in this area.

In the end, although more religious people apparently tend to say that they are more honest than less religious persons, such findings seem to be contradicted by other research showing no relationship, or even a positive relationship between lie scale scores and religiosity. More importantly, there is not much evidence from studies of actual behavior to support the position that religious people are somehow more honest, or less likely to lie or cheat, than are their less religious or nonreligious peers. In view of the clear teachings of most faiths on such issues, we are left to ponder why religion does not have a significant impact in reducing cheating *behavior*.

Substance Use and Abuse

Religious teachings across diverse groups typically oppose the abuse of such substances as alcohol and illicit drugs. One might expect, therefore, that faith would be associated with decreased substance use/abuse. And, in fact, the related literature generally does confirm this. Gorsuch and Butler (1976) noted this in their survey of studies prior to the mid-1970s, and more recent reviews (e.g., Benson, 1992b; Gorsuch, 1995) concluded that research since the mid-1970s has quite consistently confirmed the tendency for more religious persons (as defined in many different ways) to be less likely to use and abuse alcohol and drugs.

The range of studies in this area is impressive, focusing variously on alcohol, tobacco, and illicit drugs used for nonmedical purposes (e.g., cocaine, heroin, amphetamines, barbiturates, and psychedelic substances). Some studies focus on either alcohol *or* "drugs," but many investigate the impact of religion on both. Here we consider the findings of the various studies together, because their results are so similar.

The Negative Relationship between Religion and Substance Use/Abuse

In the early 1980s, Khavari and Harmon (1982) analyzed data from almost 5,000 people between the ages of 12 and 85; they concluded that there was a "powerful" negative relationship between religiousness and both alcohol consumption and the use of psychoactive drugs. People who reported that they were "not religious at all" tended to use more tobacco products, marijuana, hashish, and amphetamines, compared with people who considered themselves to be religious. Results such as these seem to suggest that religion somehow contributes to decreased use of a variety of products that have possible negative implications for health (Khavari & Harmon, 1982).

Similarly, a massive study of over 10,000 youths in Minnesota (Benson, Wood, Johnson, Eklin, & Mills, 1983) found that many indices of religious belief and behavior were negatively related to the use of such drugs as marijuana, LSD, PCP, Quaaludes, and amphetamines. More recently, congruent results were obtained by Perkins (1994) in a study of several thousand New York college students between 1982 and 1991; by Hope and Cook (2001) in their investigation of 7,661 church-affiliated young people; and by other research involving large samples (e.g., Bahr, Maughan, Marcos, & Li, 1998; Cook, Goddard, & Westall, 1997; Lee, Rice, & Gillespie, 1997; Park, Bauer, & Oescher, 2001; Sutherland & Shepherd, 2001). Moreover, T. N. Brown, Schulenberg, Bachman, O'Malley, and Johnston (2001) concluded that religiosity was consistently (negatively) linked to various types of substance abuse among high school seniors, in research conducted annually from 1976 to 1997.

Benson (1992b) has pointed out that the negative relationship between religion and substance use/abuse has been found in multiple studies of adolescents, college students, and adults, and that it seems to hold for both males and females. With few exceptions, consistent findings have been obtained in diverse parts of the United States (Donahue, 1987), as well as in countries as disparate as Canada (Hundleby, 1987), Nigeria (Adelekan, Abiodun, Imouokhome-Obayan, Oni, & Ogunremi, 1993), Scotland (Engs & Mullen, 1999), the Netherlands (Mullen & Francis, 1995), Sweden (Pettersson, 1991), Israel (Kandel & Sudit, 1982), Australia (Najman, Williams, Keeping, Morrison, & Anderson, 1988), Thailand (Assanangkornchai, Conigrave, & Saunders, 2002), Spain (Grana Gomes & Munoz-Rivas, 2000), Saudi Arabia (Qureshi & Al-Habeeb, 2000), and China (Wu, Detels, Zhang, & Duan, 1996). This effect has even been found among children of opium addicts (Miller, Weissman, Gur, & Adams, 2001). And *parental* religiosity is also apparently linked with lesser substance abuse among children (Foshee & Hollinger, 1996; Merrill, Salazar, & Gardner, 2001).

As an initial general conclusion, then, there seems to be little argument that greater religiosity is associated with lesser substance use.

The Magnitude and Generality of the Relationship. The size of the relationships noted above varies from study to study. Still, Benson (1992b) concluded that on average, correlations with alcohol, tobacco, and marijuana use are roughly −.20, and that the corresponding relationships for other illicit drugs are lower. Donahue (1987) noted some tendency for the strength of the associations to decline in the 1980s, at least among high school seniors. Although the obtained relationships are fairly weak, they often remain significant even after the effects of age, gender, race, region, education, income, and other variables are controlled for (see, e.g., Benson & Donahue, 1989; Cochran, Beeghley, & Bock, 1988).

However, we should not assume that other variables are inconsequential. Mason and Windle (2002), in a 1-year longitudinal study, found that religious attendance initially seemed to predict fewer subsequent alcohol problems. But when peer, family, and school influences were statistically controlled for, the relationship disappeared. A Finnish study of adolescents (Winter, Karvonen, & Rose, 2002) showed a negative correlation between religiousness and alcohol use only for a rural sample; there was no relationship for an urban sample. There are also suggestions that gender is important, with stronger relationships for women than for men (e.g., Templin & Martin, 1999). Race may also be a factor, with the relationship being stronger for white than for black adolescents in the United States (Amey, Albrecht, & Miller, 1996), and with different aspects of religiosity being better predictors for blacks than for whites. For example, a study of adolescents (mostly 14- and 15-year-olds) in Ohio and Kentucky found that church attendance was a better negative predictor of alcohol use among blacks, but that fundamentalism was the best negative predictor for whites (T. L. Brown, Parks, Zimmerman, & Phillips, 2001). Unfortunately, it is not clear what such differences mean, or whether they are generalizable beyond the samples in these studies. A recent study by Corwyn and Benda (2000) is highlighted in Research Box 13.2, to give the reader a better

---

Research Box 13.2. Religiosity and Church Attendance: The Effects on Use of "Hard Drugs" after Sociodemographic and Theoretical Factors Were Controlled For (Corwyn & Benda, 2000)

This questionnaire study involved 532 students in grades 9 to 12 from three inner-city public high schools in a metropolitan area on the U.S. East Coast. The authors pointed out that "church attendance" has been a favorite measure of religion in studies of religion and substance use, but because this measure is confounded by other variables, they suspected that personal religiosity might be a more appropriate measure. The authors also wondered about the extent to which the relationship between religion and substance abuse might be mediated by other variables. That is, there has been some question about whether religion is related to substance abuse simply because of its relation to other relevant variables, or whether religion makes some unique contribution to the relationship that cannot be "explained" by resorting to those other variables. Also, relatively few studies have investigated the use of "hard drugs" (e.g., cocaine, heroin) in relation to religiosity.

The results of this study led the authors to conclude that "church attendance, like attendance in a college classroom, is at best a vicarious indicator of commitment and a poor measure of performance" (p. 253). Indeed, church attendance did not show a negative association with hard drug use, but personal religiosity (e.g., private prayer, Bible study) did show the expected negative association. Indeed, the results indicated that personal religiosity was negatively correlated with self-reported hard drug use even after other strong predictors found in the literature were statistically controlled for.

This investigation is of course limited by the nature of the sample (inner-city high school students) and the measures (relatively few single items were used to generate measures of attendance and personal religiosity), as well as the use of self-reports for all dependent variable information. However, this investigation did consider a variety of other potentially influential variables, without assuming that initial correlations themselves justified the conclusion that religion is negatively related to hard drug use.

appreciation for the complexities of "controlling for other variables" and ways in which the relationship can be further specified.

It should be noted that substance use is apparently very common among young people. A survey of more than 12,000 U.S. university students in 1993–1994 revealed that 72% consumed alcohol at least once a year, and that about 20% were heavy drinkers (consuming at least five drinks per occasion at least once per week) (Engs, Diebold, & Hanson, 1996). Other estimates suggest that up to 90% of college students ingest alcohol at least once per year (Prendergast, 1994). Use of drugs such as Ecstasy is apparently much less common on university campuses, although its use is increasing dramatically. Between 1997 and 1999, Ecstasy use by college students increased by 69% (from 2.8% to 4.7%; Strote, Lee, & Wechsler, 2002). One in four U.S. college students reports having used marijuana within the past year (Bell, Wechsler, & Johnston, 1997).

New Religions. The negative association between religion and substance use/abuse is not limited to traditional religious groups, as discussed in Chapter 12. Although there is evidence that individuals who become members of "cults" often have a history of greater drug and alcohol utilization before joining (Rochford, Purvis, & NeMar, 1989), research suggests that their subsequent use of these substances often declines, sometimes dramatically (Galanter & Buckley, 1978; Richardson, 1995). In fact, these sorts of findings led Latkin (1995) to suggest that "The study of new religions may provide insights into methods of improving drug treatment programs" (p. 179). On the other hand, new or alternative religions sometimes also encourage substance use. For example, some "cults" from the 1960s and 1970s openly advocated LSD use (Gorsuch, 1995).

Why Does This Relationship Exist? It is one thing to find an association between variables, and quite another to explain *why* that relationship exists. There are probably many factors involved in the inverse correlation between religion and substance use/abuse, and various theories have been proposed to explain the association (see Cochran, 1992; Gorsuch, 1995). Benson's (1992b) review of the related empirical literature led him to infer:

> Nearly all of these efforts appeal to the social control function of religion, in which religious institutions and traditions maintain the social order by discouraging deviance, delinquency, and self-destructive behavior. Religion, then, prevents use through a system of norms and values that favor personal restraint. (p. 216)

The impact of reference and social support groups has also been isolated as one means by which religion can influence substance use (see, e.g., Cochran, Beeghley, & Bock, 1992; Mason & Windle, 2001). In addition, it has been argued that religion has its strongest influence when there is no general social consensus on the acceptability of alcohol and drugs. That is, religious norms may be particularly powerful referents when there is "social dissensus" concerning substance use, since people will then be most likely to look to their religion for guidance (see, e.g., Hadaway, Elifson, & Petersen, 1984).

Gorsuch (1995) has pointed out that at least two other mechanisms may be operating here. First, socialization processes may also decrease substance use through the internalization of (religious) antiabuse norms. Second, religion may serve as an alternative (i.e., to drugs or alcohol) means of meeting basic needs, such as the need to relieve mental anguish and suffering.

Benson (1992b) has argued that in addition to social control mechanisms, religion decreases alcohol and drug use/abuse indirectly by "promoting environmental and psychological assets that constrain risk-taking" (p. 218). He is referring here to religion's attempts to encourage positive behaviors through promoting family harmony and parental support, as well as through sponsoring prosocial values and social competence. Others have similarly concluded that religious young people are generally less likely to engage in health-compromising behaviors and more likely to engage in health-enhancing behaviors (Wallace & Forman, 1998). Research is needed to assess the extent to which such indirect mechanisms are effective deterrents to drug and alcohol use/abuse.

There are interesting variations in the relationship between religion and substance use/abuse across faith groups. Cochran (1993), for example, found that for alcohol consumption, this association was strongest for religious bodies that condemn alcohol; faiths that were silent regarding alcohol revealed little influence of religiosity. Another study (Beeghley, Bock, & Cochran, 1990) showed that when people changed religions, the effects of faith on alcohol consumption were strongest when their new religious group banned the use of alcohol. These findings confirm the importance of religion in the context of reference groups, and also mesh neatly with the important distinction between religiously proscribed and non-proscribed behavior—as conceptualized by Batson, Schoenrade, and Ventis (1993), and described in more detail in our discussion of religion and prejudice in Chapter 14.

The Role of Religion in Prevention and Treatment of Substance Abuse

Some of religion's role in inhibiting substance abuse may derive from its role in preventing abuse before it begins. For example, Stewart (2001) found that religious beliefs seemed to act as a buffer for university students, deterring them from making an initial decision to use alcohol or drugs. In this sense, religion may play a role in prevention.

Beyond the prevention effect, the many studies that show religion and substance use/abuse to be negatively related might suggest that religion could be incorporated into treatment programs to combat substance abuse. Of course, the studies illustrating this association are correlational in nature, and we cannot assume a cause-and-effect relationship. However, research has shown that individuals recovering from alcoholism and drug addiction who report higher levels of religiosity also show positive mental health characteristics, such as increased coping and optimism, greater perceived social support, and so on (Pardini, Plante, Sherman, & Stump, 2000); moreover, they are abstinent from illicit drugs significantly longer during the first 6 months of a treatment program (Avants, Warburton, & Margolin, 2001). And individuals successfully recovering from addiction have been shown to have higher levels of religious faith and spirituality, compared those who relapse (Jarusiewicz, 2000).

It is likely that some prevention, treatment, and support programs could benefit from the aspects of religion that combat substance abuse, though research is needed to clarify what those specific elements are. For example, church attendance has been found to be associated with decreased alcohol and cocaine use among participants in a substance abuse treatment program (Richard, Bell, & Carson, 2000). But we do not yet understand precisely why this and similar associations exist. Gorsuch (1995) has suggested that religion may be especially effective for religious people who want their beliefs to be considered in treatment for substance abuse, if it is within a nurturing, supportive faith context. As Benson (1992b) laments, the potential of religion has not been recognized in the general prevention and treatment literature on alcohol and drug abuse.

This is not to say that prevention and treatment approaches do not include religious elements. Some programs sponsored by churches rely heavily on a religious perspective. Alcoholics Anonymous (AA) is an organization that has had some success in treating alcoholism over the years (Oakes, Allen, & Ciarrochi, 2000), although some authors would argue that AA's success, especially as portrayed in the mass media, is overrated (see, e.g., Bufe, 1991). AA is essentially a secular organization, but it has incorporated aspects of religious experience and practices into its treatment program, especially a reliance on a higher power (God) as the source of rehabilitation (Morreim, 1991). However, the specific contribution of religion to such programs, as compared to the contribution of a treatment program's other features, is difficult to assess (Horstman & Tonigan, 2000). Also, apparently clinicians tend not to refer nonreligious clients to AA-type rehabilitation programs, even though religious and nonreligious people alike may benefit from those programs (Winzelberg & Humphreys, 1999). Research is needed that attempts to isolate the extent to which religion actually contributes to the success of prevention and treatment programs, and to show how it might better be incorporated into such attempts to improve people's lives.

Caveats

One drawback of the many studies on religion and substance use/abuse is that they typically rely on self-reports. If, as Batson et al. (1993) have suggested, religious persons (especially those who are intrinsically oriented) have an inclination toward socially desirable responses, it is possible that they are reporting a kind of ideal image of themselves, rather than an accurate assessment of actual substance use and abuse. Apparently few investigators have considered this possibility.

In addition, most of the studies in this area have examined religiousness in a very general sense, relying on such measures as church attendance and affiliation. These measures are probably overly simplistic, and studies are needed that involve more sophisticated scales of personal religiosity and religious orientation. There is evidence that in some specific contexts, the usual negative relationship between religion and substance use/abuse may disappear, or may even be reversed. For example, after conducting an extensive survey of more than 18,000 children and parents, Forliti and Benson (1986) concluded that a "restrictive" religious orientation was in fact associated with *increased* alcohol use. Makela (1975) claimed that the liberalization of alcohol policies (both religious and other) would result in increases in *moderate* alcohol consumption, but would decrease *heavy* drinking. And some studies of adolescents have revealed the usual negative relationship with substance use, but have also found a *positive* relationship between some aspects of religion (e.g., proscriptiveness) and binge or problem drinking (e.g., Kutter & McDermott, 1997), or between early (teen) religiosity and increased adult alcohol use (Galaif & Newcomb, 1999).

The results of relevant studies are correlational, leading to some difficulties in interpretation. The most obvious cause-and-effect interpretation seems to be that greater religiosity somehow protects individuals from substance use and abuse. However, it is conceivable that substance use decreases religiosity. For example, adolescents who experiment with alcohol or drugs may find less room for religion in their lives, and the "hassles" of religious proscriptions for substance use may make religious teachings seem less relevant to their lives and therefore less important. At the least, there may be a reciprocal causal relationship between religiosity and substance use (e.g., Benda, 1997; Benda & Corwyn, 2000; Corwyn, Benda, & Ballard, 1997).

In spite of repeated findings of low negative correlations between religion and substance use/abuse, there are exceptions. Some "failures" to find the expected association may reflect unique cultural or religious situations. For example, studies carried out in Iran (Spencer & Agahi, 1982), in Colombia (Marin, 1976), and among Chinese students in Singapore (Isralowitz & Ong, 1990) have shown no link between religion and alcohol or drug use. Other "failures" may simply be related to the generally weak nature of the relationships; slightly weaker correlations in some samples, or small sample sizes, might also result in "no relation-ship" results. In addition, as noted above, there have been reports of a positive relationship between religion and *problem* drinking (e.g., Alem, Kebede, & Kullgren, 1999).

Finally, we must remember that the "substances" considered in this section sometimes play a part in religious ceremonies or rituals for specific faith groups, and that within this context their use may actually be increased by religious involvement. For example, religious ceremonial use was one justification for drinking alcohol in Nigerian (Oshodin, 1983) and in Mexican and Honduran (Natera et al., 1983) samples. In the 1960s some new religious groups encouraged the use of LSD, and Clark (1969) and Siegel (1977) have argued that psy-chedelic drugs may contribute to religious experiences and behaviors. In a different vein, Westermeyer and Walzer (1975) have even suggested that drug use among young people may occur in part because it generates personal and social benefits that would formerly have de-rived from religious practice. It has also been noted that traditional religious-based festivals may serve as a vehicle for binge drinking, as well as violence against women (Perez, 2000).

Summary of the Research on Religion and Substance Use/Abuse

The vast majority of studies in this area reveal a negative link between religion and substance use and abuse. The relationship is typically rather weak; there are also confounds to consider, as well as occasional failures to replicate the effect. But, all in all, it is impressive how gen-eral and consistent the association is across diverse samples and studies. In light of this, it is somewhat surprising that the overall literature on substance use/abuse makes only token acknowledgment of religion as an important explanatory variable, and then only as one of many possible cultural influences (see, e.g., Gorsuch, 1995; Petraitis, Flay, & Miller, 1995).

Sexual Behavior

Religious institutions have attempted to control sexual behavior over the years, and one might agree with Shea (1992) that these attempts have historically resulted in a great amount of human distress and misery:

> If we consider those people prosecuted and punished for sexual sins or crimes in Christian com-munities, we might conservatively estimate the number of castrations, whippings, incarcerations, burnings, beheadings, hangings, and other executions attributable directly to Christian teach-ing to be in the millions. (p. 70)

Shea points out that such treatment has to some extent continued to the present time, but suggests that religion's active attempts to control personal sexuality go far beyond such blatant physical punishments. Religion has engendered shame, guilt, fear, and anxiety for a wide variety of sexual "sins" (e.g., see Patton, 1988). The psychological effects of religiously based conflict over sexuality are considered in Chapter 16. Here, however, we evaluate the evidence that religion does indeed influence the perceived morality of human sexuality, as well as sexual behavior itself.

Traditionally, religion has acknowledged the proper role of sexuality as being for procreative purposes within the marital relationship (see Chapter 7). Consequently, virtually any sort of sexual expression outside of heterosexual marriage has been considered inappropriate and sinful. These norms have been both strong and stable across the centuries, but recent changes in these standards have occurred, particularly in Europe and North America. The population at large and some religious groups are currently showing an increased tolerance of masturbation, premarital sex, and even some extramarital sexual behavior. As Cochran and Beeghley (1991) have pointed out,

> some churches have addressed the problem by adjusting and softening their stand, while others have steadfastly avoided such secularization. As a result, there are significant differences in the official stands taken toward nonmarital, particularly premarital sex, among mainstream religious bodies in America. (p. 46)

Apparently, it is conservative Protestant churches that have most resisted a softening of attitudes towards nonmarital sex. Petersen and Donnenwerth (1997) examined more than 14,000 cases from longitudinal data obtained from 1972 to 1993. Their results showed that, across the years, mainline Protestants and Catholics revealed less support for traditional beliefs in sex before marriage; however, conservative Protestants showed no such decline.

Religion and Nonmarital Sex

In spite of these denominational differences, research has generally found that stronger religious beliefs and involvement are associated with self-reported decreased nonmarital sexual activity, especially premarital sex, in a broad sense. A considerable research literature supports this conclusion. For example, a longitudinal New Zealand investigation revealed that for both men and women, being involved in religious activities (as measured at both age 11 and age 21) predicted abstinence from sexual intercourse until at least age 21 (Paul, Fitzjohn, Eberhart-Phillips, Herbison, & Dickson, 2000). Apparently, "religion was an important factor in decisions to delay sexual intercourse past age 20, especially for men" (p. 1). Other studies have also shown that various measures of religiosity are related to decreased premarital sexual activity (e.g., Grey & Swain, 1996; Holder et al., 2000; Lammers, Ireland, Resnick, & Blum, 2000; Woody, Russel, D'Souza, & Woody, 2000; Zaleski & Schiaffino, 2000).

The reader will recognize that cause and effect are not entirely clear in such correlational relationships. It is tempting to infer that religiousness is influencing sexual beliefs and practices. However, it is also possible that sexual beliefs and practices are affecting religious commitment. Most probably, young people are making their own decisions about both religion and sexuality at approximately the same time. But decisions to have more permissive attitudes concerning sexuality could influence people to be less frequent church attenders, possibly because religious participation is less satisfying to them (Thornton & Camburn, 1989). Of course, the bulk of the literature assumes that the causal direction is from religion to sexuality; given religious teachings about sexual morality, this is a reasonable position.

Recent work has typically found this negative association between religiousness and nonmarital sexuality, but has also tried to further specify and explain the relationship. For example, Cochran and Beeghley (1991) examined cumulative data from the National Opinion Research Center's General Social Survey series conducted in the United States between 1972 and 1989, involving almost 15,000 people. They did find an overall tendency for religious persons to disapprove more strongly of premarital sexuality, extramarital sexuality, and homosexuality than the less religious respondents did. However, there were notable variations across different religious groups (see Table 13.1), apparently indicative of the official doctrines of U.S. churches. The more strongly one's (religious) reference group condemns and prohibits various sexual acts, the more likely one is to agree. "That is, as religious proscriptiveness increases, the effect of religiosity on nonmarital sexual permissiveness increases" (Cochran & Beeghley, 1991, p. 46).

In a somewhat different vein, recent research involving 112 clergy found that clergy attitudes toward rape tended to vary, such that more fundamentalist (and sexist) clergy had more negative attitudes toward rape victims (Sheldon & Parent, 2002). More unsettlingly, these authors concluded that "most clergy blame the victim and adhere to rape myths" (p. 233).

Qualifications. The vast majority of research in this area focuses on *pre*marital sexual activity among adolescents and young adults. More investigations are needed on older populations, as is research focusing on other aspects of nonmarital sexual behavior (such as extramarital sex and noncoital activity).

It is surprising that there has not been more interest in the relationship of specific religious *orientations* to nonmarital sexual attitudes and behavior. Haerich (1992) investigated the role of intrinsic and extrinsic religiousness in the sexual attitudes of about 200 undergraduate psychology students. Consistent with other research, Haerich found that lower church attendance and religiousness were (by self-report) weakly but significantly associated with more permissive attitudes toward nonmarital sexuality, as measured by a sexual permissiveness scale. Furthermore, permissive attitudes were inversely linked to Intrinsic scale scores and positively associated with Extrinsic scale scores, usually in the .20 to .30 range. This is consistent with Woodroof's (1985) finding that extrinsically religious persons were more likely to be nonvirgins and to have had more sexual experience than intrinsically reli-

TABLE 13.1. Attitudes toward Nonmarital Sexuality: Percentages Saying Specific Behaviors Are "Almost Always Wrong" or "Always Wrong" among Different Religious Groups

Religious group	Attitude toward:		
	Premarital sexuality	Extramarital sexuality	Homosexuality
Nonaffiliated	10	66	49
Jewish	18	75	43
Catholic	36	87	77
Episcopalian	25	85	66
Presbyterian	36	89	76
Lutheran	40	90	81
Methodist	43	91	84
Baptist	49	90	89
Other Protestant	55	93	86
Total sample	40	88	79

Note. Adapted from Cochran and Beeghley (1991, pp. 54–55). Copyright 1991 by the Society for the Scientific Study of Religion. Adapted by permission.

gious persons. Haerich interpreted these findings as indicating that greater commitment to religious institutions (Intrinsic scores) is associated with decreasing permissiveness, whereas people with a religious orientation that focuses on personal comfort and security (Extrinsic scores) will, in a similar manner, use sexual intimacy to contribute to their personal comfort and security. However, this interpretation must be considered speculative, pending further research. One study, for example, found that *both* Intrinsic and Extrinsic scores were linked with decreased sexual activity (Zaleski & Schiaffino, 2000).

More religious young people also tend to be less knowledgeable about sexual issues. For example, adolescents reporting no religious affiliation were found to have the fewest misconceptions about condom use (Crosby & Yarber, 2001). We need more research on how such misconceptions and/or lack of knowledge about sexuality may affect premarital sexual activity and, for example, the likelihood of premarital pregnancy. Some authors (Zaleski & Schiaffino, 2000) have speculated that although religion helps to protect adolescents from initiating sexual activity, it does not seem to have a protective effect against practicing unsafe sex, at least among students who are already sexually active. Possibly this failure of religion to protect against unsafe sex is related to lack of knowledge or misconceptions among more religious adolescents.

The many studies that simply look for relationships between general measures of religiousness and sexual attitudes and behaviors neglect potentially important factors. For example, Reynolds (1994) has pointed out that research investigating premarital sexual experience typically assumes that early sexual activity is consensual, when in many cases it is not, especially for females. Cases of nonconsensual sex should not be included in studies of the influence of religion on sexuality, she argues, since this could distort the nature and strength of the overall relationship. Furthermore, gender differences are sometimes found with respect to the relationship between religion and sexuality. For example, research at a large public "Bible belt" university revealed that strength of religious beliefs was significantly negatively linked with engaging in risky sexual behavior for women only (Poulson, Eppler, Satterwhite, Wuensch, & Bass, 1998). Similarly, a Scottish study found that religiosity had greater influence on women's judgments about sexual standards than on men's judgments (Sheeran, Spears, Abraham, & Abrams, 1996). Clearly, gender issues are potentially important in this area.

Finally, Hammond, Cole, and Beck (1993) have noted another complicating factor in the relationship between religion and nonmarital sexuality. Their investigation indicated that at least among white Americans, young people from fundamentalist and sect-like religions are more likely to marry before the age of 20 than are mainline Protestants, even when various other factors are controlled for. They argue that this tendency may result from generally stronger pressures to avoid premarital sexual intercourse. In one sense, this is important because it emphasizes another way in which a person's religious background may influence an aspect of the transition to adulthood—namely, marriage. In another sense, this tendency could also unfairly contribute to the "religion deters premarital sexual activity" finding in many studies, because early marriages among fundamentalist groups will reduce the "opportunity" for premarital sexual interaction between highly religious young people. By definition, one cannot engage in *pre*marital sex *after* marriage.

Summary of the Research on Religion and Nonmarital Sex. There is little dispute about the typically weak but consistent tendency for religion to be negatively related to nonmarital sexual attitudes and behaviors. However, it is also evident that the relationship is not as simple as was once thought, and future research needs to consider various issues: denominational differences in sexual standards and behavior; religious orientation; knowledge and misconceptions about sexuality; and gender.

Clergy Sexual Abuse

The issue of clergy sexual abuse is a problem caught between morality and mental disturbance. We are not simply speaking about socially irresponsible and illegal behavior, but what lies behind it. Much that is counter to the law is properly excused when mental aberration that can be defined by the courts as insanity is present. In most instances, this does not appear to be true here. Therefore, we examine the topic in this chapter, in the context of religion and morality.

Many books and articles on clergy sexual abuse have appeared over the years, but often these have focused on theological or church-related issues, have offered armchair analyses of such abuse, or have been concerned with pastoral care and counseling issues. It is only relatively recently that empirical attempts to analyze and understand clergy abuse have begun to proliferate. In keeping with the theme of this book, we refer primarily to empirical work here, but necessarily sometimes mention other relevant material.

Background Information.   Recently, much more descriptive information on this topic has become available; this helps us to better understand both clergy who perpetrate abuse and their victims. Bottoms, Shaver, Goodman, and Qin (1995) reported the results of an initial survey of almost 7,000 professionals, and a detailed follow-up of 797 of these people who had encountered ritualistic or religion-related abuse. The responses of these professionals indicated that children almost always knew and trusted the abuse perpetrators. When only abuse perpetrated by a religious authority was considered, 94% of these cases were sexual in nature. And even though Catholics constitute about one-quarter of the U.S. population, in the reported cases of child sexual abuse involving religious authorities, about 54% of both victims and perpetrators were Catholic. Apparently, sexual abuse by Catholic priests and brothers occurs much more frequently than one would expect, given the number of Catholics in the United States. Finally, Bottoms et al.'s (1995) data did not support the common view that boys are more likely than girls to be targets of clergy sexual abuse. In fact, the data showed that whether or not the perpetrator was Catholic, boys and girls were about equally likely to be victims.

In light of the recent intense media coverage of the sexual abuse of children by priests, one might suspect that there is an abusing priest lurking in every parish. However, Sipe (1990, 1995) has estimated that just 2% of priests are pedophiles, and possibly 4% would be classified as "ephebophiles" (those who reveal sexual attraction and behavior toward adolescents). Also, as these figures suggest, postpubescent adolescents are more likely to be abused than are prepubescent children (see Plante, 1999). Of course, even these small percentages translate into substantial numbers of abusing priests in the United States (3,600). And if each perpetrator were to have 10 victims (probably a conservative estimate), this would suggest 36,000 young people who are victims of clergy abuse (de Fuentes, 1999). Other researchers have estimated 100,000 or more young victims of Catholic clergy abuse alone (Greeley, 1993).

Research on Clergy Abuse.   Clergy sexual abuse, especially in the Catholic Church, has been a problem for centuries (Isley, 1997). In the research literature, the potential for clergy sexual abuse may initially have been implied in a study done over 40 years ago. In that study, which used the very widely employed psychological test the Minnesota Multiphasic Personality Inventory, note was made of elevated clerical Psychopathic Deviate scores (Aloyse, 1961). This language gave way to the term "character disorder," which, as Stewart (1974) observed, appears to be increasing in the clergy as various neurotic expressions decrease. Persons so affected are not regarded as mentally disturbed, in that they know right from wrong and possess adequate control over their impulses. They may, however, be described as egocentric, immature, and narcissistic individuals, who want gratification of their desires as rapidly as possible without concern for the needs and feelings of others. The rates of such individuals in prisons tend to be high (MacDonald, 1958; White & Watt, 1981). It may therefore be argued that this condition, though it is indeed deviant, is not usually considered a form of mental disorder. Unfortunately, more time and energy has been spent in documenting the prevalence of clergy sexual abuse than in conducting research to help us understand those who have engaged in abusive behavior.

The situation is too complicated to be explained by simple reference to a pattern of personality traits. For example, it has been pointed out that the clerical profession exposes clergy to sexual temptation—women or men who "fall in love" with their pastors, or parishioners who bare their most intimate problems to ministers, rabbis, or priests. Such actions make both the clergy and those who seek their help vulnerable to exploitation. Given such encounters, it may not come as a surprise that one study of 1,500 Catholic priests over a 25-year period indicated that about half had violated their celibacy vows (Schaffer, 1990). Other work reports that between 42% and 77% of women clergy claim that they have been sexually harassed or abused (see Culver, 1994; Fortune & Poling, 1994; Simpkinson, 1996). Though some estimates suggest that up to one-third of U.S. ministers admit to having engaged in sexual misconduct (Fortune & Poling, 1994), most work indicates that about 25% of pastors have had some kind of sexual involvement with a parishioner (Culver, 1994; Lebacqz & Barton, 1991). Actual intercourse rates between 10% and 15% have been reported (Culver, 1994). In the 1983–1993 decade, one concerned organization documented over 1,150 such incidents (Fortune & Poling, 1994).

Despite these numbers, efforts at psychologically characterizing clergy who perpetrate abuse have met with limited success, in part because of the variety of such abuse. These episodes can involve heterosexual or homosexual behavior and the mistreatment of children or adults. Among other possibilities, one scheme identifies what might be termed "passive and neurotic" perpetrators and angry/impulsive perpetrators (Camargo & Loftus, 1993). Another framework distinguishes six different types (Hands, 1992). Yet another attempt was based on the statistical technique of cluster analysis, and focused on Roman Catholic priests and brothers who had been identified as child sexual offenders (Falkenheim, Duckro, Hughes, Rosetti, & Gfeller, 1999). This investigation identified four clusters of abusers, which were labeled as follows by the authors: Sexually and Emotionally Underdeveloped; Significantly Psychiatrically Disturbed; Undefended Characterological; and Defended Characterological. Unfortunately, we still do not know how to recognize any of these clerics before they do damage.

The application of psychological and psychiatric labels to clergy sexual abuse has not proven particularly useful, for although such behavior is unacceptable, individual cases often involve many unique, sometimes tragic circumstances that would also influence average people. Furthermore, especially in cases involving abuse of children, many years may pass before complaints are lodged or legal action is taken. In such cases, issues of memory accuracy and the legitimacy of so-called "repressed memory" become important (see, e.g., Loftus & Guyer, 2002; Qin, Goodman, Bottoms, & Shaver, 1998).

In any profession, perfection is an unrealizable ideal. However, people frequently look to the clergy as ideal role models, forgetting that they are subject to the same stresses, problems, motives, and shortcomings as are parishioners and congregants themselves. Clergy, especially when celibacy is expected as part of their role, may experience considerable conflict over personal sexuality (Fones, Levine, Althof, & Risen, 1999). Possibly better procedures are needed to select those who enter the religious professions; however, screening processes will undoubtedly contain a fair amount of error for some time to come. Psychological and character disorders will therefore persist in religious institutions. Little, however, can be done about such difficulties until they become evident, and the tragedy is that when they do come to light, there will be victims—clerics and laypersons alike.

What about the Victims? Celibacy pressures may also stimulate sexual exploitation of nuns by priests and other nuns, indicating both heterosexual and homosexual abuse (Chibnall, Wolf, & Duckro, 1998). In this work, the overall incidence of such harassment and exploitation of nuns was reportedly 12.5%. The results of these traumatic experiences were often extreme, necessitating psychotherapy, and many negative effects persisted throughout the victims' lives. Higher rates of abuse have been reported by Protestant and Jewish female clergy: 77% of Methodist clergywomen and 75% of female rabbis indicate sexual abuse by male clergy (Chibnall et al., 1998). The problem is so severe that a number of organizations have been created to aid the victims of sexual coercion by clergy (Chibnall et al., 1998). Apparently, too, important gender differences exist in the perception of sexual harassment. A study of United Methodist clergy (Frame, 1996) revealed that females were more likely than males to perceive interaction between a senior pastor and an associate as sexual harassment, in each of several different scenarios.

In a discussion of clergy abuse such as this, it is easy to lose sight of the victims, given our desire to understand the perpetrators. Studies of course indicate that the victims of such abuse reveal serious emotional and psychological consequences (e.g., Disch & Avery, 2001; Goodman, Bottoms, Redlich, Shaver, & Diviak, 1998). Furthermore, reduced trust in the priesthood and church, as well as in relationship to God, was found among Catholics who were sexually abused as children by priests (Rossetti, 1995; see also Hall, 1995). Finally, the consequences of abuse extend far beyond the victims themselves. Family, relatives, friends, and others may all suffer adverse effects when someone is abused.

Summary of the Research on Clergy Sexual Abuse. The term "clergy sexual abuse" covers considerable territory, with victims involving children, adolescents, adults, and other clergy. Abuse can range from harassment and psychological threats or innuendo, through inappropriate physical contact, to sexual intercourse. As we have seen, research often focuses on describing perpetrators and victims, or attempts to dissect the psychological type or makeup of perpetrators. We have learned much from these investigations. Unfortunately, we are still a long way from a clear understanding of abusers and the effects on victims, and especially in being able to predict (and thereby prevent) clergy abuse before it happens.

Criminal Behavior and Delinquency

Statistics concerning rising crime rates are commonly reported by the media; this was especially true during the 1960s and 1970s (Putnam, 2000). There have even been projections that crime and delinquency will continue to increase, perhaps to "epidemic" proportions (Walinsky,

1995). As is the case for alcohol and drug use/abuse, and to some extent nonmarital sexuality, churches and synagogues typically take strong stands against criminal and delinquent behavior. One might hope that religion could act as a powerful deterrent to such acts.

First, we should consider a few points of clarification. The phrase "criminal and delinquent behavior" covers considerable territory, some of which is discussed elsewhere in this chapter. (For example, it covers clergy sexual abuse, as well as serious cases of cheating/dishonesty.) Also, there is sometimes confusion regarding where to draw a line between mental disorder and criminal behavior. Furthermore, crime statistics themselves may be unreliable. Definitions of crimes may vary from one jurisdiction to the next; some governments and police agencies may be more zealous in enforcing laws; and much crime surely goes unreported. Also, the methodological and statistical challenges in teasing out religion–delinquency relationships are considerable. In light of such problems, it is not surprising that studies in this area often generate conflicting findings.

Finally, a comment about terminology is in order. It is not entirely clear how "delinquency" differs from "criminality," though typically the former refers to a younger age group of perpetrators (as in "juvenile delinquency"), who may or may not be tried in adult court. Delinquency is sometimes considered "less serious" than adult criminality, possibly because of its association with juveniles. But there is considerable overlap in the use of these terms in the literature. Here, where appropriate, we use the term used in the original research being discussed. Otherwise, we often simply refer to "crime" or "criminality" in our discussion.

Do Crime Rates Vary with Degree of Religious Involvement?

The Historical Context.   The theoretical underpinnings of the expectation that low religious involvement may be associated with higher crime rates can be traced to the early years of this century—particularly Durkheim's (1915) emphasis on the social roots of religion, and his social integration theory of deviance and religion's place in society. Durkheim felt that religion is integrally tied to the social order, playing an important role in legitimizing and reinforcing society's values and norms. Deviance may then stem from a breakdown in the church's role in this regard. Consistent with what many people would consider "commonsense" reasoning, the Durkheimian tradition links strong religious ties with decreased crime rates. In fact, many of the relevant data available to us come from sociologists who have carefully scrutinized crime statistics and their relationship to church attendance, denominational affiliation, religious commitment, and so on. The majority of this work has focused on adolescent delinquency, with relatively few investigations of adult crime.

Contradictions and Inconsistencies.
"There Is No Relationship." Some early research did indeed show the expected negative religion–crime correlations (see Jensen & Erickson, 1979). However, a widely cited paper with the provocative title "Hellfire and Delinquency," published in the late 1960s by Hirschi and Stark (1969), reported that there was little or no association between religiousness and delinquency among several thousand California adolescents. The authors suggested that earlier findings of a negative relationship had been weak and were probably spurious. Possibly because this finding was unexpected, it stimulated numerous subsequent investigations of this topic. Some of the follow-up research seemed to replicate Hirschi and Stark's original finding (e.g., Burkett & White, 1974). However, other investigators challenged this conclu-

sion, finding that religion was indeed negatively correlated with some kinds of delinquency (see, e.g., Elifson, Petersen, & Hadaway, 1983; Peek, Curry, & Chalfant, 1985).

"Yes, There Is." In a notable study, Jensen and Erickson (1979) reanalyzed Hirschi and Stark's data, and concluded that the original authors had reached erroneous conclusions because of their methodology. There was actually a negative relationship between religion and delinquency, they claimed, which had remained hidden because of the statistical analyses carried out by Hirschi and Stark. Their own findings, based on several thousand Arizona high school students, confirmed the general inverse religion–delinquency relationship, though specific comparisons were often weak and did not always achieve statistical significance. Furthermore, Jensen and Erickson noted that the importance of religious variables in "explaining" crime statistics was greater for Mormons than it was for Catholics and Protestants. This tendency for correlations to be stronger, relatively speaking, within samples of Mormon adolescents has been replicated by Chadwick and Top (1993). That is, denominational variations may affect the results obtained.

"No, There Isn't." To complicate things even more, Cochran, Wood, and Arneklev (1994) studied more than 1,500 Oklahoma high school students. They observed, much as Hirschi and Stark (1969) had done 25 years earlier, that for most categories of delinquency the effect of religiosity was reduced to nonsignificant levels when nonreligious control variables were also considered. This led Cochran et al. to assume that in most cases, the religion–delinquency relationship is spurious.

Resolutions and More Contradictions. Based on a review of the relevant research, Bainbridge (1992a) concluded that there has been some tendency for studies carried out in areas where organized religion is weak to show no relationship. But work conducted in areas where organized religion is relatively strong usually generates the negative religion–delinquency findings. Thus, consistent with previous inferences by Stark (1984), Bainbridge suggested that the religious community context is critical in explaining the contradictory findings in this area. Religion is more likely to act as a deterrent to delinquency if religious social support exists (e.g., if one's friends are also religious).

More recently, Stark (1996) provided further evidence that social context is important. That is, stronger (negative) religion–delinquency relationships are typically found within more religious samples. Stark felt that studies generating findings inconsistent with this argument had erred in the way they defined social context. He backed up his arguments with data from an extensive survey of high school seniors. These data showed a weak religion–delinquency correlation in the relatively weak religious context of the U.S. West, but a stronger association in the more religious East. Admittedly, this is a very general, oversimplified way to define (religious) social context, but the data are supportive and fit with some other findings (e.g., stronger correlations within highly religious Mormon samples, as discussed above). Still, other researchers have not found support for the social context distinction (e.g., Junger & Polder, 1993).

In an extensive investigation, Bainbridge (1989) examined data from 75 U.S. metropolitan areas. After taking into account some possible intervening variables (e.g., social mobility, poverty), he claimed that larceny, burglary, and assault were apparently deterred by religion, but that murder, rape, and possibly robbery were not. Pettersson (1991) investigated the relationship between religion and a variety of criminal behaviors by analyzing data from almost 1,000 Swedes. He noted that relationships varied, depending on the type of crime at issue, but the pattern differed somewhat from that found by Bainbridge in the United States. A negative association was found between church involvement and crimes associated with violence, violations of public order and safety, and alcohol abuse; however, there was no substantial relationship for property, narcotic, or moral offenses.

Such inconsistencies across studies are common. Studies on the relationships between religion and crime/delinquency continue to appear regularly, especially in the sociological literature, and one is struck by the extent to which the specific types of crime found to be related to religion in one study are found to be nonsignificant in another investigation. Or the measure of religion that is related to delinquency in one study is the very measure that is *not* related to it in the next research report. And so on. In addition, theory-based explanations of religion's link to crime and delinquency continue to be controversial. What are we to make of this research, apparently so full of contradictory findings and lack of clarity?

Making Sense of the Contradictions. A recent review and meta-analysis of 60 investigations published from 1967 to 1998 led to the conclusion that in general, religious beliefs and behaviors were moderately negatively related to individuals' criminal behavior (Baier & Wright, 2001). However, it was noted that results varied, depending on the conceptual and methodological approaches in individual studies. This is an important point; operational definitions of crime and religion vary substantially across studies, as do samples, data collection techniques, statistical analyses, and controls for potentially confounding factors. It is not surprising that studies in this area generate conflicting results, given the tendency for "apples and oranges" to be thrown into the same bowl as if they are identical (see also Benda & Corwyn, 1997a).

Virtually all of the published studies on crime and religion are correlational. Thus they are able to say little about cause and effect. It is generally assumed, however, that negative correlational relationships must mean that religion somehow prevents or reduces crime in individuals—and, in fact, some authors use this kind of causal wording in their articles. But it also makes some sense that causality (if indeed there is any direct causality in the relationship) could be in the opposite direction. That is, as individuals begin to participate in criminal activities and to establish friendships with criminals, they may be less and less inclined to attend church, hold religious beliefs, and so on. Multiple studies with longitudinal data would help to sort out this issue (see, e.g., Benda, 1995). In addition, it is clear that basic correlations between gross measures of religion and delinquency can be quite misleading, since the removal of the effects of other social and cultural variables often reduces these associations considerably or even entirely (see, e.g., Benda & Corwyn, 1997a).

However, as a generalization, studies have tended to find various aspects of religion to be negatively related to different categories of criminality. This has been confirmed in a number of recent investigations (e.g., Benda & Corwyn, 1997b; Johnson, Jang, Larson, & Li, 2001; Johnson, Jang, Li, & Larson, 2000; McKnight & Loper, 2000), although other studies report nonsignificant relationships or correlations that become nonsignificant when other factors are controlled for (e.g., Benda & Corwyn, 1997a; Rodell & Benda, 1999). There has also been reasonable support for the Bainbridge–Stark proposal that social context and religious community are important in explaining some seemingly conflictual findings. That is, relationships between religion and crime are stronger in areas where religious social context is more pronounced.

Also, Bainbridge (1992a) has drawn an important distinction between "hedonistic" or "antiascetic" acts and other forms of deviance. His own research (as well as that of others) suggests that religion is negatively associated with drug and alcohol use, promiscuous sexuality, and similar hedonistic acts, regardless of the religious community context. It is when deviant acts such as theft, assault, and murder are examined that the religious social context apparently becomes important in qualifying the religion–delinquency relationship. Again, there is not complete agreement on this "antiascetic" distinction (especially the operational definition of the term), and specific results do vary across studies (see, e.g., Benda, 1995; Benda & Corwyn, 1997a).

No doubt we will continue to see study after study published in this area. But it will be some time before there is any general agreement among social scientists on precisely which aspects of crime are related to which components of religion, how strong these associations are, the role of confounding factors, just what is causing what, which measures should be used in research, and so on. In the meantime, we must sometimes settle for vague generalizations and sometimes incorrect conclusions, as the increasing volume of research gradually teases out the specifics of the relationship.

Summary of the Research on Religion and Crime Rates. The literature on religion and rates of crime is somewhat contradictory and ambiguous. Although some studies do show a negative relationship, it tends to be weak and inconsistent. As in some other areas, there has been a tendency to use very general measures of religion (e.g., church attendance, denominational affiliation), and to ignore the important but subtle differences that may be based on religious *orientation*, rather than simple attendance or affiliation. When this deficiency is combined with the unreliability of crime statistics and other problems, it becomes almost impossible to reach firm conclusions.

Benson, Donahue, and Erickson's (1989) survey of the literature on adolescence and religion led them to conclude that the weight of the evidence supports the existence of a weak to moderate negative relationship between religion and delinquency. But, along with others (Burkett & Warren, 1987; Cochran et al., 1994; Elifson et al., 1983; Welch, Tittle, & Petee, 1991), they point out that much of this association may be attributable to social environment factors rather than to religion itself. "After accounting for whether they have friends who engage in deviant behaviors, the adolescents' closeness to their parents, and how important it is for them to do what their parents say, religion contributes little independent constraining effect" (Benson et al., 1989, p. 172).

In general, the negative relationship seems most likely to appear for "victimless activities" (e.g., the use/abuse of alcohol and drugs, consensual premarital sexual activity), rather than other delinquent behavior (Chadwick & Top, 1993). It is important to go beyond simple correlational relationships, as indicated in research carried out by Peek et al. (1995). They found evidence that over time, higher delinquency rates appeared among students who declined in religiousness, compared to those who were low in religiousness throughout the same period. Such longitudinal trends may provide the basis for future investigations of adolescent delinquency.

Religion and Domestic Abuse

There has been increasing concern with the issue of domestic violence toward both spouses/partners and children. Some studies have focused on partner or child abuse that is apparently related to religious beliefs. Similar violence related to religion has been documented across cultures and through time, so we are not witnessing a phenomenon indigenous to our own time and social order (Girard, 1977). In the past, like clergy abuse, domestic abuse was often "hushed up"; people seemed to prefer to believe that it did not exist. However, more recently such abuse has generally been considered to be criminal in nature, and more and more cases are appearing before the courts. Therefore, we have included our discussion of religion and domestic abuse here, in the section on criminal behavior.

As we consider the material in this section, it is to be noted that it is not always clear in related research whether or not abuse is domestic. Some studies simply ask respondents whether they were abused, without distinguishing between domestic or other abuse. We sometimes refer to research that does not make this distinction. Also, in our consideration of the research on domestic abuse, it is important to be aware that such abuse is almost always determined via self-reports. Such personal accounts may be biased for many reasons (e.g., reluctance to admit to abuse, having heard overly positive or negative stories about one's childhood from parents or others). Exploratory research has even indicated that the *belief* that one was abused may be more important than *actual* abuse history in predicting some effects of abuse (Webb & Otto Whitmer, 2001).

Religious "Justification" for Abuse. Apparently religion may be seen by some people as "justifying" child or partner abuse, in the sense that it may encourage physical punishment of children or violence against one's partner (Capps, 1992, 1995; de Jonge, 1995; Greven, 1991; Kroeger & Beck, 1996; Volcano Press, 1995). These authors point to numerous Biblical passages, as well as books and articles written by Christian authors, that may be interpreted as encouraging the use of physical force, especially in disciplining children. It is argued that this could serve as a justification for various forms of abuse (e.g., "It is for the child's own good," "The man is the head of the household"). Furthermore, Bottoms et al. (1995) suggested that religious beliefs can threaten the welfare of children in various ways, including the withholding of medical care and attempts to rid children of evil, as well as direct physical and psychological abuse that adults see as religiously justified. At the same time, religious institutions have usually taken strong positions against domestic abuse (Volcano Press, 1995).

Research on Religion and Domestic Abuse. Research in this area has generated unclear results because of influencing factors such as education, denial that abuse has taken place, reluctance to admit to having endured or perpetrated abuse, and differing definitions of abuse. For example, we might be tempted to conceive of domestic violence as only physical or sexual. But the Volcano Press (1995), for instance, has listed 98 forms of domestic abuse, including 29 that are considered physical, 16 sexual, 17 financial, 16 verbal, and 20 emotional. The research that has been carried out on this topic, however, has generally been confined to more straightforward operational definitions of domestic abuse.

One summary of this literature indicated that those who attended church frequently were half as likely as infrequent attenders to experience physical violence themselves, or to use physical aggression against their partners (Mahoney, Pargament, Tarakeshwar, & Swank, 2001). Similarly, Ellison and Anderson (2001) recently found a negative relationship between church attendance and domestic violence (see also Ellison, Bartkowski, & Anderson, 1999), and Lown and Vega (2001) reported that regular church attendance was associated with decreased physical abuse by a partner for Mexican American women. In a somewhat different vein, Makepeace (1987) found religion to be negatively associated with courtship violence among college students. A Canadian investigation of more than 1,000 adults reported that more frequent church attenders were the least violent (Brinkerhoff, Grandin, & Lupri, 1992). Initially, then, the research evidence seems to show a link between higher religiosity (generally speaking) and reduced domestic abuse.

Is There a Link between Fundamentalist Religion and Domestic Violence? Brinkerhoff et al. (1992) found that their hypothesis that the more fundamentalist, conservative Protestants would be more abusive "because of the stereotypes surrounding their value of patriarchy" (p. 28) received mixed support. Conservative Protestant women (but not men; could this represent a self-serving bias or a reluctance to admit to abuse?) reported the highest rates of violence (37.8%), compared to mainline Protestants (28.1%), Catholics (23.9%), and nonaffiliated respondents (30.8%).

There have been other suggestions that family abuse, generally speaking, has roots in the strong patriarchal family structure espoused by some conservative religions, as mentioned by Brinkerhoff et al. (1992). This patriarchal system is sometimes interpreted as justifying the subordination of women, particularly in terms of their subjection to powerful male authority (Clarke, 1986; Pagelow & Johnson, 1988), though some women may turn to religion as a source of personal empowerment in other ways (Ozorak, 1996). The problem may be confounded by some clergy, who counsel women to remain with abusive husbands because it is their religious duty and responsibility to stay with and obey their spouses (Alsdurf & Alsdurf, 1988). Indeed, women from such patriarchal environments whose intimate partners have sexually abused their children may experience intense value conflict over the need to preserve the family, and their loyalty to both their abusive partners and their victimized children (Alaggia, 2001). This patriarchal issue may cross cultural boundaries. Higher levels of religiosity among Arab women in Israel were associated with the attitude that abused women should assume more personal responsibility for their husbands' violent behavior (Haj-Yahia, 2002).

There have been other indications that more conservative Christians, especially men, may be more prone to using domestic violence. Neufeld (1979) and Steele and Pollock (1968) have suggested that fundamentalist religious parents may be especially prone to punish their children physically, and also possibly to abuse them. Hull and Burke (1991) have proposed that members of the "religious right" may be more likely to tolerate family abuse in general. The study by Brinkerhoff et al. (1992) supports this conjecture, as does the literature review by Mahoney et al. (2001). It is possible that this latter finding was a function of religious differences in conservatism between the husband and wife: If the wife was liberal and the husband conservative, there was a higher incidence of domestic violence than when the spouses had similar religious views (Ellison et al., 1989; Mahoney et al., 2001). However, some studies fail to find any such differences. For example, an investigation of 1,440 married couples in the United States did not reveal any differences in intimate partner violence across denominational groups, nor did such violence vary when partners had the same or different denominational affiliations (Cunradi, Caetano, & Schafer, 2002). Indeed, specifically male-to-female partner violence was highest in liberal religions and lowest in fundamentalist groups. Of course, measures and ways of grouping religions differed across the studies discussed above, and one must be careful not to assume that the same factors govern child violence and partner abuse.

An investigation involving self-reports of first-year university students suggests that type of religion is related to whether child sexual abuse was initiated by a relative or nonrelative.

Students who reported being sexually abused by a relative were more likely to be affiliated with a fundamentalist Protestant religion. But students who reported being sexually abused by a nonrelative were more likely to be nonreligious or to be affiliated with a liberal religious denomination (Stout-Miller, Miller, & Langbrunner, 1997). Thus religion may be related in rather complex ways to sexual abuse of children and the perpetrators of the abuse.

Consequences for the Victims of Abuse. Studies have shown that child sexual abuse has both religious and nonreligious consequences for those who are abused. Doxey, Jensen, and Jensen (1997) investigated more than 5,000 women, including more than 600 who reported being sexually abused when they were growing up. Those reporting abuse also reported higher rates of emotional and psychological problems (e.g., depression, lower self-esteem), as well as lower levels of religiousness. Pritt (1998) looked at the effects of sexual abuse on Mormon women and noted that it was spiritually disruptive. Among other things, such abuse created alienation from self and God, resulting in a sense of powerlessness and meaninglessness in a woman's life. The effects of domestic violence on children and women, especially when religiously justified, are profound and long-lasting (Volcano Press, 1995). A study of 1,207 male veterans reported that those who had a history of sexual abuse did report greater spiritual injury, but abuse was not related to an overall measure of current religious behavior (Lawson, Drebing, Berg, Vincellette, & Penk, 1998).

However, there are also indications that religion can help people to deal with the effects of domestic abuse possibly through a mechanism such as social support (Coker et al., 2002). Elliott (1994) investigated child sexual abuse among almost 3,000 professional women. She could find no evidence that its prevalence was related to family religious affiliation, but there was a tendency for adult religious practices to mediate the severity of symptoms for those victimized as children. Similarly, Reinert and Smith (1997) found that their sample of women who had been sexually abused as children often looked to faith for support. Another investigation compared about 1,000 female teenagers who had been sexually abused to a sample of 1,000 female teenagers who had not been abused (Chandy, Blum, & Resnick, 1996). Results indicated that greater religiosity seemed to act as a protective factor against a variety of adverse outcomes. And Giesbrecht and Sevcik (2000) found that abused women from a conservative evangelical background could allow their faith either to engender shame and guilt or to provide a vehicle for hope and change. Studies such as this underline the potential of religion to help some adult survivors to cope with their earlier abuse.

Perceptions of Abuse. One's religious orientation is apparently linked to how one views partner abuse in others. Burris and Jackson (1999) experimentally varied scenarios depicting a woman who was abused by her boyfriend. They found that their undergraduate students' ratings of the abused woman and her abuser changed, depending on whether the woman was depicted as upholding or as violating religious values (see Research Box 13.3).

Summary of the Research on Religion and Domestic Abuse. This is another area where it is difficult to come to firm conclusions, based on the relevant research. It is challenging to carry out research on domestic abuse for many reasons, such as potentially biased self-reports from respondents, difficulties in operationalizing concepts, lack of agreement regarding measures to be used, and so on. In spite of these problems, the most common finding has been a negative relationship between measures of religion and domestic violence. There is also some support for the claim that some domestic violence may seem to be justified by

---

ã

Research Box 13.3. Hate the Sin/Love the Sinner, or Love the Hater?: Intrinsic Religion and Responses to Partner Abuse (Burris & Jackson, 1999)

The authors of this study began by noting inconsistencies in the little research that exists on the relationship between religion and partner abuse. Past research, they pointed out, was limited by a possible social desirability bias (intrinsically religious people may be more prone to this bias and attempt to present themselves in a more positive light), crude measures of religiosity, and a failure to take contextual influences into account. They attempted to deal with all of these problems in their investigation of how an intrinsic religious orientation would be associated with reactions to the perpetrator and the victim of abuse, under different conditions.

Ninety undergraduate volunteers responded to the Allport–Ross Intrinsic and Extrinsic religious orientation scales, and were then randomly assigned to one of three conditions in which they read a vignette about a woman who was abused by her partner. The vignettes were mostly the same for all conditions, describing a situation where, after dating for 9 months, Rob asked Cheryl to marry him. She asked for a week to think about his proposal, after which they had dinner together at a restaurant. The vignettes diverged at this point. In one condition ("value-affirming"), Cheryl told Rob that their religious differences were too great; she "would not feel right about marrying outside of my faith" (p. 165), and therefore regretfully said no to his marriage proposal. In a second ("value-neutral") condition, Cheryl admitted that she did not think that she was in love with Rob, and therefore could not accept his proposal. In the final condition ("value-violating"), Cheryl said that the reason she could not marry Rob was that she needed time to resolve issues about her sexual orientation, especially her concern that she might be a lesbian. All vignettes ended with Rob throwing a glass of ice water in Cheryl's face and storming out of the restaurant, leaving Cheryl alone and crying.

Participants indicated their liking for both Cheryl and Rob on a 9-point response format, from "not at all" (1) to "very much" (9). A check indicated that after reading the vignette, all respondents did remember Cheryl's reason for turning down Rob's marriage proposal.

As expected, people with higher Intrinsic scale scores tended to like the victim more when she based her decision to decline the marriage proposal on her religious values. However, when the victim (Cheryl) based her decision on value-violating concerns (that she might be a lesbian), those with higher Intrinsic scores actually liked the abuse perpetrator (Rob) more. These relationships are especially interesting because the perpetrator's behavior was identical in all conditions, the victim suffered precisely the same abuse in all conditions, and these two correlations were not found for any of the other conditions.

The authors reasoned that Cheryl's rationale for saying no to the marriage proposal gave more intrinsically religious persons a sort of contextual justification to express what otherwise would probably have been socially undesirable responses, in actually expressing liking for an abusive person. This rather subtle shift from loving the person who was abused to expressing more positive attitudes toward the abuser is disturbing, since it seems to fly in the face of intrinsically oriented individuals' "claim to endorse positive attitudes toward women and to reject many patriarchal beliefs. . . . The present research suggests that the commitment underlying their profession may be tenuous and undercut by other value commitments (e.g., 'family values'), however" (p. 171). The findings of this study are especially relevant to our discussion of partner abuse, because they might help to explain why victims of abuse do not always receive the expected love and sympathy from their religious group, and why sympathy for the perpetrator can sometimes override concern for the victim among religious persons.

the patriarchal family structure found most often in fundamentalist or conservative religious groups. Also, victims of abuse can potentially suffer serious adverse effects for many years. Often victims become less religious, but there is evidence that religion can serve as a positive resource as well in their coping with abuse. Finally, some perpetrators of abuse may be viewed sympathetically, especially if "value violation" might have contributed to the abuse. In spite of these findings, this area of study is still in its infancy, with many research contradictions and anomalies to be resolved.

Does Religion Sometimes Contribute to Crime?

Although some studies show that religion and crime are negatively (albeit weakly) associated, we must consider the possibility that religion may also *contribute* to criminal behavior, at least in some situations. Some religions might emphasize the importance of standing up for one's rights ("an eye for an eye"), or a particular religious group may stress that members of this group are superior to various others; either of these factors could potentially incline individuals to act aggressively in some situations. In a study of regional differences in crimes against persons in the United States, Ellison (1991a) concluded that there was some evidence that "the public religious culture" of the South plays a role in legitimizing this kind of violence. That is, an emphasis on the "an eye for an eye" approach to the world, instead of "turn the other cheek," may contribute both to greater tolerance of physical force and to personal justification for retaliatory violent acts. There have been few investigations of this issue, however, and research is needed to clarify the specific contexts (if any) in which religion might actually exacerbate such acts. As we shall see in Chapter 14, certain kinds of religious orientation are associated with intolerance of some outgroups.

In recent years, there has been much publicity concerning physical and sexual abuse of children, adolescents, and sometimes adults by members of the clergy. It has been suggested that religion may be a contributing factor to such abuse because of celibacy requirements, rigid rules and expectations concerning sexuality, support for patriarchal family structure, and so on. Also, religious teachings may in some cases be used to justify domestic violence or excessive physical punishment of children. Most mainstream churches take a strong public stand against such religion-based deviance and criminality; however, this does not seem to stop some individuals and religious groups from using religion to justify antisocial behavior.

OVERVIEW

We have had something of a roller-coaster ride in this chapter. Religion does indeed seem to be related to some aspects of moral attitudes and behaviors, although there are almost always studies with contradictory findings. We have seen that in the areas of substance use/abuse, nonmarital sexual behavior, and (to a lesser extent) crime and delinquency, more religious persons generally report that they have stricter moral attitudes and are less likely to engage in behaviors that contravene societal (and especially religious) norms. The relationships are not always strong, but they do seem to be reasonably consistent, albeit qualified by various relevant factors as research progresses. However, faith is surprisingly unrelated to some other behaviors, such as cheating/dishonesty. There are indications that religious people *say* they are more honest, but the data do not bear this out for actual behavior in a secular setting. And religion may even be seen to justify some domestic violence, or to contribute to clergy abuse of children—for example, by dictating conditions such as celibacy that may lead some clergy to find inappropriate outlets for their sexual tension.

These findings deserve a moment of reflection. Religious persons may derive some consolation from studies showing that personal faith is negatively associated with substance use/ abuse, nonmarital sexual behavior, and some criminal acts. However, these associations tend to be relatively weak when found, and usually must be qualified by other findings. We might wonder why the correlations are not much larger, given the strength and consistency of religious teachings on these moral issues, and why the nonreligious qualifying factors sometimes reduce the correlations or make them disappear. In addition, there is the failure of religion to relate consistently to honesty versus cheating.

One drawback to most of the research discussed in this chapter is that it relies very heavily on self-reports of moral attitudes and behaviors. We have warned that such self-reports may be inaccurate and unreliable. However, in most cases it is very difficult to measure actual moral behavior, and few studies have attempted to do so—especially in highly sensitive domains such as honesty–cheating, crime, and domestic abuse. In consequence, we must rely on self-reports as "the next best thing," since in many cases they probably give us a reasonable impression of people's attitudes and behaviors. However, we must recognize the weakness inherent in this approach; we must strive wherever possible to supplement these measures with convergent reports (e.g., from parents, friends, teachers), and especially with actual behavioral measures.

We are left to puzzle over many things. Why do obtained relationships vary so much for different moral behaviors? Why doesn't religion have a stronger impact in *all* of these areas? How do we explain the "no relationship" findings? Can religion really be a source of criminal behavior, such as child sexual abuse or domestic violence? If so, can religion "right itself" and find within itself the cure for such problems? These questions are difficult to answer, but they may serve as stimuli for future research efforts.

Chapter 14

HELPING BEHAVIOR
AND PREJUDICE

> [Religion] makes prejudice and it unmakes prejudice. . . . Some people say the only cure for prejudice is more religion; some say the only cure is to abolish religion.
>
> . . . history, down to the present day, is a melancholy record of the horrors which can attend religion: human sacrifice, and in particular the slaughter of children, cannibalism, sensual orgies, abject superstition, hatred as between races, the maintenance of degrading customs, hysteria, bigotry, can all be laid at its charge. Religion is the last refuge of human savagery.
>
> . . . being helpful is a scriptural criterion of true religion (James 1:27), and humans will ultimately be judged on their efforts on behalf of those in need of aid or comfort (Matthew 25:31–46).
>
> Religious involvement is an especially strong predictor of volunteering and philanthropy.
>
> . . . terrorism is religious because religion provides the moral justification for killing and the images of cosmic warfare that impact a heady illusion of power. . . . every major religious tradition has served as a resource for violent actors.[1]

HELPING BEHAVIOR

"Help those in need." "Love one another." "Treat others as you would have them treat you." These are simple yet powerful imperatives, and similar themes are espoused by all of the world's major religions (Coward, 1986). Religion has been identified with humanity and community through such terms as "love," "justice," "compassion," "mercy," "grace," and "charity." The scriptural writings of most religions provide many examples of religious persons being kind to and helping others in need. And even in contemporary society, religious organizations and individuals sometimes stand out in their efforts to assist others. Churches become involved in relief efforts to ease the effects of famines, earthquakes, wars, and other disasters. Religious groups organize and fund soup kitchens in cities large and small; they help refugees to escape from unbelievable horrors and to become established in a new land;

---

1. These quotations come, respectively, from the following sources: Allport (1954, p. 444); Whitehead (1926, p. 37); Ritzema (1979, p. 105); Putnam (2000, p. 67); and Juergensmeyer (2000, p. xi).

they become actively involved as peacemakers in the world's "hot spots." Interviews with hundreds of people who rescued Jews in Nazi Europe revealed some who attributed their behavior to their religious values (Oliner & Oliner, 1988). The list of such religiously sponsored helping efforts is a long one.

Yet many nonreligious and even antireligious persons assist others as well. Present-day society offers unlimited opportunities to aid others in a secular context, and many people accept this challenge; "religion" apparently has little or nothing to do with their good will. Of course, this is why anecdotes are of little use in clarifying our understanding of the relationship between religion and helping behavior. Examples can be marshaled to show that both religious and nonreligious individuals and organizations assist others, and that they can also act with callous neglect when people cry out for assistance. Our challenge is to move beyond rhetoric and anecdotal material—to examine more general links between religion and helping, as revealed in the empirical literature.

Measurement and Definitional Problems

As in many areas of the psychology of religion, psychometric, methodological, and definitional issues are important in the study of helping behavior. Norms for helping can differ across cultural or religious groups (e.g., Kanekar & Merchant, 2001). Also, in keeping with many psychological studies of religion generally, much research in this area relies on questionnaires, asking for self-reports of religiousness and helping behavior. This raises concerns about "self-presentation" issues. For example, religious persons may be concerned that they should appear to be good representatives of their faith, and therefore may be inclined to exaggerate the extent to which they help others. Fortunately, there are also some studies in this area that utilize behavioral measures, and these serve as an important counterbalance to the many questionnaire studies on helping.

The literature on religion and helping is generally distinct from that on religion and prejudice, and therefore these topics are considered separately in this chapter. However, there is some overlap in the relevant issues. For example, a less-than-average inclination to help specific minority group members could be interpreted as prejudice. Also, helping behavior has been investigated when the target of help is described as tolerant or intolerant of some minority group members (Batson, Eidelman, Higley, & Russell, 2001); in this research, therefore, issues of helping and prejudice are intertwined. Does failure to help indicate the presence of prejudice? Is intolerance of intolerance a good thing, or is it a kind of prejudice itself?

In this section we purposely use the term "helping" rather than "altruism," in order to avoid the thorny issue of whether all helping behavior is egoistically motivated, or whether at least some helping behavior is motivated purely by the ultimate goal of benefiting someone else (i.e., altruistic behavior). Readers interested in pursuing this issue further might consult Batson's (1991) book on altruism, which addresses philosophical, theoretical, and empirical aspects of this distinction.

Early Questionnaire Studies

Early survey studies in this area tended to rely on measures of frequency of church attendance as the primary measure of religiousness, with occasional forays into measures of such factors as belief in God, affiliation, or religious involvement. Assessment of "helping" typically involved self-reports (and occasionally others' reports) of one's inclination to assist others. These studies were fairly "primitive," in the sense that the measures of both religion and helping were quite simple and basic, and investigators merely looked for correlations between such general measures. These studies typically reported low to moderate positive correlations between religiousness and helping (see, e.g., Langford & Langford, 1974; Nelson & Dynes, 1976; Rokeach, 1969), with some investigations reporting mixed or qualified associations (see, e.g., Cline & Richards, 1965; Friedrichs, 1960). More recent investigations concluded that conservative Christians were more likely to report volunteering and giving in both religious and secular realms (Lam, 2002; Regnerus, Smith, & Sikkink, 1998; Uslaner, 2002).

Most of these studies failed to take other factors into account. They did not, for example, control for church-related helping as opposed to helping outside the "church walls." Nelson and Dynes (1976) found low but significant associations between religiousness and helping through social service agencies; however, when these relationships were corrected for some other factors (e.g., helping through one's church, income, age), the correlations essentially disappeared. Similarly, Hunsberger and Platonow (1986) found that although religiously orthodox students reported that they were more likely to volunteer to help in religion-related contexts, there was no evidence that they were more helpful in a nonreligious context. As Putnam (2000) has concluded, "People active in religious organizations volunteer for ushering in church or visiting shut-in parishioners, whereas people active in secular organizations are most likely to work on cleaning up the local playground" (p. 119). Furthermore, when we turn to studies that incorporate actual behavioral measures of helping, there is little evidence that religious people are more helpful than less religious or nonreligious people.

Early Behavioral Studies

Batson, Schoenrade, and Ventis's (1993) review of the literature to that date on religion and helping led them to conclude that there is a considerable difference between "pencil-and-paper" and "behavioral" studies of helping. The early questionnaire investigations often showed at least some positive connection between religion and helping. However, consistent with studies indicating that the positive correlations from questionnaire studies tended to disappear when possible confounding variables were controlled for, Batson et al.'s (1993) review of six early studies employing behavioral measures showed that five of the six found no evidence that more religious individuals were more helpful.

These early studies were creative in their employment of behavioral measures. Forbes, TeVault, and Gromoll (1971) "lost" addressed letters near different churches and examined the extent to which people "helped" by putting these letters into mailboxes. Smith, Wheeler, and Diener (1975) gave people the opportunity to volunteer to work with a retarded child. Annis (1975, 1976) put people in a situation where they apparently heard a woman in distress after a ladder fell. McKenna (1976) measured the extent to which people would call a garage for a stranded woman motorist without any money. Yinon and Sharon (1985) examined financial contributions to help a needy family.

Only the last of these studies (i.e., Yinon & Sharon, 1985) showed any inclination for more religious individuals to be more likely to help than their less religious counterparts, and even this finding held only when the request came from a religious person. After reviewing these six studies, Batson et al. (1993) concluded that "this evidence strongly suggests that the more religious show no more active concern for others in need than do the less religious. The more religious only present themselves as more concerned" (p. 342).

Dimensions of Religion and Helping

The reader will observe that the studies discussed above did not take into account possible differences in helping tendencies associated with varying religious *orientations*. The dimensions and accompanying measures of Intrinsic (I) and Extrinsic (E) religious orientations proposed by Allport and colleagues (see Chapter 2 and Research Box 14.3, below), for example, would lead one to expect that persons with an intrinsic orientation should be more helpful since they tend to "live" their religion, and that persons with an extrinsic orientation should be less helpful because their religion derives from self-interest. Batson and colleagues, on the other hand, have proposed that intrinsic religiousness relates only to the *appearance* of being more helpful (Batson, 1976, 1990; Batson, Floyd, Meyer, & Winner, 1999; Batson, Schoenrade, & Pych, 1985; Batson et al., 1993, 2001). However, a measure of the Quest (Q) dimension, a flexible, questioning approach to religion, has proved to be the best and most direct predictor of helping behavior. Batson (who developed the standard version of the Q scale) has carried out a series of investigations to test these proposals, and we describe this program of research shortly.

First, however, other researchers have tended to focus on the extent to which helping may be associated with I and E religious orientations, typically based on self-reports of helping-related values and religious orientation. These investigations have usually revealed positive correlations between I scores and self-reports of *values* associated with aiding others (Bernt, 1989; Chau, Johnson, Bowers, Darvill, & Danko, 1990; Johnson et al., 1989; Tate & Miller, 1971; Watson, Hood, Morris, & Hall, 1984; Watson, Hood, & Morris, 1985). Batson et al. (1993) have argued that this kind of study does not resolve the issue of whether intrinsic persons are really more helpful, because such persons are simply trying to "look good" by agreeing with altruistic values (a social desirability interpretation).

Other studies have produced significant correlations between I-E scores and self-reported helping. For example, Benson et al. (1980) found that "nonspontaneous helping," as measured by self-reports of the kinds of charitable activities that people engaged in to assist others, was positively related to I scores ($r = .30$). Unfortunately, we do not know the extent to which social desirability might have played a role in this relationship, and Benson et al. did not distinguish between church-related helping and secular charitable situations. Hunsberger and Platonow (1986) studied participants' inclination to volunteer for *secular* charitable work in their study, and found that there was a weak but significant correlation between such volunteering and I scores ($r = .17$), as well as a negative association for E scores ($r = -.27$). Furthermore, a measure of social desirability was *not* related to I scores ($r = .02$) in this study, but it was significantly correlated with E scores ($r = .22$).

The evidence presented above suggests that more religious persons, especially more intrinsic individuals, tend to help others through their religious organizations in a variety of ways. Also, it would appear that intrinsic religiosity is positively but weakly related to an inclination to *say* one helps others, and possibly the tendency actually to volunteer in a charitable context. There is some evidence that social desirability does not explain this relationship, though the relevant studies have relied to a large extent on self-reports. The situation is certainly not clear-cut, since the associations that have appeared tend to be weak, and they are not entirely consistent from one study to the next. However, Batson et al. (1993) have argued that only behavioral studies can resolve the controversy over a possible religion–helping relationship.

Batson's Research Program

C. Daniel Batson and his students have reported a series of investigations on the relationship between religion and helping. Much of this work has focused on the controversy concerning how religious *orientation* is related to assisting others, and these researchers have introduced a number of important behavioral measures of helping that have allowed this area to address some of the problems associated with investigations based solely on self-reports.

The Good Samaritan Study

An early behavioral study in this area attempted to place the parable of the good Samaritan in an experimental context (Darley & Batson, 1973; see Research Box 14.1). Essentially, this experiment revealed no tendency for scores on Means (similar to E), End (similar to I), or Q measures to be related to helping behavior.

Darley and Batson (1973) concluded that among those who did not offer to help, the more orthodox intrinsic persons might be helping for their own reasons, instead of being sensitive to those needing aid. This interpretation has been challenged (Gorsuch, 1988;

Research Box 14.1. Situational and Dispositional Variables in Helping Behavior (Darley & Batson, 1973)

In the parable of the good Samaritan, Jesus described a man who was robbed, beaten, and left for dead at the side of the road. Two "religious" individuals, a priest and a Levite, passed by but did not stop to help. However, a Samaritan (a religious outcast), at some cost to himself, gave the robbery victim the help he needed. Jesus apparently wanted to make the point that people should model their behavior after the Samaritan, not after "religious" people who may be so caught up in their thoughts that they do not see the needs of people around them.

Would the results differ if this situation were to occur in contemporary society? Darley and Batson attempted to construct a similar "help-needed" situation at Princeton University. Sixty-seven seminary students first completed questionnaires to assess their religious orientation, among other things. Then, one at a time, 40 of them showed up for a follow-up experimental session. They were asked to prepare a short talk based on either (1) the parable of the good Samaritan, or (2) jobs that seminary students might pursue. After having a few minutes to prepare for their forthcoming talk, participants were given a map to show them how to get to a room in another building where they would give their talk. Half of the participants were told that they would need to hurry, since they were late for their appointment.

As these students passed down an alley, they met a man who clearly seemed to be in need of help. A confederate of the experimenters was slumped in a doorway, head down,

continued

Research Box 14.1. *continued*

eyes closed, not moving. As each seminarian passed, the victim coughed and groaned; given the geographical setting, it was virtually impossible to miss him. The key dependent measure in this study was whether or not the students stopped to offer any kind of help. In fact, just 16 of the 40 seminarians (40%) offered assistance. And religious orientation scores—Means (similar to E), End (similar to I), or Quest (Q)—did not predict who would stop to offer aid.

However, among those who did stop, an interesting finding emerged. When a seminarian offered help, the victim indicated that he had just taken his medication, he would be fine if he just rested a few minutes, and he would like to be left alone. Some of the "good Samaritans" were quite insistent, however. In spite of the victim's objections, some participants insisted on taking him into a nearby building and pouring some coffee and/or religion into him. Among only those who did stop to help, scores on the intrinsic measure correlated positively with this "I know what is best for you" helping style ($r = .43$), but scores on the Q measure were negatively associated with such insistent aid ($r = -.54$). Darley and Batson concluded that the more I-oriented seminarians seemed to be guided by a "preprogrammed" helping response, which was not affected by the expressed needs of the victim. It was almost as if the "super helpers" were satisfying their own internal need to help, rather than meeting the needs of the victim. However, those with a Q orientation had a more tentative helping style, sensitive to the person needing help, since they tended to accept the victim's statement that he really just wanted to be left alone and everything would be fine.

Before we leave our consideration of this study, there are some loose ends to tie up. Contrary to expectations, it did not make any difference whether the participant was preparing to give a speech on the parable of the good Samaritan or on jobs for seminary graduates. Apparently, thinking about helping in a Biblical context did not make participants more likely to offer aid in a similar situation. Finally, those participants in the "hurry up, you're late" condition were significantly less likely to stop and offer any kind of help than were those with no "hurry up" instructions. Apparently, the most powerful variable in determining helping behavior overall in this study was a nonreligious one—whether or not the participant was in a hurry.

Watson et al., 1985). Possibly those with higher Q scores helped "tentatively" because they really weren't very committed to helping in the first place, and the more assertive assistance of those with higher I scores reflected more genuine caring and concern on their part. Furthermore, we may wonder about the generalizability of findings from the relatively homogeneous and religious sample of seminary students. Another study (Batson & Gray, 1981) extended the original Darley and Batson findings in a very different context.

"Helping Janet"

In the follow-up investigation by Batson and Gray (1981), 60 female introductory psychology students at the University of Kansas, all of whom reported being at least moderately religious, were placed one at a time in an experimental situation involving an exchange of written notes. "Janet," supposedly another participant, was a fictitious person who indicated that she was feeling lonely and needed to work through some problems. Half of the time Janet expressly asked the real participant to meet with her again for further conversation, and the other half of the time Janet indicated quite clearly that she was resolved to work out her problems on her own. How did the participants respond to Janet's clear request for help or no help? I scores were positively correlated with participants' previously obtained self-reports of helpfulness and concern for others. But when Batson and Gray examined actual helping responses, I scores were correlated about .27 with helping, *whether or not* Janet wanted any help. Q scores, however, were positively associated with helping ($r = .37$) when Janet said she wanted help, and negatively related to helping ($r = -.32$) when Janet indicated she wanted to work things through on her own. This finding supports Darley and Batson's (1973) earlier suggestion that individuals with high Q scores are sensitive to the expressed needs of others with respect to help needed, but that people with an intrinsic (end) orientation are rather indiscriminately inclined to help, whether the other person wants help or not.

Altruism or Egoism?

Three further studies by Batson and his colleagues have pursued the "altruism versus egoism" issue concerning underlying motivation for helping by people with different religious orientations. These investigations have provided additional valuable data concerning the relationship of the I and Q orientations to helping behavior.

In the first of two studies reported by Batson et al. (1989), participants were told that they could volunteer to help a 7-year-old boy with a rare genetic disorder—but that even if they were willing to help, they would have to pass a sort of physical fitness qualifying task before they could participate in a walkathon. Some participants were led to believe that the qualifying standard was relatively easy; others were told that it was "extremely stringent." Batson et al. reasoned that when the standard was described as difficult, it would be easy to volunteer because there wasn't much chance that a participant would actually have to follow through with the volunteer commitment. The researchers found that, as expected, E scores were negatively correlated with volunteering for both the easy and difficult qualifying standards ($r = -.37$, on average). I scores, however, did not correlate with volunteering when the standard was easy, but they were positively correlated ($r = .50$) when the standard was difficult. Although other interpretations are possible, Batson et al. suggested that the results support their contention that intrinsically inclined people want to *look* like helpers, but only if there is actually just a small chance of their having to carry through with the assistance. Q scores did not correlate with helping in either the easy or difficult conditions.

Furthermore, those who volunteered were actually asked to proceed with the qualifying task (stepping up and down from a block for 30 seconds). There was evidence that those with high I scores tried harder in the difficult condition only if they had *not* volunteered to help. Q scores, on the other hand, were positively related to performance on the qualifying task only for those who *had* volunteered to help. Batson et al. interpreted these rather complex results as being consistent with their earlier research findings. First, intrinsic persons' motivation for helping stemmed from a personal need to appear helpful (without actually having to help), rather than from the needs of others. Second, questers' motivation for helping was generated by the needs of others, since they worked hardest when they thought it would be difficult to qualify to help.

A second investigation reported in the same article focused on a different helping context—an undergraduate who was coping with family tragedy and needed help from others to support her siblings. The pattern of correlations suggested that those with high E scores were less likely to volunteer, that those with high Q scores were more likely to volunteer when there was little pressure to do so, but that I scores were unrelated to offering assistance under either high- or low- pressure conditions. Thus the findings for both studies reported by Batson et al. (1989) were interpreted as being consistent with expectations that intrinsic-based helping is motivated by concern for "appearances," and quest-based assistance stems from genuine sensitivity to others' needs.

Batson and Flory (1990) subsequently attempted to manipulate the extent to which research participants thought they would "look good," by employing a cognitive interference task (involving the Stroop effect) and an appeal involving a family tragedy similar to that in the second Batson et al. (1989) study above. As they expected, Batson and Flory found that high I scores were associated with "looking good," and that there was a weak (but nonsignificant) tendency for Q scores to be linked with helping stemming from concern for the victim's welfare.

Intrinsic and Quest Religion as a Source of Universal Compassion?

Batson et al. (1999, 2001) recently carried out two studies to investigate more thoroughly the role of the I and Q religious orientations in helping behavior—specifically, when a target person's behavior violated or threatened one's values. These studies are described in Research Box 14.2. Batson et al. (1999, 2001) argued that in combination, these studies showed that a high Q orientation—but not a high I orientation—was associated with broadly based compassion. Their investigations overlap the two foci of this chapter (helping and prejudice), and are included here because they speak directly to the underlying motivation of religious people's helping behavior. Specifically, the authors investigated people's inclination to help, depending on the extent to which helping might violate their values. An intrinsic orientation was found to be associated with less help being offered for people who violated values. That is, intrinsic people's antipathy was not limited to value violators' (sinful) behavior, but was apparently directed at the value-violating person as well (i.e., the sinner). High Q scores, on the other hand, were associated with less help being offered to aid value-violating behavior, but there was not greater antipathy toward the value-violating person (the sinner).

In a recent investigation, Goldfried and Miner (2002) attempted to replicate and extend Batson et al.'s (2001) work, but were led to a rather different conclusion. The "target" for helping/prejudice in Goldfried and Miner's study was a "religious fundamentalist" rather than the "gay person" targeted by Batson et al. (2001). Goldfried and Miner concluded that the quest orientation is not indicative of a universally compassionate religious style. Rather, even those with a quest orientation demonstrate discrimination against (i.e., a lesser tendency to help) someone (here, a "religious fundamentalist") whose values threaten the central beliefs of those who score higher on a quest scale.

Summary of Batson's Research

This series of studies has provided substantial but not entirely consistent support for Batson's interpretation of tendencies to help, and motivation for assisting others, depending on religious orientation. These investigations all involved small samples of university students, and

---

Research Box 14.2. Intrinsic and Quest Religion as a Source of Universal Compassion (Batson et al., 1999, 2001)

Batson et al. (1999) studied 30 male and 60 female introductory psychology students at the University of Kansas, all with a Christian background and all at least moderately interested in religion. These people were told that the investigation was about self-disclosure, and they were randomly assigned to one of three experimental conditions by means of (self-disclosing) notes, supposedly from another student who was always of the same sex as the recipient. The notes indicated that (1) the discloser was gay and needed money to visit his or her grandparents in Santa Fe; (2) the discloser was not gay and needed money to visit his or her grandparents in Santa Fe; or (3) the discloser was gay and needed money to attend a gay pride rally in San Francisco. The discloser made it clear that he or she wanted to win a raffle to help support the travel outlined above. Participants were then given 2 minutes to work on one of two tasks. By working on Task A, the participant could in effect give raffle tickets (toward a $30 gift certificate) to the discloser. By working on Task B, the participant could give raffle tickets to an unknown student.

Overall, more than 80% of participants' time was spent on Task A, which would in effect help the discloser. However, the rate of helping varied across conditions. A median split was used to divide people into groups with high and low I scores. Of particular interest here was a significant tendency for those with high I scores to help less whenever the discloser said that he or she was gay, regardless of whether the discloser needed money to help promote homosexuality (i.e., to travel to San Francisco gay pride rally) or simply to visit grandparents. Those with low I scores, on the other hand, tended to help the discloser more if he or she intended to visit grandparents, but less if the discloser intended to travel to the gay pride rally. That is, the latter participants were more likely to help the gay discloser if doing so did not promote homosexuality. However, those with high Q scores tended to help the discloser at the same relatively high level regardless of whether he or she was gay, and regardless of whether the discloser intended to visit grandparents or a gay pride rally. Batson et al. concluded that

> devout, intrinsic religion appeared to be associated with tribal rather than universal compassion; there seemed to be antipathy toward the homosexual person, not just toward promoting homosexuality. Instead of intrinsic religion breeding Good Samaritans who saw any person in need as neighbor, as Allport (1966) claimed, it seemed to breed priests and Levites whose concept of neighbor was restricted to the right kind of person. (1999, p. 455)

The second study (Batson et al., 2001) was similar to the first, but it focused on Q, and there were some important variations from the previous investigation. Sixty female undergraduate students at the University of Kansas participated; again all were from Christian backgrounds and expressed at least a moderate interest in religion. They were led to believe that the study dealt with disclosure of personal information (though notes), and again they understood that their choice of Task A or B would generate raffle tickets for the discloser, also a female undergraduate. But in this study the discloser was portrayed as either intolerant or not intolerant of gay persons. Furthermore, the intolerant discloser said that she needed money either to travel to visit her grandparents or to attend a rally of people opposed to giving jobs to gays. The not-intolerant discloser always said that she needed money to visit her grandparents. This manipulation therefore generated three

continued

Research Box 14.2. *continued*

experimental conditions: not-intolerant/grandparents, intolerant/grandparents, and in-tolerant/rally. A median split divided people into groups with high and low Q scores, thus generating a 2 (Q scores) × 3 (condition) design.

Results indicated that those with high Q scores were approximately equally likely to help the discloser when she needed money to visit her grandparents, whether or not she tended to be intolerant of gays, but that these participants were much less likely to help the intolerant discloser who intended to attend a rally that promoted intolerance of gays. Those with low Q scores, on the other hand, distinguished between the intolerant and the not-intolerant discloser who wanted to visit grandparents, giving more assistance to the not-intolerant discloser than the intolerant discloser (and even less help to the intol-erant discloser who wanted to attend the rally). Batson et al. (2001) concluded that the group with high Q scores seemed to distinguish between the sin and sinner, showing an-tipathy toward value-violating behavior, but not toward the value-violating individual as a person. This is especially interesting, because it has been argued by others that the I (not Q) orientation is the one should contribute to a distinction between sin and sinner (see Fulton, Gorsuch, & Maynard, 1999). Batson et al. found no such tendency for those with high I scores to direct their antipathy toward the sin (i.e., to be less likely to help), but not toward the sinner.

These two studies do have limitations, such as the small and unique samples of under-graduates. Also, the first study revealed surprisingly high rates of helping behavior in all conditions. One might argue that the experimental context was contrived, although evi-dence from manipulation checks suggested that the intolerance manipulation was effec-tive. And the focus of helping and intolerance in these studies was homosexuality, which may be unique compared to other domains where helping and intolerance come into play. Batson et al. (2001) also pointed out that it is not entirely clear what "tolerance of intol-erance" means. However, this research constitutes the most direct assessment of helping behavior in a "sin–sinner" context, as it relates to the I and Q religious orientations. Batson et al. concluded that "the combined results . . . suggest that those scoring high on the Intrinsic scale are value-violation vigilant, inclined to judge and reject those who stray from the straight and narrow in any direction. . . . The compassion—even the tolerance—of those scoring high on the Intrinsic scale seems circumscribed" (2001, p. 48).

the generalizability of the findings may be questioned. The expected correlational relation-ships did not always achieve significance in specific studies, and the weak psychometric prop-erties of the version of the Q scale used in the earlier studies is a concern. Specific findings are open to alternate interpretations. However, the combined impact of these investigations suggests that the tendency for those with an I orientation to be helpful may stem to some extent from personal need rather than from the needs of others. Moreover, the Q orienta-tion has predicted helping under some circumstances, and the evidence indicates that the resulting assistance is motivated by the needs of others rather than by personal reward or appearance. In this sense, quest-related helping may approach "altruistic" assistance, whereas intrinsic-related helping has a more "egoistic" basis (Batson et al., 1989), although this interpretation has been questioned (Goldfried & Miner, 2002).

More on Helping and Value Threat

Jackson and Esses (1997) also investigated the extent to which religious orientation was related to helping behavior under different value-threatening circumstances, but focused on religious fundamentalism (RF) rather than the I, E, and Q religious orientations. (An RF orientation, as discussed here, involves an inflexible belief that one's religious beliefs represent absolute truth that *must* be followed.) Jackson and Esses suspected that when other people threatened the values of individuals high in RF, these individuals would be more likely to attribute responsibility for problems to the other people themselves, and this in turn would affect the *type* of help that they felt was appropriate.

In particular, it was predicted that in value-threatening situations, individuals high in RF would be inclined to help the threatening others by simply reminding or admonishing them about the need to take personal responsibility for their (personally caused) problems ("moral model")—or possibly by going a step further and encouraging the other people in need to accept personal responsibility, as well as to seek help from a recognized authority ("enlightenment model"). Value-threatened people scoring high on a measure of RF were also expected to be less likely to offer direct help ("medical model") or to attempt to empower others to help themselves ("compensatory model"). Jackson and Esses noted that the medical and compensatory models assume that persons in need are not responsible for causing the problem, but the moral and enlightenment models do assume that needy persons are personally responsible for their situation. We might add that the moral model in particular does not really offer help in the usual sense.

Two investigations were conducted with Canadian undergraduate students, who read short paragraphs about unemployment in Canada suggesting that unemployment was disproportionately high among target group members. In Study 1, the value-threatening target group was homosexuals, and the nonthreatening group Native Canadians; in Study 2, the groups were single mothers and students, respectively. Manipulation checks indicated that these groups were indeed perceived as threatening or nonthreatening to the values of those high in RF, as expected. The research participants then completed attribution and helping measures.

Results from both studies indicated that religious fundamentalism was related to attributions of responsibility for value-threatening groups (who were felt to be more personally responsible for their plight), and also to the type of help thought to be appropriate (i.e., endorsement of personal change), but only when the target involved a value-threatening group. This makes sense, because high RF scores are indicative of both strong values and belief in the ultimate truth of one's own religious values. Thus a group that threatens one's (strongly held) values might be seen as more salient, and also as "wrong" or "sinful," by those with high RF scores. This in turn could incline high-RF individuals to see value-violating others as both morally incorrect (and therefore responsible for their problems), and also in need of personal change in order to deal with those problems. This interpretation should be viewed as tentative, pending further research.

The Jackson and Esses (1997) research thus indicated that RF predicts a tendency to admonish (rather than to help directly) value-threatening groups in need, apparently because of a tendency to attribute personal causes for problems of needy target groups. RF did not predict types of helping for non-value-threatening needy groups.

One might wonder whether similar tendencies to favor specific approaches to helping might be characteristic of other religious orientations (e.g., I, E, Q, and religiously orthodox). As Jackson and Esses pointed out, we do not know to what extent their findings are unique to their samples, target groups, and value threats. How would findings differ for groups that promote rather than threaten one's values? Given that right-wing authoritarianism (RWA) is closely associated with RF (e.g., Altemeyer & Hunsberger, 1992), as we discuss later in this chapter, is it RF or RWA that is the critical variable in the obtained relationships? Do other variables (e.g., stereotypes, affect) mediate the relationship between RF and helping style for value-threatening groups? Do these findings hold at the individual as well as the group level? Such questions offer rich research opportunities.

Given the apparent central role of values in highly religious people's lives, we might also wonder whether their religious values could be used in a more positive way. Could a direct appeal to religious values increase helping behavior—for example, by increasing perceived personal moral obligation to help among religious persons? Recent research suggests that such an approach might be productive, at least in the context of blood donations as helping behavior (Ortberg, Gorsuch, & Kim, 2001). However, this same study found that an appeal based on (nonreligious) attitude was even more productive in terms of blood donation behavior. This investigation reminds us that values not only serve as a potential source of threat; they may also provide a means of increasing helping behavior for religious persons.

Conclusions about Religion and Helping Behavior

The study of religion and helping behavior is especially interesting because of the availability of both self-report questionnaires and investigations of actual and anticipated behavior. Furthermore, few areas have seen extensive use of theory accompanied by a systematic research program, such as that provided by Batson and his coworkers. Not all authors are prepared to accept Batson's conclusions that intrinsic religion is related to the *appearance* of helping, and that the assistance provided by such individuals is likely to be a preprogrammed, self-serving type of aid. Nor is there complete acceptance of the finding that the Q orientation is a good predictor of *actual* (behavioral) helping, and that quest-based assistance is motivated by the needs of others—a kind of source of universal compassion (see, e.g., Gorsuch, 1988; Watson et al., 1984). Specific criticisms have also been directed at the measures of religion used, as well as the context for helping (Ritzema, 1979). However, Batson has provided a systematic program of research, the results of which provide support for his conclusions. It is to be hoped that those who prefer alternate interpretations of the Batson findings will carry out their own multiple-study programs of research to test these interpretations. Until such investigations are forthcoming, the increasing body of empirical evidence produced by Batson and his coworkers continues to favor his interpretations as outlined above.

Also, Jackson and Esses (1997) have given us much to think about in their unique investigations of religion and helping. Apparently Religious Fundamentalism scores predict a tendency to attribute personal causes for need, at least to value-threatening groups. Those with high RF scores seem inclined to conclude that members of such value-threatening groups need to change personally, and therefore feel that direct helping of such groups might be less appropriate. These issues and related questions await additional research.

PREJUDICE, DISCRIMINATION, AND STEREOTYPING

Since most world religions espouse a common theme of "love one another," it might be expected that this teaching would have a powerful effect in reducing prejudice among the members of these religions. But research has not been supportive of this generalization. In fact, many studies have linked various aspects of religiousness with *increased* discriminatory attitudes. Glock and Stark (1966) even built a case that Christianity contributes directly to anti-Semitic prejudice; in spite of challenges to this position, it has been confirmed by other researchers (e.g., Eisinga, Konig, & Scheepers, 1995). Indeed, the relationship between religion and prejudice has possibly generated more interest, research, and controversy than any other domain in the psychology of religion.

Recently, religion and religious extremism have been prominently linked with terrorism (see, e.g., Juergensmeyer, 2000)—particularly in the wake of the terrorist attacks on the World Trade Center in New York City and the Pentagon in Washington, D.C., on September 11, 2001. World leaders who led the subsequent war against terrorism in Afghanistan repeatedly emphasized that their war was against terrorism, not any particular religion. But the immediate targets of their aggression were the Muslim Taliban government of Afghanistan and the fighters who supported the Taliban. Politics, the military, and religion are sometimes intertwined to an extent that it is almost impossible to tease apart their separate effects.

Moreover, after the terrorist attacks of September 11, religious extremism was seen in the United States as well. The Christian fundamentalist preacher Jerry Falwell went so far as to blame the American Civil Liberties Union, abortionists, feminists, and gay and lesbian persons for removing God's protection from the United States and thereby allowing the terrorist attacks to occur (*The Globe and Mail*, 2001). In light of such examples, one might well wonder whether religion does not directly contribute to intolerance, injustice, and even violence.

Of course, religiously based prejudice and conflict are disturbingly evident all over the world, even if one ignores the 2001 terrorism attacks on the United States and the subsequent U.S. "war on terrorism." In spite of attempts to resolve disputes peacefully, different religious groups engage in major, bloody conflicts in virtually every corner of the earth. In addition to the many blatant examples of this, extensive but often more subtle discrimination against minority groups may also be rooted in religion, as elaborated below. How are we to understand the links between prejudice and religious groups that preach love and kindness toward others?

As noted of the beginning of this chapter, Gordon Allport—one of the 20th century's most prominent authorities on prejudice—concluded that the effect of religion on prejudice is paradoxical, because "it makes prejudice and it unmakes prejudice" (Allport, 1954, p. 494). The reasoning behind this paradox was that different religious orientations might be differentially related to prejudice. First, let us consider the related research in historical perspective. In reviewing the work on religion and prejudice, we do not offer an exhaustive review of the literature that has accumulated in the area (see, e.g., reviews by Gorsuch & Aleshire, 1974; Batson et al., 1993; Hunsberger, 1995; Hunsberger & Jackson, in press; Spilka, Hood, & Gorsuch, 1985). Rather, we attempt to summarize different stages in the development of our understanding of the religion–prejudice relationship. We ultimately focus on promising developments that have occurred in the past decade or so, involving religious fundamentalism and quest orientations, right-wing authoritarianism, and intergroup conflict perspectives.

Early Studies

Many studies over the years have found that people's responses to measures of religion and prejudice are related. In light of his review of the literature, Wulff (1997) was led to conclude:

> Using a variety of measures of piety—religious affiliation, church attendance, doctrinal ortho-
> doxy, rated importance of religion, and so on—researchers have consistently found positive cor-
> relations with ethnocentrism, authoritarianism, dogmatism, social distance, rigidity, intolerance
> of ambiguity, and specific forms of prejudice, especially against Jews and blacks. (p. 223)

Others have similarly concluded that as a broad generalization, the more religious an individual is, the more prejudiced that person is (Batson et al., 1993; Dittes, 1969; Gorsuch &
Aleshire, 1974; Meadow & Kahoe, 1984; Myers & Spencer, 2001; Paloutzian, 1996; Spilka,
Hood, & Gorsuch, 1985). However, most of these authors are quick to qualify this inference
in terms of a possible curvilinear relationship, and also in terms of religious orientation (see
below).

Research showing a religion–prejudice link has a long history. It dates at least to the
1940s, when Adorno, Frenkel-Brunswik, Levinson, and Sanford's (1950) famous studies of
the authoritarian personality disclosed a positive association between religion and prejudice.
Batson et al. (1993) reviewed much work on religion and prejudice, and found that for investigations published in 1960 or earlier, 19 of 23 findings confirmed the positive relationship between religion and prejudice; there was no clear relationship in 3 studies; and just 1
revealed a negative relationship. Similarly, of 24 additional studies published between 1960
and 1990, 18 showed that religion was positively related to prejudice, and just 1 investigation revealed a negative association. It is unusual for so many efforts in the social sciences to
converge on such a clear conclusion. However, the generalization that religion is positively
correlated with prejudice is more complex than it might first appear.

Is the Religion–Prejudice Relationship Curvilinear?

There have been suggestions that this religion–prejudice relationship may actually be curvilinear, at least when church attendance is the measure of religiousness (e.g., Gorsuch, 1993;
Gorusch & Aleshire, 1974; Wulff, 1997). It has been proposed that those who do not attend
church are relatively unprejudiced; that those attending infrequently to moderately frequently
are the most prejudiced persons; and that "Active church members [are] among the least prejudiced in society" (Gorsuch, 1988, p. 212). This curvilinear relationship is sometimes idealisti-
cally portrayed as a smooth bell-shaped curve (e.g., Spilka, Hood, & Gorsuch, 1985, p. 271).
Although the curvilinear relationship has apparently been readily accepted in the relevant
literature, there is in fact limited empirical evidence to support it, and authors often do not
acknowledge the many weaknesses and qualifications associated with the relevant findings.
Some researchers have even reported data suggesting that the relationship is in fact a reasonably strong linear one (e.g., Altemeyer, 1996; Altemeyer & Hunsberger, 1993). Altemeyer
(2003), for example, concluded that "the general finding appears plain and linear: The more
one goes to church, the more likely one will be prejudiced against a variety of others" (p. 18).

Some of the confusion concerning curvilinear findings may have resulted from the fact that some investigators did not distinguish between weakly religious and nonreligious persons (e.g., they combined church members who attended seldom or never with non-members); others did not include nonreligious persons at all, and therefore their research can shed no light on this aspect of the proposed curvilinear relationship. Furthermore, there is no agreement in the literature on what constitutes "high," "moderate," and "low" religiosity or church attendance, and different studies may use unique reference points in comparing these groups. Hunsberger (1995) pointed out that there exists little empirical evidence to support the conclusion that very frequent church attenders are any less prejudiced than *non*religious persons (see Eisinga, Felling, & Peters, 1990; Scheepers, Gijsberts, & Hello, 2002), who have in fact been found to be the *least* prejudiced persons in some investigations (e.g., Adorno et al., 1950; Altemeyer & Hunsberger, 1992; Fisher, Derison, Polley, Cadman, & Johnston, 1994).

Altemeyer (1996) reexamined the 27 studies that served as the basis for Gorsuch and Aleshire's (1974) curvilinear conclusion. Fifteen of these studies reportedly did not distinguish between completely unaffiliated persons and church members who seldom attended. Of the remaining 12 studies, Altemeyer found that just 1 (Hoge & Carroll, 1973) showed "a significant up-and-down curvilinear relationship" (p. 150). Furthermore, Gorsuch and Aleshire's "moderate" church attender category overlapped with both the "low" and "high" categories.

Given the problems with early studies that purportedly showed the curvilinear effect, the lack of recent studies to confirm such an effect, and the existence of some studies that looked for but could not find a curvilinear effect, it is questionable today whether such an effect does indeed exist. However, a focus on simple measures of religion, such as frequency of church attendance or "being religious," is likely to obscure the influence of potentially important factors, such as religious orientation, in the religion–prejudice relationship.

Does Religious Orientation Make a Difference?

Early research on religion and prejudice did not often take religious *orientation* into account. Indeed, much of this initial work was conducted before the conceptualization and measurement of various personal religious orientations began in the mid-1960s and later. We might hope that such refinements in our thinking about religion would help to resolve the issue of a possible link between religion and prejudice.

Allport and Ross (1967) addressed this issue head-on when they published their famous article outlining the formulation of the I and E religious orientations, as well as the scales developed to measure the concepts, since this work was done in the context of their study of prejudice. Ultimately, Allport and Ross concluded that more intrinsic persons were, as expected, less prejudiced than those with an extrinsic religious orientation, who in turn were less prejudiced than those with an "indiscriminately pro" (IP) orientation (i.e., those who scored high on both the I and E scales). This finding concerning prejudice levels (i.e., I < E < IP) has become firmly embedded in the literature (see, e.g., Gorsuch, 1988). In fact, in light of these and subsequent findings, the first edition of the present text concluded in 1985 that "the problem of religion and prejudice seems to be essentially solved" (Spilka, Hood, & Gorsuch, 1985, p. 273)

However, as several authors (e.g., Altemeyer, 1996; Donahue, 1985b; Hunsberger, 1995; Kirkpatrick, 1989; Kirkpatrick & Hood, 1990; Laythe, Finkel, & Kirkpatrick, 2001) have pointed out, there were numerous problems with the original intrinsic and extrinsic concepts and scales as presented by Allport and Ross (1967). In Research Box 14.3, we describe their study and its findings; In Research Box 14.4, we critically reevaluate this influential study and its conclusions.

ॐ

Research Box 14.3. Personal Religious Orientation and Prejudice
(Allport & Ross, 1967)

In light of previous research that they thought showed a curvilinear relationship between church attendance and prejudice, Allport and Ross developed their I and E scales to assess whether people with an extrinsic religious orientation were more prejudiced than people with an intrinsic orientation. This, it was felt, would help to explain why some "religious people" are prejudiced while others are not; it also fit neatly with Allport's (1954, 1966) earlier work, in which he had distinguished between "immature" and "mature" religious orientations. It seemed to make sense that intrinsic persons, with a committed, interiorized faith, would live their religion and be less prejudiced, but that extrinsic persons, with a consensual, exteriorized, utilitarian religious orientation, would be more prejudiced.

Both direct and indirect questionnaire measures of prejudice were included; the former tapped prejudice against blacks, Jews, and other minorities, whereas the latter measured a lack of sympathy with mental patients, as well as a generalized distrust of people. These instruments were administered to 309 Christian churchgoers from six faiths, including 94 Roman Catholics from Massachusetts, 55 Lutherans from New York, 44 Nazarenes from South Carolina, 53 Presbyterians from Pennsylvania, 35 Methodists from Tennessee, and 28 Baptists from Massachusetts.

Allport and Ross initially conceptualized the I and E orientations as opposite ends of a single dimension, but found a positive correlation between various measures of prejudice and *both* the E scale and a "total Extrinsic–Intrinsic scale" (p. 437), whereas they had expected to find a *negative* correlation between prejudice and the I scale. They did not report the correlation between their prejudice measures and the I scale alone.

After contemplating these initial results, which did not support their expectations, the authors decided that a "reformulation" was necessary. Instead of simply examining the correlations between I-E scores and prejudice, Allport and Ross decided that it might be better to categorize people according to four types determined by median splits on the I and E scales: consistently I, consistently E, "indiscriminately pro" (IP; high scores on both scales—also referred to as "religious muddle-headedness"), and "indiscriminately anti" (IA; low scores on both scales). Since they did not include any nonchurchgoers in their sample, they were not able to examine the IA category. Reanalyzing their data for the remaining three religious types (with each of the three types constituting very roughly one-third of the sample), they reported that the extrinsic type was more prejudiced on both direct and indirect measures of prejudice, and also that IP persons were more prejudiced than either the consistently I or consistently E types.

Allport and Ross concluded that prejudice is often part of personality structure, and that this is intertwined with the individual's religious orientation:

> One definable style marks the individual who is bigoted in ethnic matters and extrinsic in his religious orientation. Equally apparent is the style of those who are bigoted and at the same time indiscriminately proreligious. A relatively small number of people show an equally consistent cognitive style in their simultaneous commitment to religion as a dominant, intrinsic value and to ethnic tolerance. (p. 442)

Thus it seemed that the intrinsic–extrinsic distinction would be a valuable tool in clarifying links between religion and prejudice. In order of decreasing prejudice came IP individuals, extrinsic persons, and finally intrinsic persons.

Problems in this investigation (and in some subsequent research) make us reluctant simply to accept the Allport and Ross conclusion at face value. Furthermore, Hunsberger (1995) has argued that "although the findings of some other studies have paralleled Allport and Ross' results . . . the [I-E] conceptualization has not lived up to expectations in identifying or reducing prejudice" (p. 117). Similarly, Donahue's (1985b) review and meta-analysis of the I-E literature led him to conclude that the I scale "is uncorrelated, rather than negatively correlated, with prejudice across most available measures. [The E scale] is positively correlated with prejudice, but not nearly so strongly as Allport's writings might have predicted" (p. 405). The many problems with the E scale make its apparent link with prejudice difficult to interpret, and Hoge and Carroll (1973) even concluded that the only thing we could be sure about was that the E scale "is not tapping extrinsic religious motivation" (p. 189).

Research Box 14.4. A Critical Reevaluation of "Personal Religious Orientation and Prejudice" (Allport & Ross, 1967)

A close examination of the Allport and Ross study calls into question its basic conclusions. First, the switch from using one continuous I-E scale to examining discrete orientation categories involved some data analysis "gymnastics," resulting in the final "I < E < IP" conclusion, which served as the basis for further research and conclusions that appeared regularly in the literature. This is not a minor point; as Donahue (1985a) has observed, few studies in the literature have actually used the four-way categorization recommended by Allport and Ross. Rather, most studies have simply reported correlations between each of the I and E scales and other measures—precisely what the original authors decided they should *not* do. In fact, some later authors seem to have incorrectly concluded that Allport and Ross reported a positive correlation between I scores and either humanitarian attitudes (Vergote, 1993) or lower prejudice (Koenig, 1992). But all of this aside, if we ignore the reformulations and reanalyses that were necessary to reach the conclusion that extrinsic persons are more prejudiced than intrinsic ones, and instead focus on the research itself, what do we find?

For one thing, although overall comparisons were significant, inconsistencies appeared for the different religious subgroups. For example, just one of Allport and Ross's six religious denominational groups actually showed the I < E < IP pattern for the "anti-Negro prejudice" measure. In the other five groups, either the mean for the IP participants was lower than that for the E participants, or the E group's mean was lower than that for the I group.

Questions can be raised concerning the prejudice measures used, especially their theoretical and psychometric strength, since such properties were typically not reported in the 1967 paper. One must wonder about potential biases such as those that might be stimulated by what Allport and Ross called an "indirect" measure of prejudice. It described the attempts of a young black woman to rent a room in an all-white neighborhood, then asked "If you had been Mrs. Williamson, would you have rented to the Negro girl?" We suspect that a proreligious and possibly nondiscriminatory bias might have been aroused in participants by these sorts of measures, especially since apparently all participants knew that they were in this study because they attended a specific church.

continued

Research Box 14.4. *continued*

We have noted the many problems with the I scale and especially the E scale. In fact, an entire subliterature has evolved, arguing the pros and cons of these two scales. At one extreme, Kirkpatrick and Hood (1990) have suggested, as one of several possibilities, that the scales might be abandoned because of their many problems. Altemeyer (1996) concluded that the E and I scales "plainly failed to measure what they were supposed to measure . . . [and] plainly failed to show what they were supposed to show" (p. 154), and that the sizeable literature based on these two scales can be safely ignored.

Certainly the psychometric properties of the scales vary from study to study, and are sometimes less than convincing. Cronbach's alpha (a measure of internal consistency) tends to be somewhat erratic, and Donahue (1985a) has concluded that the E scale especially suffers from low internal consistency and item–total correlations. It is tempting to speculate that the problems with these scales contributed to Allport and Ross's decision not to report any psychometric information on the scales in their 1967 article. A number of authors have attempted to deal with the scales' problems by rewording, rewriting, reconceptualizing, or restructuring them. Most researchers who use the I and E scales today rely on a consistent Likert-type "agree–disagree" response format, although the original scale used different response formats across items. Attempts to consider subdimensions (personal vs. social well-being) of the E scale have offered some promise (Kirkpatrick, 1989; Gorsuch & McPherson, 1989).

It might be argued that, regardless of the problems with the scales and the original Allport and Ross report of a link between prejudice and intrinsic-extrinsic religiosity, so many subsequent studies have confirmed their initial conclusions that we should not over-concern ourselves with problems in the initial investigation. That is, the "weight of the evidence" suggests that IP individuals are more prejudiced than are extrinsic individuals, who in turn are more prejudiced than intrinsic persons—and that this in turn justifies the I-E conceptualization. But others are concerned about the scales' psychometric shortcomings, the lack of conceptual clarity, the inconsistency in Allport and Ross's results and some subsequent findings, and indeed the difficulty in making sense of these findings in light of the problems mentioned above.

Finally, we have offered this critique of a classic study for several reasons. We do not in any way wish to belittle the work and contributions of Gordon Allport, who stimulated a tremendous amount of psychological research and theory about religion. Rather, it is important to consider all research, including "classic studies," with a critical eye. Scientific progress depends on such criticality. The critical approach is especially important because flawed research sometimes becomes firmly embedded in the literature as fact, even when subsequent evidence does not support the initial findings. Also, the conclusions of the Allport and Ross study in particular have had a huge influence on the psychology of religion in general, and on work on religion and prejudice in particular. We might have saved ourselves a lot of trouble, and had a clearer view of religion and prejudice years ago, if researchers had more carefully considered the problems inherent in the Allport and Ross (1967) research.

Is Social Desirability a Confounding Variable?

There have been attempts to reinterpret the findings regarding I-E religious orientations and prejudice. For example, Batson et al. (1993) argued that social desirability may be acting as an intervening variable, confusing the relationship between prejudice and I-E religiosity. They suggested that social desirability and the I orientation are positively correlated, making it difficult to assess the real relationship between intrinsic religiosity and prejudice. Intrinsic persons may *seem* to be less prejudiced because they are also concerned with "looking good," and therefore they respond to questionnaire items on prejudice in a biased manner, making themselves look less prejudiced than they actually are. Batson et al. suggested that if we could just control for these social desirability effects among intrinsic individuals the negative correlation between I scores and prejudice that sometimes appears may disappear or may even be reversed. Batson and his colleagues carried out two studies that seem to support this interpretation.

Batson, Flink, Schoenrade, Fultz, and Pych (1986) and Batson, Naifeh, and Pate (1978) reported that I scores were negatively correlated with overt prejudice, but this relationship was not apparent when the effects of social desirability were controlled for in the first study, or when a covert behavioral measure of prejudice was used in the second study. E scores were unrelated to all measures of prejudice. These findings differ from previous research in important ways. As Donahue (1985b) pointed out, previous studies have typically revealed little or no relationship between I scores and prejudice, but have shown a weak positive correlation between E scores and prejudice. The two Batson et al. studies apparently reveal very different trends—positive associations between I scores and prejudice, but no relationship for E scores.

Batson et al. (1978) reported a link in one study between I scores and social desirability (.36), whereas other authors have been unable to find a significant relationship in this regard (e.g., Hunsberger & Platonow, 1986; Spilka, Kojetin, & McIntosh, 1985) or have reported a significant but very low correlation (.12; Duck & Hunsberger, 1999). Also, two studies (Duck & Hunsberger, 1999; Morris, Hood, & Watson, 1989) found that controlling for social desirability did not change prejudice–religion relationships. Furthermore, it has been argued (Watson, Morris, Foster, & Hood, 1986) that weak positive correlations between I scores (or scores on a similar religiousness dimension) and social desirability are unique to the Crowne–Marlowe Social Desirability scale (Crowne & Marlowe, 1964; the measure used by Batson et al., 1978, and Duck & Hunsberger, 1999). That is, such correlations are not a result of social desirability, but appear because the Crowne–Marlowe Social Desirability scale "has a substantial number of items confounded by a religious relevance dimension" (Watson et al., 1986, p. 230). However, Leak and Fish (1989) have challenged Watson et al.'s conclusions in this regard. The reader will understand why these discrepancies make it difficult to come to firm conclusions regarding the role of social desirability in the relationship between intrinsic religiousness and prejudice.

The assertions of many psychology of religion articles and texts notwithstanding, the relationship between prejudice and the I-E dichotomy is at best tenuous and difficult to interpret. At times it seems that the I-E distinction, which was intended to help us understand Allport's paradoxical assertion that religion both makes (the E religious orientation) and unmakes (the I religious orientation) prejudice, has instead led us into a psychometric and empirical morass of confusion. Certainly, not all authors agree with this rather bleak assessment of the research on I-E religiosity and prejudice, and some see more potential for these concepts in the future. Studies focusing on the I-E orientations continue to appear regularly in the literature. However, other approaches to religious orientation may offer more promise in explaining the religion–prejudice connection.

Proscribed versus Nonproscribed Prejudice

It seems logical that for religious people, the stand of their church on issues of prejudice would have some effect on their own attitudes and behavior. However, it has been noted that the existing research on religion and prejudice rarely considers the potential impact of the formal or informal stance of one's religious group on such issues (Batson et al., 1993; Batson & Burris, 1994). If religious communities make serious attempts to eliminate prejudiced attitudes ("proscribed prejudice"), it is argued that highly religious (e.g., intrinsic) individuals will at least give the appearance that they are unprejudiced on overt measures of prejudice, such as pencil-and-paper questionnaires. They see themselves as religious persons. Their church teaches that a specific prejudice is wrong. Therefore, they say that they do not hold that particular prejudice.

But there may be situations in which a religious group does not attempt to negate prejudice, and in fact may even formally or informally support specific prejudice ("nonproscribed prejudice"). In such cases, the same religious (e.g., intrinsic) persons will be likely to admit to their prejudice because it is sanctioned by their church. That is, people who try to live their religion will openly include discriminatory attitudes as part of their approach to the world around them. Furthermore, Batson et al. (1993) argued that even if prejudice is condemned, religious persons will admit to their discriminatory attitudes if the measure of prejudice is "covert," as in the case of subtle behavioral measures.

Other researchers (e.g., Fisher et al., 1994; Griffin, Gorsuch, & Davis, 1987; Herek, 1987; McFarland, 1989) have made similar suggestions, though Batson et al. (1993) have most clearly articulated the potentially important distinction between proscribed and nonproscribed prejudice. But how do we decide which prejudices are proscribed and which are not? One might argue that all prejudice is proscribed by Christian and some non-Christian religions, which teach that people should be sensitive, caring, and helpful to *all* other people. But specific religious individuals and groups have used religious teachings as justification for many discriminatory attitudes and behaviors. Even within Christianity, interpretations of Biblical passages vary from denomination to denomination, from church to church, and even from individual to individual within a given church. It is not always easy to ascertain whether specific prejudice is proscribed or not, partly because of such variations.

Batson et al. (1993) have argued that some prejudice (e.g., racial) is now generally proscribed by mainline North American Christian churches, but that prejudice against homosexuals and Communists is not. Certainly the link between religion and negative attitudes toward homosexuality is well established (e.g., Fisher et al., 1994; Gentry, 1987; Herek, 1988; Kunkel & Temple, 1992; Marsiglio, 1993; VanderStoep & Green, 1988; see also Chapter 7). Unfortunately, most studies on religion and homosexuality have not attempted to assess the proscribed–nonproscribed distinction. Duck and Hunsberger (1999) examined this issue by asking undergraduate students directly about church teachings related to prejudice. Their results indicated that, as predicted by Batson and his colleagues, racial prejudice was typically proscribed by students' religious groups, but intolerance toward gay and lesbians persons was generally not proscribed.

Importantly, Duck and Hunsberger's (1999) results mostly supported Batson et al.'s (1993) predictions about the role of proscription and nonproscription in the relationship between religious orientation and prejudice. For example, I scores were negatively related to proscribed prejudice (racism), but positively associated with nonproscribed prejudice (negative attitudes toward homosexuals) in two separate studies. Also, as predicted, Q scores were negatively correlated with both proscribed and nonproscribed prejudice (although one of four correlations was not statistically significant). Apparently, the position of one's church vis-à-vis specific prejudices is potentially important, and future research should focus on related issues.

Religious Fundamentalism and Quest

Recent evidence suggests that there may be other ways of assessing religious orientation that are more productive in explaining religion's link with prejudice than the traditional I-E. Of particular interest are the concepts of quest and religious fundamentalism. Both of these approaches to religious orientation avoid focusing on the content of beliefs; rather, they emphasize the ways in which beliefs are held, as well as the openness of people to changes in their beliefs.

Defining Quest

In the 1970s, Batson proposed the existence of a quest religious orientation, quite distinct from the then-popular I-E dichotomy (see, e.g., Batson et al., 1993). The quest (Q) orientation involves a questioning, open, flexible approach to religious issues—and, importantly for this chapter, it is theoretically associated with a tolerant, nonprejudiced view of the world. Questions about the conceptual and methodological underpinnings of quest have been raised (e.g., Donahue, 1985b). Also, an early version of a Q scale was criticized on psychometric grounds (see, e.g., Altemeyer, 1996). Batson and Schoenrade (1991a, 1991b) subsequently developed a 12-item revised Q scale that addressed the earlier problems, and that generated Cronbach's alphas of .81 and .75 in two samples. Other Q scales have also been developed (e.g., Altemeyer & Hunsberger, 1992; alpha = .88). But we must be careful in comparing different Q scales; there is little item overlap, and it is not clear to what extent different scales might tap different conceptualizations of quest. Batson's 12-item revised Q scale has become the instrument of choice in much related research.

Defining Fundamentalism

Early in the 20th century, William James (1902/1985) anticipated the importance of going beyond the content or orthodoxy of a person's beliefs. He argued that a rigid, dogmatic style of religious belief might be associated with bigotry and prejudice. Over the years, some investigators have used the term "religious fundamentalism" (RF) to capture this rigid, dogmatic way of being religious. In this context, some researchers reported a positive relationship between fundamentalism and prejudice. However, the definition of the term "fundamentalism" was quite variable, and often did not correspond to religious use of the word. In fact, early researchers often used the term interchangeably with "orthodoxy of belief," "intense interest in religion," or "considerable religious involvement."

Altemeyer and Hunsberger (1992) have offered a conceptualization of RF that is theoretically distinct from these other aspects of religion:

the belief that there is one set of religious teachings that clearly contains the fundamental, basic, intrinsic, essential, inerrant truth about humanity and deity; that this essential truth is fundamentally opposed by forces of evil which must be vigorously fought; that this truth must be followed today according to the fundamental, unchangeable practices of the past; and that those who believe and follow these fundamental teachings have a special relationship with the deity. (p. 118)

This definition, which is consistent with other theoretical work on fundamentalism (e.g., Kirkpatrick, Hood, & Hartz, 1991), is potentially applicable to most major world religions— unlike much previous work on fundamentalism. Also, the reader will recognize that we might expect this conceptualization to be negatively related to Batson et al.'s (1993) Q orientation, which involves a questioning approach to religion; openness and flexibility; and a resistance to clear-cut, pat answers. Altemeyer and Hunsberger (1992; see Research Box 14.5, below) developed a 20-item RF scale to measure their conceptualization. The RF scale is balanced against response sets and generated Cronbach's alphas of .91 to .95 in different studies.

Relationships with Prejudice

The RF and Q scales have been found to correlate significantly with measures of prejudice. Batson et al. (1993) cited five studies that revealed significant negative relationships between Q scores and prejudice (Batson et al., 1978, 1986; McFarland, 1989, 1990; Snook & Gorsuch, 1985). Two other studies (Griffin et al., 1987; Ponton & Gorsuch, 1988) did not replicate this negative association. However, all of these studies apparently used the earlier, psychometrically weaker version of Batson's Q scale (Batson & Ventis, 1982).

More recent studies using Batson and Schoenrade's (1991a, 1991b) revised Q scale have sometimes replicated the significant negative associations between quest and intolerance (Duck & Hunsberger, 1999), as did research by Altemeyer and Hunsberger (1992) with their own version of the Q scale. Similarly, the research on helping (Batson et al., 1999, 2001) discussed earlier in this chapter (see Research Box 14.2) seems to support the link between Q and tolerance. However, still other investigations (often with different versions of the Q scale) have obtained rather mixed results (Fisher et al., 1994; Fulton et al., 1999; Jackson & Hunsberger, 1999; Kirkpatrick, 1993).

Altemeyer and Hunsberger (1992) reported that their RF and Q scales were strongly negatively correlated ($r = -.79$ in an adult sample), as expected. They also found that RF scores were significantly and positively correlated with four measures of prejudice and authoritarian aggression (r's ranged from .23 to .41), and that Q scores were significantly negatively associated with the same prejudice measures (r's ranged from $-.26$ to $-.39$). The positive relationship between fundamentalism and prejudice has apparently been essentially replicated elsewhere (e.g., Fulton et al., 1999; Kirkpatrick, 1993; McFarland, 1989) in studies involving somewhat different measures of fundamentalism that had a more Christian focus, as well as in studies involving the original RF scale or a variation (Altemeyer, 2003; Hunsberger, 1996; Hunsberger, Owusu, & Duck, 1999; Jackson & Esses, 1997; Laythe et al., 2001; Wylie & Forest, 1992).

Can Prejudice Be Reduced by Decreasing Fundamentalism?

In light of the consistently strong relationships between fundamentalism and prejudice, one might wonder whether we might be able to reduce prejudice if only we could effectively weaken tendencies toward RF (see, e.g., Hunsberger, 1996). Given the correlational nature of findings, we must be cautious about such cause-and-effect implications.

However, Billiet (1995) argued that among his sample of Flemish Catholics, "sociocultural Christianity" tended to prevent fundamentalism, a religious orientation that he felt could encourage ethnocentrism. He defined sociocultural Christianity as "the values of solidarity, charity, and social justice, which have been emphasized in the legitimations and the collective identity of the Catholic social organizations [in Belgium] since the late sixties" (p. 231). Thus Billiet posited that a pattern of specific faith values (sociocultural Christianity), when taught and emphasized by churches, might actually reduce ethnocentrism by counteracting the development of RF. Billiet pointed out that Flemish "Catholic church leaders and prominent Catholics declared openly that they favored the integration of immigrants, and Catholic organizations promoted the idea" (p. 232). This is consistent with the suggestion that the proscribed–nonproscribed distinction is important in the study of religion and prejudice.

Summary of the Fundamentalism–Quest Research

In the end, these relationships between RF and Q on the one hand, and prejudice on the other, emphasize the potential importance and utility of these two approaches to religious orientation in explaining the historical religion–prejudice relationship. However, it is appropriate to consider an additional concept, right-wing authoritarianism (RWA), in this regard.

The Link with Right-Wing Authoritarianism

Religion, Authoritarianism, and Prejudice

Over 50 years ago, it was noted by Adorno et al. (1950) that religiousness was related to authoritarianism, as measured by the California F scale. For example, it was rare for religious people also to score low on authoritarianism. However, Adorno et al.'s work has received considerable criticism on methodological and conceptual grounds (see, e.g., Altemeyer, 1981), and these authors used rather unsophisticated operationalizations of religion (e.g., frequency of attendance, importance of religion).

Work by Altemeyer (1981, 1988, 1996) has confirmed that RWA may help us to understand the relatively high levels of prejudice found among religious persons scoring high on RF and low on Q. Altemeyer's reconceptualization of authoritarianism focuses on three attitudinal clusters (authoritarian submission, authoritarian aggression, and conventionalism), instead of Adorno et al.'s nine components. As Duckitt (1992) has noted, Altemeyer's conceptualization of authoritarianism and his development of a reliable and valid Right-Wing Authoritarianism (RWA) scale to measure this construct "finally seem to have made it possible for the study of authoritarianism to move beyond the unresolved methodological controversies and inconclusive findings that have thus far plagued it" (p. 209).

Adding Fundamentalism and Quest to the Equation

Altemeyer and Hunsberger (1992) conducted a study to assess the links among RF, Q, prejudice, and RWA (see Research Box 14.5). They found that people who scored high on the RWA scale tended also to score high on RF ($r = .68$), as well as to be prejudiced in a variety of ways (r's $= .33$ to $.64$). This is not to imply that all high-RWA individuals are high on RF, or the reverse. However, "off-quadrant" cases (i.e., those high on RWA and low on RF, or vice versa) were quite rare, and Altemeyer (1988) concluded that RF and RWA do seem to "feed" each other. That is, they both encourage obedience to authority, conventionalism, self-righteousness, and feelings of superiority.

Given these relationships, and Billiet's (1995) argument that fundamentalism is a cause of ethnocentrism, we might wonder whether fundamentalism or authoritarianism (or neither) is the more basic "causative agent" with respect to prejudice. This is not an easy matter to resolve, especially with the available correlational data, but the evidence leans toward authoritarianism as the more basic factor. For example, in Altemeyer and Hunsberger's (1992) central study of almost 500 adults, partialing out the effects of RWA from the sizeable RF–prejudice relationship reduced these correlations to nonsignificant levels. But removing RF from the RWA–prejudice associations reduced them only slightly. These findings were confirmed by multiple-regression analyses in work carried out by Laythe et al. (2001). Although not definitive, this suggests that RWA is the more basic contributor to prejudice. In other words, RF correlates with measures of prejudice because those high in RF tend also to be high in RWA. Possibly, as Hunsberger (1995) has suggested, "fundamentalism might be viewed as a religious manifestation of right-wing authoritarianism" (p. 121). If this is true, one might expect people with RWA personalities to become high in RF and RF would be expected to encourage and reinforce this (authoritarian) personality.

We have focused here on links among RWA, prejudice, and RF, but RWA is also an important variable when other aspects of religion are considered. For example, Duck and Hunsberger (1999) concluded that RWA was a stronger predictor of prejudice than was proscription status; furthermore, RWA was significantly correlated with I scores (.39), but negatively related to E (–.23) and Q (–.27) scores. Indeed, controlling for RWA scores in relationships between I scores and prejudice eliminated a positive correlation for attitudes toward homosexuals (nonproscribed prejudice) and increased the negative association in the case of racial (proscribed) prejudice. These authors speculated that RWA scores might act as a moderating variable between different religious orientations (especially the I orientation) and prejudice, and they recommended that a reconceptualization of the I orientation take into account the RWA component.

Differing Perspectives

The findings described above have not gone without comment in the psychology-of-religion literature. Gorsuch (1993) questioned several aspects of the Altemeyer and Hunsberger (1992) study, and the authors provided additional data and arguments that supported their original conclusions (Altemeyer & Hunsberger, 1993).

Leak and Randall (1995) have suggested that RWA's positive association with religion is limited to measures of "less mature faith development" (p. 245). They found that such measures of "less mature" religion (e.g., a scale assessing Christian orthodoxy, measures of Fowler's second and third stages of faith development [see Chapter 4], and church attendance) were positively related to RWA scores, but that measures of "more mature" religion (e.g., Batson's Q scale, measures of Fowler's fourth and fifth faith stages, and a Global Faith Development scale) were negatively correlated with RWA.

The real issue here may be semantics. Just what *is* "mature faith"? Leak and Randall have chosen to regard a quest sort of orientation as "mature" (see also Kristensen, Pedersen, & Williams, 2001). Their Global Faith Development scale included items such as "It is very

❧

Research Box 14.5. Authoritarianism, Religious Fundamentalism, Quest, and Prejudice (Altemeyer & Hunsberger, 1992)

Based on their conceptualization of religious fundamentalism (see text), the authors developed a 20-item RF scale, including items such as "God will punish most severely those who abandon his true religion." They developed this measure, as well as a 16-item Q scale, in several studies of university students in Manitoba and Ontario. Satisfied that their new measures were reliable and interrelated as expected among students, the authors then carried out an investigation of 491 Canadian parents of university students.

In addition to the RF and Q scales, these adults completed a 12-item Attitudes Toward Homosexuals scale (e.g., "In many ways, the AIDS disease currently killing homosexuals is just what they deserve"); a 20-item Prejudice scale (e.g., "It is a waste of time to train certain races for good jobs; they simply don't have the drive and determination it takes to learn a complicated skill"); the RWA scale; and two additional measures of prejudice—a Posse–Radicals survey (in which participants indicated the extent to which they would pursue radicals outlawed by the government), and a Trials measure (in which respondents "passed sentence" in three court cases involving a dope pusher, a pornographer, and someone who spit on a provincial premier). The resulting web of relatively strong and significant correlations led these authors to conclude the following about the answer to the question "Are religious persons usually good persons?":

> [It] appears to be "no," if one means by "religious" a fundamentalist, nonquesting religious orientation, and by "good" the kind of nonprejudiced, compassionate, accepting attitudes espoused in the Gospels and other writings. But the answer is "yes" if one means by "religious" the nonfundamentalist, questing orientation found most often in persons belonging to no religion. Which irony gives one pause. (pp. 125–126)

The authors cautioned against overgeneralizing these findings, since there were inevitably exceptions to the rule—people scoring high on the RF scale and low on the Q scale who showed nonprejudiced, accepting attitudes; or people scoring low on RF and high on Q who were bigoted. But the correlations that emerged were quite strong and clear-cut. Apparently individuals who scored high on RF and low on Q, as defined here, tended to be prejudiced in a variety of ways. The authors speculated that fundamentalist beliefs can be linked to some of the psychological sources of authoritarian aggression (e.g., fear of a dangerous world and self-righteousness), as well as the tendency for high-RWA individuals to reduce guilt over their own misdeeds through their religion.

---

important for me to critically examine my religious beliefs and values" (p. 248), and in this respect it bears some resemblance to Q scales. It is not surprising that such measures have a negative association with authoritarianism, as previously reported by Altemeyer and Hunsberger (1992). However, it seems a moot point to define, for example, global faith development and a quest orientation as "mature," and religious orthodoxy and fundamentalism as "less mature." Religiously orthodox persons and those with a fundamentalist orientation may feel that *their* religion is the mature one, and that questing is immature. Of course, Gordon Allport considered an I orientation to be mature and an E orientation to be immature (Allport, 1954; Allport & Ross, 1967). In any case, we would suggest that Leak and Randall's findings, aside from the maturity issue, are consistent with earlier findings of relationships among RF, Q, RWA, and prejudice.

Laythe et al. (2001) suggested that in addition to RWA, there is a second component of RF that predicts prejudice. They nominated "belief content."

> Christian religious teaching may indeed "unmake prejudice" in the most direct way: Strength of orthodox Christian belief, stripped of authoritarian trappings, predicts decreased levels of racial prejudice. Unfortunately (at least from our perspective), such beliefs evidently are coupled with authoritarianism more often than not . . . given the well-documented positive correlation between measures of RWA and [Christian orthodoxy]. (p. 9)

Finally, it is worth noting that the relationships described here are not unique to the specific measures and North American samples reported above. Research from Europe, using very different measures of religiousness, authoritarianism, and prejudice, have found links among these measures that are quite consistent with the findings reported above (e.g., Billiet, 1995; Eisinga et al., 1995). Apparently the findings on religion, prejudice, and authoritarianism cut across differing variables and cultural contexts, at least within Christianity.

What about Non-Christian Religions and Samples outside North America?

Hunsberger (1996) assessed RF–RWA–prejudice relationships in small samples of people from non-Christian religions in Canada. The psychometric properties of the RF scale, as well as its relationship to prejudice and RWA, remained relatively stable in small samples of adult Hindus, Muslims, and Jews. Cronbach's alpha for RF ranged from .85 to .94; its correlations with (negative) attitudes toward homosexuals were .42 to .65; and correlations between RF and RWA ranged from .45 to .74. The strength of these relationships is similar to those found in samples of mostly Christian adults and university students in Canada (Altemeyer & Hunsberger, 1992) and college students in the United States (Laythe et al., 2001). These associations have also been essentially replicated with Muslim and Christian university students in Ghana (Hunsberger et al., 1999). These results seem to confirm the links among RF, RWA, and prejudice across various religious groups in North America and elsewhere. However, further research is needed to assess the relationships in larger samples, and particularly for non-Christian groups outside North America.

Aside from the investigations just described, cross-cultural and cross-religious studies on religion and prejudice have been uncommon. Some work has been carried out in non-Christian settings and outside North America, but it typically does not include cross-cultural or cross-religious comparisons—and partly because of the diversity of measures involved, such studies cannot be directly compared with each other.

A series of investigations has been carried out in Belgium and the Netherlands by a group of European researchers, focusing on religious beliefs, authoritarianism, and prejudice (Billiet, 1995; Duriez & Hutsebaut, 2000; Eisenga, Billiet, & Felling, 1999; Eisenga et al., 1990; Konig, Eisenga, & Scheepers, 2000), although they did not include any standard religious orientation measures (the commonly used I, E, Q, and RF scales). Consistent with some North American research (e.g., Altemeyer & Hunsberger, 1992; Jacobson, 1998; Laythe et al., 2001), these investigations have typically revealed little or no relationship between ethnic prejudice and measures of Christian belief or attendance, although there are occasional exceptions of positive (e.g., Duriez & Hutsebat, 2000) or negative (e.g., Billiet, 1995) relationships. Also, the influence of third variables (e.g., age, education, localism, authoritarianism, and anomie) apparently could statistically "explain" most of the positive religion–prejudice associations. An exception involved links between Christian beliefs and anti-Semitism, which could not similarly be "explained" by third variables.

Outside Europe and North America, several relevant investigations have been reported. Griffin et al. (1987) found that on the Caribbean island of St. Croix, members' commitment to the Seventh-Day Adventist Church and their intrinsic orientation were positively correlated with prejudice (withholding human rights from Rastafarians). However, the authors pointed out that church members perceived the church itself to be relatively prejudiced in this regard; therefore, this could be an instance of a positive link between an I orientation and prejudice when such prejudice is nonproscribed by one's church. In Venezuela, Ponton and Gorsuch (1988) reported a negative link between I religiosity and (ethnic) prejudice, as well as a positive association for E religiosity. The Q orientation was uncorrelated with prejudice. Of course, the proscription of specific prejudice may be specific to cultural, religious, and temporal context. For example, Lafferty (1990) argued that in South Africa racial prejudice was (until the abolition of apartheid) religiously nonproscribed, but others have pointed out that it is proscribed in North America (e.g., Batson et al., 1993; Duck & Hunsberger, 1999).

A study at a university in northern India showed a "reverse prejudice" (Murphy-Berman, Berman, Pachauri, & Kumar, 1985, p. 33), in that Hindu students allocated more money to Muslim (than to Hindu) targets in a hypothetical situation. The authors speculated that a social desirability effect might have influenced the results. Hassan and Khalique (1987) reported a tendency for Muslim college students to be more prejudiced than Hindus. In Bangladesh, Hewstone, Islam, and Judd (1993) had Muslims (the majority group) and Hindus (the minority group) evaluate targets of different religion (Muslim or Hindu) and nationality (Bangladeshi or Indian). They concluded that religion and nationality were both important predictors of outgroup discrimination.

Such studies are important in broadening the investigation of religion and prejudice to different cultural and religious groups in the world. However, these studies often do not include comparison groups; their measures and samples vary considerably; results are sometimes seemingly contradictory; and it is therefore very difficult to compare their results and make sense of them in a systematic way. Comprehensive cross-cultural research is needed—especially investigations that compare the same measures and similar samples across cultures and religious groups, while controlling for other important variables such as proscription status, demographic aspects of the sample, and the cultural context of the research (e.g., majority vs. minority status of participants).

The Target of Prejudice

Earlier in this chapter, we have concluded that the position of one's church on specific prejudices (i.e., proscribed vs. nonproscribed) may have important implications for self-reported personal prejudice. Possibly related to the proscribed–nonproscribed distinction, the target of prejudice seems to be important. In particular, some authors have noted different religion–prejudice relationships when the target of prejudice involves racial groups compared to groups based on sexual orientation (e.g., Herek, 1987; Laythe et al., 2001).

Hunsberger and Jackson (in press) constructed a table to show relationships between four religious orientations (I, E, Q, and RF) and measures of prejudice directed toward specific targets (racial/ethnic groups, gay or lesbian persons, women, Communists, and religious outgroups), as well as the RWA scale (as a measure often associated with prejudice). They included only studies published from 1990 to the time their paper was written in 2003, and only investigations that used the well-accepted I, E, Q, and RF scales. They included 16 different papers[2] that reported studies of 25 distinct samples involving more than 5,800 adults and undergraduate students. The results of their survey are shown in Table 14.1.

If one were simply to examine the total scores in the bottom row of this table, one would conclude that I, E, and RF were all associated with intolerance. The reader will recall that the literature typically portrays the I orientation as linked to tolerance rather than intolerance, however. Furthermore, Table 14.1 shows that Q was usually associated with increased tolerance in these studies, as expected. However, the relationships sometimes changed markedly for different targets of prejudice. If we consider only ethnic and racial targets, the historical expectation of a negative correlation with I scores was evident in 4 of 4 studies. But in 7 of 9 samples, I scores were *positively* related to intolerance directed toward gay men and lesbians. This difference apparently supports the proscribed–nonproscribed distinction (e.g., Batson & Burris, 1994) when the I religious orientation and prejudice were considered.

Studies involving the E and Q scales were more mixed, but there was some tendency for the E scale to be positively related to both racial/ethnic prejudice (3 of 4 studies) and gay/lesbian prejudice (4 of 8 investigations), and also for the Q scale to be linked to more tolerant attitudes toward racial/ethnic groups (2/5, but no correlations were negative) and gay/lesbian persons (7/9). The most consistent predictor of prejudice, regardless of target, was the RF scale, which in every case was linked to negative attitudes toward gay/lesbian persons, women, Communists, and religious outgroups, as well as to RWA (39/39 findings in total). Only the relationship between RF and racial/ethnic prejudice was less clear (5 positive relationships, 6 nonsignificant findings).

TABLE 14.1. Relationships between Four Religious Orientations and Measures of Intolerance: A Survey of Studies from 1990 to 2003

	Religious orientation measure											
	I			E			Q			RF		
Type of intolerance	+	0	–	+	0	–	+	0	–	+	0	–
Racial/ethnic groups	0	0	4	3	1	0	0	3	2	5	6	0
Gay/lesbian persons	7	1	1	4	2	2	0	2	7	17	0	0
Women	0	1	0	0	1	0	0	1	0	3	0	0
Communists	1	0	0	0	1	0	0	1	0	3	0	0
Religious outgroups	1	0	0	1	0	0	0	1	0	3	0	0
RWA	2	0	0	0	0	2	0	0	4	13	0	0
Total	11	2	5	8	5	4	0	8	13	44	6	0

Note. Sixteen studies, some with multiple samples and/or multiple measures, are included. "+," significant positive relationship between religious orientation and intolerance; "0," no relationship; "–," significant negative relationship. Adapted from Hunsberger and Jackson (in press). Copyright by Blackwell Publishing, Ltd. Adapted by permission.

2. Altemeyer (2003); Altemeyer and Hunsberger (1992); Batson et al. (1999); Duck and Hunsberger (1999); Fisher et al. (1994); Fulton et al. (1999); Griffiths, Dixon, Stanley, and Weiland (2001); Hunsberger (1996); Hunsberger et al. (1999); Jackson and Esses, (1997); Jackson and Hunsberger (1999); Kirkpatrick (1993); Laythe et al. (2001, 2002); Leak and Randall (1995); and Wylie and Forest (1992).

Unfortunately, there have been few studies involving prejudice toward such target groups as women, Communists (or other political or ideological groups), or religious outgroups—including both prejudice toward nonreligious individuals (Hunter, 2001; Jackson & Hunsberger, 1999) and more general "religious ethnocentrism" (Altemeyer, 2003). Work is needed to assess links between such specific types of prejudice and religious orientation measures, and also to assess the extent to which antipathy toward such targets is religiously proscribed.

Relatedly, the specific measure of prejudice can also be important. Many different pencil-and-paper instruments have been used to measure prejudice; unfortunately, some self-report scales suffer from such problems as weak or unreported psychometric properties, the fact that they are obviously tapping prejudice, social desirability effects, and so on. Although more subtle and more valid pencil-and-paper indices of prejudice have been proposed (e.g., McConahay, 1986; Rudman, Greenwald, Mellott, & Schwartz, 1999), such measures have seldom been used in religion–prejudice investigations. More subtle measures may be necessary to identify prejudice against targets that tend to be protected by religious or other societal standards. For example, studies have found that more subtle (implicit) measures draw out evidence of greater anti-Semitism in both the United States (Rudman et al., 1999) and Italy (Franco & Maass, 1999) than do more explicit measures.

Distinguishing between Sin and Sinner

In the section on helping and religion, we have referred to a distinction that is sometimes made between "sin" and "sinner." In the context of prejudice, it has been argued that anti-homosexual sentiment may stem partly from Biblically based moral judgments (e.g., Leviticus 18:22), which committed Christians such as those high in I orientation or RF would take very seriously as the word of God (Fulton et al., 1999; Gorsuch, 1993). The implication seems to be that Christians high in RF and/or I would distinguish between the perceived sin (i.e., homosexual behavior) and the perceived sinner (i.e., the gay person), such that they would "hate the sin, but love the sinner."

Fulton et al. (1999) reported some support for this position from an investigation of students at a conservative Christian college with a Seventh-Day Adventist affiliation. The researchers attempted to categorize negative attitudes toward gays and lesbians into morally rationalized (sin) and nonmorally rationalized (sinner) groups. Examples of items representing these two categories are "Homosexuality is a perversion," and "A person's homosexuality should not be a cause for job discrimination," respectively (Fulton et al., 1999, p. 17). The authors concluded that their results indicated that the I orientation in particular was correlated with morally rationalized but not nonmmorally rationalized antipathy: "Intrinsics appear to be relatively accepting of homosexual people, but not of homosexual behavior" (p. 19). This study was limited by the unique (e.g., relatively high-RF) and homogeneous nature of the sample, and the use of an unpublished RF scale (we do not know how it compares to other measures of this concept). Also, the authors did not report the internal consistency of the measures used—for example, for the moral and nonmoral subscales—and some of the items drawn from the original Herek (1987) scale to measure attitudes toward homosexuals do not fall neatly into "morally rationalized" and "nonmorally rationalized" categories. These issue could have affected the results of the investigation.

The few other studies that speak to this issue have not supported Fulton et al.'s (1999) conclusion. Indeed, Altemeyer and Hunsberger (1993) pointed out that fundamentalism was associated with condemnation of both sin and sinner on an item-by-item basis in their study of attitudes toward gay persons. Research by Batson et al. (1999, 2001), discussed earlier in this chapter in the "Helping Behavior" section, led to the conclusion that intrinsic individuals do *not* distinguish between sin and sinner. Burris and Jackson (1999) interpreted their findings in a study of attributions regarding partner abuse as inconsistent with the sin–sinner interpretation proposed by Fulton et al.

Given the fact that few studies have investigated this sin–sinner issue, the limitations of the existing studies, and the lack of consistency in their results, the issue deserves further empirical attention.

Is Cognitive Style Relevant?

Since religions offer people a particular view of the world, potentially giving meaning to their existence and offering answers to questions about the universe and the world around them, one might wonder whether religions influence people to think in similar ways (see Hunsberger & Jackson, in press). Some evidence does point in this direction. For example, RF is apparently related to complexity of thought about existential issues (e.g., Hunsberger, Alisat, Pancer, & Pratt, 1996; Hunsberger, Pratt, & Pancer, 1994). "High and low fundamentalists may actually perceive and deal with their own (and others') religious experiences in different ways" (Hunsberger et al., 1996, p. 218); that is, high-RF persons may tend to incorporate new information into an existing religious schema, whereas low-RF persons may be more likely to adapt their religious beliefs to accommodate religious doubts or new information. Also, the Q orientation has been associated with increased complexity of thought (Batson & Raynor-Prince, 1983) and openness to different perspectives (McFarland & Warren, 1992).

It has been suggested that such unique cognitive styles, associated with religious orientation, might help us to understand the religion–prejudice connection (Hunsberger & Jackson, in press). Specifically, those high in RF may tend to cling to existing stereotypes rather than changing their views in light of new information. Conversely, those with a Q orientation may be inclined to think more complexly about both religion and, for example, cultural diversity, contributing to greater tolerance of such diversity. Similarly, these individuals' tendency toward greater cognitive complexity may incline them to be less influenced by group or social norms that tolerate prejudice. However, these possibilities remain speculation, awaiting empirical test.

Beyond Personal Religion to Group Effects

Several recent papers have argued that research on religion and prejudice needs to expand to focus more on intergroup issues (Altemeyer, 2003; Hunsberger & Jackson, in press; Jackson & Hunsberger, 1999). Historically, research on religion and prejudice has been dominated by work involving an individual-difference perspective (especially that of religious orientation), as reflected in much of our discussion so far in this chapter. However, it has been argued that a group perspective could help us to understand religion–prejudice relationships.

Some theories of intergroup relations suggest that group members are susceptible to prejudice against outgroup members. For example, social identity theory (e.g., Tajfel & Turner, 1986) posits that personal self-esteem may be bolstered when group members compare themselves with other groups. In terms of religious groups, if individuals believe that their religion is the source of absolute truth, this could enhance their self-esteem (and ingroup attachment); it could also serve as a source of prejudice against members of other religions, who are seen as belonging to inferior groups. In general, it could seemingly justify intolerance of people who do not adhere to divinely revealed morality (Hunsberger & Jackson, in press).

Similarly, realistic group conflict theory (e.g., Sherif, 1966) argues that the perception of being in competition with other groups for valued resources can exacerbate intergroup tension and prejudice. Perceived threat to values can apparently engender greater discrimination against disadvantaged groups by some religious people (Jackson & Esses, 1997). So, for example, the perception that immigrants compete for jobs with established members of a society can foster prejudice against those immigrants' religion in particular (Jackson, 2001), even if the original perceptions of job competition are incorrect. In a similar vein, Struch and Schwartz (1989) reported that perceived conflict of interest among different Jewish groups in Israel was associated with intergroup negativity and endorsement of antagonistic behaviors toward outgroups. In this context, it has been argued that stronger religious group identification is characteristic of especially devout persons—for example, those who score high on such measures of religious orientation as I, orthodoxy, or RF scales (Hunsberger & Jackson, in press). Indeed, I scale scores have been found to be strongly correlated (+.70) with religious group identification (Burris & Jackson, 2000), as have RF scores (+.46) and scores on a measure of Christian orthodoxy (+.51) (Jackson & Hunsberger, 1999).

Jackson and Hunsberger (1999) reported two studies that investigated these intergroup conflict proposals in a religious context. Research Box 14.6 summarizes these studies, which led to the conclusion that there was quite pervasive prejudice against religious outgroup members. Similarly, Altemeyer (2003) found that both RF and emphasis on religious identity in childhood were associated with "religious exclusiveness," a kind of religious ethnocentrism involving a tendency to reject atheists as well as persons of other faiths (including faiths with rather similar beliefs to their own). These studies provide evidence that religious group membership per se can contribute to intergroup prejudice, especially intolerance of religious outgroup members.

Further Thoughts on Why Religion Is Sometimes Associated with Prejudice

Much of the literature on religion and prejudice attempts to describe how religion (particularly religious orientation) and prejudice are related, but does not explore in depth the underlying reasons for obtained links. That is, little work has addressed the issue of *why* religion and prejudice are associated. Hunsberger and Jackson (in press) have recently considered possible explanations for links. Several of these have been mentioned in our previous discussion of religion and prejudice, and are briefly summarized here.

1. Cognitive style (e.g., convergent vs. divergent thinking, integrative complexity of thought) may differ by religious orientation. The way people think about intergroup and interpersonal relationships may have some influence on their conclusions in this regard, and therefore their prejudice.

2. Personal goals and motives associated with one's religiosity may be linked with prejudice. For example, the religion of extrinsic individuals was traditionally thought to be a source of utilitarian benefits such as social status, while intrinsic persons were thought to be moti-

---

Research Box 14.6. An Intergroup Perspective on Prejudice
(Jackson & Hunsberger, 1999)

Both studies reported by these authors involved Christian and religiously nonaffiliated undergraduate students who were asked to complete measures of their religious orientation, as well as their attitudes toward various religious outgroups. Using an "evaluation thermometer" with labels describing every 10-degree change, participants indicated their evaluation of various groups: 0 degrees indicated "extremely unfavorable," 50 degrees was "neither favorable nor unfavorable," and 100 degrees was "extremely favorable." This measure has been used successfully in other research on intergroup attitudes and relations (see Haddock, Zanna, & Esses, 1993).

Results suggested that measures of RF, orthodoxy, I, E, and Q were *all* associated with more favorable attitudes toward ingroup members (Christians, "believers") and greater intolerance of religious outgroups (atheists, "nonbelievers"). It is particularly interesting that all religious orientation measures were associated with negativity toward outgroups, when it has been argued in the past that the I and particularly Q orientations should be associated with tolerance of others (see earlier discussion in this chapter). The authors concluded that "prejudice against religious outgroups is pervasive . . . religious intergroup relations are no different from any other form of intergroup relation, and . . . for a variety of reasons, group identifications can generate intergroup antagonism" (p. 521). Interestingly, people who identified themselves as atheists or nonbelievers did not show the same degree or pervasiveness of outgroup negativity toward religious groups (i.e., believers and Christians—"religious outgroups," from their perspective).

One might wonder about replicability with broader adult samples, since the original investigations involved undergraduates. However, the findings do suggest that analyses of religion and prejudice at the group level may hold considerable promise in clarifying religion–prejudice links, and researchers might be advised to focus more attention in this direction.

---

vated by "more mature" concerns, such as making religion a part of their lives. Such motivations should theoretically lead I persons to be more likely to accept religious teachings about brotherhood and tolerance (see Allport & Ross, 1967). Apparently this "explanation" has never been directly tested, and problems with the I-E approach noted earlier leave its validity in question.

3. The proscribed–nonproscribed distinction is possibly based on a desire to be seen as in good standing with one's religion (Batson & Burris, 1994). That is, church members who wish to be seen as "good" members (e.g., intrinsic persons) may be likely to accept church teachings related to tolerance, and therefore may be inclined to be relatively tolerant of members of other racial groups (typically a proscribed prejudice) but intolerant of gay or lesbian persons (typically a nonproscribed prejudice).

4. Religious group identification may promote ingroup glorification and outgroup derogation as a means of enhancing the self-esteem of group members, possibly through downward group comparisons. Intergroup conflict can also be promoted by perceived con-

flict with other (e.g., religious) groups over valued resources—ranging from material goods, economic benefits, and territory, to voting power and political influence.

5. As part of the group identification process, groups or individuals that threaten one's religious (or other) values may be especially open to derogation. Several studies have found that "value threat" may be an important stimulant or magnifier of prejudice (e.g., Batson et al., 2001; Jackson & Esses, 1997).

Several additional ideas about why religion might be linked with prejudice, not yet discussed in this chapter, have also been suggested by Hunsberger and Jackson (in press):

6. Religion might contribute to a legitimization of the status quo, even when inequalities exist between groups of people, possibly in part because of religion's tendency to be linked with conservative values (Hunsberger & Jackson, in press). For example, it has been found that intrinsic religiosity is associated with such values as "freedom" and "heritage" in the United States (Burris, Branscombe, & Jackson, 2000). Given that an emphasis on freedom may correspond to a lack of support for members of underprivileged groups (McConahay, 1986; Sears, 1988), religion may unwittingly contribute to such societal inequity by confirming the reality and importance of "freedom." This might be partly because people then incorrectly assume that the ideal of freedom of opportunity is actually a reality.

7. Prejudice does not always entail clearly negative attitudes toward others. Sometimes attitudes that seem to be positive may actually be a form of prejudice because they legitimize the unequal treatment of groups (see Glick & Fiske, 1996; Jackman, 1994). For example, some religions promote the apparently benign teaching that "men and women are different but equal." However, such teachings, especially when couched in positive, affectionate terms (e.g., "Women are especially loving and nurturant"), can serve as a basis for restricting women to low-status domestic roles and preventing them from assuming roles of leadership or power.

8. Prejudice can occur unconsciously (Greenwald & Banaji, 1995), and religious teachings against such bias might not be sufficient to counteract unconscious bias. Consequently, some people may hold an egalitarian self-image that is quite consistent with religious teachings, yet engage in stereotyping and discrimination. That is, such people may not realize that their attitudes and behavior could contribute to discrimination, at least in part because the discrimination can be rationalized in apparently genial ways.

9. Religious teachings may actually justify some intolerance, directly or indirectly. For example, it has been suggested that religious teachings justify negative attitudes toward same-sex sexuality (i.e., the behavior itself—Fulton et al., 1999), but these same teachings advocate loving the "sinner" (i.e., gay and lesbian persons). However, it is not clear that religious people who claim that the sin–sinner justification for antipathy toward same-sex sexuality actually make the distinction between sin and sinner in their everyday attitudes. Indeed, most prejudices do contain subjective justification, however authoritative or erroneous the source of justification may be construed by proponents and critics. In extreme form, acts of terrorism, war, and genocide have been justified in the name of religious ideals (Hunsberger & Jackson, in press).

Summary of the Religion–Prejudice Research

Clearly, the religion–prejudice link is more complicated than the initial suggestion of a linear relationship between church attendance and prejudiced attitudes indicated. We are not as convinced as some authors that the I-E dichotomy has been very helpful in understanding the relationship between religion and prejudice. Furthermore, we now know that it was premature to conclude that Gorsuch and Aleshire's (1974) review of the prejudice–religion literature "marked the end of an era, [since] by the early 1970s, mainstream American culture no longer countenanced blatant prejudice. The casual church attender thus stopped admitting to bigoted outlooks, and results became nonreplicable" (Spilka, Hood, & Gorsuch, 1985, p. 274). Developments in the 1990s have shown that we have much to learn about this area. High RF and low Q scores are apparently linked to prejudice and discrimination; there is also some evidence that it is not RF per se that causes prejudice, but rather the tendency for those high in RF to be high in RWA as well.

We have also emphasized that many other factors are important in the religion–prejudice relationship. These include cross-cultural and cross-religious issues, specific targets of prejudice, measurement problems, cognitive factors, and especially group dynamics and intergroup issues. We have summarized some reasons *why* religion may be associated with prejudice, but little research has been conducted to assess most of these possibilities.

It is disconcerting to some that those who make the strongest claims to being "true believers" of religious traditions, and who reportedly follow religious teachings most scrupulously, also tend to be the most intolerant of others. That is, prejudice seems relatively unrelated to the content of people's beliefs, but it is associated with the ways in which people hold their religious beliefs, possibly through the influence of RWA and group dynamics. These conclusions need further investigation, and work from the past decade in particular suggests considerable promise for these new approaches to help us understand the religion–prejudice relationships.

OVERVIEW

In Chapter 13, we have seen that religion does indeed seem to be related to some aspects of moral attitudes and behaviors. However, as noted in this chapter, faith is surprisingly unrelated to helping behavior. There are indications that religious people *say* they are more helpful, but the findings do not bear this out for actual behavior in a nonreligious setting. Within a religious context, the more faithful do indeed help more by giving money, time, and talent to religiously based causes. However, outside such a context, it becomes very difficult to distinguish helpers from nonhelpers on the basis of their religion. Batson and his coresearchers have tried to build a case that I religiousness is only related to the *appearance* of helpfulness, not to actual behavior; however, some studies failed to find any association between I scores and self-reported helping. Also, the Q religious orientation is usually positively associated with behavioral measures of giving assistance to others.

Furthermore, when people do help others, there is some evidence that persons with high I scores may offer a kind of preprogrammed, self-serving aid, whereas individuals scoring high on Q offer a more flexible and victim-focused assistance. Although there are arguments against this interpretation, some recent evidence confirms that a Q orientation tends to be linked with universal compassion, but that an I orientation is more likely to be associated with helping guided by the values of the helper (Batson et al., 1999, 2001).

The tendency for questers to demonstrate more universal compassion is perplexing, in the sense that the Q orientation bears little similarity to what most people think of as religion in a traditional sense. For example, persons with high Q scores tend to score low on measures of religious orthodoxy (Altemeyer & Hunsberger, 1992; Batson et al., 1993).

Possibly more troubling than this, however, is what we find in the area of prejudice. The evidence indicates that in some ways, religion is *positively* related to prejudice. This association has been researched and debated over the years, but in the end it seems that it is not religion per se that is linked to prejudice; rather, it is the ways in which one holds one's faith, the importance of one's religious *group* affiliation, and so on. Thus RF is positively, and Q negatively, associated with various measures of prejudice, and stronger identification with religious groups seems to be associated with more negative views of religious outgroups.

As with the research reviewed in Chapter 13, one drawback to most of the research discussed in this chapter is that it relies very heavily on self-reports—in this case, self-reports of religion, helping, and prejudice. Such self-reports may be inaccurate and unreliable, and possibly biased in socially or religiously desired ways. However, in most cases it is difficult to measure relevant helping or discriminatory behavior, and little research has attempted to do so, especially in highly sensitive domains such as prejudice. In consequence, we must once again rely on self-reports as "the next best thing"; they probably usually give us a fair idea of people's attitudes and behaviors. However, we must remain aware of the weakness inherent in this approach. We must attempt wherever possible to supplement these measures with reports from others (e.g., from parents, friends, teachers), and especially with actual behavioral measures.

Our knowledge of *how* religion is related to both helping and prejudice has advanced considerably in the last decade or two. Recent findings should serve as takeoff points for more studies. Also, speculation and limited evidence concerning *why* religion is sometimes associated with more intolerance deserve increased empirical attention.

Chapter 15

RELIGION, COPING, AND ADJUSTMENT

> When misery is the greatest, God is the closest.
>
> While I am sick, I desire the love of religion.
>
> God helps them that help themselves.
>
> A mighty fortress is our God,
> A bulwark never failing;
> Our helper He amid the flood
> Of mortal ills prevailing.
>
> We turn to God only to obtain the impossible.
>
> A little girl repeating the Twenty-Third Psalm said it this way: "The
> Lord is my shepherd, that's all I want."[1]

September 11, 2001 posed a huge and unexpected problem with which U.S. residents had to cope. The destruction of the World Trade Center in New York City, and the attack on the Pentagon in Washington, D.C., still reverberate in U.S. society. A war on terrorism was proclaimed, and the nation was immediately put on guard. Air passenger inspections were extensively tightened. The government mobilized a variety of resources for sensitizing the American people to the dangers posed by terrorism. Home preparedness became the watchword. At this writing, the United States continues to be bombarded with alarms and warnings of possible new attacks from enemies. How have people dealt with these changes?

In the week following the September 11 tragedy, U.S. national polling organizations reported anywhere from a 6% to a 24% increase in church attendance (Walsh, 2002). This trend continued through October into November. Members of many religious bodies sensed a revival of faith. People were turning to their deity for support and comfort. *The Boston Globe* reported that religious education programs were stimulated by "many of these new, terrorism-inspired seekers" (quoted in Walsh, 2002, p. 27). Was this indeed a new revival of faith? Apparently not, as 3 months later, the influx of churchgoers had receded to pre-September 11 levels. Coping by means of religion had subsided. Does this imply that religious coping is little more than a "passing fancy"? Even though we must await more definitive studies of who was affected by the September 11 disaster and how personal resources were marshaled, let

---

1. These quotations come, respectively, from the following sources: Gross (1982, p. 242); Theobaldus, quoted in Benham (1927, p. 843); Benjamin Franklin, quoted in Bartlett (1955, p. 330); Martin Luther, quoted in Bartlett (1955, p. 86); Albert Camus, quoted in Peter (1977, p. 213); Mead (1965, p. 166).

us examine the fact that religion often serves as a major bulwark in the way we handle the stress of living.

Coping is at the heart of life. From its biological and evolutionary roots to complex human social behavior, it is the essence of living. In individualistically oriented Western society in particular, people are usually judged on their ability to cope with what is demanded of them. In many cases, personal trials prompt people to turn to their faith for help. Religion may be an especially important resource when individuals must deal with those "times that try men's souls"—when crisis strikes and options are limited.

THEORETICAL APPROACHES TO COPING AND RELIGION

"Coping" means resolving the difficulties that confront us as human beings. This can be done in any of three ways—changing the environment, changing ourselves, or changing both to some degree. "Adaptation" involves the second or third possibility; "adjustment" more strictly implies self-modification to meet situation requirements.

In order to understand how people handle life's problems, some researchers have emphasized coping *styles* or *traits*—relatively long-lasting, if not permanent, characteristics of individuals. Others have looked to the *process* of coping, and to change in the way difficulties are handled (Lazarus & Folkman, 1984). Though it may be argued that personal religiosity is commonly treated as if it were an aspect of personality, those who have studied the role of religion in coping are mostly concerned with it as a process variable, asking what it does for the person and how it functions when problems arise.

The Process of Coping: Pargament's Theory

Probably the foremost scholar in research on the role of faith in relation to coping behavior is Kenneth Pargament of Bowling Green State University. For a number of years, he has been meticulously defining and assessing the contributions of religion to the various facets of the coping process. His book *The Psychology of Religion and Coping* (Pargament, 1997) is the definitive work in the field. With a colleague, he has asserted:

> People do not face stressful situations without resources. They rely on a system of beliefs, practices, and relationships which affects how they deal with difficult situations. In the coping process, this orienting system is translated into concrete situation-specific appraisals, activities, and goals. Religion is part of this general orienting system. A person with a strong religious faith who suffers a disabling injury, must find a way to move from the generalities of belief to the specifics of dealing with the injury. (Silverman & Pargament, 1990, p. 2)

Building upon the work of Lazarus and Folkman (1984), Pargament (1997) identifies the initial step in the coping process as "appraisal." First, when an event takes place, the person implicitly asks, "What does this mean to me?" In other words, is it irrelevant, positive, or negative? If the answer is that it is negative and stressful, the next question becomes "What can I do about it?" This brings to the fore additional judgments of "harm/loss," "threat," or "challenge." In the case of harm/loss, the individual has already suffered some adverse effects, such as illness or injury. Threat focuses on anticipated difficulties, whereas in challenge the person sees the likelihood of future growth and development. This form of appraisal has also been termed "primary appraisal." Pargament notes the differential role of religion in such appraisal, as a person can view what is happening as an intentional action of God to teach a lesson, or possibly to reward or punish via everyday success or failure.

The apparent clarity of the challenge, harm/loss, and threat conceptualization has not resulted in consistent findings, however. Two studies found that religious coping was more likely to be employed in threat and harm/loss situations than in challenge ones (Bjorck & Cohen, 1993; Bjorck & Klewicki, 1997). McRae (1984) observed that of 28 coping possibilities, religion ranked 2nd when harm/loss occurred to others, but only 13th when it was personally experienced. Faith came in 2nd and 7th, respectively, for threat to others and to the self; it ranked 14th and 10th, respectively, for other-directed and self-directed challenge situations. Though the findings of Bjorck and colleagues and of McRae imply that responses are state- rather than trait-dependent, Maynard, Gorsuch, and Bjorck (2001) failed to find any differences among the three stressor scenarios, suggesting that traits are also part of religious coping behavior. An interesting alternative that might be introduced into this area is to assess the degree of ambiguity and self-doubt in the respondent for each of these stress possibilities. Moreover, instead of utilizing religion as a means of coping, a person under stress might turn to materialistic possibilities (Chang & Arkin, 1999). More research is obviously needed to resolve these questions.

Dealing with the problem is the next step in the coping process, and the act of deciding how to do this has been labeled "secondary appraisal." In secondary appraisal, an assessment of personal resources for dealing with the difficulty occurs. A religious person may do a number of things, one of which is praying—a behavior that Holahan and Moos (1987) view as an active, cognitive coping strategy. The praying person is doing something, making an appeal to the highest power possible for help in overcoming misfortune and suffering. This may be constructive, in that it can spur the individual to adopt new means to solve a problem. Prayer, however, may also be dysfunctional if it causes the person to avoid actively seeking to confront the predicament by trusting passively in God to solve the dilemma.

When people assess ways of dealing with various difficulties, they face two obstacles: the problem itself, and the emotions that the problem arouses. Chances are that both will be dealt with, but to different degrees. Attention is initially directed more toward one of these concerns than the other, suggesting that an individual's style of coping may be primarily "problem-focused" or "emotion-focused" (Lazarus & Folkman, 1984). Moreover, the person may deal with the problem by using either "approach" or "avoidance" strategies, and the latter can be indicative of poor adjustment to the situation. Though emotion-focused coping may be beneficial and may manage anxiety constructively (i.e., it may be a form of "approach", the general tendency has been to regard this concern as largely avoiding the problem (Holahan & Moos, 1987). We sometimes see this emotion-focused avoidance when life is especially trying, as among elderly persons who are ill (Conway, 1985–1986). Whether or not religion is distracting under such circumstances, it does seem to stress the reduction of unpleasant emotions first.

Evidence suggests that people are likely to use problem-focused cognitions and behaviors when a situation is considered changeable. If circumstances can't be modified, the tendency is to resort to emotion-focused coping. Those who turn to prayer and religious methods frequently consider the problems toward which these means are directed as changeable. At the same time, particularly among younger people, religion may counter undesirable emotions (disgust and anger) while enhancing pleasure and happiness (Folkman & Lazarus, 1988). In other words, turning to one's faith in times of difficulty is helpful and constructive in dealing with both problems and emotions.

Pargament (1997) caps his theory of coping with the notion that people engaged in coping are gaining or searching for a "sense of significance" (p. 92). This is especially cogent for a theory that emphasizes religious coping, since religion is an exclusively human venture. "Significance" is really a complex composite of values, beliefs, feelings, and conceptual schemas that defines the phenomenological essence of a person. Significance is thus a unified, holistic pattern of orientations toward oneself, others, and the world. Pargament (1997) also speaks of an "orienting system, a frame of reference, a blueprint of oneself and the world that is used to anticipate and come to terms with life's events" (p. 100). It therefore contributes to and is part of the search for significance. Needless to say, religion, for many if not most people, is an important part of this orienting system. Given the detailed nature of his perspective, it is understandable how Pargament has been able to carry on an extensive research program on religion and coping.

The Coping Functions of Religion

In our view, stress, whether it involves harm/loss, threat, or challenge, reflects a situation in which meaning and control are in jeopardy. We may have difficulty making sense out of a situation, or be unable to master it. Religion is one way these needs are met, and the worldwide prevalence of religion may testify in part to the success of faith in attaining these goals. In Chapters 1 through 3, we have offered a framework for conceptualizing the psychology of religion in terms of meaning and control. We now further enlarge the scope of this framework, in order to understand the functions of religion for coping with life.

The Need for Meaning

Baumeister (1991) simply and directly tells us that religious meanings help people cope with the trials of life. Like Lazarus and Folkman (1984), he views meaningful explanations as helping to solve problems and regulate emotions. Similarly, Fichter (1981) asserts that "religious reality is the only way to make sense out of pain and suffering" (p. 20). That this struggle to understand tragedy via religion may last for a long time is evidenced by one extensive study (Echterling, 1993). Interviews with flood disaster survivors over a 7-year period led the researcher to infer that "they became theologians by asking how God could have allowed such tragedies to occur to them and their loved ones. They became philosophers by asking the meaning of life when they knew how frail and ephemeral life could be" (Echterling, 1993, p. 5). In other words, they searched for meaning in their moment of trial.

Simply put, being able to comprehend tragedy—to make it meaningful—probably constitutes the core of successful coping and adjustment. For most people, religion performs this role quite well, especially in times of personal crisis.

Faith habitually conveys the meaning that life's difficulties can be overcome. Whether or not people control objective conditions may be less important than their belief that even insurmountable obstacles can be mastered. As noted in earlier chapters, in much of life the sense of control is really an illusion; yet it is one that can be a powerful force supporting constructive coping behavior (Lefcourt, 1973).

The Importance of Control

When we apply our framework to religious coping, we find that the concept of "control" takes on new dimensions. These, of course, enrich our theory's structure: They make it more applicable to religion, and they enhance our understanding of the importance of control in human life.

With regard to control and religious coping, Pargament (1997) has posited three approaches that he began researching in 1988, and that have proven quite useful. If a "deferring" mode of relationship is adopted—for example, praying in order to put the problem totally in the hands of God—this does not appear to be as helpful as when a "collaborative" mode of relationship is manifested, in which God and the supplicant work together. Here prayer may keep the individual working on the problem while seeking the support of the deity. In a "self-directive" approach, God is acknowledged, but the problem is regarded as requiring personal rather than divine solution. Gorsuch and his colleagues have proposed a fourth style, which they term "surrender" (Maynard et al., 2001; Wong-MacDonald & Gorsuch, 1997). This is similar to the deferring approach, but the deferring mode is akin to assigning *all* control to the external power of God, whereas the surrender style occupies a middle ground (some or most personal control is "surrendered" to God. In both self-direction and collaboration, by contrast, internal control is present. Petitioning for aid from God (i.e., the collaborative approach) is best for the individual who feels that personal responsibility cannot be deferred or surrendered.

A considerable research literature indicates that for adaptation and coping, an internal locus of control is better than an external locus of control (Phares, 1976). In Pargament's scheme, the self-directive and collaborative coping modes are more internally oriented than the deferring, which is clearly external. On the average, the collaborative and self-directive modes relate to more positive coping outcomes than does the deferring approach (Harris, Spilka, & Emrick, 1990; McIntosh & Spilka, 1990; Pargament et al., 1988).

Coping and Forms of Control.   The idea of control is complex—so complex that Skinner (1996) was able to identify 88 control constructs. There is great overlap among these concepts, but one elemental scheme that is pertinent to our concern speaks of two basic forms: (1) "primary control," or "being in charge" (i.e., having the ability to change the situation); and (2) "secondary control," or being able to effect change in oneself. The famous writer Nikos Kazantzakis (1961) noted this latter potential when he quoted a mystic's prescription: "Since we cannot change reality, let us change the eyes which see reality" (p. 45). Faith may play an important role in stimulating both primary and secondary forms of control, and the two forms are probably not independent of each other. In psychological circles, however, religion is largely regarded as functioning as a form of secondary control.

Meaning as Control.   In most cases, information gives people the feeling that we can do something about whatever is troubling them. As Sir Francis Bacon put it, "knowledge is power" (quoted in Bartlett, 1955, p. 118). Baumeister (1991) adds that "meaning is used to predict and control the environment" (p. 183), and religious meaning can help people regulate their emotions. In other words, simply having information may reduce stress (Andrew, 1970). A wonderful anecdotal example of how religion can realize this role was provided by a patient with breast cancer, who stated, "I had no idea that God could answer so many of my questions" (Johnson & Spilka, 1988, p. 12). Though we may call this "informational" control, it is intimately tied to three forms of secondary control that have been theorized by Rothbaum, Weisz, and Snyder (1982). These are termed "interpretive," "predictive," and "vicarious" control, and are especially significant for understanding how religion helps people deal with the problems they confront both in everyday living and in troubled times.

Interpretive Control.   When people are in great difficulty, it is natural for them to feel that there is no way out of their predicament. In seeking to understand such an event and to achieve some degree of control over what seems hopeless, people often reinterpret what is taking place. They exercise interpretive control and construe a distressing situation in less troubling or even positive terms. For example, they may claim that "things could be worse" or that "I have it better than a lot of other people." For example, in one study a patient with cancer concluded, "I looked upon cancer as a detour in the road, but not a roadblock" (Johnson & Spilka, 1988, p. 13). Through such interpretations, people gain control over their emotions and may thus become better able to handle their difficulties in a constructive way. In other words, they may become increasingly problem-focused.

Predictive Control.   The perpetual human dream is to foretell the future. The idea of precognition fascinates people. If they could predict what would happen on future rolls of dice, who would win horse races, what the stock market might do, or whether their efforts in general would result in success or failure, they would expect to become the beneficiaries of unlimited wealth and happiness. The Bible has said that "The Lord himself shall give you a sign" (Isaiah 7:14).

Predictive control, as a form of secondary control, assures a person that things will turn out all right in the end. For example, another patient with cancer stated, "Because of my relationship with God, I had faith that this cancer was not going to take my life" (Johnson & Spilka, 1988, p. 12). There is a poignant example of predictive control in Eliach's *Chassidic Tales of the Holocaust* (1982). Eliach tells the story of a devout Jew who during World War II was brought by the Nazis into the death camp at Auschwitz. The number 145053 was tattooed on his arm. He looked at it and suddenly concluded that he would live. He reached this conclusion by adding the digits together and finding that they totaled 18; 18 is a number that within Judaism means life, and thus he felt assured of survival. It was as if God had offered an omen signifying a secure future. Such predictive control gives the person confidence that the morrow will be good. We must keep in mind, however, that the critical element here is *perception* of the future; what actually occurs is independent of this aspiration.

Vicarious Control.   When people feel that they may not be able to cope with their troubles—particularly in cases of serious illness, where death is a possibility—they often turn to their God, and vicariously, the deity becomes a support or substitute for their own efforts. The essence of such vicarious control was stated by one woman with cancer, who declared, "I could talk to my God and ask for his help in healing" (Johnson & Spilka, 1988, p. 12). Identifying with her God gave her the strength to face potential death through her perceived divine connection. She thus attained a measure of vicarious control over her circumstances.

To illustrate the role of control in relation to faith and coping with health problems, Research Box 15.1 presents a significant study.

ɝ

Research Box 15.1. Religion and Physical Health
(McIntosh & Spilka, 1990)

Treating religion and control as multidimensional constructs, the authors hoped to objectify a primarily anecdotal literature. To accomplish this, they administered a number of questionnaires to 69 college students and 7 adult church members.

Religious orientation was assessed with the Allport–Ross (1967) Intrinsic and Extrinsic scales, and with a revised version of the Quest measure (Batson & Ventis, 1982). In addition, a brief, highly reliable Meaning from Religion scale was developed. Frequency of prayer was also determined.

Control was evaluated by the Levenson (1973) and Kopplin (1976) questionnaires. These yielded scores for internal control, control by chance, control by powerful others, and control by God. The first three constructs were also assessed specifically in relation to health via a measure created by Wallston, Wallston, and DeVillis (1978). Finally, a measure assessing Pargament's "collaborative" mode of relationship with the deity (active person, active God) was also utilized.

The participants' health was evaluated via two measures: (1) health habits (an 8-item checklist), and (2) health status (a 57-item symptom checklist). A factor analysis of the symptom list resulted in four subscales: Emotional, Somatic, Visceral, and Respiratory. These labels indicate the symptomatic content of the measures.

Though considerable statistical significance was observed among the measures, the relationships tended to be weak. The indices of traditional religious commitment (e.g., the Intrinsic scale, the Meaning from Religion scale, the frequency of praying) were associated with better health, whereas Extrinsic scale scores were correlated with signs of poorer health status. With regard to health and control, the external forms of control (chance, powerful others) were found to be related positively to a few indicators of poorer health. The religion scales can be considered aspects of secondary control that reflect coping with stress. Since Intrinsic scale scores were correlated positively with control by God plus a collaborative God–person approach, and negatively with the external forms of control, this suggests further evidence of secondary control. In other words, religion as secondary control beneficially affects health.

What Factors Prompt People to Turn to Religion?

The availability hypothesis or heuristic raises the question of why, in specific circumstances, certain things have a higher likelihood than others of coming to people's minds (Fiske & Taylor, 1991). Among the many factors that might stimulate the selection of religion as a means of coping, the fact that mainstream North American culture and child-rearing practices inculcate a readiness to turn to religion or exercise spirituality in times of distress is undoubtedly the most important. A less obvious point is that religious cues in the immediate situation are apt to be significant. For example, one often sees people (especially in the United States) wearing religious medals, crucifixes, Stars of David, and the like. St. Christopher medals frequently hang from rearview mirrors in cars. Catholics may carry rosary beads with them. Small Bibles are not uncommon. The meaning of such symbols has been nicely demonstrated in one investigation (Antkowiak & Ozorak, 2000). These researchers studied the use of sacred "objects as means of comfort" (p. 1), and confirmed Lamothe's (1998) view that these objects "not only provide comfort and solace but a sense of identity and cohesion" (quoted in Antkowiak & Ozorak, 2000, p. 7). Such referents may go far toward arousing religious and spiritual thoughts and feelings that calm, refresh, and strengthen distressed individuals.

People also turn to religion because it works for them. Levin and Schiller (1987) raise the interesting possibility that "perhaps the nervous system represents the locus of a mechanism by which religious faith or religious beliefs . . . promote well-being" (p. 24). The mechanism may well be the sense of control that is often promoted by religion (McIntosh, Kojetin, & Spilka, 1985). Specifically, the perceptions that one is personally in control of life situations and that God is in overall control (i.e., Pargament's "collaborative" mode) relate to good health (Loewenthal & Cornwall, 1993; McIntosh & Spilka, 1990). Another possibility has been advanced by Benson (1975)—namely, that certain religious rituals (prayer, meditation, etc.) may stimulate a "relaxation response" that is broadly healthful (Goleman, 1984). In other words, not only may religion promote an increased sense of control; its rituals themselves may reduce stress and tension.

Finally, Bjorck and Cohen (1993) claim that the greater the stress, the more religious coping takes place. Further threats (defined as the anticipation of more damage) elicit greater use of religion than actual harm/losses, which require acceptance. Since events that challenge people call upon personal effort and resources, they are seen as most controllable. Resort to faith as a coping aid is thus least often employed in these situations (Bjorck & Cohen, 1993).

Varieties of Religious Coping

Religion provides many possible ways of coping with the stresses of life. Table 15.1 mainly includes the work of Pargament, Poloma, and Tarakeshwar (2001), yet permits a consideration of various religious devices and roles.

Pargament et al.'s (2001) approach is one way in which the various coping functions may be described. Others may see many of these devices as aspects of prayer, such as confession, thanksgiving, pleading, meditation, or self-improvement (David, Ladd, & Spilka, 1992; see also the discussion of prayer below). An excellent example of coping research in this tradition is presented in Research Box 15.2.

Unhappily, translating concepts into their operational equivalents often runs into difficulty. Pargament, Koenig, and Perez (2000) attempted to develop a comprehensive measure of religious coping. This resulted in seven "negative religious coping scales" and nine "positive religious coping scales." Direct overlap with the varieties of religious coping listed in Table 15.1 appeared to be present in six of the measures. The other notions might have been included in the remaining scales, but were not definitive enough to be distinguished in the respondents' answers to the various questions. This is a very common problem in scale construction.

PRAYER AND FORGIVENESS AS COPING METHODS

Among the many ways religion can be used in coping, two merit special recognition—namely, prayer, because it occupies such a central and significant role in the lives of most people; and forgiveness, which has only very recently been recognized as an important coping mechanism. Interest and research in both realms have been increasing rapidly and cannot be overlooked.

TABLE 15.1. Various Means of Using Religion for Coping with the Stresses of Life

Variety of coping	Typical statement
Self-directive coping	"It's my problem to solve, not God's."
Collaborative coping	"God helps those who help themselves."
Deferring coping	"It's in God's hands."
Pleading religious coping	"Please, God, help me through this terrible time."
Benevolent religious reappraisal	"God gives me these trials to test me."
Punishing God reappraisal	"I have sinned and deserve to suffer."
Demonic reappraisal	"It is the work of the Devil."
Reappraisal of God's powers	"Nothing is too small for God not to notice and help."
Seeking spiritual support	"I know I can rely on God's love."
Spiritual discontent	"How could God do this to me?"
Seeking congregational support	"I know I can depend on my minister and other church members for help."
Interpersonal religious discontent	"I feel as if the church has deserted me."
Religious forgiving	"Father, help me be a better person; let me not be angry and afraid."
Rites of passage	"Now I am a man."
Religious conversion	"I have seen the light; I have found the way; I am born again."

Note. Adapted from Pargament, Poloma, and Tarakeshwar (2001, Table 13.1), Copyright 2001 by Oxford University Press. Adapted by permission.

Prayer

Prayer has often been viewed as the core of faith (Brown, 1994; Buttrick, 1942; Heiler, 1932). It is easy to perform, intensely personal, can be kept private, and is widely employed. Approximately 90% of U.S. residents indicate that they pray, and 76% regard it as very important in everyday life (McCullough & Larson, 1999; Poloma & Gallup, 1991). As Trier and Shupe (1991) have observed, "prayer [is] the most often practiced form of religiosity" (p. 354). We suggest that it is so popular because of how well it helps people cope with their problems.

Religious activities, especially prayer, are usually regarded as positive coping devices directed toward both solving problems and facilitating personal growth (Folkman, Lazarus, Dunkel-Schetter, De Longis, & Gruen, 1986). Some psychologists, however, see religious ritual, including prayer, as a means of controlling one's emotions (Koenig, George, & Siegler, 1988). Others see it as an effective problem-focused mechanism, in that praying may be the only practical way of dealing with many tragedies, such as the death of a loved one (Bjorck & Cohen, 1993). Apparently, it can perform both problem- and emotion-focused functions (Carver, Scheier, & Pozo, 1992).

Forms of Prayer

This simple concept and word, "prayer," covers many possibilities. Foster (1992) conceptually identified 21 different forms of prayer. A survey of seven empirical efforts resulted in from four to nine kinds of prayer (Ladd & Spilka, 2002). The most stable types identified

---

Research Box 15.2. God Help Me: I. Coping Efforts as Predictors of the Outcomes to Significant Negative Life Events (Pargament et al., 1990)

In this landmark research, a very basic question was addressed: "What kinds of religious coping are helpful, harmful, or irrelevant to people dealing with significant negative events?" (p. 798). The authors also attempted to find out whether measures of religious coping techniques would predict outcomes of coping better than measures of nonreligious coping techniques.

A sample of 586 Christian church members responded to questionnaires assessing religious and nonreligious coping activities and outcomes in regard to negative events that they had experienced during the preceding year. Six kinds of religious coping and four kinds of nonreligious coping were identified. Three outcome measures were assessed: mental health status, general outcome of the negative event, and its religious outcome. The religious variables, to varying degrees, predicted all three of the outcomes. This was most evident for spiritually based activities and for faith and trust in God. Religious discontent and concern with punishment from God hindered coping and adjustment. Positive effects were predictable from perceptions of a just, loving, and supportive deity; involvement in religious rituals, such as attendance at services; prayer; Bible reading; focusing on the afterlife, living a good life; and having support from clergy and church members. It was also observed that an extrinsic, utilitarian faith was helpful. The authors concluded that at least among church members, religious coping is an important and beneficial part of the overall process of coping with stress.

---

have been "petitionary," "ritualistic," "meditational," "confessional," "thanksgiving," "intercessory," "self-improvement," and "habitual." All have been confirmed and measured by separate, reliable scales (David et al., 1992). One U.S. national study discussed "contemplative," "conversational," "colloquial," "ritual," "petitionary," and "meditative" prayers (Poloma & Gallup, 1991). There is considerable overlap among the various proposed schemes—a condition that has not been helped by the lack of a coordinating theory. If any generalities may be inferred from the data on prayer, it would appear that the more people pray, the more forms of prayer they utilize (David et al., 1992). In addition, frequency of prayer goes with praying for more things—health, interpersonal concerns, and financial matters (Trier & Shupe, 1991).

In order to provide some theoretical footing for conceptualizing prayer, Ladd and Spilka (2002) surveyed the literature and attempted to create a categorizing structure for the forms of prayer that have been empirically identified. This work is detailed in Research Box 15.3.

Usage and Efficacy of Different Forms of Prayer

People are selective in their praying, and the different forms of prayer they use may be employed in different circumstances. For example, patients who have survived more than 5 years since an initial diagnosis of breast cancer are likely to stress prayers of thanksgiving (Ladd, Milmoe, & Spilka, 1994). Petitionary prayers, which are said to be the oldest and most common prayers, are employed to counter frustration and threat, whereas contemplative prayers

---

**Research Box 15.3. Inward, Outward, and Upward:
Cognitive Aspects of Prayer (Ladd & Spilka, 2002)**

Using the framework suggested by Foster (1992), these researchers first hypothesized that all specific kinds of prayer derive from one underlying basic general factor—namely, a connection between the person who is praying and the deity toward which the prayer is directed. The first level above this underlying factor suggests three main types of prayer. "Inward" prayers are simple, spontaneous, uncensored efforts to connect with the divine. In a sense, the person "bares the soul" and desires to grow. "Outward" prayers shift to the world and needs to be satisfied from outside the person. Here are petitionary and intercessory prayers, hopes to enhance interpersonal relations, and wishes to transform external forces. "Upward" prayers recognize the superior position of God and the inferior status of people. This recognitioni results in meditation, contemplation, adoration, and thanksgiving as possible efforts to experience the divine.

The initial factor analysis, utilizing 309 responders to 153 items, resulted in eight factors. These item composites distinguished a number of inward, outward, and upward forms of prayer.

A second-order factor analysis of the first-order factors was undertaken. Three factors resulted, one of which was clearly composed of outward prayer content; however, the other two combined inward and outward, and inward and upward, possibilities. Even though the first-order factors revealed the three theorized prayer directions, these became mixed in the second-order analysis.

A final, third-order factor analysis did not result in the hoped-for general factor. One wonders whether the three hypothesized directions might be better delineated with a larger sample and a more careful selection of test items. Even though this research was not fully successful, theoretically guided work like this opens the door to more refined and systematic thinking and work in the realm of prayer.

(attempts to relate deeply to one's God) seem to aid internal integration of the self (Janssen, de Hart, & den Draak, 1989; Poloma & Gallup, 1991). Meditational prayers (which are concerned with one's relationship to God) seem to reduce anger, to lessen anxiety, and to aid relaxation (Carlson, Bacaseta, & Simanton, 1988). Contemplative prayers have also been shown to aid psychotherapy by lessening distress and specific kinds of complaints (Finney & Malony, 1985a). By contrast, there is some suggestion that mechanical, ritualized prayers may relate negatively to well-being (McCullough & Larson, 1999).

Little coping research has been done with most forms of prayer; however, a few, such as intercessory and petititionary prayer, are deserving of further exploration.

Intercessory Prayer.   Intercessory prayer is a particularly controversial issue. The idea that prayers in behalf of another person can influence the health of that other person has a long history. It has been subjected to research, but this generally leaves much to be desired.

In 1965, Joyce and Weldon matched patients with chronic or progressively deteriorating rheumatic or psychological illness on gender, age, and clinical diagnosis. Two groups of

19 patients each were created. The "treatment" group participants were prayed for by members of a prayer group. The "nontreatment" group served as a control. Each patient in the "treatment" group was the recipient of a total of 15 hours of prayer over a 6-month period. This was a double-blind study in which neither the patients nor their physicians knew of the prayer "treatment." After 6 months of intercessory prayer, no differences between the two groups could be demonstrated.

Within a few years, another intercessory prayer study was reported by Colipp (1969). This involved 18 children with leukemia, 10 of whom were randomly chosen to be the objects of prayer by the author's friends and church members. After 15 months of prayer, the treatment group seemed to have a slight advantage over the control group in survival at the 10% level of confidence.

More recently, an attempt was made to see whether intercessory prayer might favorably reduce alcohol consumption by individuals with alcohol abuse or dependence. A control/comparison group was employed, but after 6 months, no differences between the groups were observed (Walker, Tonigan, Miller, Comer, & Kahlich, 1997).

McCullough and Larson (1999) cite an unusual finding in a study comparing the "agents" of prayer (those who request God's intercession) with the "subjects" (those needing God's intervention). That is, the agents revealed greater improvements in their mental state than did the subjects for whom intercessory prayers were offered.

A fourth study utilizing 393 patients with coronary disease was undertaken by Byrd (1988). Patients, doctors, and the author were all kept "blind" (i.e., unaware of which patients were assigned to which conditions) in this work. The results seemed to support the power of intercessory prayer, as the treatment group appeared to do better than the controls. Though this work looks impressive on the surface, many serious questions may be posed regarding its design, the data analysis, the results, and their interpretation. In fact, strong challenges to virtually all of these studies can be advanced, based on the nature (and often size) of the samples, evaluation procedures, methodology, and statistical analyses. If scientific doubts are not enough, many theologians should be able to mount their own criticisms of this kind of work. We must conclude that at this stage of research on intercessory prayer, its power and significance have yet to be demonstrated.

Petitionary Prayer.   As noted above, petitionary prayer is the most common kind of prayer offered, and though it is often treated negatively by religionists, it has repeatedly been averred that "petition is the heart of prayer" (Capps, 1982, p. 130). Capps (1982) further terms it "the crux of the psychology of religion" (p. 131). Simply said, prayers of petition ask for something. One content analysis of 227 petitionary prayers (Brown, 1994) showed that most requested something for family members (37%); next came prayers for alleviation of illness (21%). (The latter, though petitionary, were also intercessory when the illness was that of someone else, not the person doing the praying.) In third place were petitionary prayers for persons who had died (Brown, 1994). Obviously, people can plead for anything—one reason for the popularity of petitionary prayers. Earlier work by Brown (1966) with children and adolescents led to the conclusion that on the average, the more serious a situation is, the more strongly young people feel petitionary prayer is appropriate. An egocentric belief in the direct efficacy of petitionary prayer decreases with increasing age. There is reason to believe that as the belief in the material effectiveness of these prayers lessens, it is replaced by a belief in nonspecific effects, such as "granting courage, improving morale or producing other psychological changes" (Brown, 1968, p. 77).

Forgiveness

Even though the theme of forgiveness is central in all of the world's major religions, it has only recently been recognized by psychologists as a means of coping with distress when another person has wronged someone (or a third party) or has behaved in an unjust way (Pargament & Rye, 1998; Sanderson & Linehan, 1999). We include here not only personal injury, but also the negative feelings that are aroused when one reads about the mistreatment of others through the immoral use of power, which occurred during the Holocaust of World War II and continues to occur in the atrocities perpetrated upon innocent and helpless people at all too many places in the world. Theologies differ in terms of who may forgive—the victims or uninvolved others—but emotionally there is little doubt that people may be aroused by injustice anywhere. The result is often that such people harbor enmity and hatred of the perpetrators. Simon Wiesenthal's significant book *The Sunflower* (1976) poignantly discusses the issues raised by crimes against humanity, and presents a variety of religious perspectives related to the forgiveness of such transgressions.

Conditions for Forgiveness

Sanderson and Linehan (1999) claim that "all religious traditions offer similar practical instructions for forgiveness" (p. 210). The perpetrator of the injustice or wrong must do the following:

1. Accept personal responsibility for the act.
2. Express honest regrets.
3. Where possible, make appropriate reparation.
4. Make assurances that the offending action will cease.
5. Request forgiveness.

Forgiveness, however, is a two-way process; it includes both an offender and a victim. Both parties may suffer shame, anger, and injury, and both may be greatly distressed. Often, however, only one party may look to faith for understanding and the alleviation of pain and suffering. In cases such as this, where either the offender or the victim does not participate fully in the process, the position of the other party is exceptionally difficult. Pargament and Rye (1998) conceive of forgiving as a transformation. In coping with the wrong, the person who was hurt must shift from desiring revenge to desiring peace. (The perpetrator may be in a similar position.) What has been done must now be seen in a new light in order to reduce guilt and other negative feelings. Within a religious framework, pastoral counseling and therapy may be necessary to resolve the difficulty.

The Effects of Forgiveness: Empirical Studies

Given the place of forgiveness in institutional faith, it is no surprise that an emphasis on forgiveness usually accompanies being religious (Gorsuch & Hao, 1993). Even though research fails to show any direct effect by forgiveness on health, the potential for indirect effects exists. For example, as noted in Chapter 3, forgiveness is antithetical to hostility; it decreases both subjective and objective indicators of stress; and it also lowers blood pressure (an outcome that may reflect the previous two findings). Coyle and Enright (1997) have similarly shown reductions in hostility along with depression and anxiety.

In an effort to explain these findings, Worthington, Berry, and Parrott (2001) speak of a trait of "unforgiveness," which is associated with emotional, cognitive, and behavioral responses known to correlate negatively with health. We see the situations that arouse unforgiveness as threatening an individual's sense of control. The reaction is one of anger and/or fear. A religious or spiritual framework, via forgiveness, reduces inappropriate emotions and enhances the sense of control.

THE STATE OF RESEARCH ON RELIGION AND COPING

Nothing is ever as simple as we wish it were. The idea of research carries with it the notion of definitive answers—which is a myth. So often, studies are weak in controls, design, and data analysis. Chance also enters the picture and is especially pertinent when statistics are employed. Too many findings fail to be replicated. Unfortunately, overviews and meta-analyses of the work done in a field are rarely undertaken, but when they are carried out, we may be shocked to see how tenuous our assumptions are. In the realm of religion and coping, Pargament and Brant (1998) have done yeoman work that brings the necessity of caution to the fore. Table 15.2 summarizes this work.

Our basic hypothesis is of a positive association between some religious expression and the outcome of negative events. A positive relationship says that the situation worked out well; a negative finding indicates that the results were undesirable; and, of course, no relationship tells us that nothing could be inferred one way or the other. For example, in Table 15.2, 34% of the studies yielded positive results with religious orientations (e.g., individual religious expressions such as prayer, religious beliefs, church activity, intrinsic, extrinsic, and other faith forms). Only 4% were meaningfully negative, but 62% failed to provide any significant information. When we consider religious coping (e.g., seeking spiritual support, expressing spiritual discontent, participating in religious rituals), the studies revealed a higher percentage of positive than negative outcomes, but again nonsignificant relationships predominated.

These findings may shake one's confidence in the research, and we must rely on our own judgments of what the best work tells us. With regard to Table 15.2 and the role of religious orientations, our choice is between significant positive findings and nonsignificant ones. Overall, significant negative relationships seem to be too minor to be considered. The situation is not so clear regarding religious coping, and we are again left to our own resources. The tables in Pargament and Brant (1998) from which these summaries were derived do provide additional direction, as they further subdivide and detail studies under each of these

TABLE 15.2. A Summary of Studies on Different Aspects of Religion and Coping: Significant and Nonsignificant Findings

	Significant positive results	Significant negative results	Nonsignificant results
Religious orientations and negative event outcomes	34% (130)	4% (14)	62% (233)
Religious coping and negative event outcomes	32% (151)	21% (98)	47% (219)

Note. The numbers in parentheses are numbers of studies. Adapted from Pargament and Brant (1998). Copyright 1998 by Academic Press. Adapted by permission.

headings, and thus offer further guidance to scholars. Still, it is evident that the research waters are muddied, and that caution and questioning are the best guides.

CONTEXTUAL COPING CONCERNS

The concept of coping seems to have no limits. The content of this field varies from dealing with one's own outlook on life, to handling relations with others at home, work, school, and play, to dealing with the most tragic crisis situations that may be encountered. One person's petty annoyances can be another's sources of deep distress and depression. Therefore, it is necessary to consider contextual issues (both external and internal) that affect coping.

Faith and Coping with Daily Hassles

Coping begins with the needs of daily living, and is not restricted to handling crises. Some researchers have thus asked whether faith might play a role in adapting to the "hassles" of everyday life (Belavich, 1995). Noting that a number of adaptive coping strategies might be utilized, Belavich administered a carefully selected battery of tests to over 200 college students, and controlled for a variety of demographic variables. Sophisticated data analyses revealed that "religion plays a significant role in a person's experience with minor stressors on a day-to-day basis" (p. 24). Specifically, faith aids coping by diverting individuals from stress, and by enabling them to call upon the social support provided by other religious people and figures. Some aspects of religious coping were, however, related to poorer adjustment. The latter indicators—pleading and spiritual coping—implied a negative function. Conceptual efforts to explain these adverse findings call for further research.

The Effects of Contextual Consonance and Dissonance

The "hassles" of daily living may sometimes be implicit in one's life circumstances. We should therefore be sensitive to the social context of faith. Rosenberg (1962) studied consonance and dissonance between people's religious identification and the religious identifications of others in their surroundings. For example, a dissonant context would exist if a person was Jewish but his or her neighborhood was predominantly Christian. Consonance would, of course, mean that all neighborhood residents shared the same faith. Studying Catholics, Protestants, and Jews, Rosenberg observed that in a dissonant religious context, a person usually felt isolated from coreligionists and therefore lacked their support. Discrimination was also apt to occur. The long-range effects of contextual dissonance were likely to be low self-esteem, depressive feelings, and psychosomatic symptoms. A variation on this theme that merits study is dissonance in degree of religious commitment (i.e., the situation that exists when one's residence area is uniform in religious orientation, but the person is either more or less religiously involved than others).

Spirituality and Coping

Some valuable insights may be derived from the recent work of Socha (1999) on spirituality and coping. Emphasizing the "human existential situation," Socha goes beyond religion to a broader spiritual scheme. (See the discussions of "religion" versus "spirituality" in several previous chapters.) He offers a holistic, growth-oriented view, in which a person recognizes the transitory nature of situations and acknowledges his or her own coping limits. Such awareness implies knowing when to define circumstances in terms of "sacredness"—a religious or secular notion of placing things in broader perspective. Belavich's (1995) work indicates what is done on a day-to-day basis; Socha's outlook suggests why, and introduces a different theoretical frame—a phenomenological approach that emphasizes how the individual perceives and explains the situation. This takes us back to the question of the meanings that precede the actions people take (another direction for research on coping and religion).

In other work relating to spirituality, Kennedy, Rosati, Spann, Neelon, and Rosati (n.d.), like Socha (1999), broaden the notion of coping from a focused pattern of responses to a broader approach based on making lifestyle changes. Working within a medically based program, these workers felt that their therapeutic procedures would constructively affect well-being and spirituality. Though they did not distinguish between religion-based and non-religion-based spiritualities, half of the participants in their program evidenced an increase in spirituality, and close to 100% reported an increase in their subjective sense of well-being. Positive and significant correlations were obtained among spirituality, well-being, and meaning. Distinguishing between faith-oriented and non-faith-oriented spiritualities should provide a substantive direction for further research, and may enable participants to utilize such avenues more effectively to make the desired lifestyle changes.

Religion and Positive–Negative Life Orientation

Another factor that contributes to effective coping behavior is whether a person takes a generally positive or generally negative perspective on life and its problems. This dimension is often treated as a general characteristic that includes attitudes toward both oneself and the world (Myers, 1992). Primarily viewed as trait-dependent, it is largely conceptualized in terms of optimism–pessimism. Its significance is well illustrated by a longitudinal study in which a pessimistic explanatory style manifested in early life predicted poor health in middle and old age (Peterson, Seligman, & Vaillant, 1988). Faith has been shown to be a significant component of optimism.

The association of religion with personal happiness is apparently a major function of faith in general (Ellison, 1991b). Extensive surveys of thousands of people in 14 countries have also shown a positive association between religiousness and feelings of well-being (Myers, 1992). Utilizing a variety of religious measures in national samples in the United States, Pollner (1989) concluded that "relations with a divine other are a significant correlate of well-being" (p. 100). In his system, religion's effectiveness results from the following: (1) It brings a sense of order and coherence to stressful situations; (2) it has been found to counter feelings of shame or anger that are aroused by stress; (3) it also creates positive feelings about oneself, simply as a result of having a perceived relationship with the deity; lastly (4) religion fosters a general tendency to see the self and the world in positive terms. In addition, there is strong evidence that religion, in offering a sense of meaning, control, and esteem, does support an optimistic outlook. This in turn helps people deal constructively with life, and seems to have long-range beneficial effects

Optimism–Pessimism and Fundamentalism

A common hypothesis is that a negative self-concept and low self-esteem should be associated with fundamentalist views, because of their emphasis on personal sin and guilt (Hood,

1992). To date, no consistent support has been found for this view. In fact, there is some indication that the opposite may be true.

Sethi and Seligman (1993) compared members of three different religious groups (liberal, moderate, and fundamentalist) on a variety of measures from which they derived indices of optimism and pessimism. Optimism was greatest among the members of the fundamentalist group, followed by those from the moderate group. The members of the liberal group evidenced the least optimism. Religious leaders were interviewed with regard to distinguishing the prayers and hymns typically used by the different faiths. A content analysis of these materials showed that theory paralleled the level of group optimism. In other words, the fundamentalist group was exposed to the most optimistic religious content, and the liberal group to the least. In related work, it was concluded that fundamentalism stresses the most hopefulness, the least hopelessness, and the least self-blame for negative happenings (Sethi & Seligman, 1994). There is a need to repeat this work with different procedures, however, since Kroll (1994) has raised questions about the validity of the optimism–pessimism measures used.

Religion, Self-Esteem, and Life's Meanings

We shift now to the related work on self-esteem and similar concepts. A recent large-scale study of almost 1,000 people in Australia found that belief in God, attending church, and praying correlated positively with self-esteem and well-being (Francis & Kaldor, 2002).

In a rather sophisticated effort, a deep personal identification with religion was found to be affiliated solidly with high scores on a measure of global self-esteem. This finding also held for scores on the measure of Intrinsic religious orientation, but not for either Extrinsic or Quest scores (Ryan, Rigby, & King, 1993). More recent work focusing exclusively on the Intrinsic measure confirms the foregoing finding (Laurencelle, Abell, & Schwartz, 2002).

Other fairly large-sample research (Delbridge, Headey, & Wearing, 1994) examined whether religious practice is directly associated with a favorable outlook on life, or whether there is an intervening factor. Specifically, does one's faith endow a person with a sense of purpose or meaning for life? This study points out that many different social and cultural referents offer meaning to people. For those who are religious, one's faith performs this role directly, and it may also do this indirectly in various ways. For instance, in addition to religious/spiritual resources, churchgoing provides social support—which, through its community integrative function, contributes to the feeling that life has a purpose.

Images of God and a Positive or Negative Sense of Self

Benson and Spilka (1973) showed that a positive outlook toward oneself corresponds to a similar perception of God. It is, however, well established that God concepts are multidimensional (Gorsuch, 1968; Spilka, Armatas, & Nussbaum, 1964). One long-standing dichotomy that is basic to Western religion is the one between notions of a loving God and a controlling God (Benson & Spilka, 1973; Spilka, Addison, & Rosensohn, 1975). Examining this dichotomy, Culbertson (1996) expected these images to relate to one's sense of personal shame. A controlling God concept was found to be positively affiliated with shame, but a loving God concept was independent of shame. Pargament et al. (1990) have observed that viewing God in a positive and benevolent light can buttress meaning, self-esteem, and one's sense of control in life.

Foster and Keating (1990) conducted a rather ingenious investigation into the relationships between male and female God images for men and women. They observed greater self-esteem when women interacted with a female God, while males viewed themselves more favorably when their God was masculine.

Religious Coping, Self-Esteem and Well-Being: Are They State- or Trait-Related?

Competence and success are the normal precursors to well-being, satisfaction with life, happiness, optimism, and self-esteem. This notion raises the question of whether competence and success in coping are functions of situations or more basic aspects of personality. In other words, are they state- or situation-dependent, or are they trait-dependent (Spielberger, 1966)? We may further ask whether the same is true of well-being and optimism. It appears that religion can be a part of this picture. In other words, using religion to cope successfully with life should relate positively to one's subjective sense of well-being, and, as implied above, the research literature overwhelmingly supports this hypothesis. According to Maynard et al. (2001), both state and trait considerations are pertinent when religious coping occurs.

Jones (1993) further notes that "extensive studies have found the presence of religious beliefs and attitudes to be the best predictors of life satisfaction and a sense of well-being" (p. 2). This is also the essence of the message that Pargament (1997) provides in his definitive volume on religion and coping.

RELIGION AND COPING WITH MAJOR STRESS

We have pictured living as a process of continuous coping. Clearly, religion can play a constructive role in handling the problems of daily life, but the real test of faith comes when common hassles are supplemented by the major trials of human existence—aging, illness, or disability; family, social, and economic difficulties; the loss of loved ones; and, of course, confronting our own death. In Chapter 8, we have looked at the last two issues.

The stress-buffering role of faith seems to have very broad application. Maton (1989) has shown that it relates positively to college adjustment among first-year students who have experienced high stress during the preceding 6 months. Newman and Pargament (1990) observed that religion also provides emotional support for college students and helps them redefine their problems. The need for new and positive meanings may be met this way. This redefining or "reframing" is a coping strategy that can be quite constructive. For example, caregivers of patients with dementia—who are placed in an extremely trying role—utilize their faith to redefine their situation and thus to make it more acceptable and manageable (Wright, Pratt, & Schmall, 1985).

Park, Cohen, and Herb (1990) point out that members of various faiths may differentially focus on prayer, seek group support, resort to sacred writings, or utilize positive thinking to cope with stress. They conducted a comparison of Catholics and Protestants, and found differences suggesting that religion may both alleviate and exacerbate stress. Given the fact that over 200 Protestant bodies exist in the United States alone, plus the strong ethnic variations that often parallel denominational distinctions, there is a need for additional work in this area to examine more exactly defined religious bodies and the relative success of their approaches.

Hypothesizing that entering a university constitutes a very stressful experience for young people, Hunsberger, Pancer, Pratt, and Alisat (1996) attempted to get a large group of incoming first-year students to take a broad range of psychological tests. These were adminis-tered in blocks: prior to coming to the university, early in the first term, and late in the first year. Though a variety of religious measures (including one on fundamentalism) failed to relate to indices of adjustment, indices of religious doubt were consistently and negatively linked to indices of adjustment, including poorer relationships with parents and increased stress. Hunsberger et al.'s work suggests that the usual measures of religious belief and be-havior may not be enough in studying coping behavior; the issue of religious doubt per se may need to be considered. Rejection of religion and religious doubt may well be different phenomena, and research illustrating their differential significance would make a nice con-tribution to the literature.

Having examined some of the major parameters surrounding the issue of religion and coping with major stress, and considering that Pargament (1997) wrote over 500 pages on this topic, it behooves us to focus on a few specific areas. To this end, we look first at the role of religion in enabling elderly persons to cope with the various stressors they confront (as well as religion's possible effects on longevity). We then select from the vast literature dealing with religion and health. Finally, we consider what is probably the most catastrophic stressor parents can face—the death of a child—and the ways religion can help parents deal with this tragedy.

Religion, Stress, and Elderly People

The Stressors of Old Age

Old age, the final stage in life, involves a number of particularly significant stressors. In a society such as ours that values individuality and progress, those who have retired and/or developed the infirmities of old age often find it difficult to avoid negative self-views and loneliness. Elderly persons are likely to interact less and less with younger people and may withdraw from social interactions in general. Again we confront the issue of disengagement, which we have mentioned in Chapter 8. Personally, socially, and economically, life for older individuals becomes increasingly problematic.

Erik Erikson (1963), the first modern thinker to develop a lifespan developmental psy-chology, pictured these last years as a struggle between ego integrity and despair. The indi-vidual must confront multiple issues of loss—the loss of various skills; the loss of personal significance through work after retirement; the loss of friends through death; and finally the knowledge that his or her own life may shortly conclude. As a 90-year-old Papago woman said some 70 years ago to an anthropologist, "It is not good to be old. Not beautiful. When you come again, I will not be here" (Underhill, 1936, p. 64).

In addition to the psychological difficulties of old age, elderly persons are increasingly beset by physical infirmities. Former strengths and capabilities are supplanted by weaknesses and the loss of muscle. Youthful beauty is replaced by wrinkles and white hair. There is a growing sus-ceptibility to a wide variety of illnesses, such as cancer, heart disease, and arthritis. New aches and pains keep appearing as the years pass. All create new sources of unavoidable stress.

Religious Coping with Age-Related Stressors

Research has consistently revealed that religious coping mechanisms, especially prayer, are most frequently employed when senior citizens are dealing with health-related stress

(Conway, 1985–1986; Manfredi & Pickett, 1987). Turning to a deity for support appears to be the most effective strategy available to elderly persons with health problems. This holds true for persons of different ethnic groups, socioeconomic statuses, and widely varying levels of education (Koenig, George, & Siegler, 1988; Krause & Van Tranh, 1989).

Furthermore, whether the religious variables examined are attendance at services, beliefs, prayer, or church social support, all correlate negatively with depression and loneliness among elderly persons (Johnson & Mullins, 1989; Koenig, Kvale, & Ferrel, 1988; Pressman, Lyons, Larson, & Strain, 1990). Faith not only fosters long-range hope, but also creates optimism for the short-term future (Myers, 1992). Among senior citizens, religious involvement is a solid correlate of happiness (Myers, 1992).

One study of religiosity and time perspective found that religious people are more willing to look into the distant future and confront their eventual death than their nonreligious peers are (Hooper & Spilka, 1970). One's own impending demise is obviously a threat, and thinking about personal death is positively correlated with participation in religious activities by elderly persons (Fry, 1990). In addition, the salience of an individual's religion to self-image increases with age (Moberg, 1965a).

To sum up, the data are clear: religion is a powerful buffer against stress among the elderly. As Myers (1992) puts it, "the happiest of senior citizens are those who are actively religious" (p. 75).

Religion and Longevity

One may argue that the final test of the relationship between religion and aging may be found in longevity. Do religious people live longer than their less religious counterparts? A surprisingly large number of studies have addressed this issue. Even though most of this work indicates that religious involvement is associated with low mortality, the problem has proven to be far more complex than it appears on the surface. Because many variables confound the religion–longevity relationship, much research that has dealt either directly or indirectly with this issue has not produced clear or consistent results. For example, the tie between gender and faith shows that correlations between mortality and religion are stronger for women than for men. We cannot take this finding at face value, however, because women tend to outlive men. In addition, they use health facilities more often than men, insuring faster treatment for problems (Taylor, 1991). Clearly, researchers need to correct for gender.

The subtle influence of socioeconomic status may also complicate the religion–longevity issue. Higher status is associated with joining more organizations, and churches may be included in this picture (Chalfant, Beckley, & Palmer, 1981). Higher socioeconomic status also means more knowledge about health, greater use of medical services, and better quality healthcare. These factors will have an obvious impact on longevity. Similarly, indices of public religious involvement such as church attendance have been found to relate positively to longevity, but this might be due to the likelihood that nonattenders have poorer health that prevents them from going to church. These are only a few of many possible confounds; thus it is understandable that the more such variables are controlled for, the weaker the association between faith and longevity becomes.

Research on a sample of institutionalized chronically ill elderly persons claimed that those who died within the year were less religious (Reynolds & Nelson, 1981). This picture is muddied by the fact that they also had poorer prognoses and were more cognitively impaired. Another group of researchers reported that religion was positively correlated with longevity, but only among elderly persons who were in poor health (Zuckerman, Kasl, & Ostfeld, 1984).

Richardson (1973) studied over 1,300 octogenarians and found religion to be unrelated to 1-year survival rates. More recent work by Koenig (1995) confirmed this finding. Idler and Kasl (1992), by contrast, found that public religiousness was related to lower disability and that private religiousness was linked to lower mortality. Moreover, for both Christians and Jews, there were significantly fewer deaths in the 30 days prior to a major religious holiday than for the same period afterwards (see Research Box 15.4).

Recognizing the need for a meta-analysis of data on this issue, McCullough, Hoyt, Larson, Koenig, and Thoreson (2000) conducted such an analysis on studies with samples totaling almost 126,000 people. (Remember that meta-analysis is a methodological/statistical procedure in which one gathers a great many data on a topic and analyzes them in order to resolve discrepancies and conflicting findings.) After considering some 15 possible confounding factors, these scholars found that religious involvement and longevity were positively related, but that the association was rather weak. For example, if we had two groups of 100 people each—one group being high in religiosity, the other less religious—we could expect to find at a later follow-up that 53 people in the less religious group had died, while only 47 in the more religious group had died. This outcome apparently held for public religious activity (e.g., church attendance), but not for private devotions. The association between religion and mortality was also stronger for women than men. McCullough (2001) offers a number of possibilities to account for these observations, opening the door to further research.

Research Box 15.4. Religion, Disability, Depression, and the Timing of Death (Idler & Kasl, 1992)

In this interesting study, the authors examined the effects of public and private religiosity on health, the ways in which these varied for Christians and Jews, and mortality rates around religious holidays. Starting with a sample of 2,812 people over 65 in 1982, Idler and Kasl reinterviewed the members of this group in 1983, 1984, and 1985.

By means of sophisticated data analyses, public religious participation in 1982 was found to be related to low functional disability in the following 3 years. Things were more complex with private religiousness: This was associated with greater disability in 1984, but an examination of who died and those who lived revealed that those engaging in private religiosity seemed to be protected against mortality.

Studying who lived and who died in the 30 days preceding and following religious holidays showed very strong effects relative to Easter for the Christian groups; the death rate was significantly lower prior to this holiday than after it. As expected, this did not occur for Jews relative to the Christian holiday, but was found for the Jewish holidays of Passover, Rosh Hashanah (the New Year), and Yom Kippur (the Day of Atonement). The pattern of reduced deaths prior to the holidays held for Jewish males but not for females. This variation was seen as a function of the greater role and investment of Jewish males than females in these holidays. This work shows a considerable potential for religious influence on both the health and mortality of elderly people.

Religion and Health

Religion, Stress, and the Immune System

Even though many illustrations and studies in the preceding pages have dealt with health, we now focus on this issue per se. Health is intimately connected to the defenses mobilized by the body when illness and infection are encountered. These stressors activate the body's immune system. One response is the release of a steroid hormone, cortisol. Secreted by the adrenal glands, cortisol has been called the "stress hormone." Too much or too little cortisol can be harmful to a broad spectrum of physiological activities. The negative effects of most interest here are elevated blood pressure, increased heart rate, indirect release of glucose for energy into the bloodstream, and possible problems with emotional control (Purves, Orian, & Heller, 1995; Stoppler, n.d.; Weber, n.d.). Especially in relation to the psychological effects, high levels of cortisol are considered undesirable.

Koenig, McCullough, and Larson (2001) review an immense medical literature in their *Handbook of Religion and Health.* They report research indicating that persons engaging in Buddhist meditation showed significant reductions in cortisol levels. In other work, female patients who resorted to prayer and religion while awaiting breast biopsies for possible cancer revealed less cortisol production than those not employing these methods. A study of women with metastatic breast cancer who evidenced religious activity and who considered faith important also showed lowered evening cortisol levels, but not reduced overall levels. In a number of other researches, the contributors to the *Handbook* found religion to be beneficial to the immune system with regard to other physiological indicators, such as interleukin. Apparently, therefore, religious and spiritual coping can reduce bodily expressions of stress.

Religion, Health, and Illness in General

We proceed now from the work on immune system function to the broader realm of health and illness in general. Levin and Schiller (1987) reviewed over 200 studies that related faith and health–illness, and concluded that the two domains are positively associated. However, a more recent survey of a portion of this literature for the year 2000 claimed that only 17% of 266 articles dealing with religion and cardiovascular disease showed such a relationship (Sloan & Bagiella, 2002). Criticizing the methodology of much of this research, these workers believe that the claims of religion's beneficial effects are greatly exaggerated. Obviously more meta-analytic studies need to be undertaken in this area, and over a broader range of illness.

This is another area where relationships are not simple, for even though some research finds "direct" connections between physical well-being and religion, these may work indirectly by fostering good health habits. Among these, faith (particularly an intrinsic religious orientation) counters the use of tobacco, drugs, and alcohol, and supports the use of seat belts, among other possibilities. Beliefs about prevention may also relate to religious commitment. A comparison of highly religious mothers with their less committed counterparts revealed that the former were significantly more likely to engage in active illness prevention behaviors than the latter group (Ameika, Eck, Ivers, Clifford, & Malcarne, 1994). Still, the more religious mothers felt that they had less control over illness. Since a major prevention category was to "go to the doctor," there might be an inclination here for religion to promote deference both to God and to medical authorities. This possibility merits further assessment, as it may also imply a more general obeisance to authority. Finally, churches often actively sponsor a wide variety of healthful practices (e.g., dietary restrictions, prohibitions against alcohol and smoking); these are often adopted by believers (King, 1990; Levin & Schiller, 1987; Sarafino, 1990).

Even though religious groups may differ in vulnerability to certain illnesses because of diet and cultural factors, faith is associated with a low incidence of a number of cardiovascular conditions, hypertension, stroke, and different forms of cancer (Levin & Schiller, 1987). Another possibility is that since religiosity correlates positively with optimism, life satisfaction, and purpose in life, more religious people may be less inclined to report symptoms of illness and therefore downplay their possible significance (Kass, Friedman, Leserman, Zuttermeister, & Benson, 1991). This, of course, would work to their detriment, and does not appear to be generally true.

Another possible reason for the positive tie between faith and overall health may come from the observation noted earlier that religion seems to enhance one's sense of control, and that this is associated with better health (Loewenthal & Cornwall, 1993; McIntosh et al., 1985). This has been shown earlier in Research Box 15.1, with reference to a study on control, religion, and health (McIntosh & Spilka, 1990). In a large-scale community investigation, these results were further supported, but it was noted that religion was of particular benefit when people were dealing with either chronic illness or the death of loved ones (Mattlin, Wethington, & Kessler, 1990). In another study, resorting to one's faith was found to be the most useful coping device when dealing with such issues (McRae & Costa, 1986), which are addressed in more detail below.

Despite much research in these areas, there remain many unanswered questions. The mechanisms through which faith may operate in overall health and illness have yet to be identified. There is also a definite need for studies that control for religious affiliation, cultural differences, and behaviors that promote or damage health (King, 1990; Levin & Schiller, 1987). In addition, issues of response biasing have yet to be addressed. This is a fertile topic for further study.

Religion and Serious Illnesses

Hayden (1991) researched the utility of religion in helping patients with arthritis cope with pain—an important feature of this illness. He noted tendencies for a conservative religiosity and a sense of meaning in life to counter pain perceptions. These worked best with individuals who were not very depressed to begin with, and who believed that their faith could address their pain effectively. That there is a significant psychological component in the perception of pain goes without saying. Physical and psychological pain often go together, and a strong faith combined with being religiously active seems to counter pain-related distress, depression, and anxiety (Ross, 1990).

When serious, potentially fatal illness strikes, one can expect religion to be invoked rapidly and with telling effect. This is especially true when the problem is cancer. There is apparently a pervasive tendency to avoid blaming God for the bad things that happen to people, and to credit God for positive possibilities and outcomes (Johnson & Spilka, 1991; Spilka & Schmidt, 1983b). To the degree that patients with cancer view God as being in control of things, their sense of threat to life lessens, and their self-esteem improves (Jenkins & Pargament, 1988). An intrinsic religious orientation also counteracts feelings of anger, hostility, and social isolation (Acklin, Brown, & Mauger, 1983). In addition, patients may receive much so-cial support from their coreligionists. We discuss cancer in greater depth below.

When the issue is hypertension, a review of the literature avers that high religious in-volvement seems to counter high blood pressure (Levin & Vanderpool, 1989).

Religion and Cancer: A Closer Look

The literature on the role of faith in serious illness clearly covers a broad range of maladies. In order to gain some perspective, let us confine ourselves to the literature on religion and cancer, particularly since the public identifies cancer with death. Though this association is markedly overdrawn in today's world, it is usually the first idea that comes to mind. In ad-dition, though much research deals with people without reference to their sociocultural framework, let us also situate patients with cancer within their families, as this more poi-gnantly allows us to recognize the seriousness of cancer in its natural context (Spilka & Hartman, 2000). Keep in mind that terms such as "patients," "people," and so on are ab-stractions that lose sight of the real meaning of the ramifications of the disease. Can anyone doubt this when we translate people, individuals, and persons into children, mothers, fathers, and other family members?

If a child contracts cancer, for instance, how do the child, siblings, parents, and other family members react? The child victim is likely to experience hospitalizations involving sepa-rations from others, as well as to experience much pain (both from the illness and from ef-forts to counter it). The effects of possible surgical procedures and chemotherapy can be particularly devastating. The predominant child responses are depression and anxiety (Spilka, Zwartjes, & Zwartjes, 1991). Though the age of the child is a factor, fear of death and a wide variety of other anxieties indicate extreme stress. The basic problems have been pictured as those of meaning and mastery (Hart & Schneider, 1997; Spinetta, 1977), and religion appears to meet these needs rather well (Spilka et al., 1991). Psychiatrist Robert Coles (1990) has written of the efficacy of prayer, religious ritual, and Biblical readings in helping children with cancer cope with their trials. Pargament (1997) points out how religion may also construc-tively deal with the mechanism of denial—a common factor in these circumstances.

Religion plays a role in helping parents and siblings cope as well. With regard to par-ents, the list of reactions to children's cancer is extensive, ranging from anxiety and fear to extreme marital distress and breakup (Enskar, Carlsson, Golsater, Hamrim, & Kreuger, 1997; Grootenhuis & Last, 1997; Leyn, 1976). Church social support and religion's potential for meaning and control can provide strong backing to parents in dealing with their children's ill-ness and their own reactions (Zwartjes, Spilka, Zwartjes, Heideman, & Cilli, 1979).

Siblings may be plagued with anxiety about death, as well as guilt over their conflicted feelings toward their afflicted brother or sister. Anger toward parents may be also present as the parents shift their attention and concern to their ill child (Zwartjes et al., 1979). Faith, possibly with the aid of pastoral counseling, can work to resolve these sibling concerns and strengthen family ties in general.

When a parent is diagnosed with cancer, some different concerns are confronted. There is always fear of death; however, when a mother contracts cancer, the most common condi-tion is breast cancer. In such a case, a daughter often worries about carrying the gene for the condition. The mother's response is often guilt, while both mother and daughter become anxious about the mutilation of mastectomy. Frequently religion is employed to cushion the blow (Johnson & Spilka, 1991).

Though more research needs to be done on religion and the effects on a family when a mother develops cancer, none seems to have been reported about what happens when a father receives a cancer diagnosis. Since he is usually the primary breadwinner, apprehension about economic matters may well be added to uneasiness about other disease-related issues. Extreme distress among the children is commonly observed under these circumstances (Hart & Schneider, 1997).

Whether the issue is serious illness in general or cancer in particular, when people feel that they can be active (e.g., do something constructive) in coping with their disease, they appear to benefit. Prayer, as has already been noted, is an active, cognitive coping strategy (Holahan & Moos, 1987), and patients with cancer who pray feel it is helpful both in reducing their pain and in aiding them to deal with their disease (Meyer, Altmeier, & Burns, 1992; Yates, Chalmer, St. James, Follansbee, & McKegney, 1981). The objective evidence supports such a position.

Religion and Coping with Disability

One of the earliest studies in the literature on religion and coping examined young people who were coping with paraplegia or quadriplegia, primarily as the result of accidents (Bulman & Wortman, 1977). This classic study is detailed in Research Box 15.5.

Religion and Coping with the Death of a Child

Our primary discussion of religion in connection with various aspects of death, including grief and bereavement, has occurred in Chapter 8. However, we feel that our discussion here of religion in relation to coping and adjustment would be incomplete without at least some

---

Research Box 15.5. Attributions of Blame and Coping in the Real World: Severe Accident Victims React to Their Lot (Bulman & Wortman, 1977)

In a noteworthy research study, Bulman and Wortman interviewed 29 young people with paraplegia or quadriplegia, whose spinal injuries had occurred 12 months or less prior to their interviews. Objective measures of religiosity, internal–external control, and the concept of a "just world" ("people get what they deserve") were also administered to the sample. The interviews focused on who or what was to blame for the accidents that resulted in the spinal injuries, whether the accidents were avoidable, and how seriously the victims perceived what happened to them.

Those most likely to blame themselves tended to be highly religious and also felt that the accident could have been avoided. These individuals coped best with their condition. The most frequent explanation for an accident was that "God had a reason" for what occurred. Those who handled their problem best seemed to hold a "just world" view—a finding that is generally true of religious people. The authors emphasize the need for people to search for explanations that reflect an "orderly and meaningful world [more] than a need for a controllable one" (p. 362).

consideration of the greatest disaster that can befall any parent—the death of a child. Indeed, religion may be of the utmost importance in coping with this most major of stressors.

Religion and Sudden Infant Death

We expect the old to die; we painfully acknowledge that younger people do die, mostly by accident; but the death of youngsters is something we want to deny. Still, it occurs, and the death of infants who have not yet had a chance to enjoy life is particularly upsetting. With all the publicity that sudden infant death syndrome (SIDS) has gotten in recent years, new parents often worry about such a possibility. (Fortunately, however, the death rate from SIDS has slowly declined from 1.5 per 1,000 in 1980 to 0.7 per 1,000 infants in 1998; U.S. Bureau of the Census, 2001.)

McIntosh, Silver, and Wortman (1993) have examined the role of faith following the death of an infant from SIDS (see Research Box 15.6). They found that religious participation elicited social support, and that religion helped bereaved parents for whom it was important to derive meaning from this calamity. In other words, parental faith supported the parents' efforts at cognitively processing the death of their child.

Other Studies of Religion and the Death of Children

The McIntosh et al. (1993) study suggests that religion as a coping device may be especially important when a devastating, uncontrollable event such as the death of a child occurs. Naturalistic explanations of a child's death are unsatisfactory for most people, because they imply no future, no hope—simply complete and total termination. In contrast, religious interpre-

---

છ&

Research Box 15.6. Religion's Role in Adjustment to a Negative Life Event: Coping with the Death of a Child (McIntosh, Silver, & Wortman, 1993)

This significant study examined how religion helped parents who lost an infant to SIDS adjust to this tragedy. A sample of 124 parents was studied; each set of parents was interviewed within 15 to 30 days after their child's death, and reinterviewed 18 months later. Adjustment and coping were related to four factors: religion, social support, cognitive processing, and meaning. The researchers hypothesized that religious participation would promote perceptions of social support and adjustment. They also expected that when religion per se was important to the parents, it would help them find meaning in the loss and aid cognitive processing of the event, and would enhance adjustment through these avenues. These hypotheses were supported. In addition, religious participation helped the parents derive meaning from their loss.

This study revealed that religion may not affect adjustment and distress directly; rather, it may work indirectly by bolstering perceptions of social support, aiding cognitive processing, and increasing the meaningfulness of an infant's death, probably by putting it in the context of a positive religious framework. Research such as this indicates the complexity of the role of religion in the coping process, and clarifies some of the mechanisms that are operative when a person's faith is tested by crisis and tragedy.

tations offer the potential of future life and other-worldly gratification for the deceased, and this-worldly answers that offer a measure of contentment for survivors. Mcintosh et al.'s (1993) study indicates this for parents who suddenly lose an infant to SIDS, and it has also been demonstrated for those who anticipate the death of a child from illness (Friedman, Chodoff, Mason, & Hamburg, 1963). Similar findings hold when parents have to deal with the deaths of premature and newborn infants (Palmer & Noble, 1986).

Maton (1989) offered evidence that spiritual support was particularly effective in countering depression and bolstering the self-esteem of parents who had recently lost a child as opposed to those whose offspring had died more than 2 years previously. Rollins-Bohannon (1991) found that church attendance was associated with a reduction in death anxiety for both parents and particularly for mothers, for whom it seems to lessen grief "related to feelings of anger, guilt, loss of control, rumination, depersonalization, and optimism/despair" (Cook & Wimberly, 1983, p. 237). In addition, there are indications that religious beliefs are strengthened by such tragedy when one already has a religious commitment.

Three different theodicies have been observed among bereaved parents: "1) reunion with the deceased in an afterlife; 2) death as a purposive event; and 3) death as punishment for wrong-doing on the part of survivors" (Cook & Wimberly, 1983, p. 237). These are regarded as attempts to make the death meaningful, and even to experience guilt feelings. Attributions to a purposeful God are also invoked when a friend dies, but people with an intrinsic religious orientation may undergo much cognitive restructuring in order to understand what has occurred, possibly because of their positive image of the deity. There is also the possibility that it is cognitively easier to deal with one's own death than that of another valued person (Park & Cohen, 1993; Schoenrade, Ludwig, Atkinson, & Shane, 1990).

OVERVIEW

A central theme in this chapter, if not this book, is that religion "works" because it offers people meaning and control, and brings them together with like-thinking others who provide social support. We have also suggested that these needs are satisfied through religious beliefs, experiences, and practices. These appear to constitute a system of meanings that can be applied to virtually every situation a person may encounter. Often premised upon scripture and/or a popular or civil religion, one finds God images that have the potential to explain both world and personal events (Spilka, Shaver, & Kirkpatrick, 1985). The deity is at one and the same time forgiving, loving, merciful, blessed, wrathful, involved in all human affairs, and simultaneously uninvolved since people have been "given free will" (Gorsuch, 1968). The many concepts of God that are held can be called upon as needed to explain occurrences that seem to defy naturalistic interpretations. People are loath to rely on chance. Fate and luck are poor referents for understanding, but the deity in all its possible manifestations can fill the void of meaninglessness admirably. There is always a place for one's God— simply watching, guiding, supporting, or actively solving a problem. In other words, when people need to gain a greater measure of control over life events, the deity is there to provide the help they require.

To hold a belief is to "know" something. As Herbert Benson (1975) has claimed, "the faith factor" is a powerful force in coping. It makes everything meaningful and strengthens our hand in dealing with the world. The internal mechanisms by which such beliefs work have not been determined, but no one can doubt that they can have profound effects.

Chapter 16

RELIGION AND MENTAL DISORDER

Religion is comparable to a childhood neurosis.

There is a madness which is the special gift of heaven.

Religious anxiety is rarely, if ever, a cause of insanity. The sublime faith of Christianity is rather a safeguard against it.

Religion as we know it today serves as an institutionalized defense against anxiety.

She wore a crown of thorns. She scarred her face with pepper so no man would find her attractive. Someone had the bad taste to praise her hands, so she dipped them in lye.[1]

PAST AND PRESENT: CONFUSION, CONFLICT, RESOLUTION

Religion and mental disorder have had a long and troubled relationship. For most of this period, one might even call them "intimate enemies." Whether the relationship was noted in the Bible, in ancient Greece and Rome, or in China and India, there seemed to be a tug-of-war over whose word was final with regard to abnormality. In the West until the last four to five centuries, power was vested in the church, and the medical profession took its orders from ecclesiastical authorities (McNeill, 1951; Zilboorg & Henry, 1941). The operating principle from the Bible was that "the Lord shall smite thee with madness" (Deuteronomy 28:28) for disobeying God's commandments—and, by extension, church leaders' pronouncements. In reacting to mental disturbance during its first 1,500 years, the Christian tradition combined kindness and compassion with cruelty and punishment. Initially, tolerance and sympathy were united with prayer and supportive religious practices (McNeill, 1951; Zilboorg & Henry, 1941). Challenges to church power in the late Middle Ages and the Renaissance paralleled a growing concern with sin, confession, repentance, and punishment. Reformation and Enlightenment ideas further threatened religious institutions, which often hardened their position even further in response. An increasing emphasis on witchcraft, demons, and the influence of Satan resulted in the suffering and death of many thousands of mentally disturbed persons (Bromberg, 1937).

Established religion reluctantly ceded power to medicine and psychiatry. With similar reluctance, medicine has slowly yielded some control to psychology and social work. Yet the earlier notions of sin are still with us, though they are usually now more subtly hidden (Borinstein, 1992; Hall, Zilboorg, & Bunker, 1944; Reisman, 1991; Rotenberg, 1978).

---

1. These quotations come, respectively, from the following sources: Freud (1927/1961, p. 53); Jowett (1907, p. 549); Caplan (1969, p. 132); Symonds (1946, p. 187); and McGinley (1969, p. 129).

Suspicion of and concern about religion within the psychological/psychiatric community are abating. Historically, psychoanalysis and positivistic behaviorism either were openly antithetic toward religion or simply had no place for it in their views of mental life (Burnham, 1985; Farberow, 1963; Wulff, 1997). However, classic behaviorism has faded into psychological history, and psychoanalytic ideas (often in new garb) have become integral to the psychological study of religion and often the work of the clergy (Beit-Hallahmi, 1995; McDargh, 1983; Smith & Handelman, 1990). A new and growing level of cooperation now characterizes religion–psychology relationships.

But all is still not peace and harmony. The notion that sin and wrongdoing are the causes of mental problems remains in the popular mind, and such themes even persist among the helping professions (Kirk & Kutchins, 1992; Nunnally, 1961). Though the cruder versions of these ideas seem to be fading, some still prevail in certain religiously conservative quarters, particularly in relatively isolated groups. In contrast, however, we find conservative mainstream religious bodies such as the American Baptist Churches (1992) formally adopting sophisticated approaches to mental illness.

The third edition of the *Diagnostic and Statistical Manual of Mental Disorders* (DSM-III; American Psychiatric Association, 1980) was said to contain "an implicit and sometimes explicit tendency to devalue experiences common to many religions and to cast them into the pale of psychopathology" (Kilbourne & Richardson, 1984b, p. 2). This appears to have changed, however. The fourth edition of the DSM (DSM-IV; American Psychiatric Association, 1994) recognizes "religious and spiritual difficulties as a distinct mental disorder deserving treatment" (Sleek, 1994, p. 8). As part of this new awareness, religion and spirituality can be considered psychotherapeutic tools. Antireligious statements, such as Ellis's (1980) view that "the less religious [patients] are, the more emotionally healthy they will tend to be" (p. 637), are becoming passé. Ellis (2000) now feels that "religious beliefs which [he] once saw as irrational, are potentially helpful to some clients. Religious believers embrace some rational, self-helping beliefs as well" (p. 277).

For the last several decades, therefore, psychologists and religionists have been replacing previous doubts and antagonisms with a new spirit of mutual concern and support. The resulting integration of contemporary religion and psychology supports Hiltner's (1962) religious position that "psychology [is] a theological discipline internal to theology itself" (p. 251). We have come full circle, to the realization that cooperation between religion and the behavioral sciences is essential to human betterment.

CONCERNS, CAUTIONS, AND DIRECTIONS

Problems of Definition

Since research on religion and abnormality spans many decades, the language employed in earlier work may not be in use any more. Translating older mental health terminology into terms that are acceptable today is rarely done, and in some cases may not even be possible. In addition, those who have worked with one DSM classification system for psychopathology are frequently reluctant to adopt new frameworks, and may mix older concepts and ideas with the latest categories. In other words, the application of diagnostic labels is less precise than is desirable from either a research or an applied perspective (Kirk & Kutchins, 1992).

When one reviews the religious facets of work in this area, the definition and use of terms are no more precise. Most studies simply designate their respondents as "Catholic," "Protestant," "Jewish," and "other" (Hollingshead & Redlich, 1958; Rose, 1955; Srole, Langner, Michael, Opler, & Rennie, 1962). Little or no explanation is provided for variations among these broad groups. Confounding factors such as socioeconomic status or ethnic groups are ignored, though both of these factors are significant correlates of mental disorder (Dohrenwend & Dohrenwend, 1969; Hollingshead & Redlich, 1958). These confounding factors affect psychiatric diagnoses as well (Dohrenwend & Dohrenwend, 1969; Rose, 1955). That is, diagnosticians unknowingly apply more severe diagnoses to patients who differ more from them culturally, economically, and ethnically (Hollingshead & Redlich, 1958). Needless to say, clients/patients suffer from such biasing.

In addition, issues such as degree of religious commitment and church or synagogue participation are not considered. It must also be noted that the four broad religious classifications given above are simplifications. Are Jews Orthodox, Conservative, or Reform? Italian Catholics can sometimes be very different from Irish Catholics in background and religious expression. And just what does it mean to be Protestant? The *Yearbook of American and Canadian Churches and Megachurches* lists about 260 religious bodies, of which about 220 are said to be Protestant (Lindner, 2003). The futility of conducting research when the religious variable is poorly defined is obvious. Furthermore, the habit has developed of providing demographic information such as gender and age without a theory that makes such data meaningful.

In Chapter 2, we have discussed the complexity of the religious domain, suggesting that categories such as the Intrinsic and Extrinsic or Committed and Consensual dimensions and measures (among other possibilities) might be useful. Simplistic indicators of religion often mask researchers' poor understanding of this highly complex realm. Still, consistency over multiple studies suggests reliable findings, and even where respondents have been poorly classified, clues may be present that stimulate better research. Unfortunately, this is a costly and a time- and energy-consuming path to follow. A much more efficient approach entails the development of adequate theory to guide such studies; more exacting definitions on both sides of the religion-and-mental-disturbance issue are essential prerequisites in such work.

Possible Relationships of Religion and Mental Disorder

The purpose of this chapter is to show the many ways in which faith and psychological problems may be related. Among these possibilities are the following:

1. Religion may be an expression of mental disorder.
2. Institutionalized faith can be a socializing and suppressing force, aiding people to cope with their life stresses and mental aberrations.
3. Religion can serve as a haven—a protective agency for some mentally disturbed people.
4. Spiritual commitment and involvement may perform therapeutic roles in alleviating mental distress.
5. Religion can be a stressor, a source of problems; in a sense, it can be "a hazard to one's mental health."[2]

---

2. With the exception of the last role for religion, we are deeply indebted to James E. Dittes for this framework, which was first used in Spilka and Werme (1971).

In addition to these five relational patterns, much research has been conducted on connections between personal faith and a variety of behavioral disturbances, such as substance abuse and crime/delinquency (see Chapter 13 regarding these problems); mild to severe forms of psychopathology; and particular areas of concern, such as mental disorder among women, elderly individuals, and persons who affiliate with what are pejoratively termed "cults." Moreover, there are few matters in the social psychology of religion more complex and controversial than the relationship of religion to what are most accurately termed "psychosocial disorders" (e.g., sexual abuse). At the outset, however, let us say that the overwhelming mass of research evidence suggests more beneficial associations than adverse effects between religion and mental well-being.

This last assertion gains support from an older meta-analysis of 24 researches relating indices of religion and psychopathology. Because of multiple samples and relevant variables in these studies, a total of 30 effects were assessed. Fourteen of these showed a favorable relationship between religion and mental health; nine evidenced no association; and seven indicated religion and abnormality to be affiliated (Bergin, 1983). Bergin (1983) reviewed a number of other studies supporting the view that faith and mental health are positively associated.

A POSSIBLE THEORETICAL DIRECTION

In Chapter 15, we have applied our integrative framework to religion, coping, and adjustment. Extending these ideas to the realm of mental disorder, we encounter a new set of issues. Not the least of these concern biological factors. More specifically, genetic influences are increasingly found in many mental conditions that were previously considered functional products of experience. Even though the translation of their expression into the domain of social conduct is our main concern, we must remember that genetic factors only suggest probabilities; they do not wholly determine mental disorders or other conditions (see Chapter 3). For example, schizophrenia has long been known to be a genetically involved disturbance. Current work focuses on two genes on chromosomes 6 and 8 as involved in this disorder. However, if one identical twin manifests schizophrenia, the other twin will develop the selfsame condition only 30–50% of the time, despite having exactly the same genetic endowment (Wade, 2002). Of course, this implies that 50–70% of the incidence of schizophrenia is due to environmental influences.

With regard to our conceptual framework, mental abnormality entails (1) distortions of meaning, such as delusions of grandeur and persecution; (2) the feeling that one lacks control, as occurs in depression; and (3) a lack of social connection that results from deviant thinking and behavior and adversely affects social relationships. We will see in this chapter that religion can function to enforce meanings that more accurately describe reality, enhance one's sense of personal control, and improve social relationships.

RELIGION AS AN EXPRESSION OF MENTAL DISORDER

Many years ago, when Bernard Spilka was an undergraduate, he and his fellow students were regularly harassed and challenged by two street corner evangelists. Actually, only one was capable of presenting his Biblically based arguments; the other stood to the side, reading from a large open Bible in an unintelligible mumble. The students never saw him do anything else.

It was evident that his contact with reality was extremely poor. Spilka now thinks of him as a person with poorly integrated schizophrenia. He illustrated what has often been demonstrated in books on psychopathology—namely, that any aspect of religious belief, experience, or behavior can be meaningful to a seriously disturbed mind.

Disturbed Beliefs

It is not uncommon that a person suffering from major mental illness who is delusional and possibly hallucinating feels chosen by God to do certain things. Delusions may be manifested in the belief that one is an angel of God—or, on the other side of the coin, that one is cursed by God. An excellent example is the famous study by Milton Rokeach (1964), in which he studied three men who variously identified themselves as Jesus Christ and God. Though none felt victimized by God, all illustrated how religion might be a part of severe mental disorder.

Scrupulosity: Disturbed Religious Thought and Behavior

One form of mental pathology that is manifested in religious thinking and behavior has been termed "scrupulosity" (Mora, 1969). Askin, Paultre, White, and Van Ornum (1993, p. 3) call it "the religious manifestation of Obsessive–Compulsive Disorder," which is defined in DSM-IV as an anxiety disorder. They specifically define scrupulosity as "a condition involving continuous worry about religious issues or compulsions to perform religious rituals" (Askin et al., 1993, pp. 3–4). Askin and her colleagues have developed a short objective measure of scrupulosity that correlates very strongly with indices of obsessions–compulsions. Similar behavior has been reported for a group of disturbed Catholic children (Weisner & Riffel, 1960).

Primary among the expressions associated with scrupulosity are a fear of sin and compulsive doubt (Nolan, 1990; Overholser, 1963). Those suffering from this disorder continually seek assurances from religious authorities and tend to reject psychotherapy. It is possible, however, for an involved cleric to work with a therapist to help alleviate the problem (Nolan, 1990). In addition, scrupulous persons engage in rigid ritualistic observances and practices in order to gain some sense of purification—something they can never accept. They can never feel clean and accepted by God, due to attributions to themselves as bad and sinful and to the deity as unforgiving and tolerating no deviation from extreme religious strictures. Freudian theory suggests that scrupulosity relates to sexual impulse control; in support of this theory, there is evidence that its peak period of occurrence in life is adolescence (Nolan, 1990; Wulff, 1997). It is not restricted to the teenage years, however.

Religious and Mystical Experience

The often extremely unusual and graphic nature of religious or mystical experiences can easily lead one to conclude that they are signs of mental disturbance. However, before we too readily label these experiences as indicating mental deviance, let us first accept a well-established survey research finding that is detailed in Chapter 10 on mysticism: namely, that considerable proportions of the U.S. and British populations report such encounters. Depending on the way the question eliciting this information is phrased, 25–50% of those sampled indicate having had such experiences (Greeley, 1974; Hardy, 1979; Hay & Morisy, 1978; Thomas & Cooper, 1978). If one selects religiously active people, the incidence is usually in the 70–

80% range (Spilka, Ladd, McIntosh, & Milmoe, 1996). In fact, certain religious bodies, usually quite conservative ones, expect their members to have these episodes and to disclose them publicly. In these groups, such experiences help integrate people into the church and therefore support their adjustment. In addition, in both Western and other cultures, reports of such occurrences frequently contribute to the reputations of spiritual figures such as saints (Prince, 1992). In other words, having a religious or mystical experience is often seen as quite normal and may aid adjustment.

Despite these facts and findings, it has been acknowledged that "some mystics are badly disoriented personalities" (Greeley, 1974, p. 81). In fact, a committee of the Group for the Advancement of Psychiatry (GAP) (1976) indicated that it was unable "to make a firm distinction between a mystical state and a psychopathological state" (p. 815). The committee did feel that mysticism "serves certain psychic needs, or that it constitutes an attempt to resolve certain ubiquitous problems" (p. 715). Even though this GAP committee offered some comments on the possibly favorable outcomes of mystical experiences and attempted to distinguish them from schizophrenic episodes, its members were still too strongly attached to classic psychoanalytic and psychiatric views to overcome their traditional view of such experiences as signs of illness. They identified mystical behaviors as "intermediate between normality and frank psychosis; a form of ego regression" (p. 731). Other psychiatrists, however, have suggested that mystical experience can represent a rejection of aggression or even be a suicide preventative (Horton, 1973; *Roche Report*, 1972). Without definitive success, some research has also attempted to distinguish between mystical states and schizophrenic thinking and behavior (Siglag, 1987).

The association of religious and mystical episodes with the use of drugs has been widely noted (Batson, Schoenrade, & Ventis, 1993; Bridges, 1970; see also the discussion of entheogens in Chapter 9). Insofar as drug use may reflect abnormality, psychedelic experiences with a religious flavor can be regarded as expressing deviance in personality. Hood (1995a), however, details a wide variety of avenues to religious experience, further suggesting that such experience is not a common result of psychopathology.

Over 70 years ago, Leuba (1929) looked at the role of epilepsy in mystical expression, inferring that aberrant neural function might underlie such experiences in many people. He spoke of "the presence in our great mystics of nervous disorders, perhaps of hysteria" (p. 191). Leuba also felt that mental problems such as "neurasthenia" and depression might predispose one to have mystical experiences.

In a highly significant theoretical and research paper, Rodney Stark (1965) offered a breakdown of religious and mystical experiences ranging from the normal to the possibly pathological. For example, his "salvational" type is said to be motivated by a sense of "sin and guilt" (p. 102). Of a more extreme nature, with much potential for illustrating mental disturbance, is Stark's "revelational" experience. It is the rarest and most deviant form he discusses, and is expressed in visual and auditory hallucinations that the individual regards as messages from the divine, angels, or Satan. It has also received some confirmation from work showing that personality and adjustment problems may be associated with religious experiences involving extreme physical–emotional reactions and/or hallucinations (Jackson & Spilka, 1980). Similar connections have been offered by other scholars (Boisen, 1936; Spilka, Brown, & Cassidy, 1993).

Summarizing the research literature, Lukoff, Lu, and Turner (1992) note that those reporting mystical experiences score more favorably on measures of abnormality and psychological well-being than members of control groups do. That religious and mystical encounters may reflect mental disturbance, there is no doubt; however, the weight of the evidence suggests that most such experiences are not pathological, and that many even have beneficial effects (Clark, Malony, Daane, & Tippett, 1973; McCallister, 1995).

Glossolalia

A cousin of religious experience and behavior, glossolalia or "speaking in tongues" can be quite impressive in its effects, and may be expressive of mental disorder. It is discussed at length in Chapter 9. Not too many years ago, it easily led to interpretations of psychopathology; in some instances, when it was observed outside its approved religious setting, recommendations for psychiatric intervention were likely to occur (Prince, 1992). One fairly recent estimate suggests that at least 2 million persons in the United States engage in glossolalia (Greenberg & Witztum, 1992).

The question "Is glossolalia a normal or abnormal behavior?" has been with us for some time. Clinical psychological and psychiatric professionals are inclined toward explanations that stress deviance. Researchers emphasize either minor personality differences or, more commonly, find no distinctions between glossolalic and nonglossolalic people. Kildahl (1972) viewed the former as suggestible, passive, submissive, and dependent. In contrast, Teshome (1992) found glossolalic individuals to be more independent and to rely on others less than nonglossolalic persons, but observed little else.

Taking the deviance perspective, Pattison (1968) claimed that glossolalic individuals demonstrate "overt psychopathology of a sociopathic, hysterical, or hypochondriacal nature" (p. 76). If so, this would certainly indicate serious disorder. Kelsey (1964) noted an implied correlation with schizophrenia, but rejected such an identification. He was more willing to accept glossolalia as a lesser neurotic symptom, but also expressed doubt about applying such a label to these people. There is evidence that speaking in tongues usually follows a period of crisis and works to resolve the resulting anxiety (Kildahl, 1972). In a similar way, Preus (1982) has described glossolalia as a "release from tension and an answer to personal stress and trauma . . . and can be accomplished by almost any person who really wants to" (p. 290). These last views are more moderate than the extreme position of Pattison, but still maintain some potentially aberrant motivation due to stress and anxiety. Goodman (1972) used the phrase "hyperarousal dissociation" to imply abnormality, but this phrase is really a better description of an altered state of consciousness, such as that found in mystical experience.

Glossolalia is a worldwide phenomenon (Bourguignon, 1992; Greenberg & Witztum, 1992). Psychiatry and psychology are slowly accepting the idea that it is normal (i.e., not pathological) behavior. There is currently little doubt that it is learned behavior, which is reinforced in certain group settings into which glossolalic individuals are socialized (Goodman, 1972; Samarin, 1959). Schumaker (1995) speaks of the dissociation of learned associations, but then identifies dissociation with a broad range of mental problems. At worst, glossolalia might be termed a "mild psychopathological disorder" (Greenberg & Witztum, 1992, p. 306), but this may be more the exception than the rule. A representative example of research in this area is presented in Research Box 16.1.

Conversion

Chapter 11 discusses and defines conversion. Historically, it has often been the object of clinical and psychiatric concern (especially when a person affiliates with a religiously deviant

---
ða

Research Box 16.1. The Psychology of Speaking in Tongues (Kildahl, 1972)

In this study, two groups—one of 20 persons who spoke in tongues, the other of 20 people who did not—were interviewed in depth about their lives and tongue-speaking experiences. The groups were equated for religiosity, which was evidently high. Three projective tests (the Rorschach ink blot, the Thematic Apperception Test, and the Draw-a-Person) and one objective test (the Minnesota Multiphasic Personality Inventory) were administered to the participants.

It was observed that the nonglossolalic individuals tended to be more independent and autonomous, but more depressed than their glossolalic peers. Speaking in tongues was associated with strong trust in a religious group leader. Though no real differences existed between the two groups in well-being, the glossolalic participants were characterized as being more dependent on the guidance of a valued religious authority. They were inclined to relinquish personal independence and control to this leader, and usually ceased engaging in glossolalia when they lost faith in their spiritual guide.

Kildahl cited one researcher who asserted that "more than 85 percent of tongue-speakers had experienced a clearly defined anxiety crisis preceding their speaking in tongues" (p. 57). In this study, the glossolalia seemed to be constructive and anxiety-reducing.

---

group usually described as a "cult"; see Chapter 12). We are concerned here with only one part of the multifaceted phenomenon termed "conversion."

Without question, most conversions are not symptomatic of mental disturbance (Bainbridge, 1992b; Rambo, 1992, 1993). Personal problems may set the stage for conversion, and it can be a constructive solution to those difficulties. Probably the earliest major study was conducted by E. D. Starbuck (1899) in the late 1890s. High among the motives he found to motivate conversion were "fear of Death or Hell" and "Remorse, Conviction for Sin, etc." (p. 52). The most common emotional states he found to be associated with conversion were "depression, sadness, pensiveness," with "restlessness, anxiety, uncertainty" following closely (p. 63).

In another classic study of over 2,000 people, E. T. Clark (1929) reported three kinds of "religious awakening." Two of these, the "definite crisis awakening" and the "emotional stimulus awakening," were judged to have the highest potential of expressing psychological problems. They were generally accompanied by feelings of sin, guilt, and depression, and were frequently affiliated with sexual problems. Clark's "gradual awakening" type was a more positive form of conversion, a normal process that slowly occurred over a long period of time. In three separate samples, Clark classified 53–77% of the converts in this "gradual" category. A number of later studies have suggested that rapid conversions follow major personal and social upheavals (Rambo, 1992).

Other work revealed that persons suffering from affective disorders (the earlier name for DSM-IV mood disorders, such as depressive and bipolar disorders) showed an increased likelihood of having conversion and salvational experiences (Gallemore, Wilson, & Rhoads,

1969). This was explained by noting the heightened emotional responsiveness of such individuals. The outcomes of such religious manifestations spanned the range from pain and depression to increased maturation.

Relative to our framework (see Chapters 1–3), Ullman (1982) initially theorized that a need for meaning might stimulate conversion, but found that emotional and relational difficulties (often involving childhood distress) provided the motivation. The issue may not have been a lack of meaning, but a deficiency in control plus difficulties in social relationships.

The research of Starbuck (1899) and Clark (1929) brought to the fore the question of sudden versus gradual conversion. The literature usually indicts the former as an expression of underlying pathology, while suggesting that the latter form implies mental health and well-being. The general position has been that, on average, those who convert suddenly tend to be emotionally unstable and are likely to relapse. They may also engage in repeated conversions, particularly in revival-type situations. A follow-up of persons who made such "decisions" during a Billy Graham crusade in Great Britain revealed that about half had religiously lapsed during the subsequent year (Argyle, 1959). Another investigation reported that 87% of these converts had reverted within 6 months to their former religious behavior (Argyle, 1959). Some of these people had converted up to six times. Psychiatrist Leon Salzman (1953) termed these sudden and superficial conversions "regressive–pathological," and viewed them as related to conflicts with paternal authority. The same theme pervaded the work of Allison (1969), whose study of converts also stressed the role of alcoholic, absent, or weak fathers. Christensen (1963) similarly reported parent–child difficulties prior to conversion, particularly among persons with early fundamentalist training.

Though claims such as these have been made by knowledgeable clinicians, it is sometimes difficult for the outside reader to reach the same conclusions from the data as those reporting such work. Still, this kind of thinking is popular in certain psychological/psychiatric quarters. Illustrative is an extensive and informative case history in which Levin and Zegans (1974) viewed the conversion of a young man as a substitution for a weak father. This theme of conversion reflecting paternal problems has commonly been found among psychoanalytically oriented scholars, but needs confirmation by more exacting research. Such workers often hold a negative view that connotes conversion as "generally a regressive, disintegrative, pathological phenomenon" (Rambo, 1982, p. 155). This position has failed to gain any substantial support in almost a century of research.

Research on the sudden–gradual distinction has fairly consistently shown that rapid conversion is associated with higher anxiety and poorer chronic adjustment than the gradual form (Kildahl, 1965; Roberts, 1965; Spellman, Baskett, & Byrne, 1971). Severe depression and the potential of suicide have also been components in these sudden conversions (Cavenar & Spaulding, 1977). However, as popular as the image of the sudden conversion is in the public mind, the evidence suggests that it is relatively uncommon, affecting under 10% of converts (Clark, 1929; Starbuck, 1899).

We may say that conversion, though often impressive, is infrequently a manifestation of psychological disturbance. The rapid acquisition of a new religious faith is more likely than its gradual counterpart to reflect problems in coping with one's impulses and relations with others and the world. However, most large-scale studies demonstrate that conversions are constructive events (Srole et al., 1962).

RELIGION AS A SOCIALIZING AND SUPPRESSING AGENT

The Control Functions of the Religious Community

Marty (1975) details how "religious America has been and is conducive to the building of human community" (p. 35). Churches and congregations thus strive to create and strengthen a natural human desire to belong; this is sociality (as described in Chapters 1–3) par excellence. To maintain and reinforce the group's bonds, a religious community actively functions to socialize, suppress, and inhibit what the community considers deviant and unacceptable behavior—whether these functions emanate from scriptural guidance, clerical pressure, or the social reinforcement of congregants (Koenig, McCullough, & Larson, 2001).

Churchgoers overwhelmingly represent the more conservative and conforming members of the North American social order (Glock & Stark, 1965; Herberg, 1960; McGuire, 1992; Stark & Glock, 1968). Stark and Glock (1968) refer to "churches as moral communities" (p. 163); as such, mental deviance is often redefined as a moral problem, since it threatens social cohesion. Whether a religious institution is liberal or conservative, it attempts to suppress conflict among its adherents, even if this increases dissension in the larger community (McGuire, 1992). This suppression can extend into all aspects of an individual's life, not the least of which are child-rearing practices that attempt to control displeasing and socially inappropriate behavior such as aggression (Bateman & Jensen, 1958).

Studying maladaptive behavior among mainline Protestants, MacDonald and Luckett (1983) suggested that failure to adapt may result from early exposure at home to overly strong and repressive controls. Such experiences, rather than aiding adjustment to reality, foster rigid identifications with ideals that cannot be realized in modern life. Thinking of this nature works against community, and adherents to religious doctrines are likely to counter such views. We need to recognize that groups form within churches based on similarities in age, shared interests and outlooks, and similar goals (Fichter, 1954). Variance in attitudes and behavior from these norms creates pressures to conform.

Social disapproval and ostracism are strong weapons for shaping thought and action. If these fail, contact with the offender is reduced until the latter is socially isolated from other group members (Schachter, 1951). By such means, the religious community becomes a learning environment that can direct abnormal thinking and activity into approved channels. This is mediated both through the social values and responses of the church members and through religious doctrines.

These socializing forces will be effective to the degree that mentally disturbed persons attend religious services and have contact with others in this setting, and become exposed to their traditional outlooks. The research supports such an inference: Improvements in mental health go along with church or temple attendance (Strawbridge, Shema, Cohen, & Kaplan, 2001). Specifically, most studies show that those who attend church, especially elderly individuals, reveal fewer depressive symptoms than nonattenders do (Levin & Chatters, 1998; Plante & Sharma, 2001). In addition, such associations apparently strengthen impulse controls and counter a variety of deviant tendencies (Rohrbaugh & Jessor, 1975). This is evidently true even for Hare Krishna members, whose overall adjustment improves with the length of time that they are affiliated with this group. The social controls exercised by this cult constitute a learning environment for its adherents (Ross, 1983).

More in line with the mainstream, Stark (1971) has shown that mentally disturbed persons who live outside a hospital setting assign less personal importance to religion and are less religiously active than nondisturbed citizens are. He has theorized that "psychopathology seems to *impede* the manifestation of conventional religious beliefs and activities" (p. 175; emphasis in original). This notable study is detailed in Research Box 16.2. It confirms other findings indicating that the faith of mentally disordered individuals is itself disturbed and deviant (Hardt, 1963; Lowe, 1955; Lowe & Braaten, 1966; Reifsnyder & Campbell, 1960). There are also indications that the more severe an individual's psychopathology is, the less the individual is involved in both personal and organized religious activity (MacDonald & Luckett, 1983).

The Control Functions of Religious Ideas and Institutions

In the preceding section, we have looked at the control functions of religion that emanate from church affiliation. As Pruyser (1971) noted, religion is "a perennial form of wish-fulfillment and need gratification . . . it condones [infantile wishes] by symbolic satisfactions" (p. 79). The implication is that mental disturbance may be socially shaped and focused by religious ideas and the ways churches present them.

Institutionalized faith lives by both formal and informal rules and referents—the Ten Commandments, the Golden Rule, the Bible, Papal statements, interpretations and decisions of denominational conclaves, and so forth. Scripture is replete with statements that associate religious devotion with bodily and mental health (Koenig et al., 2001). The ecclesiastical climate also sponsors notions of how a "good Jew" or a "good Christian" thinks and acts. These notions are supported by images of God's love, mercy, or vengeance—which are not

Research Box 16.2. Psychopathology and Religious Commitment (Stark, 1971)

Theorizing that conventional religious involvement would be incompatible with deviant thinking and behavior, Rodney Stark hypothesized a negative relationship between these two variables. In his study, 100 mentally disturbed persons were carefully matched with 100 nondisturbed individuals and compared on a variety of religious items. The basic findings were as follows.

Percentage claiming:	Mentally disturbed	Nondisturbed
No religious affiliation	16	3
Religion not important at all	16	4
Not belonging to any church	54	40
Never attending church	21	5

Note. Adapted from Stark (1971). Copyright 1971 by the Religious Research Association. Adapted by permission.

The hypothesis was clearly confirmed, as the mentally disturbed persons demonstrated less conventional religious involvement than the nondisturbed sample. In another part of this study, Protestants and Catholics from a national sample who scored low on indices of psychic difficulties were more likely to be religiously orthodox and to attend church frequently than those revealing such problems. Again, the hypothesis was supported.

taken lightly by faithful people, whether they be nondisturbed or disturbed individuals. When adopted as guides for personal action, these rules and referents may be very effective forces for the suppression and socialization of abnormal impulses.

Even if psychopathology comes to the surface, the argument has often been made that the use of religion may prevent worse things from happening. One paper suggests that "occasionally religiosity in paranoid schizophrenia might itself be a mechanism to control underlying hostility and aggressive behavior" (MacDonald & Luckett, 1983, p. 33). In a case study, two psychiatrists claimed that a patient's "religious conversion enabled him to find a new and potentially viable self-definition" (Levin & Zegans, 1974, p. 80). It apparently functioned as a substitute for the "overwhelming panic of his acute psychosis" (p. 79). Similarly, Allison (1968) referred to intense religious experiences and conversion as "adaptive regression" that may "help reorganize a weakened ego" (p. 459).

There is no need to document the very negative attitude of Western religious institutions toward suicide. Dublin (1963) has emphasized that "suicide . . . is infrequent where the guidance and authority of religion are accepted without question, where the church forms the background of communal life, where duties are rigidly prescribed" (p. 74). This relationship is most evident in such bodies as Roman Catholicism, Greek Orthodoxy, and Orthodox Judaism. Countries in which these faiths predominate report the lowest suicide rates. The greater emphasis of Protestantism on individualism and personal freedom may work to set a troubled person adrift in an anomic world; hence suicide rates for Protestants are two to three times higher than for Jews and Catholics (Argyle, 1959).[3]

Despite these historical and sociological considerations, mostly small-sample studies have not consistently found negative relationships between religious variables and suicide attempts (Koenig et al., 2001). There is a clear need for meta-analytic studies tying religion to suicide attitudes, ideation, and attempts.

In summary, Mowrer (1958) quoted Feifel on the socializing function of religious doctrine: "Religion . . . tries to school us in those wise restraints—self-discipline, the capacity for sacrifice and service to others—that make the repressive control of impulses unnecessary" (p. 579). This is an ideal that many disturbed people attempt to realize.

Religious Role Models

Both children and adults often learn how to behave by modeling themselves after people whom they admire or who purvey ideas and ideals that speak to success in attaining desired goals. In other words, they learn by observing others and emulating their thoughts and behavior. These others may be people with whom they interact or about whom they read, hear, or are informed. Social learning theory suggests that "the power of a moral model . . . can be an important component in the development of self-control" (Casey & Burton, 1986, p. 82). Within limits, people can learn to be what is generally defined as "normal" or "abnormal" by emulating others.

Ministers, priests, rabbis, Biblical heroes, Jesus and his apostles, saints, and so forth stand as sanctified models to be imitated. Explicitly and implicitly, these figures enact roles that

---

3. There is, of course, this confounding factor: A religious setting that condemns suicide is not likely to produce medical and civil authorities who are willing to define a death as suicide, except where the evidence is irrefutable and/or has become public knowledge (Gibbs, 1966).

may significantly influence the behavior and thinking of religious people along approved lines. In local settings, clergy may stand as greatly admired models. In one study of over 3,000 children and adolescents, clerics were rated as more supportive than parents, suggesting the potential of priests and ministers as positive role models (Nelsen, Potvin, & Shields, 1976). In all likelihood, these images can be meaningful referents for some mentally disturbed individuals. As Bandura (1977) has affirmed, "modeling influences can strengthen or weaken inhibitions over behavior" (p. 49).

Such a behavioral role model approach has been formalized by the Swedish scholar Hjalmar Sundén. As noted in earlier chapters, his role theory appears applicable to religious behavior in general, since it stresses experience, perception, motivation, and learning. Holm (1987a) notes that "when an individual in a certain religious tradition absorbs descriptions from sacred history, he learns models for his attitudes toward the supernatural" (p. 41); he adds that "this description will function as a structuring role pattern" (p. 41). Here is a theoretical framework that usefully connotes religious role models with the socialized control of thinking and behavior on the part of mentally distressed persons.

Religion and the Disturbed Self

Another approach to understanding abnormality relates to the way people view themselves. Since deviant behavior may both result from and contribute to the social ostracism of disturbed persons, it is to be expected that such people possess negative views of themselves. We also know that unfavorable self-attributions parallel similar outlooks toward the deity and religion (Benson & Spilka, 1973). In some instances, this pattern might prevent these individuals' getting help either from their personal faith or from association with others in religious institutions. Jensen and Erickson (1979) suggest that strict religious group attitudes, along with the positive role models provided by clergy and coreligionists, may jointly act to socialize and restrain deviant thinking and behavior.

It is evident that religious systems and their supporters can suppress abnormal thinking and behavior, and can help mentally disordered people become part of the larger community. Such social and ideological sustenance may also contribute to ego strength and integration. Stated differently, adherence to a faith that is in line with cultural norms can constructively influence psychopathology.

RELIGION AS A HAVEN

Religion can offer mentally distressed individuals refuge from the stresses of daily life—a safe harbor from the turmoil and turbulence of living. This can take place in three ways: (1) Everyday existence may be circumscribed and controlled by rules that leave little doubt about how to behave; (2) being part of a religious organization may alleviate fears of social isolation and rejection; and (3) strong identification with a religious body can provide the perceived security of divine protection. These processes can also take place within three different types of religious organizations: (1) groups or movements that are out of the religious mainstream (so-called "sects" or "cults"); (2) encapsulated religious communities, such as the Amish and the Hutterites; and (3) separate communities within mainline religions, such as sisterhoods of nuns.

Groups or Movements That Are Out of the Mainstream

Though many reasons exist for the formation of new religious bodies, particularly sects and cults, such movements can attract mentally disturbed individuals. As noted earlier, if such persons are not socialized by mainline churches, they may become estranged from traditional religion. This is a two-way street: The average churchgoer is probably sympathetic to the plight of mentally disordered individuals, but may still prefer not to be associated with such people. The inability of mentally disturbed persons to fit in may cause them to respond in a reciprocal manner and to reject conventional beliefs and believers. They may, however, find a home in religious or spiritual subcultures that are out of the mainstream (i.e., sects or cults). Since members of these bodies often feel that they are ostracized by society (and in many instances they actually are), they may find common cause with others who are similarly rejecting or rejected for reasons of individual mental deviance.

It is important to recognize that the majority of members of what are socially regarded as deviant religious groups are quite "normal" and mentally healthy (Richardson, 1995). Some disturbed individuals may, of course, find a haven that functions as a source of meaning and a framework of needed control in these religious groups, but this is probably the exception and not the rule (Ross, 1983).

Alienated individuals may be attracted by a wide variety of religious and ecclesiastical elements. Unquestioning attachment to a spiritual leader may reflect emotional immaturity and strong dependency needs. The charismatic quality of some of the founders of these groups can also entice persons whose reality contacts are weak. One study of the Unification Church (pejoratively called "the Moonies") revealed that over 40% admitted having had mental difficulties prior to joining the church, many of these had sought professional help, and a few had been hospitalized (Galanter, Rabkin, Rabkin, & Deutsch, 1979). As Research Box 16.3 (see below) notes, the outcome of affiliation with the Unification Church was psychologically beneficial.

Snelling and Whitley (1974) studied four of what they termed "problem-solving groups," including a Hare Krishna temple. They suggested that, instead of obvious abnormality predominating, there seemed to be "a noticeable strain or predisposition toward reductionism in the sense of cutting down or narrowing the 'size' of the world in order to make it more manageable" (p. 331). Though such a reaction may indicate some coping difficulties, especially in relation to control, it may be a wise choice on the part of some devotees. Also, since the great majority of these individuals return to mainstream society, their experience in such "manageable" environments may permit them needed time to develop better ways to adjust to the world.

Another example of the way in which sects or cults may serve a temporary haven function is implied by work showing that some young people who affiliate with these bodies come from troubled homes and families (Schwartz & Kaslow, 1979). Such a religious group acts as a substitute family, offering needed social and psychological backing until the person is able to cope with a North American milieu that highly values personal autonomy.

The haven role not only offers a defense against a possibly unappreciative and potentially threatening society outside the chosen religious group; it also usually provides much positive acceptance and support. We see this in Kildahl's (1972) description of the fellowship among glossolalic individuals. He described them as exhibiting "a tremendous openness, concern, and care for one another . . . they bore each other's burdens . . . were with each other in spirit and in physical presence" (p. 299).

A variation on this theme may exist among the Jehovah's Witnesses, a religiously conservative and strongly proselytizing group. Said to have an incidence of schizophrenia three to four times higher than that found in the general population (a finding that needs further confirmation), this group may appeal to some distressed people who feel they require a spiritual foundation that incorporates a very strict moral code (Spencer, 1975). This may protect such individuals from life stresses and temptations, while aiding them to internalize necessary controls that permit a modicum of adjustment. The research of Galanter and his associates, which illustrates such a tendency in the Unification Church, is presented in Research Box 16.3.

Finding a spiritual haven is not easy. Particularly among the cults and sects, troubled people move rather easily from one such group to another. The unstable membership of these bodies is well documented (McLoughlin, 1978; Sasaki, 1979; Wood, 1965). There are, however, data suggesting that these shifts of commitment increase with the severity of mental problems (Galanter et al., 1979). Still, such moving about may also benefit seekers in their search for meaning, control, and esteem. Sometimes satisfactory answers are elusive.

Encapsulated Religious Communities: The Amish and the Hutterites

Though they are usually considered sects, their long histories of relative isolation and yet reasonable acceptance by the general society make groups like the Amish and the Hutterites of special interest to mental health researchers. The quality of their separation allows social scientists to regard them as "laboratory-like" sociocultural cases, worthy of much study. Neither group has attempted to bring in new members by proselytizing. People are born into these groups; rarely do they seek to join from the outside. Because of these bodies' isolation and the formal and informal controls they exercise over their adherents, they manifest the haven functions of religion well. They also provide information on some of the causes of various mental disorders.

Among the Amish, the doctrine of separation is evident in the proscription against marrying outsiders or even entering business partnerships with non-Amish persons. Basi-

---

Research Box 16.3. The Moonies: A Psychological Study of Conversion and Membership in a Contemporary Religious Sect (Galanter, Rabkin, Rabkin, & Deutsch, 1979)

With the cooperation of the Unification Church, an extensive questionnaire dealing with mental health issues was administered to 237 church members. A pattern of disruption and emotional difficulties preceded their joining the church in many instances; about one-third had sought professional help for these problems, and 6% had been hospitalized. Psychological distress scores for the time prior to church affiliation were 48% higher than at the time the testing took place. In addition, church members still showed more personal disturbance than was found in the general population. Though there were indications that adjustment initially declined when conversion to the church took place, as religious and communal ties to the group increased, so did psychological well-being. The greater a person's religious involvement and commitment, the less distress was evidenced.

cally, this view holds for any deep or long-lasting social involvement or contact with any outsider (Hostetler, 1968). Such self-segregation, when combined with very strict internal controls on behavior, creates great stress for many Amish. The expectations these rules engender have been cited as a cause of anxiety, and may in part account for an incidence of suicidal tendencies above the national average among Amish hospitalized for mental problems. Unfortunately, there is not enough information available to indicate whether the incidence of neurotic or psychotic disorders is unusual. The community acts as a haven, preferring to care for its own whenever possible.

The Hutterites are a different matter; good observational data have been collected from them. Eaton and Weil (1955) carried out a highly regarded study on religion and mental disorder with this group many years ago. Like the Amish, the Hutterites are a separatist Anabaptist sect; they live in relatively isolated communities in southern Canada and along the northwest tier of the United States from the Dakotas westward. Because the group is a close-knit and highly supportive communal organization, the authors expected low rates of mental disturbance. Where such disturbance does occur, as with the Amish, a loving community with its own constructive therapeutic views is present to aid the distressed individual.

Eaton and Weil (1955) found that the frequency of the less severe neurotic states tended to be low, particularly those in which aggressive or antisocial expressions predominated. In lieu of these symptoms, guilt and depression were commonly found; these seemed to be products of both the highly controlling social milieu and failure to live up to the strict expectations of the community. Moreover, the low neurotic rates were countered by a high incidence of severe psychotic disorders. Four centuries of relative isolation may have concentrated the genetic and constitutional potential for such illnesses; these propensities could also have been activated by the often inflexible demands of daily life. Furthermore, Eaton and Weil (1955) had reason to believe that the Hutterite communities they studied might operate much better as refuges for the less disturbed group members than for their more seriously affected counterparts.

Separate Communities within Mainline Religious Groups

Some mentally disturbed persons may believe that they are "called" to a religious vocation, and subsequently may find a haven in a religious community that separates them from the world. This view has been confirmed by Kelley (1958), who studied nuns. Finding a variety of disordered states among Catholic sisters, she concluded that these states were a function of preexisting difficulties rather than of the religious life. Reference has also been made to a high frequency of hypochondriacal complaints (Sister Margaret Louise, 1961). Similar findings have been reported in other studies of nuns (Jahreiss, 1942; Kurth, 1961). More recent similar work in North America is generally lacking. Research Box 16.4 describes Kelley's significant work.

Additional work on disturbed sisters in Italy attributed their motivation to enter orders to needs for security because of emotional starvation and/or a view of the world as dangerous. These needs were thought to be frustrated by organizational pressures and restraints which exacerbated the nuns' often tenuous grip on reality (De Maria, Giuliani, Annese, & Corfiati, 1971). Kurth (1961) has claimed that two factors may contribute to such a situation. First, "many mentally ill individuals seek to enter religious life. Such neurotic and prepsychotic individuals are especially attracted to cloistered life which, by its very nature caters to the needs of schizoid individuals" (p. 20). Second, Kurth maintained "that too many è.

Research Box 16.4. The Incidence of Hospitalized Mental Illness among Religious Sisters in the United States (Kelley, 1958)

Kelley, a nun herself, gathered data from 357 U.S. private and public mental hospitals on 783 Catholic sisters who were hospitalized for mental disorders in 1956. High rates of depression and schizophrenia were observed; yet, prior to being committed, the sisters had spent an average of 17–20 years in their order.

The incidence of severe disorders among sisters who performed domestic functions was over seven times higher than among those involved in teaching. The rates for cloistered nuns were also higher than for those in noncloistered orders. Among hospitalized nuns, 80% suffered from psychoses, 65% of which were schizophrenic. Depressive symptomatology was also quite common. Kelley theorized that the highly structured life in these religious communities often led to feelings of failure and ensuing breakdown on the part of those unable to handle the stringent demands of such an existence.

Superiors of convents in the United States think that all their candidates are psychologically sound and enjoy good mental health" (p. 23).

Somewhat to the contrary, a few studies suggest that elderly Catholic nuns may score low on emotional maturity, but still reveal good affective adaptation and a positive outlook (Huck & Armer, 1995). In a study involving Tibetan nuns who had been tortured in Tibet, the negative effects of torture and status as refugees were mitigated by Buddhist spirituality (Holtz, 1998). It is abundantly clear that the few existing studies of this topic are not enough to establish the significance of the haven function of religion. There is a need for an organized research program in this area.

In some instances, the requirement of chastity and celibacy is too much of a psychological burden for Catholic priests and nuns to bear, and abnormal expressions of anxiety and other undesirable behaviors may result (Gratton, 1959, cited in Menges & Dittes, 1965; Sipe, 1990; Slawson, 1973). The widely publicized recent reports of molestations by priests speak to these pressures. Their problems may involve mental health considerations, but our culture views their actions primarily through a moral lens. We have discussed this topic at greater length in Chapter 13.

RELIGION AS THERAPY

For the last half century, the role of faith as therapeutic has been increasingly recognized on a number of levels. Not only do religious and spiritual practices exercise such a role, but clergy themselves are now explicitly undertaking psychological training as therapists. As part of what has become known as "clinical pastoral education," churches have been able to avail themselves of theologically sophisticated counselors and therapists who can utilize the doctrines of their faith when working with mentally disturbed parishioners. We describe this and similar developments in greater detail later in the chapter (see "Religion and Psychotherapy" under "Topics of Special Concern," below).

We have seen that the suppression/socialization functions of religion may work to inhibit deviant mental expression, if not to improve disordered mental states. However, moving beyond the suppression/socialization functions of religion can be actively therapeutic. Activities and phenomena such as ritual, prayer, religious experience, glossolalia, and conversion may perform remedial roles. Sometimes these work directly; at other times, they work indirectly by involving friends and congregants as socializers and suppressors.

Ritual

That ritual is central to religion goes without saying. Its role in ceremony and prayer cannot be minimized, for it is considered a means of contacting the supernatural and concurrently oneself and others. It is often a call for vicarious control by a deity when a supplicant is unable to exercise mastery (Brown, 1994). Even though the following comments present ritual in the broadest perspective, let us keep in mind that these remarks are fully appropriate to religion per se.

Since the evidence overwhelmingly confirms that the roots of ritual run deep in both biology and the evolutionary process, it is easy to believe that it must perform some important function (Huxley, 1966, 1968). This inference is further supported by the apparent fact that there are no known cultures without ritual (Helman, 1994). Wulff (1997) cites Lorenz to the effect that ritualization is involved in "communicating, restricting aggression, and increasing pair and group cohesion" (p. 155). All of these may involve facets of mental disturbance. Rituals are also said to manage life's uncertainties (Horner & Dobb, 1997). They counter ambiguity, increase control over oneself and the environment, enhance meaning, reduce stress, decrease anxiety, and curb impulsivity (Erikson, 1966). Social bonding is also facilitated. A number of noted clinical scholars add that rituals channel destructive and extreme emotions into controllable forms (Benson & Stark, 1996; Pargament, 1997; Pruyser, 1968). Kiev (1966) has pointed out that ritual explicitly promotes "therapeutic emotional reactions" via the opportunity to "express in socially approved ways ordinarily inhibited impulses and desires" (p. 170). Pruyser (1968) has suggested that ritual is adaptive when it creates a "structure for emotional expression" or performs "dynamically as a defense against the intensity of any emotion or the unpleasantness of some" (p. 143). Through its emotion-regulating and control functions, ritual (and specifically religious ritual) works to increase self-control and to counter disordered thinking and behavior.

The early psychoanalytic approach to religion identified ritual with abnormality. Ritual was regarded as an expression of religion as "obsessional neurosis," designed to alleviate unconscious guilt (Freud, 1907/1924; Reik, 1946). This view has since been strongly rejected by most psychologists of religion, some of whom have recognized that religious ritual performs healing and beneficial roles (Argyle, 1959; Scobie, 1975). Its compulsive cathartic nature, the implication of appeasement, and the exercise of control are seen as reducing fear and anxiety. Repressed motives are said to be worked through, expressed, and dispelled (Heelas, 1985).

A study committee of the GAP has analogized ritual to psychoanalytic therapy, in that both have the "intention of facilitating growth. . . . Ritual not only stimulates regression, but controls and guides it" (GAP, 1968, p. 704). Erik Erikson (quoted in Couture, 1990, p. 1089) spoke of ritualization as "creative formalization" that controls both impulsiveness and compulsive restrictiveness, such as in constructive play. Because of such channeling, parallels have been drawn between pastoral care and counseling and ritualistic expression (Couture, 1990).

The ubiquitous nature of religious ritual is well demonstrated by Moberg (1971), who covers the range from the individual level through family, churches, and synagogues to literally nationwide forms that utilize the mass media. Given such possibilities, the healing and therapeutic possibilities inherent in rites and ceremonies appear quite impressive.

There can be little doubt about the importance of ritual. The observations of astute anthropologists and clinicians concerning its effects are quite striking; however, objective empirical work in this realm is lacking. It is a topic worthy of much study by rigorous research psychologists.

Prayer

Prayer is, of course, a form of ritual. Public ritual prayer has been established by churches, while people pattern their own individual prayers. In Chapter 15, we have described the essentially supportive and therapeutic place of prayer in one's personal armamentarium. Because of this, only a few major points need to be made here. Publicly and privately, prayer is probably the most commonly employed religious rite, with approximately 90% of the U.S. population engaging in this activity (Poloma & Gallup, 1991). We accept the view of Holahan and Moos (1987) that prayer is an "active, cognitive, coping strategy" (p. 949). In other words, it is most often an attempt to deal with distress—a kind of self-therapy. Much research has been conducted on the beneficial uses of prayer by elderly individuals, seriously ill people, and average persons in a wide variety of circumstances (see Chapter 15).

Psychiatrist Kenneth Appel (1949) claims that prayer plays a personality-integrative role in life. Kidorf (1966) views the *shiva*, a collective Jewish ceremony of mourning and prayer, as a form of group therapy. Research has found that private prayer is negatively correlated with signs of depression (Kendler, Gardner, & Prescott, 1997; Koenig, Pargament, & Nielsen, 1998). When depression is related to stress, religious activity (including prayer) is likely to increase (Koenig et al., 2001). In addition, prayer is inversely associated with anxiety, especially death anxiety (Koenig et al., 2001).

Research Box 16.5 presents Parker and Brown's (1982) study on coping with depression. The role of prayer in this work is significant.

Research Box 16.5. Coping Behaviors That Mediate between Life Events and Depression (Parker & Brown, 1982)

In an initial study, 176 general medical patients responded to items indicating factors that made them feel depressed, plus behaviors that seemed effective in reducing those stresses. After the initial measures were refined, a new sample of 103 patients was obtained. Using factor analysis, the authors found that the inclination to pray contributed strongly to a problem-solving dimension. A subsample of 20 clinically depressed patients was then compared with a control group; this revealed that the problem-solving behaviors were more likely to be used by the control group. Prayer therefore related positively to the percentage of those reporting prayer as increasing behavioral change and as effective in the process. The implication is that prayer can be a significant aid in coping with depression.

Religious Experience

Spilka, Brown, and Cassidy (1993) found that the vast majority of distressed people who reported religious experiences benefited greatly from them. This has been known for some time. Anton Boisen (1936) interpreted psychotic behavior as an effort at problem solving that is "closely related to certain types of religious experience" (p. 53). He then documented many cases that testified to the curative and restorative possibilities inherent in religious experience. Research by Bergin (1994) confirms Boisen's examples. Bergin observed that participants in his study who were not coping well "appeared to have their adjustment level boosted considerably by intense religious experiences that were like Maslow's peak experiences" (p. 88). Maslow (1964) himself analogized peak experiences to religious and mystical encounters, taking a positive view of their outcomes, and explicitly construing such events as therapeutic. Unhappily, this is not always true, as distressing and terrifying religious experiences have also been reported (Greeley, 1974; Leuba, 1929; Spilka, Brown, & Cassidy, 1993; Stark, 1965).

Recognizing the biological bases for schizophrenia, Wilson (1998) claims that the bizarre religious experiences of persons with schizophrenia are probably a function of experientially acquired content plus the motive to gain control over the psychosis. Overall, Wilson feels that religious experiences play little or no role in schizophrenia, and that spiritual interventions rarely have a beneficial effect when they occur in psychoses.

Religious experiences have, however, been associated with specific therapeutic outcomes. These include reductions in guilt feelings, a heightened sense of security and belonging, improved control of aggression and hostility, and suicide prevention (Hartocollis, 1976; Trew, 1971). Drug-induced religious experience has also been cited as having a positive influence on patients with alcoholism, narcotic addiction, neuroses, and terminal cancer (Clark, 1968; Pahnke, 1969). Clark (1968) feels that these positive effects are enhanced when the experiencers explicitly denote these events as religious. Mystical encounters have further been likened to creative experiences as "attempts at integration or reintegration by people who have not achieved satisfying results in identity formation" (GAP, 1976, p. 819).

Considering the social context, Prince (1992) notes that religious experiences may be defined as pathological or therapeutic, depending on culture and group values. In situations where such experiences are valued, he claims that some "may be channeled into socially valuable roles" (p. 289). This is true among Pentecostal sects that encourage religious mysticism. Hine (1969) suggests that these experiences aid adjustment and integrate people into their groups, which also provide quite supportive environments.

Glossolalia

Attempting to develop a theory of how religion relates to psychopathology, Schumaker (1995) turns to the concept of "dissociation," of which glossolalia is one form. Dissociation is tied to a splitting of consciousness in which one manifests various streams of thought—some dealing with reality, others varying in the degree to which they may be conscious and/or reflect fantasy. Included here are hypnosis, mysticism, trance states, hallucinations, and other forms of what Schumaker considers irrationality.

Like mystical experience and conversion, however, glossolalia may be indicative of mental disorder or may operate therapeutically, as discussed earlier. For example, many open-minded observers subscribe to what Brown (1987) calls "a benign form of the 'abnormal theory'" (p. 158)—namely, that speaking in tongues is adaptive. In addition to its social function of integrating a glossolalic individual into an approving religious group, it has been associated with increased well-being, social sensitivity, religious maturity, the resolution of neurotic conflicts, and the reduction of anxiety and tension (Hutch, 1980; Kelsey, 1964; Kildahl, 1972; Pattison, 1968). It would therefore appear to be therapeutic. Although such a possibility must not be dismissed, some research has failed to support any of these findings (Lovekin & Malony, 1977). Much good work has already been undertaken in this area, but the pathology–therapy issue still needs to be resolved.

Conversion

The beneficial and therapeutic effects of conversion have been celebrated for millennia. We hear about being "born again," "twice born," "finding God," "coming home," and so forth. Over a century ago, Starbuck (1899) claimed that for converts "the joy, the relief, and the acceptance are qualities of feeling, perhaps, which give the truest picture of what is going on in conversion—the free exercise of new powers, and escape from something, and the birth into Larger Life" (p. 122). Though clinicians might employ different language, these are unquestionably therapeutic goals.

Earlier, we have discussed the negative aspects of conversion when it reflects mental disorder. Clearly, however, there is also a positive side—with indications of increased openness, better contacts with the world and others, greater emotional responsivity, a heightened sense of personal satisfaction and happiness, conflict resolution, and productive identity formation (Bragan, 1977; Gallemore et al., 1969; Gordon, 1964). Jones (1937) and Cesarman (1957) have offered illustrations of sexual and other conflicts, which conversion replaces with an "inner calm" (p. 171). Writing from a classical psychiatric/psychoanalytic stance, Woolcott (1969) perceived the troubled person as surrendering egoism and narcissism, while the energy that has been attached to unconscious conflicts is freed and permits humility to develop. Via conversion, the person is now able to have a new relationship with God and others, and to gain new insights and better contact with reality.

These beneficial effects of conversion are not restricted to mainline churches; they also extend to cults, such as the Unification Church and Hare Krishna (Kilbourne & Richardson, 1984b; Richardson, 1992). Richardson (1992) summarizes this work simply: "The personality assessments of these groups reveals that life in the new religions is often therapeutic instead of harmful" (p. 233).

In more than a few instances, conversion may be explicitly associated with, or play a role in, psychotherapy (Bergman, 1953; Levin & Zegans, 1974; Propst, 1988). Both can also be regarded as forms of cognitive restructuring (Batson et al., 1993; Propst, 1988). Though there may be many reasons for conversion, clinicians are becoming increasingly sensitive to the potential benefits of conversion experiences (Bergman, 1953; Levin & Zegans, 1974). Overall, the empirical evidence suggests that converts appear to be better adjusted than nonconverts (Bergin, 1983; Srole et al., 1962).

RELIGION AS A HAZARD TO MENTAL HEALTH

As we have already commented, the dominant traditional view of faith in psychology has been to associate it with psychopathology. We have shown that the opposite is often true; however, religious institutions and doctrines can create stress and cause psychological problems.

Indeed, there is truth in the title of one book, *Religion Can Be Hazardous to Your Health* (Chesen, 1972). Similarly, the noted psychologist Paul W. Pruyser (1977) referred in an article title to "The Seamy Side of Current Religious Beliefs." Albert Ellis (1988) indicated 11 ways religion seems to create and support mental disorder, though he has since modified his position. The problem has been considered of such magnitude that Koenig et al. (2001), in their definitive *Handbook of Religion and Health*, devote a chapter to "Religion's Negative Effects." The message is simply this: Religion does contain elements that can adversely affect the mental well-being of its adherents.

Religion as a Source of Abnormal Mental Content

The doctrines and sources of institutional faith sometimes contain the seeds of psychopathology. Though most individuals who accept religious mandates live happy and fruitful lives, there are those who misinterpret and misapply the core elements of their faith. Others are, in a sense, victimized by parents, clergy, or influential others who misuse religion to gain power and personal gratification. This can happen when people treat religious precepts in a rigid and inflexible manner (Stifoss-Hanssen, 1994). One study dealing with some mental disorder correlates of "rigid religiosity" is detailed in Research Box 16.6. In essence, clinicians believe that a strict religious upbringing contributes to the development of emotional disorders, depression, suicidal potential, and a generally fearful response to life (Culver, 1988).

The inability to adapt church tenets and scripture to modern life is an accusation usually directed at fundamentalist groups and conservative religious bodies, often in an unbalanced manner. In fact, research, particularly on fundamentalism, suffers from a wide variety of biases. At the same time, some individuals are attracted to these bodies because of what Ostow (1990) has called an "illusory defense against reality" (p. 122).

The great reliance of orthodox groups on a literalist interpretation of scripture may be one of those defenses. For example, such an interpretation has been used to justify the abuse of women and children, and support for such behavior has often come from church officials (Alsdorf & Alsdorf, 1988; Pagelow & Johnson, 1988). Spousal and child abuse has been associated with much conflict about sexual issues and with the blaming of victims. These tendencies have been invoked to explain the claim that high rates of multiple personality disorder are found in families with fundamentalist religious backgrounds (Higdon, 1986).

Research Box 16.6. Rigid Religiosity and Mental Health: An Empirical Study (Stifoss-Hanssen, 1994)

Religious bodies possess rules and regulations that people can often interpret in ways ranging from an easy flexibility to a rigid absolutism. The latter has been defined in one major study as a "law-orientation" (Strommen, Brekke, Underwager, & Johnson, 1972). In the present study, a scale assessing rigid–flexible religiosity was developed and administered to 56 volunteer hospitalized patients with neuroses and a control group of 70 nonpatients. The patients scored significantly higher than the controls on this scale, demonstrating that rigid religiosity is a correlate of severely neurotic thinking and behavior. The author also suggested a positive relationship between mental disturbance and an extrinsic religious orientation.

Fundamentalist religion is often quite authoritarian in its structure, endowing its leaders with the image of having a special relationship with the deity. Control and the suppression of dissent are seen as the natural prerogatives of those holding high church positions. These factors have been used to explain the anxiety, "guilt, low self-esteem, sexual inhibitions, and vivid fears of divine punishment" noted among individuals who leave these groups (Hartz & Everett, 1989, p. 209). The argument is made that the absolutist structure and dictates of these institutions produce a "fundamentalist mindset" that creates adjustment problems for their members (Kirkpatrick, Hood, & Hartz, 1991). This mindset has been further described as involving extreme dogmatism and a need for simplistic "quick fixes for problems involving marriage, children, sexuality, or society" (Hartz & Everett, 1989, p. 208).

Despite all of these unpleasant inferences, research supporting such ideas is rather sparse. In fact, in Chapter 15, we have noted work suggesting the association of fundamentalism with an optimistic outlook on life (Sethi & Seligman, 1993). Other research has failed to evidence any adverse effects on the ego development or the adaptive capacity of fundamentalists (Weaver, Berry, & Pittel, 1994). When such contradictions exist, the only answer is to call for more research; however, we must keep in mind that this is a troubling and controversial area, and objectivity is imperative.

Religious doctrines are rich sources of ideas for use by mentally disturbed persons. Southard (1956) showed how identification with higher powers may help such individuals to deny reality and counter therapy; he described one patient who used hymn singing to frustrate psychotherapy. The presentation of miracles and other unusual occurrences found in religious writings can stimulate magical thinking of a pathological nature.

Commonly, religious groups and doctrines offer their members meanings that make life bearable, but at a cost—namely, a "sacrifice of intellect" (Pruyser, 1977, p. 332). Complex matters are often simplified into a dichotomy of good versus evil. Difficult and intricate issues are denied attempts at understanding by reference to such clichés as "God works in mysterious ways." At times, however, objective need and cognitive dissonance may cause individuals to challenge polarized beliefs and "stop thinking" phrases. The outcome can be a serious crisis of faith, extreme personal stress, depression, and the potential for suicide (Pruyser, 1977).

Religion as a Source of Abnormal Mental Motives

Just as religion can strengthen moral commitments, enhance optimism, and stimulate ego development it may also activate disordered thinking and behavior (Andreason, 1972; Bock & Warren, 1972). We see this in religion's concern with sin. A book chapter by O'Connell (1961) asked, "Is Mental Illness a Result of Sin?", and the well-known psychologist O. H. Mowrer (1961) attempted to bring the sin concept into psychotherapy. It has thus been examined positively and negatively—as a constructive control on behavior, and as an arouser of guilt, depression, and distress. Obsession with sin and guilt seems to be a correlate of religious frameworks that stress moral perfection (Miller, 1973). Such an emphasis can incite feelings of low self-esteem and worthlessness, which have the potential of contributing to mental disorders. We also find the presence of sin and associated guilt in the motivation for mysticism, conversion, prayer, scrupulosity, confession, bizarre rituals, self-denial, and self-mutilation (Clark, 1929; Cutten, 1908; James, 1902/1985).

The need to expunge sin and reduce guilt is a powerful motive, and one may eventuate in serious mental pathology. McGinley's (1969) fascinating presentation of the behavior of saints abounds in examples of grotesque, brutal, and painful masochistic behavior, which today we would regard as indicative of profound psychopathology.

Religious institutions and leaders that demand absolute subservience and unquestioning obedience from followers frequently use punitive threats and devices to eliminate individuality. Pruyser (1977) has pointed out that those subject to such control must suspend any semblance of critical reasoning and substitute "unbridled and untutored fantasy" (p. 333). Blind faith of this sort requires an immature, if not extremely childish, denial of reality for its maintenance. The pathetic extremes to which such belief may drive people have been evidenced many times in recent years. One need only consider such tragedies as the mass suicides and deaths in the People's Temple in Guyana, the Branch Davidians in Texas, the Solar Temple group in Europe and Canada, and the Heaven's Gate group in California.

We conclude this discussion with a markedly different example, which we have already introduced in Chapter 12—namely, the situation with Christian Science and other groups that reject modern medicine. No matter how dedicated to their faith and sincere these groups are, the vast majority of people in contemporary life seek medical aid when they are ill. Not to do so suggests a deviant point of view. With the medical knowledge currently available, the idea that religious beliefs and prayer are all that are necessary to effect a cure—regardless of a person's condition—is an outlook that may well indicate some difficulty in handling reality. Probably reflecting this situation, research on large samples shows that Christian Scientists evidence higher death rates than the overall population. For example, the death rate from cancer for Christian Scientists is double the national average (Koenig et al., 2001). Unfortunately, no similar mental health data seem to have been reported, but we advance the hypothesis that similar results should be observed for conditions and outcomes such as depression and suicide.

TOPICS OF SPECIAL CONCERN

Even with all its shortcomings, a hallmark of present-day Western society has been an increasing openness and receptivity about matters to which previous generations closed their eyes. Platitudes such as "That's life," "That's the way things are," or some variation on "It's the natural scheme of things" have given way to a new awareness of matters that were formerly either ignored, denied, taken for granted, or blindly not even recognized. Among these concerns are a great many areas in which religion and mental disorder are related. The number of such areas is immense; the interested reader should examine such recent works as Koenig et al.'s (2001) *Handbook of Religion and Health*, and Plante and Sherman's (2001) *Faith and Health: Psychological Perspectives*. These noteworthy efforts extensively survey the field. Unhappily, most of the significant research is not recent, and the good work of the past often needs corroboration.

To illustrate a few of these possibilities, we select two important areas: First, the mental health of the clergy; and, second, the relatively new and expanding relationship clerics have with counseling and psychotherapy, both as purveyors and as recipients (Koenig et al., 2000; Richards & Bergin, 2000).

The Mental Health of the Clergy

Because members of the clergy are often among the most admired and respected members of their community, their congregants and others frequently view them as somehow above the daily struggle and not subject to the strains and pressures of everyday life. A closer look rapidly shatters this idyllic picture. There are two facets to this problem: (1) The clergy, like anyone else, are subject to emotional conflicts, and these appear to be increasing (Anderson, 1963; Kelley, 1961; Rayburn, Richmond, & Rogers, 1983, 1986); and (2) the clerical profession is quite stressful.

Mental Problems among the Clergy

The majority of the work on clerical mental problems has been conducted on candidates for the ministry. Recent work on this issue is rare. One small bibliography on religion and mental health, which only covered a 4-year period over 35 years ago, listed 42 research and discussion books and papers dealing with abnormality among the clergy (National Clearinghouse for Mental Health Information, 1967). Claims of deviant findings dominated this early literature. For example, Rabinowitz (1969) asserted that Catholic seminarians were poorly integrated, tended to show depressive tendencies, and possessed a variety of interpersonal and identity problems. Also noted were early parental conflicts, ambivalent attitudes of parents toward their children, possible rejection of the children, and maternal dominance and control (Christensen, 1960). Other studies of seminary students indicated that they scored higher on indices of neuroticism, were in poorer mental health than nonseminarians, and tended to be either rather aggressive or quite submissive and dependent (Ranck, 1961; Roe, 1956; Strunk, 1959; Webster, 1967). In other words, anything that implied some psychological difficulty was inferred at one time or another. Increasingly, seminaries have begun using mental tests in order to eliminate applicants with emotional problems. Finch (1965) emphasized that circumstances can lead mentally disordered individuals to feel that they should become clergy. Apparently many, if not most, troubled individuals withdraw from clerical training programs (Aloyse, 1961; Booth, n.d.; Menges & Dittes, 1965; Wauck, 1957).

With regard to active clergy, the entire gamut of findings on personality and psychological problems has been offered. In a sample of disturbed ministers, similar early-life influences were supplemented by a late-adolescence choice of a clerical future after the arousal of considerable guilt over a sexual encounter (Christensen, 1963). As noted earlier, work on nuns suggested high rates of schizophrenia, with the incidence being greater for cloistered than for active orders. Indications of depression were also noted (Kelley, 1961). The suggestion was made that a life emphasizing meditation and withdrawal from the community might appeal to certain disturbed women (Jahreiss, 1942; Kelley, 1958).

Where psychological and emotional problems have been identified among the clergy, it is not clear whether such difficulties motivate persons to become clerics, or result from the considerable stress to which this profession is subject (Moracco & Richardson, 1985; Sammon, Reznikoff, & Geisinger, 1985).

Stress and "Burnout" in the Ministry

For the last two decades, the term of choice for workers who have experienced severe job stress for a long period of time has been "burnout." Burnout is associated with a wide variety of symptoms—psychosomatic complaints, depression, alienation, emotional turmoil, weakening of impulse controls, escapist thinking and behavior, and even career changes. It appears to be a kind of "job exhaustion." Sanford (1982) has noted that the "work of the minister is never finished, for he faces a continuous onslaught of services, weddings, funerals, crises, parish conflicts, holy day celebrations, sick persons to see, shut-ins to visit, classes to teach, and administrative classes" (p. 5). Clearly, a cleric's schedule can be daunting. A time may be reached when additional stress can no longer be tolerated, and special support is required in order to regain composure and the ability to cope with ministerial tasks (Daniel & Rogers, 1981; Sanford, 1982).

Payne (1990) studied factors that might counter burnout. Utilizing a scale developed by Kobasa, Maddi, and Kahn (1982) to assess "hardiness," he was able to demonstrate that hardiness did oppose burnout. Specifically, hardy individuals showed a high sense of control over their personal situation, plus dedication to their goals and undertakings. They also viewed their life tasks as challenging, and felt secure and safe in performing those tasks.

Clerical role stress and burnout do not affect their victims equally. In all likelihood, only a minority of the clergy is greatly affected. Most clerics are able to handle their situation without any kind of breakdown, even if they are sorely tried. Still, this problem is considered serious enough by ecclesiastical authorities to justify remedial actions that will alleviate stress and improve the job circumstances of clergy (Payne, 1990; Roach, 1990).

Religion and Psychotherapy

No treatment of the domain of religion and mental disorder would be complete without recognizing the increasing role of religious ideas and practitioners in treating psychological problems.

The educational curricula of mental health professionals now include training to increase awareness of clients' and patients' religious and spiritual concerns. This is matched in the seminary training of clergy-to-be and in programs for those already working in religious institutions; both groups are now becoming extensively familiar with the psychological complexities they must confront when dealing with congregants' mental problems (Koenig et al., 2001; Richards & Bergin, 1997).

The result of these developments has been an alliance between psychiatry and psychology on the one hand, and religion on the other (Academy of Religion and Mental Health, 1959; GAP, 1960; Klausner, 1964). This alliance has resulted in serious efforts to integrate the basic principles underlying these disciplines, such as Stern and Marino's (1970) book *Psychotheology*. Those working in this fairly new interdisciplinary realm have proposed a variety of novel approaches to enhancing people's well-being and adaptive thinking/behavior. Some new themes and approaches intended particularly for clerical counselors and therapists include "pastoral counseling" (Hiltner, 1949; Wicks, Parsons, & Capps, 1985), "clinical pastoral education" (Thornton, 1970), "spiritual psychotherapy" (Karasu, 1999), "reframing in pastoral care" (Capps, 1990), "Christotherapy" (Tyrrell, 1985), and "ethical therapy" (Andrews, 1987). Psychotherapists' appreciation of the need for spiritual perspectives and understanding in their work has also been greatly enhanced (Miller, 1999; Richards & Bergin, 2000). Mutuality and coordination to realize common goals are increasingly sought as the barriers separating religious from psychological and psychiatric professionals are reduced.

Another indication of increased understanding is the fact that religious problems are now included in DSM-IV, as noted earlier in this chapter. This brings a new perspective to mainstream clinical psychology and psychiatry regarding the place of religion in personal life. Some years ago, Bergin (1980) poignantly observed the need for clinical psychology to broaden its perspective, as the religious outlooks of clients and therapists are often markedly discrepant in regard to religion. Research Box 16.7 summarizes a survey of a

---

&❧

Research Box 16.7. Religion and Psychotherapy
(Bethesda PsycHealth, 1994)

A survey dealing with religious/spiritual issues was administered to 60 professional staff members (physicians, etc.), 50 line staff members (aides, etc.), and 51 patients of a private mental health facility. Some representative questions and responses are as follows.

1. "How important to you is the inclusion of a spiritual focus as a part of the psychotherapy process?" Percentages responding "somewhat to very important": professional staff, 73%; line staff, 55%; patients, 72%.
2. "Is there a need to increase medical/professional staff's awareness of the use of a spiritual focus in psychotherapy?" Percentages responding "some to much need": professional staff, 66%; line staff, 80%.
3. "What percentage of your patients would benefit from a spiritual focus as part of the psychotherapy process?" Percentages mentioned: professional staff, 34%; line staff, 54%. (When patients were asked whether their spiritual beliefs helped in their recovery, 45% said "yes.")
4. "How important do you consider spiritual values to be?" Percentages responding "moderately to very important": professional staff, 78%; line staff, 90%.

Note that even though 73% of the medical and professional staff considered a spiritual approach important, they still felt that only 34% of their patients would benefit from this approach. This discrepancy might be worthy of further investigation.

This is only a small sampling of the questions asked. In addition, detailed open-ended responses were also obtained. For the samples obtained here, the importance of a religious/ spiritual approach in therapy is apparent.

---

private mental health facility's staff and patients in regard to such matters. This study reveals a growing recognition of the need to consider patients' religious/spiritual beliefs and values (Bethesda PsycHealth, 1994).

OVERVIEW

Mental disorder is an extremely complex topic on many levels, from cause to expression. Though genetic influences are gaining more and more credence, heredity, as noted in Chapter 3, is probabilistic rather than deterministic. In other words, even if one identical twin reveals an inherited condition, there is often a surprisingly high probability that the other will not evidence the illness. If the latter does, it is likely to occur at another time and vary in severity and content. In terms of our framework, there is little doubt that we are viewing disorders of cognition in which personal meanings are at variance with those of other people. In like manner, the thinking and behavior of disturbed individuals reveal problems in control over themselves and in relationships with others and the world. Clearly associated with these difficulties are distressed social connections. We have indicated that religion can either work to the advantage of the troubled persons or exacerbate situational stresses.

To date, research in this area has not been organized along productive theoretical lines. Those who employ coping approaches and see mental disorder as fundamentally "problems of living" seem to be establishing some potentially fruitful avenues for future exploration (Pargament, 1997; Szasz, 1960).

Serious defects that often stemmed from antireligious perspectives exist in many of the earlier studies. The more modern view is that religion functions largely as a means of countering abnormal thinking and behavior. In most instances, faith buttresses people's sense of control and self-esteem, offers meanings that oppose anxiety, provides hope, sanctions socially facilitating behavior, enhances personal well-being, and promotes social integration.

Probably the most hopeful sign is the increasing recognition by both clinicians and religionists of the potential benefits each group has to contribute. Awareness of the need for a spiritual perspective has opened new and more constructive possibilities for working with mentally disturbed individuals and resolving adaptive issues.

Chapter 17

EPILOGUE

> One of the most devastating examples of the danger of religion, is of course, September 11, 2001.
>
> Dear God, save us from the people who believe in you.
>
> For those who regard a transcendental explanation as inadequate, or feel that an appeal to supernatural explanations involves a sacrifice of intellectual integrity, the phenomena of religious observance must be aligned with what is known of other aspects of human psychological functioning.
>
> Some significant portion of traditional supernatural belief is associated with accurate observations interpreted rationally.
>
> We have yet to fully understand the profound and mysterious religious experiences of human everywhere, experiences that shape attitudes toward life and arouse hopes for transcendence and personal immortality.[1]

At the end of our review of the ever-increasing literature on the psychology of religion, it is fitting to take stock of the field—both as it is now and as it is likely to develop in the immediate future. There is a heavy dose of evaluation in the former effort, and a bit of prophecy in the latter. Yet, as in our epilogue to the second edition, we wish at least to go on record so that prophecies can be judged empirically.

The problems and possibilities of the psychology of religion continue to be functions of the notable personalities involved in the field. To this we now add the considerable influence in shaping the field by funding linked to the interests of Sir John Templeton. The rise of positive psychology, as well as studies reflecting his interests in unlimited love, forgiveness, and spiritual transformation—all these efforts are guided by the monies his foundations have provided. As has often been true in the history of this field, single individuals can be immensely important in determining not simply whether religion will be studied, but, if so, what aspects will be examined (Hood, 2000a). Even more than the second edition of this work, this third edition reveals that differences in emphasis and orientation among us authors reflect the diversity that characterizes contemporary psychology in general and the current psychology of religion in particular. This diversity may well be restrained as major funding from individuals or foundations influences the field. The future psychology of religion may largely be one of funded research projects (Coon, 1992; Hood, 2000a).

---

1. These quotations come, respectively, from the following sources: Albacete (2002, p. 166); Dowd (2002); Hinde (1999, p. 233); Hufford (1982, p. xviii); and Wiebe (1997, p. 222).

RESEARCH IN THE PSYCHOLOGY
OF RELIGION AND SPIRITUALITY

Our immediate focus has been upon the empirical psychology of religion, because it most adequately characterizes the academic study of religion in North American psychology departments. As we have seen, the empirical psychology of religion is as old as scientific psychology itself. Yet, from its inception, scientific psychology has often been more of an ideal than a fact. The term "empirical" has undergone a curious change over time, so that entire orientations historically identified as empirical are not granted that description today by mainstream psychologists. For many psychologists, classical psychoanalytic, object relations, Jungian, and phenomenological psychologies are not empirical. "Empirical" has come to mean reliance upon the triad of observation, experimentation, and measurement. This is the paradigm that, according to Gorsuch (1988), identifies the psychology of religion. Now Hill and Pargament (in press) claim the same for the psychology of religion and spirituality. These investigators place the study of both religion and spirituality within a natural-scientific framework. In the past, this has not always been the case (Hamlyn, 1967; Hearnshaw, 1987).

A Historical Reminder

The Two Stances of Wilhelm Wundt

Authorities such as Robinson (1981) remind us that psychology as a natural science emerged in the 19th century, and that its success was largely a North American phenomenon associated with professionalization of the field (Coon, 1992; Hood, 2000a; Taves, 1999). Its roots, however, had been laid down by philosophical developments utilizing natural-scientific assumptions to describe phenomena in the light of principles based upon observation, measurement, and experimentation. Textbooks commonly cite Wilhelm Wundt's establishment of his psychological laboratory at Leipzig in 1879 as the beginning of scientific psychology. This event indicated that psychology was moving from speculative philosophy to natural science. The bridge was experimentation, which involved measurement, manipulation, and observation. Yet Wundt (1901) actually fostered two psychologies—limiting the applicability of natural-scientific assumptions to some phenomena, but applying different assumptions and methods to other, more social "folk" expressions (Wundt, 1916).

From the beginning, psychology and social psychology never quite met in terms of natural-scientific assumptions. Even less could psychology maintain its grasp on the entire range and scope of religion with natural-scientific hands—aspects of religion, maybe, but not religion itself. The reduction of religion to categories of science, a persistent goal of early Enlightenment philosophers, can be judged to have failed (Bowker, 1973; Preus, 1987). The split between psychology as a natural science and social psychology is today as firmly debated as in Wundt's time (Parker, 1989). From the efforts to reconstruct social psychology proposed by Armstead (1974) to the efforts to deconstruct social psychology as advanced by Parker and Shotter (1987), the identity of social psychology as a natural science has always been and remains problematic. This is important, insofar as the major source of our contemporary measurement-based psychology of religion and spirituality is social psychology.

The Two Stances of William James

William James, a contemporary of Wundt and a founder of North American psychology, also failed to apply laboratory measurement-based methodologies to the study of religion. Twice president of the American Psychological Association, James also helped establish the American Society of Psychical Research. The two organizations made strange bedfellows. Coon (1992) reminds us that psychology gained its professional roots in North America within a population that equated psychology ("psychical") with things spiritual. The study of things psychical was a bridging concept that allowed psychologists to gain popular support for their science, while aiming to use natural-scientific methods to debunk the claims of spiritualists.

James, as in so many instances, was an exception. His most consistently psychological work, *The Principles of Psychology* (1890/1950), took a rigorous stance that psychology was to be a natural science. However, as Hood (2000a) has emphasized, James took this stance provisionally, seeking to expose its limits. These limits were both revealed and transcended in James's confrontation with religion. Religious experience was the subject matter of his Gifford Lectures and the basis for James's other undisputed classic text in the psychology of religion.

James's *The Varieties of Religious Experience* (1902/1985) explored the range and depth of religious experience, using personal documents placed within the context of their development so that their fruits could be assessed. The stress upon measurement and the use of questionnaires, already established by such notables as Hall (1900) and Starbuck (1899), were ignored by James in favor of the existential thrust of experience, defined and interpreted within a more historical, narrative context. In modern terms, James's research was qualitative, not quantitative. His psychological treatment of religion specifically expanded the boundaries of the natural-science-based psychology articulated in *The Principles* (Hood, 1995c). *The Varieties* still remains the single most frequently assigned text in the psychology of religion (Vande Kemp, 1976). This should not, however, convey the idea that the contemporary empirical psychology of religion has been heavily influenced by James.

Despite the fact that empirical psychologists of religion tend to be primarily social psychologists, they come from the *psychological* tradition of social psychology, not the *sociological* tradition. Ironically, as Schellenberg (1990) has noted, the latter has been influenced more strongly by James than the former has been. The natural-scientific assumptions of psychology remain firm for most of the psychologically oriented social psychologists who do empirical research. Those who confine themselves to natural-scientific assumptions tend to produce what Beit-Hallahmi (1991) identifies as a "psychology of religion" rather than a "religious psychology" per se. A psychology of religion places psychological categories at the forefront, and would have psychology explain religion only insofar as its phenomena can be captured within natural-scientific constructs from mainstream psychology. On the other hand, religious psychology gives supremacy to religious constructs, and expects psychology to follow from and to be constrained within the conceptual limits of a natural science whose explanatory power is superseded by religion. There is an uneasy tension between psychologists of religion and religious psychologists, which promises to persist in the foreseeable future. It is further complicated as the psychology of religion becomes entangled in efforts to tease out differences and similarities between religion and spirituality at both conceptual and measurement levels (Hill et al., 2000; Moberg, 2002).

As we have noted in this text, not simply measurement, but the ontological status assigned to what is measured, is crucial in developing theory within the psychology of religion.

William James remains the most significant figure in identifying the tensions between a psychology of religion and the tendency to move toward a religious psychology. Measurement has often been the fence that most separates these two fields.

The Measurement Paradigm in the Psychology of Religion

Hood (1994) has argued for a compromise position—neither a psychology of religion and spirituality nor a religious and spiritual psychology, but rather psychology *and* religion *and* spirituality in interactive dialogues. This stance admits the validity of concepts from all three domains and encourages their interaction. At odds is the extent to which a genuine interaction can occur, given the limited empirical characteristics of many religious and spiritual constructs. Still, one can identify the empirical consequences of many such constructs. The psychology of religion is both broadened and challenged by newer orientations such as transpersonal psychology and the human sciences—both of which accept a broader definition of "empirical," much of it compatible with religious and spiritual traditions.

The *Journal of Transpersonal Psychology* has established itself as a major journal representing spiritual phenomena studied by means of admittedly sympathetic psychological methods. Such studies and methods contrast with those of more objective measurement-based journals, such as the *Journal for the Scientific Study of Religion*, whose focus has been on mainstream social-scientific methods applied to religious (and, to a lesser extent, spiritual) phenomena. The *Review of Religious Research* stresses theory and empirical research with some relevance or application to religious institutions. The boundaries among these journals promise to become more permeable as social scientists sympathetic to both religious and spiritual phenomena begin to develop scientific theories compatible with concepts central to religion and spirituality. Likewise, as proponents of more traditionally measurement-based psychology broaden their theoretical horizons, new measurement techniques are likely to be developed to permit a more adequate assessment of variables of religious and spiritual relevance. Moreover, some of the newer journals—such as the *International Journal for the Psychology of Religion* and *Mental Health, Religion, and Culture*—emphasize by their titles alone that the psychology of religion and spirituality can no longer be simply North American. Also encouraging are the reconstitution of the International Association for the Psychology of Religion and the reappearance of the oldest yearbook in the psychology of religion, the *Archiv für Religionpsychologie* (founded in 1914) (Belzen, 2002).

The classical non-measurement-based theories of religion, many derived from psychoanalysis or its analytical and object relations offshoots, continue to spawn an immense literature (Hood, 1995b). Largely interpretative of religion (as in the case of psychoanalysis), or interpretative of spirituality (as in the case of Jungian or object relations theory), this literature promises to influence measurement-based psychology in two ways. First, it provides hypotheses that can be subjected to measurement-based tests; many of these tests are controversial, but are legitimately empirical nonetheless. Second, as competing qualitative methodologies, approaches such as these gain credibility as other narrative and interpretive psychologies emerge and influence mainstream social psychology. In addition, the long tradition of qualitative sociological social psychology, such as symbolic interactionism, is beginning to influence more measurement-based psychological social psychology. Measurement is thus on the defensive as an all-inclusive methodological claim. As Roth (1987) has noted, methodological pluralism is the emerging norm in the social sciences. The psychology of religion and spirituality promises to benefit from interchange between theories and methods that were previously perceived as mutually exclusive. As Wulff (2000) has noted, the study of a phenomenon such as mysticism, if done openly, fundamentally challenges the methods and assumptions of empirical psychology.

Measurement-based psychology is likely to rise to the challenge by articulating more meaningful and inclusive theory that is nevertheless susceptible to empirical test. Works such as that of Spilka and McIntosh (1997), which respond to the critical demand for theoretical advancement in the empirical psychology of religion, are welcome harbingers. One major challenge to a measurement-oriented psychology of religion is simply put—interest. It is not clear that the massive literature spawned in psychology in general has yielded fruits appropriate to the effort. When one considers the explosion of literature in mainstream psychology, it is obvious that no psychologist can master even a small portion of it. It has been over 15 years since Hearnshaw (1987) noted that writing in psychology since 1950 exceeded the total output of works on the subject produced since the time of the Greeks. The literature since 1987 has continued to increase exponentially, yet has produced no agreed-upon theoretical integration. There is no all-encompassing theory in general psychology, much less in the psychology of religion and spirituality. Despite the vast amount of research produced in the North American resurgence of interest in the psychology of religion since 1950, much of it is, in Dittes's (1971a) view, a "promiscuous empiricism" (p. 393). The rigors of measurement and the cleverness of experimental designs fail if at the end the result is trivial or uninformative. The psychology of religion and spirituality is likely to become more like a quilt, in which measurement will at best sew together patches derived from diverse theoretical perspectives.

THE NEED FOR THEORY IN THE PSYCHOLOGY OF RELIGION

Within the psychology of religion, the cry for good theory remains at the level of cacophony. Our guess continues to be that the older generation of researchers will want to make their theoretical contributions in light of the plea for such guidance across the disciplines concerned with the study of religion and spirituality. Likewise, a younger generation of researchers will be trained to demand good theory as a prerequisite to the collection of meaningful empirical data. The field should profit from the emerging consensus that theory congruent with the passion and interest elicited by religion is needed. Theory and measurement need not be incompatible endeavors, but the latter alone will not rise to the level of adequate theory.

Consistent with theory development in the psychology of religion is similar growth in general psychology as it is forced to confront religious issues. Religion is no longer a marginal concern of psychology; whether in the challenges of therapy or in the collective confrontation with cults, it occupies much of the center stage of general culture. Mainstream psychology will begin to confront religion in terms of its theories, if for no other reason than to show the meaningful relevance of psychology to the interests of a culture that supports and in the process seeks guidance from this science, natural or otherwise. In many cases, the vacuum left by some religions will be filled by psychology. Vitz (1977) has made the case that for some people, psychology has become a religion. Some areas, such as transpersonal psychology, blur the boundaries between psychology as science and as a spiritual discipline. In the future, religionists will probably need to be more psychologically skilled, and psychologists will need to be more religiously and spiritually sophisticated, if there are to remain identifiable but permeable boundaries between psychology on the one hand and spirituality/ religion on the other.

In a similar vein, journals devoted to a faith commitment—either by constraining their psychology within the more narrow confines of a particular faith (e.g., the *Journal of Psychology and Christianity*, the *Journal of Psychology and Judaism*), or by interrelating or integrating psychology and religion (e.g., the *Journal of Psychology and Theology*)—will assure that psychology itself appropriately reflects on its own limits. Religion and psychology may confront similar questions, but how they are asked defines what constitutes an appropriate answer. Precisely what it is within religion or spirituality that admits of an empirical answer must be more clearly theoretically determined. So, too, the limits of empiricism must be acknowledged theoretically as new empirical methods are created.

The continual debate between nomothetic and idiographic methodologies within mainstream psychology has strong parallels in the history of religion. General covering laws have long been psychology's goal, but are no longer thought to exclude the individual case. Idiographic studies are of immense value, both as unique narratives in their own right, and as instances of a general law concretely particularized. Tageson's (1982) "objective phenomenology" is not an oxymoron. Radically subjective occurrences can enter a rigorous psychology of religion. Hufford's (1982) warning that psychologists need a parallel to ethnography— a "phenomenography"—can no longer be ignored. Psychologists have yet to provide the most basic description of the experience central to the study of religion and spirituality. The discussion of mysticism in this text also indicates the interface between phenomenological and measurement psychology, in which the results of phenomenological analysis can be operationalized and fulfill the requirements of a measurement paradigm. Once again, the issue is not only that multiple methods can be of value in the psychology of religion and spirituality, but that measurement can be based upon a variety of theoretical and even alternative methodological perspectives. It is long past the time when the psychological illumination of religious issues can be assumed to deny the validity of the religious nature that is illuminated psychologically. Boundaries must be identified theoretically even if they are to be crossed.

If there is a change in the psychology of religion, it is likely to be most evident in the North American dominance of the field. The success of psychology in the United States and Canada has always been associated with its development as a profession. Contemporary psychology has witnessed a split in allegiances between the American Psychological Association, long the dominant organization for psychologists (whether teachers, researchers, or practitioners), and the more recently formed American Psychological Society (which focuses more upon research and teaching than upon practice). This apparent dichotomy suggests that even within North American psychology, tensions between research and practice, and between knowledge and application, are considerable. The tension is reflected in religion as a specialty in the American Psychological Society and religion as a division within the American Psychological Association. Practitioners are more likely to foster a religious psychology than researchers. It is unlikely that this emphasis will gain as strong an academic foothold in North American universities as a research-based empirical psychology of religion.

Compared to North American psychologists of religion, Europeans are less measurement-oriented and more receptive to phenomenological and dynamic studies. These cultures are also less overtly committed to institutional religion. Thus the European psychology of religion promises to challenge the supremacy of the North American psychology of religion, both because of European psychology's greater breadth and scope, and because of North American psychology's tendency to take apologetic religious-psychological stances. In addition, Asian studies in the psychology of religion are emerging—with much less distinct lines among psychology, religion/spirituality, and science. To date, mainly transpersonal psychologists have examined these traditions, but their influence will undoubtedly affect measurement-based psychology. Again, the challenge to a psychology of religion premised upon measurement and experimentation is for theoretical meaningfulness as well as greater breadth and scope. We prophesied in the second edition of this book that another *Annual Review of Psychology* would be unlikely to "include a review of psychology of religion in which the data base consists exclusively of convenience samples of Protestant Christians selected primarily from North American universities" (Hood, Spilka, Hunsberger, & Gorsuch, 1996, p. 448). Unfortunately, this optimistic prophecy has not been borne out. Another such review of the field has recently appeared (Emmons & Paloutzian, 2003), but its data base is very much like that of Gorsuch's (1988) earlier review. For many reasons, this situation is even less acceptable now than we found it in our second edition.

EXTREMISM, CONFLICT, AND THE PSYCHOLOGY OF RELIGION

The urgency of the need to consider the global dimensions of psychology and religion has been highlighted by recent world events. After September 11, 2001, few would disagree that we live in seriously troubled times. Perhaps for some there is a renewed call to faith, but for others it appears that religion itself may be the problem. The great faith traditions of Christianity, Islam, and Judaism find themselves in both direct and indirect conflict. Whether it be the imagery of "Onward Christian Soldiers" or the cries of "*Jihad!*", a sense of being wronged is succeeded by hate, usually legitimated by carefully selected scriptural prescriptions.

The problem extends well beyond armed violence. There is a psychology of religious extremism that has not yet been empirically understood. It appears to be associated with a sense of righteousness and the need to demonize other points of view. Virtually all of the current "anti-" trends in religion—those targeting abortion, evolution, women, homosexuality, science, medicine, and progress in general—are clothed in anti-Satan beliefs and rhetoric. In North American Christianity, this tradition began with the Salem witch trials in 17th-century colonial Massachusetts, which reflected medieval religious views of women. The title of Karlsen's (1989) history, *The Devil in the Shape of a Woman*, places the trials in a religious framework.

Extremists may take refuge in ethnocentrism, creating ingroup–outgroup distinctions and reinforcing these with alienating rhetoric. Abortion is likely to be countered with sexism; prayer in the schools may take on an anti-Semitic tint; and brotherhood can be restricted to one's fellow believers. "True believing" knows few bounds, especially when religion is an organizing force. Believers in "conspiracy" ask who is behind pornography, evolutionary theory, secular humanism, women's rights, or opposition to prayer in the schools—and the approved answers too often excite bigotry.

This is not to say that there may not be extremists on both sides of all these issues. Those who consider themselves "warriors in God's name" find their counterparts in atheistic networks. The advocates of science in *The Skeptical Inquirer* commonly take on conservative religionists. The editors, publisher, and writers in *Science and Spirit* make a commendable effort to struggle for a middle ground by subtitling their magazine as "connecting science, religion, and life." Of course, their stance may itself be regarded as extreme by those who polarize these issues.

One does not have to look far to find religious roots for the events of September 11, 2001. These illustrate the extremes to which religious traditions are able to motivate true believers (Nielsen, 2001). Unhappily, the actions of extremist Muslims on that tragic September day has created much distress among moderate Muslims in the United States. Equally extremist Christians have directed undiscriminating hate speech against Islam and its representatives (Sachs, 2002b). The Palestinian–Israeli conflict, when seized upon by extremists on either side, has often been reduced to a conflict between Islam and Judaism, but this tendency has intensified since the September 11 events (Karsh, 2002; Sachs, 2002a). Extremism blunts perception and cognition, so that unreasonable and false generalizations simplify and polarize thinking.

Perceptions of science as the enemy, particularly where evolution is concerned, seem as strong today as they were with the Scopes trial in Tennessee over 75 years ago. State school boards in Ohio, Kansas, and Georgia, among others, have generally given up on replacing Darwinian theory with creationism, and now argue for equal time in the classroom. Whereas creationism was relatively easily rejected as religion rather than science, new arguments from "intelligent design" have been introduced into this classic fray (Clines, 2002; Holt, 2002). The backers of this more sophisticated position are often highly trained scientists themselves (Nelson, 2002).

It is not difficult to give many more examples of extreme behaviors connected to religion. However, the extremism–religion association is not well understood and merits both the development of theory and the undertaking of research. It will require a global approach—one not restricted to sampling North American university undergraduates. We need to know a great deal more than is currently understood about the cognitive and motivational aspects of the kind of religious commitment that supports extreme behavior, so that we can empirically engage Dionne's (2001) question: "Is religion the cause or the solution?" (p. B11).

FINAL THOUGHTS: NEEDS FOR TODAY AND THE FUTURE

Once again, what appears the clearest need in social-scientific work that will assure the vigor, relevance, and compatibility of the psychology of religion with mainstream psychology is theory. Our prophecy that the psychology of religion will no longer be atheoretical, piecemeal, and lacking in sustained development has not yet been proven false. Mainstream psychology has proposed a variety of theories that integrate and guide meaningful empirical research, and many of them are beginning to influence the study of religion. Likewise, more restricted theories are being developed within our field that can sustain significant research. In any case, whether broad or narrow, the demand for theory will guide the future psychology of religion.

Closely related to the issue of theory is the need for more sophisticated theological literacy among researchers in the psychology of religion (Hunter, 1989). For instance, Gorsuch (1994) has emphasized that if intrinsic religion is treated as a motivational construct, then assessing it independently of belief content is essential. Low correlations between measures of general intrinsic religiousness (such as the Allport–Ross Intrinsic scale) and other variables may be due to the fact that only when specific beliefs are taken into account can more powerful predictions be made. That is, whether one is intrinsically motivated may be a less powerful predictor than one's intrinsic motivation within a particular belief context. In a similar vein, Hood (1992) has argued that empirically identified psychological processes are of little use in making predictions unless the content of specific faith traditions is taken into account. The psychology of religion and spirituality, even when it is not a "religious psychology" in Beit-Hallahmi's (1991) sense, needs to be religiously and spiritually informed in order to make meaningful empirical predictions.

Finally, concern for theory is not unrelated to training in the professional practice of psychology. The need for clinicians and counselors to be sensitive to cultural, gender, and religious differences makes the understanding of religion and spirituality necessary. Jones (1994) has made a case for the inclusion of religious values and perspectives within modern clinical psychology. At a minimum, sensitivity to clients' values, including religious ones, is an ethical imperative for clinicians and other social science providers.

In many cases, psychotherapy takes place within a religious framework (Richards & Bergin, 1997). The American Psychological Association discovered a great demand for Shafranske's (1996) significant edited volume on religion and the practice of clinical psychology. His work has been followed by several additional books published by the American Psychological Association that focus upon the global dimension of religion and spirituality, including texts on religious diversity (Richards & Bergin, 2000) and even on the use of specific spiritual strategies in psychotherapy (Richards & Bergin, in press). An awareness of religious motivations and schemas is particularly necessary for effective intervention in cases where law enforcement deals with religiously based deviance, as in confrontations with religious sects and cults over the last few decades.

It has long been established that things believed and acted upon as true have real consequences, whether they are true or not in some ultimate sense. Understanding religious perspectives, however different from our own, is another tool for effectively interacting with those whose religiously based views provide them with meaning, security, and mastery. Theory, empirically supported, ought properly to dominate the future of the psychology of religion and spirituality. Psychology is itself a product of culture, and as we remember the events of September 11, 2001, we are keenly aware that we are North American psychologists who wish greater illumination of religious and spiritual phenomena that with our current knowledge can be seen only "through a glass darkly."

REFERENCES

Aarson, B., & Osmond, H. (1970). *Psychedelics: The use and implications of psychedelic drugs.* Garden City, NY: Doubleday.

Abraham, K. G. (1981). The influence of cognitive conflict on religious thinking in fifth and sixth grade children. *Journal of Early Adolescence, 1,* 147–154.

Abrahamson, A. C., Baker, L. A., & Caspi, A. (2002). Rebellious teens? Genetic and environmental influences on the social attitudes of adolescence. *Journal of Personality and Social Psychology, 83,* 1392–1408.

Academy of Religion and Mental Health. (1959). *Religion, science, and mental health.* New York: New York University Press.

Ackerman, D. (1994). *A natural history of love.* New York: Random House.

Acklin, M. W., Brown, E. C., & Mauger, P. A. (1983). The role of religious values in coping with cancer. *Journal of Religion and Health, 22,* 322–333.

Acock, A. C., & Bengtson, V. L. (1978). On the relative influence of mothers and fathers: A covariance analysis of political and religious socialization. *Journal of Marriage and the Family, 40,* 519–530.

Acock, A. C., & Bengtson, V. L. (1980). Socialization and attribution processes: Actual versus perceived similarity among parents and youth. *Journal of Marriage and the Family, 42,* 501–515.

Acredolo, C., & O'Connor, J. (1991). On the difficulty of detecting cognitive uncertainty. *Human Development, 34,* 204–223.

Adams, G. R., Bennion, L., & Huh, K. (1989). *Objective measure of ego identity status: A reference manual* (2nd ed.). Logan: Utah State University Press.

Aday, R. H. (1984–1985). Belief in afterlife and death anxiety: Correlates and comparisons. *Omega, 15,* 67–75.

Adelekan, M. L., Abiodun, O. A., Imouokhome-Obayan, A. O., Oni, G. A., & Ogunremi, O. O. (1993). Psychosocial correlates of alcohol, tobacco and cannabis use: Findings from a Nigerian university. *Drug and Alcohol Dependence, 33,* 247–256.

Adler, A. (1935). Introduction. *Journal of Individual Psychology, 1,* 5–8,

Adorno, T. W., Frenkel-Brunswik, E., Levinson, D. J., & Sanford, R. N. (1950). *The authoritarian personality.* New York: Harper & Row.

Ahern, G. (1990). *Spiritual/religious experience in modern society.* Oxford: Alister Hardy Research Centre, Westminister College.

Ai, A. L., Bolling, S. F., & Peterson, C. (2000). The use of prayer by coronary artery bypass patients. *International Journal for the Psychology of Religion, 10,* 205–219.

Ainlay, S. C., Singleton, R., & Swigert, V. L. (1992). Aging and religious participation: Reconsidering the effects of health. *Journal for the Scientific Study of Religion, 31,* 175–188.

Ainsworth, M. D. S. (1982). Attachment: Retrospect and prospect. In C. M. Parkes & J. Stevenson-Hinde (Eds.), *The place of attachment in human behavior* (pp. 3–30). New York: Basic Books.

Alaggia, R. (2001). Cultural and religious influences in maternal response to intrafamilial child sexual abuse: Charting new territory for research and treatment. *Journal of Child Sexual Abuse, 10*, 41–60.

Albacete, L. (2002). *God at the Ritz.* New York: Crossroad.

Albert, A. A., & Porter, J. R. (1986). Children's gender role stereotypes: A comparison of the United States and South Africa. *Journal of Cross-Cultural Psychology, 17*, 45–65.

Alberts, C. (2000). Identity formation among African late-adolescents in a contemporary South African context. *International Journal for the Advancement of Counselling, 22*, 23–42.

Albrecht, S. L., & Bahr, H. M. (1983). Patterns of religious disaffiliation: A study of lifelong Mormons, Mormon converts, and former Mormons. *Journal for the Scientific Study of Religion, 22*, 366–379.

Albrecht, S. L., & Cornwall, M. (1989). Life events and religious change. *Review of Religious Research, 31*, 23–38.

Albrecht, S. L., Cornwall, M., & Cunningham, P. H. (1988). Religious leave-taking: Disengagement and disaffiliation among Mormons. In D. G. Bromley (Ed.), *Falling from the faith: Causes and consequences of religious apostasy* (pp. 62–80). Newbury Park, CA: Sage.

Alem, A., Kebede, D., & Kullgren, G. (1999). The epidemiology of problem drinking in Butajira, Ethiopia. *Acta Psychiatrica Scandinavica, 100*(Suppl. 397), 77–83.

Aleshire, D. O. (1980). Eleven major areas of ministry. In D. S. Schuller, M. P. Strommen, & M. L. Brekke (Eds.), *Ministry in America* (pp. 23–53). San Francisco: Harper & Row.

Alexander, I. E., & Adlerstein, A. (1958). Affective responses to the concept of death in a population of children and early adolescents. *Journal of Genetic Psychology, 93*, 167–177.

Alexander, M. W., & Judd, B. B. (1986). Differences in attitudes toward nudity in advertising. *Psychology: A Quarterly Journal of Behavior, 23*, 26–29.

Ali, H. K., & Naidoo, A. (1999). Sex education sources and attitudes about premarital sex of Seventh Day Adventist youth. *Psychological Reports, 84*, 312.

Al-Issa, I. (1977). Social and cultural aspects of hallucinations. *Psychological Reports, 84*, 570–587.

Allegro, J. M. (1971). *The sacred mushroom and the cross.* New York: Bantam.

Allen, R. O., & Spilka, B. (1967). Committed and consensual religion: A specification of religion–prejudice relationships. *Journal for the Scientific Study of Religion, 6*, 191–206.

Allison, J. (1961). Recent empirical studies of conversion experiences. *Pastoral Psychology, 17*, 21–33.

Allison, J. (1968). Adaptive regression and intense religious experiences. *Journal of Nervous and Mental Disease, 145*, 452–463.

Allison, J. (1969). Religious conversion: Regression and progression in an adolescent experience. *Journal for the Scientific Study of Religion, 8*, 23–38.

Allport, G. W. (1937). *Personality: A psychological interpretation.* New York: Holt.

Allport, G. W. (1942). *The use of personal documents in psychological science* (Bulletin No. 49). New York: Social Science Research Council.

Allport, G. W. (1950). *The individual and his religion.* New York: Macmillan.

Allport, G. W. (1954). *The nature of prejudice.* Cambridge, MA: Addison-Wesley.

Allport, G. W. (1959). Religion and prejudice. *The Crane Review, 2*, 1–10.

Allport, G. W. (1966). The religious context of prejudice. *Journal for the Scientific Study of Religion, 5*, 447–457.

Allport, G. W., Gillespie, J. M., & Young, J. (1948). The religion of the post-war college student. *Journal of Psychology, 25*, 3–33.

Allport, G. W., & Ross, J. M. (1967). Personal religious orientation and prejudice. *Journal of Personality and Social Psychology, 5*, 432–443.

Allport, G. W., Vernon, P. E., & Lindzey, G. (1960). *A manual for the study of values* (3rd ed.). Boston: Houghton Mifflin.

Aloyse, Sister M. (1961). Evaluation of candidates for the religious life. *Guild of Catholic Psychiatrists Bulletin, 8*, 199–204.

Alsdurf, P., & Alsdurf, J. M. (1988). Wife abuse and scripture. In A. L. Horton & J. A. Williamson (Eds.), *Abuse and religion: When praying isn't enough* (pp. 221–227). Lexington, MA: Lexington Books.

Altemeyer, B. (1981). *Right-wing authoritarianism.* Winnipeg: University of Manitoba Press.

Altemeyer, B. (1988). *Enemies of freedom: Understanding right-wing authoritarianism.* San Francisco: Jossey-Bass.

Altemeyer, B. (1996). *The authoritarian specter.* Cambridge, MA: Harvard University Press.

Altemeyer, B. (2003). Why do religious fundamentalists tend to be prejudiced? *International Journal for the Psychology of Religion, 13,* 17–28.

Altemeyer, B., & Hunsberger, B. (1992). Authoritarianism, religious fundamentalism, quest, and prejudice. *International Journal for the Psychology of Religion, 2,* 113–133.

Altemeyer, B., & Hunsberger, B. (1993). Response to Gorsuch. *International Journal for the Psychology of Religion, 3,* 33–37.

Altemeyer, B., & Hunsberger, B. (1997). *Amazing conversions: Why some turn to faith and others abandon religion.* Amherst, NY: Prometheus Books.

Alvarado, K. A., Templer, D. I., Bresler, C., & Thomas-Dobson, S. (1995). The relationship of religious variables to death depression and death anxiety. *Journal of Clinical Psychology, 51,* 202–204.

Ameika, C., Eck, N. H., Ivers, B. J., Clifford, J. M., & Malcarne, V. (1994, April 22). *Religiosity and illness prevention.* Paper presented at the annual convention of the Rocky Mountain Psychological Association, Las Vegas, NV.

American Baptist Churches. (1992, June). *Resolution on mental illness* [Online]. Available: http://www.abc-usa.org/resources/resol/mentill.htm [Retrieved June 30, 2002].

American Civil Liberties Union. (2001, July). *Crime and punishment in America: State by state breakdown of sodomy laws* [Online]. Available: http://www.aclu.org/issues/gay/sodomy.html [Retrieved August 12, 2001].

American Psychiatric Association. (1980). *Diagnostic and statistical manual of mental disorders* (3rd ed.). Washington, DC: Author.

American Psychiatric Association. (1987). *Diagnostic and statistical manual of mental disorders* (3rd ed., rev.). Washington, DC: Author.

American Psychiatric Association. (1994). *Diagnostic and statistical manual of mental disorders* (4th ed.). Washington, DC: Author.

American Psychiatric Association. (2000). *Diagnostic and statistical manual of mental disorders* (4th ed., text rev.). Washington, DC: Author.

Ames, E. S. (1910). *The psychology of religious experience.* Boston: Houghton Mifflin.

Amey, C. H., Albrecht, S. L., & Miller, M. K. (1996). Racial differences in adolescent drug use: The impact of religion. *Substance Use and Misuse, 31,* 1311–1332.

Anand, B. K., Chhina, G. S., & Singh, B. (1961). Some aspects of electroencephalographic studies on yogis. *Electroencephalography and Clinical Neurophysiology, 13,* 452–456.

Anderson, G. C. (1963). Who is ministering to ministers? *Christianity Today, 7,* 362–363.

Anderson, V. (1998, December 5). *Church changes position on birth control.* Available: http://mormons.org.uk/birth.htm [Retrieved September 17, 2002].

Andreason, N. J. C. (1972). The role of religion in depression. *Journal of Religion and Health, 11,* 153–166.

Andrew, J. M. (1970). Recovery from surgery, with and without preparatory instructions for three coping styles. *Journal of Personality and Social Psychology, 15,* 223–226.

Andrews, E. D. A. (1963). *The people called Shakers* (new enlarged ed.). New York: Dover.

Andrews, L. M. (1987). *To thine own self be true.* Garden City, NY: Doubleday/Anchor.

Andrews, R., Briggs, M., & Seidel, M. (1996). *The Columbia world of quotations.* New York: Columbia University Press.

Angelica, D. (1977). A comparative study of attitudes toward and denial of their own death of Episcopal clergymen and laymen in Connecticut. *Dissertation Abstracts International, 37,* 466B.

Annis, L. V. (1975). Study of values as a predictor of helping behavior. *Psychological Reports, 37,* 717–718.

Annis, L. V. (1976). Emergency helping and religious behavior. *Psychological Reports, 39,* 151–158.

Anthony, D., Ecker, B., & Wilbur, K. (Eds.). (1987). *Spiritual choices.* New York: Paragon House.

Anthony, D., & Robbins, T. (1974). The Meher Baba movement: Its effect on post-adolescent social alienation. In I. I. Zaretsky & M. P. Leone (Eds.), *Religious movements in contemporary America* (pp. 228–243). Princeton, NJ: Princeton University Press.

Anthony, D., & Robbins, T. (1992). Law, social science and the "brainwashing" exception to the First Amendment. *Behavioral Sciences and the Law, 10,* 5–29.

Anthony, D., & Robbins, T. (1994). Brainwashing and totalitarian influence. In U. S. Ramachdran (Ed.), *Encyclopaedia of human behavior* (Vol. 1, pp. 457–471). New York: Academic Press.

Anthony, S. (1940). *The child's discovery of death.* New York: Harcourt Brace.

Antkowiak, C., & Ozorak, E. W. (2000, October). *A very present help: Sacred objects as means of comfort.* Paper presented at the annual convention of the Society for the Scientific Study of Religion, Houston, TX.

Apolito, P. (1998). *Apparitions of the Madonna at Oliveto Citra: Local visions and cosmic drama* (A. William, Jr., Trans.). University Park, PA: Pennsylvania State University Press.

Appel, K. E. (1959). Religion. In S. Arieti (Ed.), *American handbook of psychiatry* (Vol. 2, pp. 1777–1810). New York: Basic Books.

Appelle, S. (1996). The abduction experience: A critical evaluation of theory and evidence. *Journal of UFO Studies, 6,* 29–79.

Appelle, S., Lynn, S. J., & Newman, L. (2000). Alien abduction experiences. In E. Cardeña, S. J. Lynn, & S. Krippner (Eds.), *Varieties of anomalous experience* (pp. 253–282). Washington, DC: American Psychological Association.

Archer, S. L. (1989). Gender differences in identity development: Issues of process, domain and timing. *Journal of Adolescence, 12,* 117–138.

Arendt, H. (1979). *The origins of totalitarianism.* San Diego: Harcourt Brace Jovanovich.

Argue, A., Johnson, D. R., & White, L. K. (1999). Age and religiosity: Evidence from a three-wave panel analysis. *Journal for the Scientific Study of Religion, 38,* 423–435.

Argyle, M. (1959). *Religious behavior.* Glencoe, IL: Free Press.

Argyle, M., & Beit-Hallahmi, B. (1975). *The social psychology of religion.* London: Routledge & Kegan Paul.

Aries, P. (1974). *Western attitudes toward death from the Middle Ages to the present.* Baltimore: Johns Hopkins University Press.

Armstead, N. (Ed.). (1974). *Reconstructing social psychology.* Harmondsworth, England: Penguin.

Armstrong, T. D. (1995, August). *Exploring spirituality: The development of the Armstrong measure of spirituality.* Paper presented at the annual convention of the American Psychological Association, New York.

Arnold, M. (1897). A wish. In *The poetical works of Matthew Arnold* (pp. 288–289). New York: Thomas Y. Crowell. (Original work published 1853)

Askin, H., Paultre, Y., White, R., & Van Ornum, W. (1993, August). *The quantitative and qualitative aspects of scrupulosity.* Paper presented at the annual convention of the American Psychological Association, Toronto.

Assanangkornchai, S., Conigrave, K. M., & Saunders, J. B. (2002). Religious beliefs and practice, and alcohol use in Thai men. *Alcohol and Alcoholism, 37,* 193–197.

Atchley, R. C. (1977). *The social forces in later life: An introduction to social gerontology* (2nd ed.). Belmont, CA: Wadsworth.

Austin, J. H. (1998). *Zen and the brain.* Cambridge, MA: MIT Press.

Avants, S. K., Warburton, L. A., & Margolin, A. (2001). Spiritual and religious support in recovery from addiction among HIV-positive injection drug users. *Journal of Psychoactive Drugs, 33,* 39–45.

Awn, P. J. (1994). Indian Islam: The Shah Bano affair. In J. S. Hawley (Ed.), *Fundamentalism and gender* (pp. 63–78). New York: Oxford University Press.

Azari, N. P., Nickel, J., Wunderlich, G., Niedeggen, M., Hefter, H., Tellman, L., et al. (2001). Neural correlates of religious experience. *European Journal of Neuroscience, 13,* 649–652.

Babchuk, N., & Whitt, H. P. (1990). R-order and religious switching. *Journal for the Scientific Study of Religion, 29,* 246–254.

Bach, G. R., & Wyden, P. (1969). *The intimate enemy.* New York: Morrow.

Back, K. W., & Bourque, L. (1970). Can feelings be enumerated? *Behavioral Science, 15,* 487–496.

Badcock, C. R. (1980). *Psychoanalysis of culture.* Oxford: Blackwell.

Bader, C. (1999). New perspectives on failed prophecy. *Journal for the Scientific Study of Religion, 38,* 119–131.

Badham, P. (1976). *Christian beliefs about life after death.* London: McMillan.

Bagchi, B. K., & Wenger, M. A. (1957). Electro-physiological correlates of some yogi exercises. *Electroencephalography and Clinical Neurophysiology, 2*(Suppl. 7), 132–139.

Bahr, H. M., & Albrecht, S. L. (1989). Strangers once more: Patterns of disaffiliation from Mormonism. *Journal for the Scientific Study of Religion, 28,* 180–200.

Bahr, H. M., & Harvey, C. D. (1980). Correlates of morale among the newly widowed. *Journal of Social Psychology, 110,* 219–233.

Bahr, H. M., & Martin, T. K. (1983). "And thy neighbor as thyself": Self-esteem and faith in people as correlates of religiosity and family solidarity among Middletown high school students. *Journal for the Scientific Study of Religion, 22,* 132–144.

Bahr, S. J., Maughan, S. L., Marcos, A. C., & Li, B. (1998). Family, religiosity, and the risk of adolescent drug use. *Journal of Marriage and the Family, 60,* 979–992.

Baier, C. J., & Wright, B. R. E. (2001). "If you love me, keep my commandments": A meta-analysis of the effect of religion on crime. *Journal of Research in Crime and Delinquency, 38,* 3–21.

Bailey, L. W., & Yates, J. (1996). *The near-death experience: A reader.* New York: Routledge.

Bainbridge, W. S. (1989). The religious ecology of deviance. *American Sociological Review, 54,* 288–295.

Bainbridge, W. S. (1992a). Crime, delinquency, and religion. In J. F. Schumaker (Ed.), *Religion and mental health* (pp. 199–210). New York: Oxford University Press.

Bainbridge, W. S. (1992b). The sociology of conversion. In H. N. Maslony & S. Southard (Eds.), *Handbook of religious conversion* (pp. 178–191). Birmingham, AL: Religious Education Press.

Bainbridge, W. S. (1997). *The sociology of religious movements.* New York: Routledge.

Bainbridge, W. S., & Stark, R. (1980a). Client and audience cults in America. *Sociological Analysis, 41,* 199–214.

Bainbridge, W. S., & Stark, R. (1980b). Sectarian tension. *Review of Religious Research, 22,* 105–124.

Bains, G. (1983). Explanations and the need for control. In M. Hewstone (Ed.), *Attribution theory: Social and functional extensions* (pp. 117–143). Oxford: Blackwell.

Bakalar, J., & Grinspoon, L. (1989). Testing psychotherapies and drug therapies: The case of psychedelic drugs. In S. Peroutka (Ed.), *Ecstasy: The clinical, pharmacological, and neurotoxicological effects of the drug MDMAS.* Norwell, MA: Kluwer Academic.

Baker-Brown, G., Ballard, E. J., Bluck, S., de Vries, B., Suedfeld, P., & Tetlock, P. E. (1992). The conceptual integrative complexity scoring manual. In C. P. Smith (Ed.), *Motivation and personality: Handbook of thematic content analysis* (pp. 401–418). Cambridge, England: Cambridge University Press.

Baker-Sperry, L. (2001). Passing on the faith: The father's role in religious transmission. *Sociological Focus, 34,* 185–198.

Balch, R. W. (1980). Looking behind the scenes in a religious cult: Implications for the study of conversion. *Sociological Analysis, 45,* 301–314.

Balch, R. W., Farnsworth, G., & Wilkins, S. (1983). When the bombs dropped: Reactions to disconfirmed prophecy in a millennial sect. *Sociological Perspectives, 26,* 137–158.

Balk, D. E. (1995). *Adolescent development: Early through late adolescence.* Pacific Grove, CA: Brooks/Cole.

Ballard, S. N., & Fleck, J. R. (1975). The teaching of religious concepts: A three stage model. *Journal of Psychology and Theology, 3,* 164–171.

Bancroft, A. (1987). Women in Buddhism. In U. King (Ed.), *Women in the world's religions, past and present* (pp. 81–104). New York: Paragon House.

Bandura, A. (1977). *Social learning theory.* Englewood Cliffs, NJ: Prentice-Hall.

Bao, W. N., Whitbeck, L. B., Hoyt, D. R., & Conger, R. D. (1999). Perceived parental acceptance as a moderator of religious transmission among adolescent boys and girls. *Journal of Marriage and the Family, 61,* 362–374.

Barash, D. P. (1977). *Sociobiology and behavior.* New York: Elsevier.

Barber, T. X. (1970). *LSD, marijuana, yoga, and hypnosis.* Chicago: Aldine.

Barker, E. (1983). Supping with the devil: How long a spoon does the sociologist need? *Sociological Analysis, 44,* 197–206.

Barker, E. (1984). *The making of a Moonie.* Oxford: Blackwell.

Barker, E. (1986). Religious movements: Cult and anticult since Jonestown. *Annual Review of Sociology, 12,* 329–346.

Barker, I. R., & Currie, R. F. (1985). Do converts always make the most committed Christians? *Journal for the Scientific Study of Religion, 24,* 305–313.

Barkow, J. H. (1982). Culture and sociobiology. In T. C. Weigele (Ed.), *Biology and the social sciences* (pp.59–73). Boulder, CO: Westview Press.

Barnard, G. W. (1997). *Exploring unseen worlds: William James and the philosophy of mysticism.* Albany: State University of New York Press.

Barnes, M., & Doyles, D. (1989). The formation of a Fowler scale: An empirical assessment among Catholics. *Review of Religious Research, 30,* 412–420.

Barr, H. L., Langs, R. J., Holt, R. R., Goldberger, L., & Klein, C. S. (1972). *LSD, personality and experience.* New York: Wiley.

Barrett, J. L., Richert, R. A., & Driesenga, A. (2001). God's beliefs versus mother's: The development of non-human agent concepts. *Child Development, 72,* 50–65.

Barron, F. (1953). An ego-strength scale which predicts response to psychotherapy. *Journal of Consulting Psychology, 17,* 327–333.

Barth, K. (1963). *Evangelical theology.* New York: Holt, Rinehart & Winston.

Bartlett, J. (Ed.). (1955). *Familiar quotations by John Bartlett* (13th ed.). Boston: Little, Brown.

Basow, S. A. (1980). *Sex-role stereotypes: Traditions and alternatives.* Monterey, CA: Brooks/Cole.

Bassett, R. L., Miller, S., Anstey, K., Crafts, K., Harmon, J., Lee, Y., et al. (1990). Picturing God: A nonverbal measure of God concept for conservative Protestants. *Journal of Psychology and Christianity, 9,* 73–81.

Bateman, M. M., & Jensen, J. S. (1958). The effect of religious background on modes of handling anger. *Journal of Social Psychology, 47,* 133–141.

Bateson, P. (1988). The biological evolution of cooperation and trust. In D. Gambetta (Ed.), *Trust: Making and breaking cooperative relations* (pp. 14–30). New York: Blackwell.

Bateson, P. (2000). Taking the stink out of instinct. In H. Rose & S. Rose (Eds.), *Alas, poor Darwin* (pp. 189–207). New York: Harmony Books.

Batson, C. D. (1976). Religion as prosocial: Agent or double agent? *Journal for the Scientific Study of Religion, 15,* 29–45.

Batson, C. D. (1983). Sociobiology and the role of religion in promoting prosocial behavior: An alternative view. *Journal of Personality and Social Psychology, 45,* 1380–1385.

Batson, C. D. (1990). Good Samaritans—or priests and Levites?: Using William James as a guide in the study of religious prosocial motivation. *Personality and Social Psychology Bulletin, 16,* 758–768.

Batson, C. D. (1991). *The altruism question: Toward a social-psychological answer.* Hillsdale, NJ: Erlbaum.

Batson, C. D., & Burris, C. T. (1994). Personal religion: Depressant or stimulant of prejudice and discrimination? In M. P. Zanna & J. M. Olson (Eds.), *The Ontario Symposium: Vol. 7. The psychology of prejudice* (pp. 149–169). Hillsdale, NJ: Erlbaum.

Batson, C. D., Eidelman, S. H., Higley, S. L., & Russell, S. A. (2001). "And who is my neighbor?": II. Quest religion as a source of universal compassion. *Journal for the Scientific Study of Religion, 40,* 39–50.

Batson, C. D., Flink, C. H., Schoenrade, P. A., Fultz, J., & Pych, V. (1986). Religious orientation and overt versus covert racial prejudice. *Journal of Personality and Social Psychology, 50,* 175–181.

Batson, C. D., & Flory, J. D. (1990). Goal-relevant cognitions associated with helping by individuals high on intrinsic, end religion. *Journal for the Scientific Study of Religion, 29,* 346–360.

Batson, C. D., Floyd, R. B., Meyer, J. M., & Winner, A. L. (1999). "And who is my neighbor?": Intrinsic religion as a source of universal compassion. *Journal for the Scientific Study of Religion, 38,* 31–41.

Batson, C. D., & Gray, R. A. (1981). Religious orientation and helping behavior: Responding to one's own or to the victim's needs? *Journal of Personality and Social Psychology, 40,* 511–520.

Batson, C. D., Naifeh, S. J., & Pate, S. (1978). Social desirability, religious orientation, and racial prejudice. *Journal for the Scientific Study of Religion, 17,* 31–41.

Batson, C. D., Oleson, K. C., Weeks, J. L., Healy, S. P., Reeves, P. J., Jennings, P., & Brown, T. (1989). Religious prosocial motivation: Is it altruistic or egoistic? *Journal of Personality and Social Psychology, 57,* 873–884.

Batson, C. D., & Raynor-Prince, L. (1983). Religious orientation and complexity of thought about existential concerns. *Journal for the Scientific Study of Religion, 22,* 38–50.

Batson, C. D., & Schoenrade, P. A. (1991a). Measuring religion as quest: 1. Validity concerns. *Journal for the Scientific Study of Religion, 30,* 416–429.

Batson, C. D., & Schoenrade, P. A. (1991b). Measuring religion as quest: 2. Reliability concerns. *Journal for the Scientific Study of Religion, 30,* 430–447.

Batson, C. D., Schoenrade, P., & Pych, V. (1985). Brotherly love or self-concern?: Behavioural consequences of religion. In L. B. Brown (Ed.), *Advances in the psychology of religion* (pp. 185–208). New York: Oxford University Press.

Batson, C. D., Schoenrade, P., & Ventis, W. L. (1993). *Religion and the individual: A social-psychological perspective.* New York: Oxford University Press.

Batson, C. D., & Ventis, W. L. (1982). *The religious experience: A social-psychological perspective.* New York: Oxford University Press.

Baum, A., & Singer, J. E. (Eds.). (1987). *Handbook of psychology and health: Vol. 5. Stress.* Hillsdale, NJ: Erlbaum.

Baumeister, R. F. (1991). *Meanings of life.* New York: Guilford Press.

Baumrind, D. (1967). Child care practices anteceding three patterns of preschool behavior. *Genetic Psychology Monographs, 75,* 43–88.

Baumrind, D. (1991). Parenting styles and adolescent development. In R. M. Lerner, A. C. Petersen, & J. Brooks-Gunn (Eds.), *The encyclopedia of adolescence* (Vol. 2, pp. 746–758). New York: Garland Press.

Becker, H. S. (1963). *Outsiders.* New York: Free Press.

Beckford, J. A. (1978). Accounting for conversion. *British Journal of Sociology, 29,* 249–262.

Beckford, J. A. (1979). Politics and the anti-cult movement. *Annual Review of the Social Sciences of Religion, 3,* 169–190.

Beckford, J. A., & Richardson, J. T. (1983). A bibliography of social scientific studies of new religious movements. *Social Compass, 30,* 111–135.

Bedell, K. B. (Ed.). (1994). *Yearbook of American and Canadian churches 1994.* Nashville, TN: Abingdon Press.

Beeghley, L., Bock, E. W., & Cochran, J. K. (1990). Religious change and alcohol use: An application of reference group and socialization theory. *Sociological Forum, 5,* 261–278.

Begley, S. (2001, January 29). Searching for the God within. *Newsweek,* p. 59.

Begue, L. (2000). Social practices, religion and moral judgment: New results. *Cahiers Internationaux de Psychologie Sociale,* No. 445, 67–76.

Behe, M. J. (1996). *Darwin's black box: The biochemical challenge to evolution.* New York: Free Press.

Beit-Hallahmi, B. (1977). Curiosity, doubt, and devotion: The beliefs of psychologists and the psychology of religion. In H. N. Malony (Ed.), *Current perspectives in the psychology of religion* (pp. 381–391). Grand Rapids, MI: Eerdmans.

Beit-Hallahmi, B. (1989). *Prolegomena to the psychological study of religion.* Lewisburgh, PA: Bucknell University Press.

Beit-Hallahmi, B. (1991). Goring the sacred ox: Towards a psychology of religion. In H. N. Malony (Ed.), *Psychology of religion: Personalities, problems, possibilities* (pp. 189–194). Grand Rapids, MI: Baker.

Beit-Hallahmi, B. (1995). Object relations theory and religious experience. In R. W. Hood, Jr. (Ed.), *Handbook of religious experience* (pp. 254–268). Birmingham, AL: Religious Education Press.

Beit-Hallahmi, B., & Argyle, M. (1997). *The psychology of religious behaviour, belief, and experience.* London: Routledge.

Belavich, T. G. (1995, August). *The role of religion in coping with daily hassles.* Paper presented at the annual convention of the American Psychological Association, New York.

Bell, C. (1997). *Ritual: Perspectives and dimensions.* New York: Oxford University Press.

Bell, R., Wechsler, H., & Johnston, L. D. (1997). Correlates of college student marijuana use: Results of a US national survey. *Addiction, 92,* 571–581.

Bellah, R. N. (1967). Civil religion in America. *Daedalus, 96*(1), 1–21.

Bellah, R. N., Marsden, R., Sullivan, W. M., Swidler, A., & Tipton, S. M. (1996). *Habits of the heart* (rev. ed.). Berkeley: University of California Press.

Belzen, J. A. (2002). The reconstitution of the International Association for the Psychology of Religion. *International Journal for the Psychology of Religion, 12,* 137–140.

Benda, B. B. (1995). The effect of religion on adolescent delinquency revisited. *Journal of Research in Crime and Delinquency, 32,* 446–466.

Benda, B. B. (1997). An examination of a reciprocal relationship between religiosity and different forms of delinquency within a theoretical model. *Journal of Research in Crime and Delinquency, 34,* 163–186.

Benda, B. B., & Corwyn, R. F. (1997a). Religion and delinquency: The relationship after considering family and peer influences. *Journal for the Scientific Study of Religion, 36,* 81–92.

Benda, B. B., & Corwyn, R. F. (1997b). A test of a model with reciprocal effects between religiosity and various forms of delinquency using two-stage least squares regression. *Journal of Social Service Research, 22,* 27–52.

Benda, B. B., & Corwyn, R. F. (1999). Abstinence and birth control among rural adolescents in impoverished families: A test of theoretical discriminators. *Child and Adolescent Social Work Journal, 16,* 191–214.

Benda, B. B., & Corwyn, R. F. (2000). A theoretical model of religiosity and drug use with reciprocal relationships: A test using structural equation modeling. *Journal of Social Service Research, 26,* 43–67.

Bendiksen, R., Hewitt, M., & Vinge, D. (1979, October 27). *Cancer residence for clergy: A preliminary evaluation of an institutional response to clergy involvement in cancer management.* Paper presented at the annual convention of the Society for the Scientific Study of Religion, San Antonio, TX.

Bendyna, M., Green, R. C., Rozell, M. J., & Wilcox, C. (2000). Catholics and the Christian right. *Journal for the Scientific Study of Religion, 40,* 321–332.

Bengtson, V. L., & Troll, L. (1978). Youth and their parents: Feedback and intergenerational influence in socialization. In R. M. Lerner & G. B. Spanier (Eds.), *Child influences on marital and family interaction: A life-span perspective* (pp. 215–240). New York: Academic Press.

Benham, W. G. (1927). *Putnam's complete book of quotations.* New York: Putnam.

Bennett, L., Jr. (1966). *Before the Mayflower.* Baltimore: Penguin.

Benson, H. (1975). *The relaxation response.* New York: Morrow.

Benson, H., & Stark, M. (1996). *Timeless healing: The power and biology of belief.* New York: Scribner.

Benson, P. L. (1988a, October). *The religious development of American Protestants: Overview of the National Research Project.* Paper presented at the annual convention of the Religious Research Association, Chicago.

Benson, P. L. (1988b, October). *The religious development of adults.* Paper presented at the annual convention of the Religious Research Association, Chicago.

Benson, P. L. (1992a). Patterns of religious development in adolescence and adulthood. *Psychologists Interested in Religious Issues Newsletter, 17,* 2–9.

Benson, P. L. (1992b). Religion and substance use. In J. F. Schumaker (Ed.), *Religion and mental health* (pp. 211–220). New York: Oxford University Press.

Benson, P. L., Dehority, J., Garman, L., Hanson, E., Hochschwender, M., Lebold, C., et al. (1980). Intrapersonal correlates of nonspontaneous helping behavior. *Journal of Social Psychology, 110,* 87–95.

Benson, P. L., & Donahue, M. J. (1989). Ten year trends in at-risk behavior: A national study of black adolescents. *Journal of Adolescent Research, 4,* 125–139.

Benson, P. L., Donahue, M. J., & Erickson, J. A. (1989). Adolescence and religion: A review of the literature from 1970 to 1986. *Research in the Social Scientific Study of Religion, 1,* 153–181.

Benson, P. L., & Eklin, C. H. (1990). *Effective Christian education: A national study of Protestant congregations.* Minneapolis, MN: Search Institute.

Benson, P. L., Masters, K. S., & Larson, D. B. (1997). Religious influences on child and adolescent development. In N. E. Alessi (Ed.), *Handbook of child and adolescent psychiatry: Vol. 4. Varieties of development* (pp. 206–219). New York: Wiley.

Benson, P. L., & Spilka, B. (1973). God image as a function of self-esteem and locus of control. *Journal for the Scientific Study of Religion, 13,* 297–310.

Benson, P. L., & Williams, D. L. (1982). *Religion on Capitol Hill: Myths and realities.* New York: Harper & Row.

Benson, P. L., Williams, D. L., & Johnson, A. L. (1987). *The quicksilver years: The hopes and fears of young adolescents.* San Francisco: Harper & Row.

Benson, P. L., Wood, P. K., Johnson, A. L., Eklin, C. H., & Mills, J. E. (1983). *Report on 1983 Minnesota survey on drug use and drug-related activities.* Minneapolis, MN: Search Institute.

Benson, P. L., Yeager, P. K., Wood, M. J., Guerra, M. J., & Manno, B. V. (1986). *Catholic high schools: Their impact on low-income students.* Washington, DC: National Catholic Educational Association.

Bentall, R. P. (1990). The illusion of reality: A review and integration of psychological research on hallucinations. *Psychological Bulletin, 107,* 82–95.

Berenbaum, H., Kerns, J., & Raghavan, C. (2000). Anomalous experiences, peculiarity, and psychopathology. In E. Cardeña, S. J. Lynn, & S. Krippner (Eds.), *Varieties of anomalous experience* (pp. 25–46). Washington, DC: American Psychological Association.

Berger, P. (1979). *The heretical imperative: Contemporary possibilities of religious affirmation.* Garden City, NY: Doubleday/Anchor.

Berger, P., & Luckmann, T. (1967). *The social construction of reality: A treatise in the sociology of knowledge.* Garden City, NY: Doubleday.

Bergin, A. E. (1964). Psychology as a science of inner experience. *Journal of Humanistic Psychology, 4,* 95–103.

Bergin, A. E. (1980). Psychotherapy and religious values. *Journal of Consulting and Clinical Psychology, 48,* 95–105.

Bergin, A. E. (1983). Religiosity and mental health: A critical reevaluation and meta-analysis. *Professional Psychology: Research and Practice, 14,* 170–184.

Bergin, A. E. (1994). Religious life styles and mental health. In L. B. Brown (Ed.), *Religion, personality, and mental health* (pp. 69–93). New York: Springer-Verlag.

Bergling, K. (1981). *Moral development: The validity of Kohlberg's theory.* Stockholm: Almqvist & Wiksell.

Bergman, B. (2001, April 9). The kids are all right. *Maclean's, 114*(15), 42–48.

Bergman, P. (1953). A religious conversion in the course of psychotherapy. *American Journal of Psychotherapy, 7,* 41–58.

Bergman, R. L. (1971). Navajo peyote use: Its apparent safety. *American Journal of Psychiatry, 128,* 695–699.

Berkhofer, R. F., Jr. (1963). Protestants, pagans, and sequences among the North American Indians, 1760–1860. *Ethnohistory, 10,* 201–232.

Berlyne, D. E. (1960), *Conflict, arousal, and curiosity.* New York: McGraw-Hill.

Bernard, L. L. (1924). *Instinct.* New York: Henry Holt.

Bernhardt, W. H. (1958). *A functional philosophy of religion.* Denver, CO: Criterion Press.

Bernstein, B. (1964). Aspects of language and learning in the genesis of the social process. In D. Hymes (Ed.), *Language in culture and society* (pp. 251–263). New York: Harper & Row.

Bernt, F. M. (1989). Being religious and being altruistic: A study of college service volunteers. *Personality and Individual Differences, 10,* 663–669.

Berzonsky, M. D., & Kuk, L. S. (2000). Identity status, identity processing style, and the transition to university. *Journal of Adolescent Research, 15,* 81–98.

Bethesda PsycHealth. (1994). *Results of the Bethesda professional staff chaplain support services advisory committee survey of professional staff, line staff, and patients.* Denver, CO: Author.

Bettelheim, B. (1976). *The uses of enchantment.* New York: Knopf.

Bibby, R. W. (1978). Why conservative churches are growing: Kelley revisited. *Journal for the Scientific Study of Religion,17,* 129–137.

Bibby, R. W. (1987). *Fragmented gods: The poverty and potential of religion in Canada.* Toronto: Irwin.

Bibby, R. W. (1993). *Unknown gods: The ongoing story of religion in Canada.* Toronto: Stoddart.

Bibby, R. W. (2001). *Canada's teens: Today, yesterday, and tomorrow.* Toronto: Stoddart.

Bibby, R. W., & Brinkerhoff, M. B. (1973). The circulation of the saints: A study of people who join conservative churches. *Journal for the Scientific Study of Religion, 12,* 273–283.

Bibby, R. W., & Weaver, H. R. (1985). Cult consumption in Canada: A further criticism of Stark and Bainbridge. *Sociological Analysis, 46,* 445–460.

Bieser, V. (1995, February 23). Dying of shame. *The Jerusalem Report,* pp. 30–32.

Billiet, J. B. (1995). Church involvement, individuals, and ethnic prejudice among Flemish Roman Catholics: New evidence of a moderating effect. *Journal for the Scientific Study of Religion, 34,* 224–233.

Bird, F., & Remier, B. (1982). Participation rates in new religious movements and para-religious movements. *Journal for the Scientific Study of Religion, 21,* 1–14.

Birnbaum, J. H. (1995, May 15). The gospel according to Ralph. *Time,* pp. 18–27.

Bivens, A. J., Neimeyer, R. A., Kirchberg, T. M., & Moore, M. K. (1994–1995). Death concern and religious beliefs among gays and bisexuals of variable proximity to AIDS. *Omega, 30,* 105–120.

Bjorck, J. P., & Cohen, L. H. (1993). Coping with threats, losses, and challenges. *Journal of Social and Clinical Psychology, 12,* 56–72.

Bjorck, J. P., & Klewicki, L. L. (1997). The effects of stressor type on projected coping. *Journal of Traumatic Stress, 10,* 481–497.

Black, A. W. (1985). The impact of theological orientation and of the breadth of perspective on church members' attitudes and behaviors: Roof, Moll, and Kaill revisited. *Journal for the Scientific Study of Religion, 24,* 87–101.

Blackmore, S. (1991). Near-death experiences: In or out of the body? *Skeptical Inquirer, 16,* 34–45.

Blackwood, L. (1979). Social change and commitment to the work ethic. In R. Wuthnow (Ed.), *The religious dimension: New directions in quantitative research* (pp. 241–256). New York: Academic Press.

Blaine, B. E., Trivedi, P., & Eshleman, A. (1998). Religious belief and the self-concept: Evaluating the implications for psychological adjustment. *Personality and Social Psychology Bulletin, 24,* 1040–1052.

Blazer, D., & Palmore, E. (1976). Religion and aging in a longitudinal panel. *The Gerontologist, 16,* 82–85.

Blomquist, J. M. (1985). The effect of divorce experience on spiritual growth. *Pastoral Psychology, 34,* 82–91.

Blumer, H. (1969). *Symbolic interactionism: Perspective and method.* Englewood Cliffs, NJ: Prentice-Hall.

Bock, D. C., & Warren, N. C. (1972). Religious belief as a factor in obedience to destructive demands. *Review of Religious Research, 13,* 185–191.

Bock, E. W., & Radelet, M. L. (1988). The marital integration of religious independents: A reevaluation of its significance. *Review of Religious Research, 29,* 228–241.

Bohannon, J. R. (1991). Religiosity related to grief levels of bereaved mothers and fathers. *Omega, 23,* 153–159.

Boisen, A. T. (1936). *Exploration of the inner world.* Chicago: Willet, Clark.

Boisen, A. T. (1960). *Out of the depths: An autobiographical study of mental disorder and religious experience.* New York: Harper.

Bonner, J. T. (1980). *The evolution of culture in animals.* Princeton, NJ: Princeton University Press.

Booth, C. (n.d.). *The psychological examination of candidates for the ministry.* New York: Academy of Religion and Mental Health.

Booth, H. J. (1981). *Edward Diller Starbuck: Pioneer in the psychology of religion.* Washington, DC: University Press of America.

Booth, L. (1991). *When God becomes a drug: Breaking the chains of religious addiction and abuse.* New York: Perigee.

Borinstein, A. B. (1992). Public attitudes toward persons with mental illness. *Health Affairs, 13,* 186–196.

Boswell, J. (1988). *Christianity, social tolerance, and homosexuality.* Chicago: University of Chicago Press.

Boswell, J. (n.d.). *The life of Samuel Johnson, LL.D.* New York: Modern Library. (Original work published 1791)

Bottomley, F. (1979). *Attitudes toward the body in Western Christendom.* London: Lupus.

Bottoms, B. L., Shaver, P. R., Goodman, G. S., & Qin, J. (1995). In the name of God: A profile of religion-related child abuse. *Journal of Social Issues, 51,* 85–111.

Botwinick, J. (1978). *Aging and behavior.* New York: Springer.

Bouchard, T. J., Jr., Lykken, D. T., McGue, M., Segal, N. L., & Tellegen, A. (1990). Sources of human psychological differences: The Minnesota study of twins reared apart. *Science, 250,* 223–250.

Bouma, G. D. (1979). The real reason one conservative church grew. *Review of Religious Research, 20,* 127–137.

Bourguignon, E. (1970). Hallucinations and trance: An anthropologist's perspective. In W. Keup (Ed.), *Origins and mechanisms of hallucination* (pp. 83–90). New York: Plenum Press.

Bourguignon, E. (1992). Religion as a mediating factor in culture change. In J. F. Schumaker (Ed.), *Religion and mental health* (pp. 259–269). New York: Oxford University Press.

Bourque, L. B. (1969). Social correlates of transcendental experience. *Sociological Analysis, 30,* 151–163.

Bourque, L. B., & Back, K. W. (1971). Language, society, and subjective experience. *Sociometry, 34,* 1–21.

Bouyer, L. (1980). Mysticism: An essay in the history of the word. In R. Woods (Ed.), *Understanding mysticism* (pp. 42–55). Garden City, NY: Image.

Bower, B. (2001). Into the mystic. *Science News, 159,* 104–106.

Bowker, J. (1973). *The sense of God: Sociological, anthropological, and psychological approaches to the origin of the sense of God.* Oxford: Clarendon Press.

Bowlby, J. (1969). *Attachment and loss: Vol. 1. Attachment.* New York: Basic Books.

Bowlby, J. (1973). *Attachment and loss: Vol. 2. Separation: Anxiety and anger.* New York: Basic Books.

Bowlby, J. (1980). *Attachment and loss: Vol. 3. Loss.* New York: Basic Books.

Bowman, K. (2000, January). Abortion attitudes today. In *Gallup Poll News Service* [Online]. Available: http://www.gallup.com/poll/guest scholar/gs000112.asp [Retrieved August 14, 2001].

Boyer, P. (1994). *The naturalness of religious ideas.* Berkeley: University of California Press.

Boyer, P., & Walker, S. (2000). Intuitive ontology and cultural input in the acquisition of religious concepts. In K. S. Rosengren, C. N. Johnson, & P. L. Harris (Eds.), *Imagining the impossible: Magical, scientific, and religious thinking in children* (pp. 130–156). Cambridge, England: Cambridge University Press.

Brabant, S., Forsyth, C., & McFarlain, G. (1995). Life after the death of a child: Initial and long term support from others. *Omega, 31,* 67–85.

Bragan, K. (1977). The psychological gains and losses of religious conversion. *Journal of Medical Psychology, 50,* 177–180.

Brand, H. (1954). The contemporary status of the study of personality. In H. Brand (Ed.), *The study of personality* (pp. 1–22). New York: Wiley.

Braun, K. L., & Zir, A. (2001). Roles for the church in improving end-of-life care: Perceptions of Christian clergy and laity. *Death Studies, 25,* 685–705.

Breed, M. D., & Page, R. E., Jr. (Eds.). (1989). *The genetics of social evolution.* Boulder, CO: Westview Press.

Brehm, S. S. (1992). *Intimate relationships.* New York: McGraw-Hill.

Brennan, C. L., & Missinne, L. E. (1980). Personal and institutionalized religiosity of the elderly. In J. A. Thorson & C. C. Cook, Jr. (Eds.), *Spiritual well-being of the elderly* (pp. 92–99). Springfield, IL: Charles Thomas.

Brewer, M. B. (1997). On the social origins of human nature. In C. McGarty & S. A. Haslam (Eds.), *The message of social psychology* (pp. 54–62). Cambridge, MA: Blackwell.

Brickhead, J. (1997). Reading "snake handling": Critical reflections. In S. G. Glazer (Ed.), *Anthropology of religion* (pp. 1–84). Westport, CT: Greenwood Press.

Bridges, H. (1970). *American mysticism from William James to Zen.* New York: Harper & Row.

Bridges, R. A., & Spilka, B. (1992). Religion and the mental health of women. In J. F. Schumaker (Ed.), *Religion and mental health* (pp. 43–53). New York: Oxford University Press.

Brinkerhoff, M. B., & Burke, K. L. (1980). Disaffiliation: Some notes on "falling from the faith." *Sociological Analysis, 41,* 41–54.

Brinkerhoff, M. B., Grandin, E., & Lupri, E. (1992). Religious involvement and spousal violence: The Canadian case. *Journal for the Scientific Study of Religion, 31,* 15–31.

Brinkerhoff, M. B., & Mackie, M. M. (1993). Casting off the bonds of organized religion: A religious-careers approach to the study of apostasy. *Review of Religious Research, 34,* 235–257.

Brinthaupt, T. M., & Lipka, R. P. (Eds.). (1994). *Changing the self.* Albany: State University of New York Press.

Brody, G. H., Stoneman, Z., & Flor, D. (1996). Parental religiosity, family processes, and youth competence in rural, two-parent African American families. *Developmental Psychology, 32,* 696–706.

Bromberg, W. (1937). *The mind of man.* New York: Harper.

Bromley, D. G. (1988). Religious disaffiliation: A neglected social process. In D. G. Bromley (Ed.), *Falling from the faith: Causes and consequences of religious apostasy* (pp. 9–25). Newbury Park, CA: Sage.

Bromley, D. G. (1998). Linking social structure and the exit process in religious organizations: Defectors, whistle-blowers and apostates. *Journal for the Scientific Study of Religion, 37,* 145–160.

Bromley, D. G., & Breschel, E. F. (1992). General population and institutional support for social control of new religious movements: Evidence from national survey data. *Behavioral Sciences and the Law, 10,* 39–52.

Bromley, D. G., & Richardson, J. T. (Eds.). (1983). *The brainwashing/deprogramming controversy: Sociological, psychological, legal and historical perspectives.* Lewiston, NY: Mellon.

Bronson, L., & Meadow, A. (1968). The need for achievement orientation of Catholic and Protestant Mexican-Americans. *Revista Interamericana de Psicologia, 2,* 159–168.

Brown, F. & MacDonald, J. (2000). *The serpent handlers: Three families and their faith.* Winston-Salem, NC: Blair.

Brown, F. C. (1972). *Hallucinogenic drugs.* Springfield, IL: Charles C. Thomas.

Brown, L. B. (1966). Egocentric thought in petitionary prayer: A cross-cultural study. *Journal of Social Psychology, 68,* 197–210.

Brown, L. B. (1968). Some attitudes underlying petitionary prayer. In A. Godin (Ed.), *From cry to word: Contributions toward a psychology of prayer* (pp. 65–84). Brussels, Belgium: Lumen Vitae Press.

Brown, L. B. (1987). *The psychology of religious belief.* London: Academic Press.

Brown, L. B. (1994). *The human side of prayer: The psychology of praying.* Birmingham, AL: Religious Education Press.

Brown, T. L., Parks, G. S., Zimmerman, R. S., & Phillips, C. M. (2001). The role of religion in predicting adolescent alcohol use and problem drinking. *Journal of Studies on Alcohol, 62,* 696–705.

Brown, T. N., Schulenberg, J., Bachman, J. G., O'Malley, P. M., & Johnston, L. D. (2001). Are risk and protective factors for substance use consistent across historical times?: National data from the high school classes of 1976 through 1997. *Prevention Science, 2,* 29–43.

Browning, D. S. (1973). *Generative man: Psychoanalytic perspectives.* Philadelphia: Westminster.

Browning, R. (1895). Pippa passes. In H. E. Scudder (Ed.), *The complete poetical works of Browning* (pp. 128–145). Cambridge: MA: Riverside Press. (Original work published 1841)

Bruce, S. (1999). *Choice and religion: A critique of rational choice theory.* Oxford: Oxford University Press.

Bruggeman, E. L., & Hart, K. J. (1996). Cheating, lying, and moral reasoning by religious and secular high school students. *Journal of Educational Research, 89,* 340–344.

Bryan, J. W., & Freed, F. W. (1993). Abortion research: Attitudes, sexual behavior, and problems in a community college population. *Journal of Youth and Adolescence, 22,* 1–22.

Bryer, K. B. (1979). The Amish way of death: A study of family support systems. *American Psychologist, 34*, 255–261.

Buber, M. (1965). *Between man and man.* New York: Macmillan.

Bucher, A. A. (1991). Understanding parables: A developmental analysis. In F. K. Oser & W. G. Scarlett (Eds.), *Religious development in childhood and adolescence* (New Directions for Child Development, No. 52, pp. 101–105). San Francisco: Jossey-Bass.

Bucke, R. M. (1961). *Cosmic consciousness: A study of the evolution of the human mind.* Hyde Park, NY: University Books. (Original work published 1901)

Budd, S. (1973). *Sociologists and religion.* London: Macmillan.

Bufe, C. (1991). *Alcoholics Anonymous: Cult or cure?* San Francisco: Sharp Press.

Bufford, R. K., Paloutzian, R. F., & Ellison, C. W. (1991). Norms for the Spiritual Well-Being Scale. *Journal of Psychology and Theology, 19*, 56–70.

Bullard, T. E. (1987). *UFO abductions: The measure of a mystery.* Mount Rainer, MD: Fund for UFO Research.

Bulliet, R. W. (1979). *Conversion to Islam in the medieval period: An essay in quantitative history.* Cambridge, MA: Harvard University Press.

Bulman, R. J., & Wortman, C. B. (1977). Attributions of blame and coping in the real world: Severe accident victims react to their lot. *Journal of Personality and Social Psychology, 35*, 351–363.

Buri, J. R., Louiselle, P. A., Misukanis, T. M., & Mueller, R. A. (1988). Effects of parental authoritarianism and authoritativeness on self-esteem. *Personality and Social Psychology Bulletin, 14*, 271–282.

Burke, E. (1909). Reflections on the French revolution. In *The Harvard classics: Vol. 24* (p. 239). New York: Collier. (Original work published 1790)

Burkert, W. (1996). *Creation of the sacred: Tracks of biology in early religions.* Cambridge, MA: Harvard University Press.

Burkett, S. R., & Warren, B. O. (1987). Adolescent marijuana use: A panel study of underlying causal structures. *Criminology, 25*, 109–131.

Burkett, S. R., & White, M. (1974). Hellfire and delinquency: Another look. *Journal for the Scientific Study of Religion, 13*, 455–462.

Burnham, J. C. (1985). The encounter of Christian theology with deterministic psychology and psychoanalysis. *Bulletin of the Menninger Clinic, 49*, 321–352.

Burris, C. T., Batson, C. D., Altstaedten, M., & Stephens, K. (1994). "What a friend . . . ": Loneliness as a motivator of intrinsic religion. *Journal for the Scientific Study of Religion, 33*, 326–334.

Burris, C. T., Branscombe, N. R., & Jackson, L. M. (2000). For God and country: Religion and the endorsement of national self-stereotypes. *Journal of Cross-Cultural Psychology, 31*, 517–527.

Burris, C. T., Harmon-Jones, E., & Tarpley, W. R. (1997). "By faith alone": Religious agitation and cognitive dissonance. *Basic and Applied Social Psychology, 19*, 17–31.

Burris, C. T., & Jackson, L. M. (1999). Hate the sin/love the sinner, or love the hater?: Intrinsic religion and responses to partner abuse. *Journal for the Scientific Study of Religion, 38*, 160–174.

Burris, C. T., & Jackson, L. M. (2000). Social identity and the true believer: Responses to marginalization among the intrinsically religious. *British Journal of Social Psychology, 39*, 257–278.

Burris, C. T., Jackson, L. M., Tarpley, W. R., & Smith, G. J. (1996). Religion as quest: The self-directed pursuit of meaning. *Personality and Social Psychology Bulletin, 22*, 1068–1076.

Burton, T. (1993). *Serpent-handling believers.* Knoxville: University of Tennessee Press.

Buss, D. M., Haselton, M. G., Shackleford, T. K., Bleske, A. L., & Wakefield, J. C. (1998). Adaptations, exaptations, and spandrels. *American Psychologist, 53*, 533–548.

Butcher, J. N., Dahlstrom, W. G., Graham, J. R., Tellegen, A. M., & Kaemmer, B. (1989). *MMPI-2:Manual for administration and scoring.* Minneapolis: University of Minnesota Press.

Buttrick, G. A. (1942). *Prayer.* New York: Abingdon–Cokesbury.

Byrd, K. R., & Boe, A. (2001). The correspondence between attachment dimensions and prayer in college students. *International Journal for the Psychology of Religion, 11*, 9–24.

Byrd, R. C. (1988). Positive therapeutic effects of intercessory prayer in a coronary care unit population. *Southern Medical Journal, 81*, 826–829.

Caird, D. (1988). The structure of Hood's Mysticism Scale: A factor analytic study. *Journal for the Scientific Study of Religion, 27,* 122–127.

Camargo, R. J., & Loftus, J. A. (1993, August 20). *Clergy sexual involvement with young people: Distinctive characteristics.* Paper presented at the annual convention of the American Psychological Association, Toronto.

Campbell, E. Q. (1969). Adolescent socialization. In D. A. Goslin (Ed.), *Handbook of socialization theory and research* (pp. 821–859). Chicago: Rand.

Campbell, R. A., & Curtis, J. E. (1994). Religious involvement across societies: Analyses for alternative measures in national surveys. *Journal for the Scientific Study of Religion, 33,* 217–229.

Caplan, R. B. (1969). *Psychiatry and the community in nineteenth century America.* New York: Basic Books.

Caplovitz, D., & Sherrow, F. (1977). *The religious drop-outs: Apostasy among college graduates.* Beverly Hills, CA: Sage.

Caplow, T., Bahr, H. M., Chadwick, B. A., Hoover, D. W., Martin, L. A., Tamney, J. B., & Williamson, M. H. (1983). *All faithful people: Change and continuity in Middletown's religion.* Minneapolis: University of Minnesota Press.

Capps, D. (1982). The psychology of petitionary prayer. *Theology Today, 39,* 130–141.

Capps, D. (1990). *Reframing: A new method in pastoral care.* Minneapolis, MN: Fortress.

Capps, D. (1992). Religion and child abuse: Perfect together. *Journal for the Scientific Study of Religion, 31,* 1–14.

Capps, D. (1994). An Allportian analysis of Augustine. *International Journal for the Psychology of Religion, 4,* 205–228.

Capps, D. (1995). *The child's song: The religious abuse of children.* Louisville, KY: Westminster John Knox Press.

Capps, D., & Dittes, J. E. (Eds.). (1990). *The hunger of the heart: The confessions of Augustine.* West Lafayette, IN: Society for the Scientific Study of Religion.

Cardeña, E., Lynn, S. J., & Krippner, S. (2000a). Introduction: Varieties of anomalous experience. In E. Cardeña, S. J. Lynn, & S. Krippner (Eds.), *Varieties of anomalous experience* (pp. 3–21). Washington, DC: American Psychological Association.

Cardeña, E., Lynn, S. J., & Krippner, S. (Eds.). (2000b). *Varieties of anomalous experience.* Washington, DC: American Psychological Association.

Carey, R. G. (1971). Influence of peers in shaping religious behavior. *Journal for the Scientific Study of Religion, 10,* 157–159.

Carey, R. G. (1979–1980). Weathering widowhood: Problems and adjustment of the widowed during the first year. *Omega, 10,* 163–174.

Carey, R. G., & Posavec, E. J. (1978–1979). Attitudes of physicians on disclosing information to and maintaining life for terminal patients. *Omega, 10,* 163–174.

Carlson, C. R., Bacaseta, P. E., & Simanton, D. A. (1988). A controlled evaluation of devotional meditation and progressive relaxation. *Journal of Psychology and Theology, 16,* 362–368.

Carlson, S. M., Taylor, M., & Levin, G. R. (1998). The influence of culture on pretend play: The case of Mennonite children. *Merrill–Palmer Quarterly, 44,* 538–565.

Carlsson, B. G. (1997). Religion and cultural attitudes toward homosexuality: An emancipatory study. *Nordisk Sexologi, 15,* 143–147. [Abstract used]

Carmody, D., & Carmody, J. (1996). *Mysticism: Holiness East and West.* New York: Oxford University Press.

Carroll, J. B. (Ed.). (1956). *Language, thought, and reality: Selected writings of Benjamin Lee Whorf.* New York: Wiley.

Carroll, M. P. (1983). Vision of the virgin Mary: The effects of family structures on Marian apparitions. *Journal for the Scientific Study of Religion, 22,* 205–221.

Carroll, M. P. (1986). *The cult of the virgin Mary: Psychological origins.* Princeton, NJ: Princeton University Press.

Carroll, R. P. (1979). *When prophecy failed: Cognitive dissonance in the prophetic traditions of the Old Testament.* New York: Seabury Press.

Carter, C. S. (1998). Neuroendocrine perspectives on social attachment and love. *Psychoneuroendocrinology, 23,* 779–818.

Carter, S. L. (2000). *God's name in vain.* New York: Basic Books.

Cartwright, R. H., & Kent, S. A. (1992). Social control in alternative religions: A familial perspective. *Sociological Analysis, 53,* 345–361.

Carver, C. S., Scheier, M. F., & Pozo, C. (1992). Conceptualizing the process of coping with health problems. In H. S. Friedman (Ed.), *Hostility, coping, and health* (pp. 167–199). Washington, DC: American Psychological Association.

Casey, W. M., & Burton, R. V. (1986). The social-learning theory approach. In G. L. Sapp (Ed.), *Handbook of moral development* (pp. 74–91). Birmingham, AL: Religious Education Press.

Cather, W. (1990). *My mortal enemy.* New York: Vintage. (Original work published 1926)

The Catholic Worker. (1991, May). The aims and means of the Catholic Worker Movement. p. 5.

Cattell, R. B. (1938). *Psychology and the religious quest: An account of the psychology of religion and a defense of individualism.* New York: Nelson.

Cattell, R. B. (1950). *Personality.* New York: McGraw-Hill.

Cattell, R. B., & Child, D. (1975). *Motivation and dynamic structure.* New York: Wiley.

Cavenar, J. O., & Spaulding, J. G. (1977). Depressive disorders and religious conversions. *Journal of Nervous and Mental Disease, 165,* 200–212.

Cecil, Lord D. (1966). *Melbourne.* Indianapolis, IN: Bobbs-Merrill.

Cerny, L. J., II, & Carter, J. D. (1977). *Death perspectives and religious orientation as a function of Christian faith.* Paper presented at the annual convention of the Society for the Scientific Study of Religion, Chicago.

Cesarman, F. C. (1957). Religious conversion of sex offenders. *Journal of Pastoral Care, 11,* 25–35.

Chadwick, B. A., & Top, B. L. (1993). Religiosity and delinquency among LDS adolescents. *Journal for the Scientific Study of Religion, 32,* 51–67.

Chalfant, P. H., Beckley, R. E., & Palmer, C. E. (1981). *Religion in contemporary society.* Sherman Oaks, CA: Alfred.

Chancellor, J. D. (2000). *Life in the family: An oral history of the children of God.* Syracuse, NY: Syracuse University Press.

Chandy, J. M., Blum, R. W., & Resnick, M. D. (1996). Female adolescents with a history of sexual abuse: Risk outcome and protective factors. *Journal of Interpersonal Violence, 11,* 503–518.

Chang, L., & Arkin, R. M. (1999). *Materialism as an attempt to deal with uncertainty.* Paper presented at the annual convention of the American Psychological Association, Boston.

Chang, P. M. Y. (1997a). Female clergy in the contemporary Protestant church: A current assessment. *Journal for the Scientific Study of Religion, 36,* 565–573.

Chang, P. M. Y. (1997b). In search of a pulpit: Sex differences in the transition from seminary training to the first parish job. *Journal for the Scientific Study of Religion, 36,* 614–627.

Chau, L. L., Johnson, R. C., Bowers, J. K., Darvill, T. J., & Danko, G. P. (1990). Intrinsic and extrinsic religiosity as related to conscience, adjustment, and altruism. *Personality and Individual Differences, 11,* 397–400.

Chaves, M. (1989). Secularization and religious revival: Evidence for U.S. church attendance rates, 1972–1986. *Journal for the Scientific Study of Religion, 28,* 464–477.

Chaves, M. (1990). Holding the cohort: Reply to Hout and Greeley. *Journal for the Scientific Study of Religion, 29,* 525–530.

Chaves, M. (1991). Family structure and Protestant church attendance: The sociological basis of cohort and age-effects. *Journal for the Scientific Study of Religion, 30,* 501–514.

Chaves, M. (1997). *Ordaining women: Culture and conflict in religious organizations.* Cambridge, MA: Harvard University Press.

Chaves, M., & Cavendish, J. (1997). Recent changes in women's ordination conflicts: The effect of a social movement on interorganizational controversy. *Journal for the Scientific Study of Religion, 36,* 574–584.

Chaves, M., & Cavendish, J. C. (1994). More evidence on U.S. Catholic church attendance. *Journal for the Scientific Study of Religion, 33,* 376–381.

Chesen, E. S. (1972). *Religion may be hazardous to your health.* New York: Macmillan.

Chibnall, J. T., Wolf, J., & Duckro, P. N. (1998). A national survey of the sexual trauma experiences of Catholic nuns. *Review of Religious Research, 40,* 142–167.

Christ, C. P., & Plaskow, J. (1979). *Womanspirit rising.* New York: Harper & Row.

Christensen, C. W. (1960). The occurrence of mental illness in the ministry: Family origins. *Journal of Pastoral Care, 14,* 13–20.

Christensen, C. W. (1963). Religious conversion. *Archives of General Psychiatry, 9,* 207–216.

Christian Century. (1995, July 5–12). United Methodists show age, says survey, p. 673.

Clark, E. T. (1929). *The psychology of religious awakening.* New York: Macmillan.

Clark, J. (1978). Problems in the referral of cult members. *Journal of the National Association of Private Psychiatric Hospitals, 9,* 19–21.

Clark, J. (1979). Cults. *Journal of the American Medical Association, 242,* 279–281.

Clark, J., Langone, M. D., Schacter, R., & Daly, R. C. G. (1981). *Destructive cult conversion: Theory, research and practice.* Weston, MA: American Family Foundation.

Clark, J. H. (1983). *A map of mental states.* London: Routledge & Kegan Paul.

Clark, J. M., Brown, J. C., & Hochstein, L. M. (1989). Institutional religion and gay/lesbian oppression. *Marriage and Family Review, 14,* 265–284.

Clark, R. W. (1984). The evidential value of religious experiences. *International Journal of Philosophy of Religion, 16,* 189–201.

Clark, S. L., & Carter, J. D. (1978, June 15). *Death perspectives: Fear of death, guilt and hope as functions of Christian faith.* Paper presented at the annual convention of the Western Association of Christians for Psychological Studies, Malibu, CA.

Clark, W. H. (1958). *The psychology of religion.* New York: Macmillan.

Clark, W. H. (1968). The relation between drugs and religious experience. *Catholic Psychological Record, 6,* 146–155.

Clark, W. H. (1969). *Chemical ecstasy: Psychedelic drugs and religion.* New York: Sheed & Ward.

Clark, W. H., Malony, H. N., Daane, J., & Tippett, A. R. (1973). *Religious experience: Its nature and function in the human psyche.* Springfield, IL: Thomas.

Clark, W. R., & Grunstein, M. (2000). *Are we hardwired?* New York: Oxford University Press.

Clarke, R.-L. (1986). *Pastoral care of battered women.* Philadelphia: Westminster Press.

Clemens, N. A. (1976). An intensive course for clergy on death, dying, and loss. *Journal of Religion and Health, 15,* 223–229.

Cline, V. B., & Richards, J. M. (1965). A factor-analytic study of religious belief and behavior. *Journal of Personality and Social Psychology, 1,* 569–578.

Clines, F. X. (2002, March 12). Ohio board hears debate on an alternative to Darwinism. *The New York Times,* p. A16.

Clouse, B. (1986). Church conflict and moral stages: A Kohlbergian interpretation. *Journal of Psychology and Christianity, 5,* 14–19.

Clouse, B. (1991). Religious experience, religious belief and moral development of students at a state university. *Journal of Psychology and Christianity, 10,* 337–349.

Cobb, N. J. (2001). *Adolescence: Continuity, change, and diversity* (4th ed.). Mountain View, CA: Mayfield.

Cobb, N. J., Ong, A. D., & Tate, J. (2001). Reason-based evaluations of wrongdoing in religious and moral narratives. *International Journal for the Psychology of Religion, 11,* 259–276.

Cochran, J. K. (1992). The effects of religiosity on adolescent self-reported frequency of drug and alcohol use. *Journal of Drug Issues, 22,* 91–104.

Cochran, J. K. (1993). The variable effects of religiosity and denomination on adolescent self-reported alcohol use by beverage type. *Journal of Drug Issues, 23,* 479–491.

Cochran, J. K., & Beeghley, L. (1991). The influence of religion on attitudes toward nonmarital sexuality: A preliminary assessment of reference group theory. *Journal for the Scientific Study of Religion, 30,* 45–62.

Cochran, J. K., Beeghley, L., & Bock, E. W. (1988). Religiosity and alcohol behavior: An exploration of reference group theory. *Sociological Forum, 3,* 256–276.

Cochran, J. K., Beeghley, L., & Bock, E. W. (1992). The influence of religious stability and homogamy on the relationship between religiosity and alcohol use among Protestants. *Journal for the Scientific Study of Religion, 31,* 441–456.

Cochran, J. K., Chamlin, M. B., Wood, P. B., & Sellers, C. S. (1999). Shame, embarrassment, and formal sanction threats: Extending the deterrence/rational choice model to academic dishonesty. *Sociological Inquiry, 69,* 91–105.

Cochran, J. K., Wood, P. B., & Arneklev, B. J. (1994). Is the religiosity–delinquency relationship spurious?: Social control theories. *Journal of Research in Crime and Delinquency, 31,* 92–123.

Coe, G. A. (1900). *The spiritual life: Studies in the science of religion.* New York: Eaton & Mains.

Coe, G. A. (1916). *The psychology of religion.* Chicago: University of Chicago Press.

Coffey, K. (1998, June). It's time to end the hypocrisy on birth control. *U.S. Catholic,* pp. 24–28.

Coffin, W. S. (1990, February 18). The holiness option. *The New York Times Book Review,* p. 18.

Cohen, A. B., & Rozin, P. (2001). Religion and the morality of mentality. *Journal of Personality and Social Psychology, 81,* 697–710.

Cohen, J. M., & Cohen, M. J. (Eds.). (1960). *The Penguin book of quotations.* Baltimore: Penguin.

Cohen, M. S. (1990). The biblical prohibition of homosexual intercourse. *Journal of Homosexuality, 19,* 3–20.

Coker, A. L., Smith, P. H., Thompson, M. P., McKeown, R. E., Bethea, L., & Davis, K. E. (2002). Social support protects against the negative effects of partner violence on mental health. *Journal of Women's Health and Gender-Based Medicine, 11,* 465–476.

Cole, S. O. (1995). The biological basis of homosexuality: A Christian assessment. *Journal of Psychology and Theology, 23,* 89–100.

Coles, R. (1990). *The spiritual life of children.* Boston: Houghton Mifflin.

Colipp, P. J. (1969). The efficacy of prayer: A triple-blind study. *Medical Times, 97,* 201–204.

Condran, J. G., & Tamney, J. B. (1985). Religious "nones": 1957–1982. *Sociological Analysis, 46,* 415–423.

Conn, J. W. (Ed.). (1986). *Women's spirituality: Resources for Christian development.* New York: Paulist Press.

Conrad, P., & Schnelder, J. W. (1980). *Deviance and medicalization: From badness to sickness.* St. Louis, MO: Mosby.

Conway, F., & Siegelman, J. (1978). *Snapping: America's epidemic of sudden personality change.* Philadelphia: J. B. Lippincott.

Conway, K. (1985–1986). Coping with the stress of medical problems among black and white elderly. *International Journal of Aging and Human Development, 21,* 39–48.

Cook, A. S., & Oltjenbruns, K. A. (1989). *Dying and grieving.* New York: Holt, Rinehart & Winston.

Cook, C. C. H., Goddard, D., & Westall, R. (1997). Knowledge and experience of drug use amongst church affiliated young people. *Drug and Alcohol Dependence, 46,* 9–17.

Cook, T., & Wimberly, D. (1983). If I should die before I wake: Religious commitment and adjustment to the death of a child. *Journal for the Scientific Study of Religion, 22,* 222–238.

Cook, T. D., & Campbell, D. T. (1979). *Quasi-experimentation: Design and analysis issues for field settings.* Chicago: Rand McNally.

Coon, D. J. (1992). Testing the limits of sense and science: American experimental psychologists combat spiritualism, 1880–1920. *American Psychologist, 47,* 143–151.

Coopersmith, S., Regan, M., & Dick, L. (1975). *The myth of the generation gap.* San Francisco: Albion.

Cornwall, M. (1987). The social bases of religion: A study of factors influencing religious belief and commitment. *Review of Religious Research, 29,* 44–56.

Cornwall, M. (1988). The influence of three agents of religious socialization: Family, church, and peers. In D. L. Thomas (Ed.), *The religion and family connection* (pp. 207–231). Provo, UT: Religious Studies Center, Brigham Young University.

Cornwall, M. (1989). The determinants of religious behavior: A theoretical model and empirical test. *Social Forces, 68,* 572–592.

Cornwall, M., & Thomas, D. L. (1990). Family, religion, and personal communities: Examples from Mormonism. *Marriage and Family Review, 15,* 229–252.

Corssan, J. D. (1975). *The dark interval.* Niles, IL: Argus Communication.

Cortes, A. de J. (1999). Antecedents to the conflict between religion and psychology in America. *Journal of Psychology and Theology, 27,* 20–32.

Corwyn, R. F., & Benda, B. B. (2000). Religiosity and church attendance: The effects on use of "hard drugs" controlling for sociodemographic and theoretical factors. *International Journal for the Psychology of Religion, 10,* 241–258.

Corwyn, R. F., Benda, B. B., & Ballard, K. (1997). Do the same theoretical factors explain alcohol and other drug use among adolescents? *Alcoholism Treatment Quarterly, 15,* 47–62.

Cosmides, L., & Tooby, J. (1987). From evolution to behavior: Evolutionary psychology as the missing link. In J. Dupre (Ed.), *The latest on the best: Essays on evolution and optimality* (pp. 277–306). Cambridge, MA: MIT Press.

Cota-McKinley, A. L., Woody, W. D., & Bell, P. A. (2001). Vengeance: Effects of gender, age, and religious background. *Aggressive Behavior, 27,* 343–350.

Couture, P. (1990). Ritual and pastoral care. In R. J. Hunter (Ed.), *Dictionary of pastoral care and counseling* (pp. 1088–1090). Nashville, TN: Abingdon Press.

Coward, H. (1986). Intolerance in the world's religions. *Studies in Religion, 15,* 419–431.

Cox, K. (2002, September 16). Beatings were just, court told. *The Globe and Mail* [Toronto], p. A7.

Coyle, B. R. (2001). Twelve myths of religion and psychiatry: Lessons for training psychiatrists in spiritually sensitive treatments. *Mental Health, Religion, and Culture, 4,* 147–174.

Coyle, C. T., & Enright, R. D. (1997). Forgiveness intervention with postabortion men. *Journal of Consulting and Clinical Psychology, 65,* 1042–1046.

Crooks, E. B. (1913). Professor James and the psychology of religion. *Monist, 23,* 122–130.

Crosby, R. A., & Yarber, W. L. (2001). Perceived versus actual knowledge about correct condom use among U.S. adolescents: Results from a national study. *Journal of Adolescent Health, 28,* 415–420.

Crowne, D. P., & Marlowe, D. (1964). *The approval motive: Studies in evaluative dependence.* New York: Wiley.

Culbertson, B. (1996, June). *The correlation between shame and the concept of God among intrinsically religious Nazarenes.* Unpublished master's thesis, Southern Nazarene University.

Culver, V. (1988, April 17). Emotional upset linked to strictness in religion. *The Denver Post,* pp. 1B–2B.

Culver, V. (1994, May 11). Clergy sex misconduct prevalent. *The Denver Post,* pp. 1B, 8B.

Culver, V. (2001, November 6). Methodist court bars openly gay ministers. *The Denver Post,* p. 11A.

Cumming, E., & Henry, W. E. (1961). *Growing old: The process of disengagement.* New York: Basic Books.

Cunradi, C. B., Caetano, R., & Schafer, J. (2002). Religious affiliation, denominational homogamy, and intimate partner violence among U.S. couples. *Journal for the Scientific Study of Religion, 41,* 139–151.

Cutten, G. B. (1908). *The psychological phenomena of Christianity.* New York: Scribner.

Dahl, K. E. (1999). Religion and coping with bereavement. *Dissertation Abstracts International, 3686B.*

Daniel, S. P., & Rogers, M. L. (1981). Burnout and the pastorate: A critical review with implications for pastors. *Journal of Psychology and Theology, 9,* 232–249.

Danso, H., Hunsberger, B., & Pratt, M. (1997). The role of parental religious fundamentalism and right-wing authoritarianism in child-rearing goals and practices. *Journal for the Scientific Study of Religion, 36,* 496–511.

D'Antonio, W. V., Newman, W. M., & Wright, S. A. (1982). Religion and family life: How social scientists view the relationship. *Journal for the Scientific Study of Religion, 21,* 218–225.

d'Aquili, E. G. (1978). The neurobiological bases of myth and concepts of deity. *Zygon, 13,* 257–275.

d'Aquili, E. G., Laughlin, C. D., Jr., & McManus, J. (Eds.). (1979). *The spectrum of ritual: A biogenetic analysis.* New York: Columbia University Press.

d'Aquili, E. G., & Newberg, A. B. (1993). Religious and mystical states. A neuropsychological model. *Zygon, 28,* 177–200.

d'Aquili, E. G., & Newberg, A. B. (1999). *The mystical mind: Probing the biology of mystical experience.* Minneapolis, MN: Fortress Press.

Darley, J. M., & Batson, C. D. (1973). "From Jersualem to Jericho": A study of situational and dispositional variables in helping behavior. *Journal of Personality and Social Psychology, 27,* 100–108.

Darley, J. M., & Shultz, T. R. (1990). Moral rules: Their content and acquisition. *Annual Review of Psychology, 41,* 525–556.

Darling, N., & Steinberg, L. (1993). Parenting style as context: An integrative model. *Psychological Bulletin, 113,* 487–496.

Darwin, C. (1972). *The origin of species.* New York: Dutton. (Original work published 1859)

Datta, L. E. (1967). Family religious background and early scientific creativity. *American Sociological Review, 32,* 626–635.

David, J., Ladd, K., & Spilka, B. (1992). *The multidimensionality of prayer and its role as a source of secondary control.* Paper presented at the annual convention of the American Psychological Association, Washington, DC.

Davidson, J. D. (1972a). Patterns of belief at the denominational and congregational levels. *Review of Religious Research, 13,* 197–205.

Davidson, J. D. (1972b). Religious belief as a dependent variable. *Journal for the Scientific Study of Religion, 11,* 65–75.

Davidson, J. D., & Caddell, D. P. (1994). Religion and the meaning of work. *Journal for the Scientfic Study of Religion, 33,* 135–147.

Davidson, J. D., & Pyle, R. E. (1994). Passing the plate in affluent churches: Why some members give more than others. *Review of Religious Research, 36,* 181–196.

Davidson, J. D., Pyle, R. E., & Reyes, D. V. (1995). Persistence and change in the Protestant establishment. *Social Forces. 74,* 157–175.

Davis, C. F. (1989). *The evidential force of religious experience.* Oxford: Clarendon Press.

Davis, J. A., & Smith, T. W. (1994). *General Social Surveys, 1972–1994* [Machine-readable data file]. Chicago: National Opinion Research Center [Producer]; Storrs: Roper Center for Public Opinion Research, University of Connecticut [Distributor].

Dawkins, R. (1976). *The selfish gene.* New York: Oxford University Press.

Dawson, L. (1999). When prophecy fails and faith persists: A theoretical overview. *Nova Religio, 3,* 60–82.

Day, J. M. (1991). Narrative, psychology and moral education. *American Psychologist, 46,* 167–178.

Day, J. M. (1994). Moral development, belief, and unbelief: Young adult accounts of religion in the process of moral growth. In J. Corveleyn & D. Hutsebaut (Eds.), *Belief and unbelief: Psychological perspectives* (pp. 155–173). Atlanta, GA: Rodopi.

Day, J. M. (2001). From structuralism to eternity?: Re-imagining the psychology of religious development after the cognitive-developmental paradigm. *International Journal for the Psychology of Religion, 11,* 173–183.

De Frain, J. D., Jakub, D. K., & Mendoza, B. L. (1991–1992). The psychological effects of sudden infant death on grandmothers and grandfathers. *Omega, 24,* 165–182.

de Fuentes, N. (1999). Hear our cries: Victim–survivors of clergy sexual misconduct. In T. G. Plante (Ed.), *Bless me father for I have sinned: Perspectives on sexual abuse committed by Roman Catholic priests* (pp. 135–170). Westport, CT: Praeger.

De Haan, L. G., & Schulenberg, J. (1997). The covariation of religion and politics during the transition to adulthood: Challenging global identity assumptions. *Journal of Adolescence, 20,* 537–552.

de Jonge, J. (1995). On breaking wills: The theological roots of violence in families. *Journal of Psychology and Christianity, 14,* 26–36.

De Maria, F., Giulani, B., Annese, A., & Corfiati, I. (1971). A picture of psychopathological conditions in members of religious communities. *Acta Neurologica, 26,* 79–86.

De Roos, S. A., Miedema, S., & Iedema, J. (2001). Attachment, working models of self and others, and God concept in kindergarten. *Journal for the Scientific Study of Religion, 40,* 607–618.

de Vaus, D. A. (1983). The relative importance of parents and peers for adolescent religious orientation: An Australian study. *Adolescence, 18,* 147–158.

de Vaus, D., & McAllister, I. (1987). Gender differences in religion: A test of the structural location theory. *American Sociological Review, 52,* 472–481.

De Vellis, B. M., De Vellis, R. F., & Spilsbury, J. C. (1988). Parental actions when children are sick: The role of belief in divine influence. *Basic and Applied Social Psychology, 9,* 185–196.

De Waal, F. (1996). *Good natured: The origins of right and wrong in humans and other animals.* Cambridge, MA: Harvard University Press.

Deconchy, J.-P. (1965). The idea of God: Its emergence between 7 and 16 years. In A. Godin (Ed.), *From religious experience to a religious attitude* (pp. 97–108). Chicago: Loyola University Press.

Degelman, D., Mullen, P., & Mullen, N. (1984). Development of abstract religious thinking: A comparison of Roman Catholic and Nazarene youth. *Journal of Psychology and Christianity, 3,* 44–49.

Deikman, A. (1966). Implications of experimentally produced contemplative meditation. *Journal of Nervous and Mental Disease, 142,* 101–116.

Dein, S. (1997). Lubavitch: A contemporary messianic movement. *Journal of Contemporary Religion, 12,* 191–204.

Dein, S. (2001). What really happens when prophecy fails: The case of Lubavitch. *Sociology of Religion, 62,* 383–401.

Dein, S., & Littlewood, R. (2000). Apocalyptic suicide. *Mental Health, Religion, and Culture, 3,* 109–114.

Dekmejian, R. H. (1985). *Islam in revolution: Fundamentalism in the Arab world.* Syracuse, NY: Syracuse University Press.

Delbridge, J., Headey, B., & Wearing, A. J. (1994). Happiness and religious beliefs. In L. B. Brown (Ed.), *Religion, personality, and mental health* (pp. 50–68). New York: Springer-Verlag.

Delgado, R. (1977). Religious totalism. *University of Southern California Law Review, 15,* 1–99.

Delgado, R. (1982). Cult and conversions: The case for informed consent. *Georgia Law Review, 16,* 533–574.

Demerath, N. J. (1965). *Social class and American Protestantism.* Chicago: Rand McNally.

Demerath, N. J., & Hammond, P. E. (1969). *Religion in social context.* New York: Random House.

DeNicola, K. (1997). Response to Reich's "Do we need a theory for the religious development of women?". *International Journal for the Psychology of Religion, 7,* 93–97.

The Denver Post. (2001, November 19). Church's gay pastor a first for Lutherans. p. 9A.

Dewey, J. (1929). *The quest for certainty.* New York: Minton, Balch.

Dewhurst, K., & Beard, A. W. (1970). Sudden religous conversions in temporal lobe epilepsy. *British Journal of Psychiatry, 117,* 497–507.

Dickie, J. R., Eshleman, A. K., Merasco, D. M., Shepard, A., Vander Wilt, M., & Johnson, M. (1997). Parent–child relationships and children's images of God. *Journal for the Scientific Study of Religion, 36,* 25–43.

Dienstbier, R. A. (1979). Emotion-attribution theory: Establishing roots and exploring future perspectives. In R. A. Dienstbier (Ed.), *Nebraska Symposium on Motivation* (Vol. 26, pp. 237–306). Lincoln: University of Nebraska Press.

Dionne, E. J. (2001, September 19). Is religion the cause or the solution? *The Denver Post,* p. B11.

Disch, E., & Avery, N. (2001). Sex in the consulting room, the examining room, and sacristy: Survivors of sexual abuse by professionals. *American Journal of Orthopsychiatry, 71,* 204–217.

Dittes, J. E. (1962). Research on clergymen: Factors influencing decisions for religious service and effectiveness in the vocation. *Religious Education, 57*(Research Suppl.), S141–S165.

Dittes, J. E. (1969). The psychology of religion. In G. Lindzey & E. Aronson (Eds.), *The handbook of social psychology* (Vol. 5, pp. 602–659). Reading, MA: Addison-Wesley.

Dittes, J. E. (1971a). Conceptual derivation and statistical rigor. *Journal for the Scientific Study of Religion, 10,* 393–395.

Dittes, J. E. (1971b). Psychological characteristics of religious professionals. In M. P. Strommen (Ed.), *Research on religious development: A comprehensive handbook* (pp. 422–460). New York: Hawthorn Books.

Dittes, J. E. (1971c). Typing the typologies: Some parallels in the career of church–sect and extrinsic–intrinsic religion. *Journal for the Scientific Study of Religion, 10,* 375–383.

Dobkin de Rios, M. (1984). *Hallucinogens: Cross-cultural perspectives.* Albuquerque: University of New Mexico Press.

Doblin, R. (1991). Pahnke's "Good Friday" experiment: A long-term follow-up and methodological critique. *Journal of Transpersonal Psychology, 23,* 1–28.

Dohrenwend, B. P., & Dohrenwend, B. S. (1969). *Social status and psychological disorder.* New York: Wiley.

Domino, G., & Miller, K. (1992). Religiosity and attitudes toward suicide. *Omega, 25,* 271–282.

Donahue, M. J. (1985a). Intrinsic and extrinsic religiousness: The empirical research. *Journal for the Scientific Study of Religion, 24,* 418–423.

Donahue, M. J. (1985b). Intrinsic and extrinsic religiousness: Review and meta-analysis. *Journal of Personality and Social Psychology, 48,* 400–419.

Donahue, M. J. (1987). *Religion and drug use: 1976–1985.* Paper presented at the annual convention of the Society for the Scientific Study of Religion, Lousville, KY.

Donahue, M. J. (1994). Correlates of religious giving in six Protestant denominations. *Review of Religious Research, 36,* 149–157.

Donahue, M. J. (1998, August). *There is no true spirituality apart from religion.* Paper presented at the annual convention of the American Psychological Association, Chicago.

Donahue, M. J., & Benson, P. L. (1995). Religion and the well-being of adolescents. *Journal of Social Issues, 51,* 145–160.

Donelson, E. (1999). Psychology of religion and adolescents in the United States: Past to present. *Journal of Adolescence, 22,* 187–204.

D'Onofrio, B., Eaves, L. J., Murrelle, L., Maes, H. H., & Spilka, B. (1999). Understanding biological and social influences on religious affiliation, attitudes, and behaviors: A behavior-genetic perspective. *Journal of Personality, 67,* 953–984.

Douglass, J. D. (1974). Women and the continental reformation. In R. R. Ruether (Ed.), *Religion and sexism: Images of women in the Jewish and Christian traditions* (pp. 292–318). New York: Simon & Schuster.

Dowd, M. (2002, April 7). Sacred cruelties. *The New York Times* [Online]. Available: http://www.nytimes.com/2002/04/07/opinion07DOWD.html?todaysheadlines [Retrieved April 8, 2002].

Downton, J. V., Jr. (1980). An evolutionary theory of spiritual conversion and commitment: The case of the Divine Light Mission. *Journal for the Scientific Study of Religion, 19,* 381–396.

Doxey, C., Jensen, L., & Jensen, J. (1997). The influence of religion on victims of childhood sexual abuse. *International Journal for the Psychology of Religion, 7,* 179–183.

Dublin, L. I. (1963). *Suicide.* New York: Ronald Press.

Dubose, E. R. (2000, November). Spiritual care at the end of life. *Bulletin of the The Park Ridge Center for the Study of Health, Faith, and Ethics,* p. 18.

Duck, R. J., & Hunsberger, B. (1999). Religious orientation and prejudice: The role of religious proscription, right-wing authoritarianism and social desirability. *International Journal for the Psychology of Religion, 9,* 157–179.

Duckitt, J. (1992). *The social psychology of prejudice.* New York: Praeger.

Dudley, R. L. (1978). Alienation from religion in adolescents from fundamentalist religious homes. *Journal for the Scientific Study of Religion, 17,* 389–398.

Dudley, R. L. (1999). Youth religious commitment over time: A longitudinal study of retention. *Review of Religious Research, 41,* 110–121.

Dudley, R. L., & Dudley, M. G. (1986). Transmission of religious values from parents to adolescents. *Review of Religious Research, 28,* 3–15.

Dufour, L. R. (2000). Sifting through tradition: The creation of Jewish feminist identities. *Journal for the Scientific Study of Religion, 39,* 90–106.

Durham, W. H. (1982). Toward a coevolutionary theory of human biology and culture. In T. C. Weigele (Ed.), *Biology and the social sciences* (pp. 77–94). Boulder, CO: Westview Press.

Duriez, B., & Hutsebaut, D. (2000). The relation between religion and racism: The role of post-critical beliefs. *Mental Health, Religion, and Culture, 3,* 85–102.

Durkheim, E. (1915). *The elementary forms of the religious life: A study in religious sociology* (J. W. Swain, Trans.). London: Allen & Unwin.

Durkheim, E. (1951). *Suicide: A study in sociology.* New York: Free Press. (Original work published 1897)

Durr, R. A. (1970). *Poetic vision and the psychedelic experience.* New York: Dell.

Eaton, J. W., & Weil, R. J. (1955). *Culture and mental disorders.* Glencoe, IL: Free Press.

Echterling, L. G. (1993, August). *Making do and making sense: Long-term coping of disaster survivors.* Paper presented at the annual convention of the American Psychological Association, Toronto.

Echterling, L. G., Bradfield, C., & Wylie, M. L. (1992). *Six years after the flood: Clergy's long term response to disaster.* Poster presented at the annual meeting of the American Psychological Association, Washington, DC.

Edwards, T. (1955). *The new dictionary of thoughts* (rev. & enlarged). New York: Standard Book.

Einstein, A. (1931). Religion and science. In A. M. Drummond & R. H. Wagner (Eds.), *Problems and opinions* (pp. 355–358). New York: Century.

Eisinga, R., Billiet, J., & Felling, A. (1999). Christian religion and ethnic prejudice in cross-national perspective: A comparative analysis of the Netherlands and Flanders (Belgium). *International Journal of Comparative Sociology, 40,* 375–393.

Eisinga, R., Felling, A., & Peters, J. (1990). Religious belief, church involvement, and ethnocentrism in the Netherlands. *Journal for the Scientific Study of Religion, 29,* 54–75.

Eisinga, R., Konig, R., & Scheepers, P. (1995). Orthodox religious beliefs and anti-Semitism: A replication of Glock and Stark in the Netherlands. *Journal for the Scientific Study of Religion, 34,* 214–223.

Eister, A. W. (1973). H. Reinhold Niebuhr and the paradox of religious organizations: A radical critique. In C. Y. Glock & P. E. Hammond (Eds.), *Beyond the classics? Essays in the scientific study of religion* (pp. 355–408). New York: Harper & Row.

Eliach, Y. (1982). *Hassidic tales of the Holocaust.* New York: Avon.

Elifson, K. W., Petersen, D. M., & Hadaway, C. K. (1983). Religion and delinquency: A contextual analysis. *Criminology, 21,* 505–527.

Elkind, D. (1961). The child's concept of his religious denomination: I. The Jewish child. *Journal of Genetic Psychology, 99,* 209–225.

Elkind, D. (1962). The child's concept of his religious denomination: II. The Catholic child. *Journal of Genetic Psychology, 101,* 185–193.

Elkind, D. (1964). Piaget's semi-clinical interview and the study of spontaneous religion. *Journal for the Scientific Study of Religion, 4,* 40–46.

Elkind, D. (1970). The origins of religion in the child. *Review of Religious Research, 12,* 35–42.

Elkind, D. (1971). The development of religious understanding in children and adolescents. In M. P. Strommen (Ed.), *Research on religious development* (pp. 655–685). New York: Hawthorn Books.

Elkind, D., & Elkind, S. (1970). Varieties of religious experience in young adolescents. *Journal for the Scientific Study of Religion, 2,* 102–112.

Elkins, D., Anchor, K. N., & Sandler, H. M. (1979). Relaxation training and prayer behavior as tension reduction techniques. *Behavioral Engineering, 6,* 81–87.

Elkins, D. N., Hedstrom, L. J., Hughes, L. L., Leaf, J. A., & Saunders, C. (1988). Toward a humanistic–phenomenological spirituality. *Journal of Humanistic Psychology, 28,* 5–18.

Ellenberger, H. F. (1970). *The discovery of the unconscious: The history and evolution of dynamic psychiatry.* New York: Basic Books.

Elliott, D. M. (1994). The impact of Christian faith on the prevalence and sequelae of sexual abuse. *Journal of Interpersonal Violence, 9,* 95–108.

Ellis, A. (1980). Psychotherapy and atheistic values: A response to A. E. Bergin's "Psychotherapy and religious issues." *Journal of Consulting and Clinical Psychology, 48,* 635–639.

Ellis, A. (1986). Do some religious beliefs help create emotional disturbance? *Psychotherapy in Private Practice, 4,* 101–106.

Ellis, A. (1988). Is religiosity pathological? *Free Inquiry, 18,* 27–32.

Ellis, A. (2000). Spiritual goals and spirited values in psychotherapy. *Journal of Individual Psychology, 56,* 277–284.

Ellison, C. G. (1991a). An eye for an eye?: A note on the Southern subculture of violence thesis. *Social Forces, 69,* 1223–1239.

Ellison, C. G. (1991b). Religious involvement and subjective well-being. *Journal of Health and Social Behavior, 32,* 80–89.

Ellison, C. G., & Anderson, K. L. (2001). Religious involvement and domestic violence among U.S. couples. *Journal for the Scientific Study of Religion, 40,* 269–286.

Ellison, C. G., Bartkowski, J. P., & Anderson, K. L. (1999). Are there religious variations in domestic violence? *Journal of Family Issues, 20,* 87–113.

Ellison, C. G., Bartkowski, J. P., & Segal, M. L. (1996). Do conservative Protestant parents spank more often?: Further evidence from the National Survey of Families and Households. *Social Science Quarterly, 77,* 663–673.

Ellison, C. G., & Sherkat, D. E. (1993). Obedience and autonomy: Religion and parental values reconsidered. *Journal for the Scientific Study of Religion, 32,* 313–329.

Ellison, C. W. (1983). Spiritual well-being: Conceptualization and measurement. *Journal of Psychology and Theology, 11,* 330–340.

Ellison, C. W., & Smith, J. (1991). Toward an integrative measure of health and well-being. *Journal of Psychology and Theology, 19,* 35–48.

Ellwood, R. (1986). The several meanings of cult. *Thought, 61,* 212–224.

Elms, A. C. (1976). *Personality in politics.* New York: Harcourt Brace Jovanovich.

Embree, R. A. (1964). *A factor-analytic investigation of motivations and attitudes of college students with intentions for the ministry and a comparison of persisters and non-persisters on the Theological School Inventory.* Unpublished doctoral dissertation, University of Denver.

Embree, R. A., Spilka, B., & Horn, J. (1968, May). *Special leading and natural leading: An interpretive investigation of motivation for the Christian ministry.* Paper presented at the convention of the Rocky Mountain Psychological Association, Denver, CO.

Emmons, R. A. (1995). Levels and domains in personality: An introduction. *Journal of Personality, 63,* 341–364.

Emmons, R. A. (1999). *The psychology of ultimate concerns.* New York: Guilford Press.

Emmons, R. A. (2000). Personality and forgiveness. In M. E. McCullough, K. I. Pargament, & C. E. Thoresen (Eds.), *Forgiveness: Theory, research, and practice* (pp. 156–175). New York: Guilford Press.

Emmons, R. A., & Crumpler, A. (1999). Religion and spirituality?: The roles of sanctification and the concept of God. *International Journal for the Psychology of Religion, 9,* 17–24.

Emmons, R. A., & Paloutzian, R. (2003). Psychology of religion. *Annual Review of Psychology, 54,* 377–402.

Engs, R. C., Diebold, B. A., & Hanson, D. J. (1996). The drinking patterns and problems of a national sample of college students, 1994. *Journal of Alcohol and Drug Education, 4,* 13–33.

Engs, R. C., & Mullen, K. (1999). The effect of religion and religiosity on drug use among a selected sample of post secondary students in Scotland. *Addiction Research, 7,* 149–170.

Enright, R. D., Santos, M. J., & Al-Mabuk, R. (1989). The adolescent as forgiver. *Journal of Adolescence, 12,* 99–110.

Enskar, K., Carlsson, M., Golsater, M., Hamrin, E., & Kreuger, A., (1997). Parental reports of changes and challenges that result from parenting a child with cancer. *Journal of Pediatric Oncology Nursing, 14*(3), 156–163.

Epley, N., & Dunning, D. (2000). Feeling holier than thou: Are self-serving assessments produced by errors in self- or social prediction? *Journal of Personality and Social Psychology, 790,* 861–875.

Epstein, S., & O'Brien, E. J. (1985). The person–situation debate in historical and current perspective. *Psychological Bulletin, 98,* 513–537.

Erickson, D. A. (1964). Religious consequences of public and sectarian schooling. *School Review, 72,* 21–33.

Erickson, J. A. (1992). Adolescent development and commitment: A structural equation model of the role of family, peer group, and educational influences. *Journal for the Scientific Study of Religion, 31,* 131–152.

Erikson, E. H. (1958). *Young man Luther: A study in psychoanalysis and history.* New York: Norton.

Erikson, E. H. (1963). *Childhood and society* (2nd ed.). New York: Norton.

Erikson, E. H. (1964). *Insight and responsibility*. New York: Norton.

Erikson, E. H. (1965). Youth: Fidelity and diversity. In E. H. Erikson (Ed.), *The challenge of youth* (pp. 1–28). Garden City, NY: Doubleday/Anchor.

Erikson, E. H. (1966). Ontogeny of ritualization in man. *Philosophical transactions of the Royal Society of London, Series B, Biological Sciences, 251,* 337–349.

Erikson, E. H. (1968). *Identity: Youth and crisis*. New York: Norton.

Erikson, E. H. (1969). Identity and the life cycle [Special issue]. *Psychological Issues, 1.*

Erikson, E. H., Erikson, J. M., & Kivinick, H. Q. (1986). *Vital involvement in old age*. New York: Norton.

Ernsberger, D. J., & Manaster, G. J. (1981). Moral development, intrinsic/extrinsic religious orientation and denominational teachings. *Genetic Psychology Monographs, 104,* 23–41.

Eshleman, A. K., Dickie, J. R., Merasco, D. M., Shepard, A., & Johnson, M. (1999). Mother God, Father God: Children's perceptions of God's distance. *International Journal for the Psychology of Religion, 9,* 139–146.

Ethridge, F. M., & Feagin, J. R. (1979). Varieties of "fundamentalism": A conceptual and empirical analysis of two Protestant denominations. *Sociological Quarterly, 20,* 37–48.

Etxebarria, I. (1992). Sentimientos de culpa y abandono de los valores paternos [Guilt feelings and abandoning parental values]. *Infancia y Aprendizaje, 57,* 67–88.

Evans, R., McIntosh, D. N., & Spilka, B. (1986). *Marital adjustment and form of personal faith*. Paper presented at the Convention of the Rocky Mountain Psychological Association, Denver, CO.

Eysenck, H. J. (1981). *A model for personality*. New York: Springer.

Faber, H. (1972). *Psychology of religion*. Philadelphia: Westminster.

Faber, M. B. (2002). *The magic of prayer: An introduction to the psychology of faith*. Westport, CT: Praeger.

Fahs, S. L. (1950). The beginnings of mysticism in children's growth. *Religious Education, 45,* 139–147.

Falconer, D. S. (1981). *Introduction to quantitative genetics* (2nd ed.). New York: Longmans.

Falkenheim, M. A., Duckro, P. N., Hughes, H. M., Rossetti, S. J., & Gfeller, J. D. (1999). Cluster analysis of child sexual offenders: A validation with Roman Catholic priests and brothers. *Sexual Addiction and Compulsivity, 6,* 317–336.

Farb, P. (1978). *Humankind*. New York: Bantam Books.

Farberow, N. L. (1963). *Taboo topics*. New York: Atherton.

Faulkner, J. E., & DeJong, G. F. (1966). Religiosity in 5-D: An empirical analysis. *Social Forces, 45,* 246–254.

Fecher, V. J. (1982). *Religion and aging: An annotated bibliography*. San Antonio, TX: Trinity University Press.

Feifel, H. (1974). Religious conviction and fear of death among the healthy and the terminally ill. *Journal for the Scientific Study of Religion, 13,* 353–360.

Feifel, H., & Tong Nagy, V. (1981). Another look at fear of death. *Journal of Consulting and Clinical Psychology, 49,* 278–286.

Feifel, H., Freilich, J., & Hermann, L. J. (1973). Death fear in dying heart and cancer patients. *Journal of Psychosomatic Research, 17,* 161–166.

Feldman, K. A. (1969). Change and stability of religious orientations during college: Part I. Freshman–senior comparisons. *Review of Religious Research, 11,* 40–60.

Feldman, K. A., & Newcomb, T. M. (1969). *The impact of college on students*. San Francisco: Jossey-Bass.

Fernhout, H., & Boyd, D. (1985). Faith in autonomy: Development in Kohlberg's perspectives in religion and morality. *Religious Education, 80,* 287–307.

Ferraro, K. F., & Albrecht-Jensen, C. M. (1991). Does religion influence adult health? *Journal for the Social Scientific Study of Religion, 30,* 193–202.

Festinger, L. (1957). *A theory of cognitive dissonance*. Stanford, CA: Stanford University Press.

Festinger, L., Riecken, H. W., & Schachter, S. (1956). *When prophecy fails*. Minneapolis: University of Minnesota Press.

Feuerstein, G. (1992). *Holy madness*. New York: Arcana.

Fichter, J. H. (1954). *Social relations in the urban parish*. Chicago: University of Chicago Press.

Fichter, J. H. (1981). *Religion and pain.* New York: Crossroads.

Field, C. D. (2000). Joining and leaving British Methodism since the 1960s. In L. J. Francis & Y. J. Katz (Eds.), *Joining and leaving religion: Research perspectives* (pp. 57–85). Leominster, England: Gracewing.

Filsinger, E. E., & Wilson, M. R. (1984). Religiosity, socioeconomic rewards, and family development: Predictors of marital adjustment. *Journal of Marriage and the Family, 46,* 663–670.

Finch, J. C. (1965). Motivations for the ministry. *Insight, 4,* 26–31.

Finister, A. W. (1970). Dimensions of political alienation. *American Political Science Review, 64,* 389–410.

Finke, R., & Stark, R. (1992). *The churching of America, 1776–1990: Winners and losers in our religious economy.* New Brunswick, NJ: Rutgers University Press.

Finke, R., & Stark, R. (2001). The new holy clubs: Testing church-to-sect propositions. *Sociology of Religion, 62,* 175–189.

Finkel, D., & McGue, M. (1997). Sex differences and nonadditivity in heritability of the Multidimensional Personality Questionnaire Scales. *Journal of Personality and Social Psychology, 72,* 929–938.

Finney, J. M., & Lee, G. R. (1977). Age differences on five dimensions of religious involvement. *Review of Religious Research, 18,* 173–179.

Finney, J. R., & Malony, H. N. (1985a). Empirical studies of Christian prayer: A review of the literature. *Journal of Psychology and Theology, 13,* 104–115.

Finney, J. R., & Malony, H. N. (1985b). An empirical study of contemplative prayer as an adjunct to psychotherapy. *Journal of Psychology and Theology, 13,* 284–290.

Finney, J. R., & Malony, H. N. (1985c). Contemplative prayer and its use in psychotherapy: A theoretical model. *Journal of Psychology and Theology, 13,* 172–181.

Firebaugh, G., & Harley, B. (1991). Trends in U.S. church attendance: Secularization and revival, or merely life cycle effects? *Journal for the Scientific Study of Religion, 30,* 487–500.

Fischer, R. (1969). The perception–hallucination continuum (a re-examination). *Diseases of the Nervous System, 30,* 161–171.

Fischer, R. (1971). A cartography of ecstatic and meditative states. *Science, 174,* 897–904.

Fischer, R. (1978). Cartography of conscious states: Integration of East and West. In A. A. Sugerman & R. E. Tarter (Eds.), *Expanding dimensions of consciousness* (pp. 24–57). New York: Springer.

Fishbein, M., & Ajzen, I. (1975). *Belief, attitude, intention, and behavior: An introduction to theory and research.* Reading, MA: Addison-Wesley.

Fisher, H. E. (1983). *The sex contract.* New York: William Morrow.

Fisher, R. D., Cook, I. J., & Shirkey, E. C. (1994). Correlates of support for censorship of sexual, sexually violent, and violent media. *Journal of Sex Research, 31,* 229–240.

Fisher, R. D., Derison, D., Polley, C. F., Cadman, J., & Johnston, D. (1994). Religiousness, religious orientation, and attitudes towards gays and lesbians. *Journal of Applied Social Psychology, 24,* 614–630.

Fishman, S. B. (2000). *Jewish life and American culture.* Albany: State University of New York Press.

Fiske, J. (1883). *Excursions of an evolutionist.* Boston: Houghton Mifflin.

Fiske, S. T., & Taylor, S. E. (1991). *Social cognition* (2nd ed.). New York: McGraw-Hill.

Fitzgibbons, J. (1987). Developmental approaches to the psychology of religion. *Psychoanalytic Review, 74,* 125–134.

Flannery, E. H. (1985). *The anguish of the Jews.* New York: Paulist Press.

Flatt, B. (1987). Some stages of grief. *Journal of Religion and Health, 26,* 143–148.

Flor, D. L., & Knapp, N. F. (2001). Transmission and transaction: Predicting adolescents' internalization of parental religious values. *Journal of Family Psychology, 15,* 627–645.

Florian, V., & Kravetz, S. (1983). Fear of personal death: Attribution, structure, and relation to religious belief. *Journal of Personality and Social Psychology, 44,* 600–607.

Florian, V., & Kravetz, S. (1985). Children's concepts of death: A cross-cultural comparison among Muslims, Cruze, Christians, and Jews in Israel. *Journal of Cross Cultural Psychology, 16,* 174–189.

Florian, V., & Mikulincer, M. (1992–1993). The impact of death-risk experience and religiosity on the fear of personal death: The case of Israeli soldiers in Lebanon. *Omega, 26,* 101–111.

Fogarty, J. A. (2000). *The magical thoughts of grieving children.* Amityville, NY: Baywood.

Folkman, S., Chesney, M. A., Pollack, L., & Phillips, C. (1992). Stress, coping, and high-risk sexual behavior. *Health Psychology, 11,* 218–222.

Folkman, S., & Lazarus, R. S. (1988). Coping as a mediator of emotion. *Journal of Personality and Social Psychology, 54,* 466–475.

Folkman, S., Lazarus, R. S., Dunkel-Schetter, C., De Longis, A., & Gruen, R. J. (1986). Dynamics of a stressful encounter: Cognitive appraisal, coping, and encounter outcomes. *Journal of Personality and Social Psychology, 50,* 992–1003.

Fones, C. S. L., Levine, S. B., Althof, S. E., & Risen, C. B. (1999). The sexual struggles of 23 clergymen: A follow-up study. *Journal of Sex and Marital Therapy, 25,* 183–195.

Forbes, G. B., TeVault, R. K., & Gromoll, H. F. (1971). Willingness to help strangers as a function of liberal, conservative, or Catholic church membership: A field study with the lost-letter technique. *Psychological Reports, 28,* 947–949.

Ford, H. H., Zimmerman, R. S., Anderman, E. M., & Brown-Wright, L. (2001). Beliefs about the appropriateness of AIDS-related education for sixth and ninth grade students. *Journal of HIV/AIDS Prevention and Education for Adolescents and Children, 4,* 5–18.

Forliti, J. E., & Benson, P. L. (1986). Young adolescents: A national study. *Religious Education, 81,* 199–224.

Forman, R. K. (1992). Mysticism, constructivism, and forgetting. In R. K. Forman (Ed.), *The problem of pure consciousness* (pp. 3–49). New York: Oxford University Press.

Forman, R. K. C. (Ed.). (1990). *The problem of pure consciousness: Mysticism and philosophy.* New York: Oxford University Press.

Forman, R. K. C. (Ed.). (1998). *The innate capacity: Mysticism, psychology and philosophy.* New York: Oxford University Press.

Forte, R. (Ed.). (1997). *Entheogens and the future of religion.* San Francisco: Council on Spiritual Practices.

Fortune, M. M., & Poling, J. N. (1994). *Sexual abuse by clergy: A crisis for the church* (JPCP Monograph No. 6). Decatur, GA: *Journal of Pastoral Care.*

Foshee, V. A., & Hollinger, B. R. (1996). Maternal religiosity, adolescent social bonding, and adolescent alcohol use. *Journal of Early Adolescence, 16,* 451–468.

Foster, L. (1984). *Religion and sexuality: The Shakers, the Mormons, and the Oneida community.* Urbana: University of Illinois Press.

Foster, R. A., & Babcock, R. L. (2001). God as a man versus God as a woman: Perceiving God as a function of the gender of God and the gender of the participant. *International Journal for the Psychology of Religion, 11,* 93–104.

Foster, R. A., & Keating, J. P. (1990, November). *The male God-concept and self-esteem: A theoretical framework.* Paper presented at the annual convention of the Society for the Scientific Study of Religion, Virginia Beach, VA.

Foster, R. A., & Keating, J. P. (1992). Measuring androcentrism in the Western God-concept. *Journal for the Scientific Study of Religion, 31,* 366–375.

Foster, R. J. (1992). *Prayer: Finding the heart's true home.* San Francisco: Harper.

Fowler, J. (1994). Moral stages and the development of faith. In B. Puka (Ed.), *Moral development: A compendium. Vol. 2. Fundamental research in moral development* (pp. 344–374). New York: Garland Press.

Fowler, J. W. (1981). *Stages of faith: The psychology of human development and the quest for meaning.* San Francisco: Harper & Row.

Fowler, J. W. (1991a). Stages in faith consciousness. In F. K. Oser & W. G. Scarlett (Eds.), *Religious development in childhood and adolescence* (New Directions for Child Development, No. 52, pp. 27–45). San Francisco: Jossey-Bass.

Fowler, J. W. (1991b). *Weaving the new creation: Stages of faith and the public church.* San Francisco: Harper.

Fowler, J. W. (1993). Response to Helmut Reich: Overview or apologetic? *International Journal for the Psychology of Religion, 3,* 173–179.

Fowler, J. W. (1996). *Faithful change: The personal and public challenges of postmodern life.* Nashville, TN: Abingdon Press.

Fowler, J. W. (2001). Faith development theory and the postmodern challenges. *International Journal for the Psychology of Religion, 11,* 157–172.

Fowler, R. B., & Hertzke, A. D. (1995). *Religion and politics in America.* Boulder, CO: Westview Press.

Fox, J. W. (1992). The structure, stability, and social antecedents of reported paranormal experiences. *Sociological Analysis, 53,* 417–431.

Frame, M. W. (1996). The influence of gender and gender-pairings on clergy's identification of sexually ambiguous behavior as sexual harassment. *Pastoral Psychology, 44,* 295–304.

Francis, L. J. (1979). The priest as test administrator in attitude research. *Journal for the Scientific Study of Religion, 18,* 78–81.

Francis, L. J. (1980). Paths of holiness? Attitudes towards religion among 9–11-year-old children in England. *Character Potential: A Record of Research, 9,* 129–138.

Francis, L. J. (1982). *Youth in transit: A profile of 16–25 year olds.* Aldershot, England: Gower.

Francis, L. J. (1986). Denominational schools and pupil attitude toward Christianity. *British Educational Research Journal, 12,* 145–152.

Francis, L. J. (1989a). Measuring attitude towards Christianity during childhood and adolescence. *Personality and Individual Differences, 10,* 695–698.

Francis, L. J. (1989b). Monitoring changing attitudes towards Christianity among secondary school pupils between 1974 and 1986. *British Journal of Educational Psychology, 59,* 86–91.

Francis, L. J. (1994). Personality and religious development during childhood and adolescence. In L. B. Brown (Ed.), *Religion, personality, and mental health* (pp. 94–118). New York: Springer-Verlag.

Francis, L. J. (1997a). The impact of personality and religion on attitude towards substance use among 13–15-year-olds. *Drug and Alcohol Dependence, 44,* 95–103.

Francis, L. J. (1997b). Personality, prayer, and church attendance among undergraduate students. *International Journal for the Psychology of Religion, 7,* 127–132.

Francis, L. J. (2000). The relationship between bible reading and purpose in life among 13–15-year-olds. *Mental Health, Religion and Culture, 3,* 27–36.

Francis, L. J., & Astley, J. (Eds.). (2001). *Psychological perspectives on prayer: A reader.* Leominster, England: Gracewing.

Francis, L. J., & Brown, L. B. (1990). The predisposition to pray: A study of the social influence on the predisposition to pray among eleven-year-old children in England. *Journal of Empirical Theology, 3,* 23–34.

Francis, L. J., & Brown, L. B. (1991). The influence of home, church and school on prayer among sixteen-year-old adolescents in England. *Review of Religious Research, 33,* 112–122.

Francis, L. J., & Gibbs, D. (1996). Prayer and self-esteem among 8- to 11-year-olds in the United Kingdom. *Journal of Social Psychology, 136,* 791–793.

Francis, L. J., & Gibson, H. M. (1993). Parental influence and adolescent religiosity: A study of church attendance and attitude toward Christianity among adolescents 11 to 12 and 15 to 16 years old. *International Journal for the Psychology of Religion, 3,* 241–253.

Francis, L. J., & Greer, J. E. (2001). Shaping adolescents' attitudes towards science and religion in Northern Ireland: The role of scientism, creationism and denominational schools. *Research in Science and Technological Education, 19,* 39–53.

Francis, L. J., & Johnson, P. (1999). Mental health, prayer and church attendance among primary schoolteachers. *Mental Health, Religion and Culture, 2,* 153–158.

Francis, L. J., Jones, S. H., Jackson, C. J., & Robbins, M. (2001). The feminine personality profile of male Anglican clergy in Britain and Ireland: A study employing the Eysenck Personality Profile. *Review of Religious Research, 43,* 14–23.

Francis, L. J., & Kaldor, P. (2002). The relationship between psychological well-being and Christian faith and practice in an Australian population sample. *Journal for the Scientific Study of Religion, 41,* 179–184.

Francis, L. J., & Katz, Y. I. (1992). The relationship between personality and religiosity in an Israeli sample. *Journal for the Scientific Study of Religion, 31,* 153–162.

Francis, L. J., & Lankshear, D. W. (2001). The relationship between church schools and local church life: Distinguishing between aided and controlled status. *Educational Studies, 27,* 425–438.

Francis, L. J., Pearson, P. R., & Kay, W. K. (1982). Eysenck's personality quadrants and religiosity. *British Journal of Social Psychology, 21,* 262–264.

Francis, L. J., Pearson, P. R., & Kay, W. K. (1983a). Are children bigger liars? *Psychological Reports, 52,* 551–554.

Francis, L. J., Pearson, P. R., & Kay, W. K. (1983b). Are introverts still more religious? *Personality and Individual Differences, 4,* 211–212.

Francis, L. J., Pearson, P. R., & Kay, W. K. (1988). Religiosity and lie scores: A question of interpretation. *Social Behavior and Personality, 16,* 91–95.

Francis, L. J., & Wilcox, C. (1996). Prayer, church attendance, and personality revisited: A study among 16- to 19-year-old girls. *Psychological Reports, 79,* 1266.

Francis, L. J., & Wilcox, C. (1998). Religiosity and feminity: Do women really hold a more positive attitude towards Christianity? *Journal for the Scientific Study of Religion, 37,* 462–469.

Franco, F. M., & Maass, A. (1999). Intentional control over prejudice: When the choice of the measure matters. *European Journal of Social Psychology, 29,* 469–477.

Frank, J. (1974). *Persuasion and healing: A comparative study of psychotherapy* (rev. ed.). New York: Schocken Books.

Franks, K., Templer, D. I., Cappelletty, G. G., & Kauffman, I. (1990–1991). Exploration of death anxiety as a function of religious variables in gay men with and without AIDS. *Omega, 22,* 43–50.

Freud, S. (1919). *Totem and taboo* (A. A. Brill, Trans.). London: Routledge. (Original work published 1913)

Freud, S. (1943). *A general introduction to psychoanalysis.* Garden City, NY: Garden City. (Original work published 1917)

Freud, S. (1961a). *Civilization and its discontents* (J. Strachey, Trans.). New York: Norton. (Original work published 1930)

Freud, S. (1961b). *The future of an illusion* (J. Strachey, Trans.). New York: Norton. (Original work published 1927)

Friedenberg, E. (1969). Current patterns of a generation conflict. *Journal of Social Issues, 25,* 21–38.

Friedman, E. H. (1985). *Generation to generation: Family process in church and synagogue.* New York: Guilford Press.

Friedman, M., & Rosenman, R. H. (1974). *Type A behavior and your heart.* New York: Knopf.

Friedman, S. B., Chodoff, P., Mason, J. W., & Hamburg, D. A. (1963). Behavioral observations on parents anticipating the death of a child. *Pediatrics, 32,* 610–625.

Friedrich, C., & Brzezinski, Z. (1956). *Totalitarian dictatorship and autocracy.* New York: Praeger.

Friedrichs, R. W. (1960). Alter versus ego: An exploratory assessment of altruism. *American Sociological Review, 25,* 496–508.

Friedrichs, R. W. (1973). Social research and theology: End of the detente? *Review of Religious Research, 15,* 113–137.

Fromm, E. (1950). *Psychoanalysis and religion.* New Haven, CT: Yale University Press.

Fry, P. S. (1990). A factor analytic investigation of home-bound elderly individuals' concerns about death and dying, and their coping responses. *Journal of Clinical Psychology, 46,* 737–748.

Fugate, J. R. (1980). *What the Bible says about . . . child training.* Tempe, AZ: Alpha Omega.

Fulton, A. S. (1997). Identity status, religious orientation, and prejudice. *Journal of Youth and Adolescence, 26,* 1–11.

Fulton, A. S., Gorsuch, R. L., & Maynard, E. A. (1999). Religious orientation, antihomosexual sentiment, and fundamentalism among Christians. *Journal for the Scientific Study of Religion, 38,* 14–22.

Furnham, A. (1990). *The Protestant work ethic.* New York: Routledge.

Furnham, A. F. (1982). Locus of control and theological beliefs. *Journal of Psychology and Theology, 10,* 130–136.

Gadamer, H.-G. (1986). *Truth and method* (G. Barden & J. Cumming, Trans.). New York: Crossroad.

Galaif, E. R., & Newcomb, M. D. (1999). Predictors of polydrug use among four ethnic groups: A 12-year longitudinal study. *Addictive Behaviors, 24,* 607–631.

Galanter, M. (1980). Psychological induction into the large group: Findings from a large modern religious sect. *American Journal of Psychiatry, 137,* 1574–1579.

Galanter, M. (1983). Group induction techniques in a charismatic sect. In D. G. Bromley & J. T. Richardson (Eds.), *The brainwashing/deprogramming controversy: Sociological, psychological, legal and historical perspectives* (pp.182–193). Lewiston, NY: Edwin Mellon.

Galanter, M. (1989a). *Cults: Faith, healing, and coercion.* New York: Oxford University Press.

Galanter, M. (Ed.). (1989b). *Cults and new religious movements.* Washington, DC: American Psychological Association.

Galanter, M., & Buckley, P. (1978). Evangelical religion and meditation: Psychotherapeutic effects. *Journal of Nervous and Mental Disease, 166,* 685–691.

Galanter, M., Rabkin, R., Rabkin, J., & Deutsch, A. (1979). The Moonies: A psychological study of conversion and membership in a contemporary religious sect. *American Journal of Psychiatry, 136,* 165–169.

Gallemore, J. L., Jr., Wilson, W. P., & Rhoads, J. M. (1969). The religious life of patients with affective disorders. *Diseases of the Nervous System, 30,* 483–487.

Gallup, G., Jr. (1978). *The Gallup Poll: Public opinion 1972–1977.* Washington, DC: Scholarly Resources.

Gallup, G., Jr. (1992). *The Gallup Poll: Public opinion 1991.* Wilmington, DE: Scholarly Resources.

Gallup, G., Jr., & Lindsay, D. M. (1999). *Surveying the religious landscape: Trends in U.S. beliefs.* Harrisburg, PA: Morehouse.

Gallup, G., Jr., & Proctor, W. (1982). *Adventures in immortality.* New York: McGraw-Hill.

Gallup, G., Jr., & Simons, W. W. (2000, October). Six in ten Americans read Bible at least occasionally. *The Gallup Poll Monthly,* No. 421, 51–52.

Gallup Poll Monthly. (1992, December). No. 327, pp. 32–39.

Gallup Poll Monthly. (1993, December). No. 339, pp. p. 43–58.

Gallup Poll Monthly. (1994, July). No. 346, pp. 32–53.

Galton, F. (1869). *Hereditary genius: An inquiry into its laws and consequences* (2nd ed.) London: Macmillan.

Gambetta, D. (Ed.). (1988). *Trust: Making and breaking cooperative relations.* New York: Blackwell.

Gange-Fling, M., Veach, P. M., Kuang, H., & Houg, B. (2000). Effects of childhood sexual abuse on client spiritual well-being. *Counseling and Values, 44,* 84–91.

Gardella, P. (1985). *Innocent ecstasy.* New York: Oxford University Press.

Gardner, H. (1978). What we know (and don't know) about the two halves of the brain. *Harvard Magazine, 80,* 24–27.

Gardner, M. (1999, July–August). The religious views of Stephen Gould and Charles Darwin. *Skeptical Inquirer,* pp. 8–13.

Garrett, W. R. (1974). Troublesome transcendence: The supernatural in the scientific study of religion. *Sociological Analysis, 35,* 167–180.

Garrett, W. R. (1975). Maligned mysticism: The maledicted career of Troeltsch's third type. *Sociological Analysis, 36,* 205–223.

Gartner, J., Larson, D. B., & Allen, G. D. (1991). Religious commitment and mental health: A review of the empirical literature. *Journal of Psychology and Theology, 19,* 6–25.

Gartrell, C. D., & Shannon, Z. K. (1985). Contacts, cognitions, and conversions: A rational choice approach. *Review of Religious Research, 27,* 32–48.

Garvey, M. (1998). *Searching for Mary: An exploration of Marion apparitions across the U.S.* New York: Plume.

Gaustad, E. S. (1966). *A religious history of America* (rev. ed.). San Francisco: Harper & Row.

Geffen, R. M. (2001, March–April). Intermarriage and the premise of American Jewish life. *Congress Monthly,* pp. 6–8.

General Social Survey (GSC). (1999). *GSS cumulative datafile 1972–1998* [Online]. Available: http://www.sda.berkeley.edu/:7502 [Retrieved May 4, 2000].

Genia, V. (1991). The Spiritual Experience Index: A measure of spiritual maturity. *Journal of Religion and Health, 30,* 337–347.

Genia, V. (1997). The Spiritual Experience Index: Revision and reformulation. *Review of Religious Research, 38,* 344–361.

Gentry, C. S. (1987). Social distance regarding male and female homosexuals. *Journal of Social Psychology, 127,* 199–208.

Gerlach, L. P., & Hine, V. H. (1970). *People, power, change: Movements of social transformation.* Indianapolis, IN: Bobbs-Merrill.

Gershoff, E. T., Miller, P. C., & Holden, G. W. (1999). Parenting influences from the pulpit: Religious affiliation as a determinant of parental corporal punishment. *Journal of Family Psychology, 13,* 307–320.

Gerson, G. S. (1977). The psychology of grief and mourning in Judaism. *Journal of Religion and Health, 16,* 260–274.

Gerth, H. H., & Mills, C. W. (Eds. and Trans.). (1946). *From Max Weber: Essays in sociology.* New York: Oxford University Press.

Geyer, A. F. (1963). *Piety and politics.* Richmond, VA: John Knox Press.

Gibbons, D. E., & Jarnette, J. (1972). Hypnotic susceptibility and religious experience. *Journal for the Scientific Study of Religion, 11,* 152–156.

Gibbs, J. P. (1966). Suicide. in R. K. Merton & R. A. Nisbet (Eds.), *Contemporary social problems* (pp. 281–321). New York: Harcourt, Brace & World.

Gibbs, J. P. (1994). *A theory about control.* Boulder, CO: Westview Press.

Giesbrecht, N. (1995). Parenting style and adolescent religious commitment. *Journal of Psychology and Christianity, 14,* 228–238.

Giesbrecht, N., & Sevcik, I. (2000). The process of recovery and rebuilding among abused women in the conservative evangelical subculture. *Journal of Family Violence, 15,* 229–248.

Gilbert, J. (1997). *Redeeming culture.* Chicago: University of Chicago Press.

Gilbert, K. (1992). Religion as a resource for bereaved parents. *Journal of Religion and Health, 31,* 19–30.

Gill, R., Hadaway, C. K., & Marler, P. L. (1998). Is religious belief declining in Britain? *Journal for the Scientific Study of Religion, 37,* 507–516.

Gillespie, D. P. (1983). *An analysis of the relationship between denominational affiliation and religious orientation and death perspectives of the clergy.* Unpublished doctoral dissertation, Western Michigan University.

Gillespie, V. B. (1991). *The dynamics of religious conversion: Identity and transformation.* Birmingham, AL: Religious Education Press.

Gilligan, C. (1977). In a different voice: Women's conceptions of self and morality. *Harvard Educational Review, 47,* 481–517.

Gillings, V., & Joseph, S. (1996). Religiosity and social desirability: Impression management and self-deceptive positivity. *Personality and Individual Differences, 21,* 1047–1050.

Gilmore, N., & Sommerville, M. A. (1994). Stigmatization, scapegoating and discrimination in sexually transmitted diseases: Overcoming "them" and "us." *Social Science and Medicine, 39,* 1339–1358.

Girard, R. (1977). *Violence and the sacred.* Baltimore: Johns Hopkins University Press.

Glamser, F. D. (1987). The impact of retirement on religiosity. *Journal of Religion and Aging, 4,* 27–37.

Glass, J., Bengtson, V. L., & Dunham, C. C. (1986). Attitude similarity in three-generation families: Socialization, status inheritance or reciprocal influence? *American Sociological Review, 51,* 685–698.

Glick, I. O., Weiss, R. A., & Parkes, C. M. (1974). *The first year of bereavement.* New York: Wiley.

Glick, P., & Fiske, S. T. (2001). An ambivalent alliance: Hostile and benevolent sexism as complementary justifications for gender inequality. *American Psychologist, 56,* 109–118.

Globe and Mail [Toronto]. (2001, September 15). US got what it deserves, Falwell says. p. A2.

Glock, C. Y. (1962). On the study of religious commitment. *Religious Education, 57*(Research Suppl.), S98–S110.

Glock, C. Y. (1964). The role of deprivation in the origin and evolution of religious groups. In R. Lee & M. E. Marty (Eds.), *Religion and social conflict* (pp. 24–36). New York: Oxford University Press.

Glock, C. Y., Ringer, B. R., & Babbie, E. R. (1967). To *comfort and to challenge.* Berkeley: University of California Press.

Glock, C. Y., & Stark, R. (1965). *Religion and society in tension.* Chicago: Rand McNally.

Glock, C. Y., & Stark, R. (1966). *Christian beliefs and anti-Semitism.* New York: Harper & Row.

Glover, R. J. (1997). Relationships in moral reasoning and religion among members of conservative, moderate, and liberal religious groups. *Journal of Social Psychology, 137,* 247–255.

Gochman, E. R. G., & Fantasia, S. C. (1979). *The concept of immortality as related to planning one's life.* Paper presented at the annual convention of the American Psychological Association, New York.

Godin, A. (1968). Genetic development of the symbolic function: Meaning and limits of the work of R. Goldman. *Religious Education, 63,* 439–445.

Godin, A. (1985). *The psychodynamics of religious experience.* Birmingham, AL: Religious Education Press.

Godin, A., & Hallez, M. (1964). Parental images and divine paternity. *Lumen Vitae, 19,* 253–284.

Goldfried, J., & Miner, M. (2002). Quest religion and the problem of limited compassion. *Journal for the Scientific Study of Religion, 41,* 685–695.

Goldman, R. (1964). *Religious thinking from childhood to adolescence.* New York: Seabury Press.

Goldman, R. (1970). *Readiness for religion.* New York: Seabury.

Goldsen, R. K., Rosenberg, M., Williams, R. M., Jr., & Suchman, E. A. (1960). *What college students think.* Princeton, NJ: Van Nostrand.

Goldstein, S., & Goldscheider, G. (1968). *Jewish-Americans.* Englewood Cliffs, NJ: Prentice-Hall.

Goleman, D. (1977). *The varieties of meditative experience.* New York: Dutton.

Goleman, D. (1984, May). The faith factor. *American Health,* pp. 48–53.

Goleman, D. (1988). *The meditative mind: The varieties of meditative experience.* Los Angeles: Jeremy Tarcher/Perigee Books.

Golsworthy, R., & Coyle, A. (1999). Spiritual beliefs and the search for meaning among older adults following partner loss. *Mortality, 4,* 21–40.

Good, D. (1988). Individuals, interpersonal relations and trust. In D. Gambetta (Ed.), *Trust: Making and breaking cooperative relations* (pp. 31–48). New York: Blackwell.

Goodall, J. (1971). *In the shadow of man.* Boston: Houghton Mifflin.

Goode, E. (1968). Class styles of religious sociation. *British Journal of Scoiology, 19,* 1–16.

Goode, E. (2000, January/February). Two paranormalisms or two and a half? An empirical formulation. *Skeptical Inquirer, 24*(1), 29–35.

Goodman, F. D. (1969). Phonetic analysis of glossolalia in four cultural settings. *Journal for the Scientific Study of Religion, 8,* 227–239.

Goodman, F. D. (1972). *Speaking in tongues: A cross-cultural study of glossolalia.* Chicago: University of Chicago Press.

Goodman, F. D. (1988). *Ecstasy, religious ritual, and alternate reality.* Bloomington: University of Indiana Press.

Goodman, F. D. (1990). *Where the spirits ride the wind: Trance journeys and other ecstatic experiences.* Bloomington: University of Indiana Press.

Goodman, G. S., Bottoms, B. L., Redlich, A., Shaver, P. R., & Diviak, K. R. (1998). Correlates of multiple forms of victimization in religion-related child abuse cases. *Journal of Aggression, Maltreatment and Trauma, 2,* 273–295.

Goodwill, K. A. (2000). Religion and the spiritual needs of gay Mormon men. *Journal of Gay and Lesbian Social Services, 11,* 23–27.

Gordon, A. I. (1967). *The nature of conversion.* Boston: Beacon Press.

Gordon, D. F. (1984). Dying to self: Self-control through self-abandonment. *Sociological Analysis, 5,* 41–56.

Gordon, S. (1964). Personality and attitude correlates of religious conversion. *Journal for the Scientific Study of Religion, 4,* 60–63.

Gorelick, S. (1981). *City College and the Jewish poor.* New Brunswick, NJ: Rutgers University Press.

Gorsuch, R. L. (1968). The conceptualization of God as seen in adjective ratings. *Journal for the Scientific Study of Religion, 7,* 56–64.

Gorsuch, R. L. (1976). Religion as a significant predictor of important human behavior. In W. J. Donaldson, Jr. (Ed.), *Research in mental health and religious behavior* (pp. 206–221). Atlanta, GA: Psychological Studies Institute.

Gorsuch, R. L. (1984). Measurement: The boon and bane of investigating religion. *American Psychologist, 39,* 228–236.

Gorsuch, R. L. (1988). Psychology of religion. *Annual Review of Psychology, 39,* 201–221.

Gorsuch, R. L. (1993). Religion and prejudice: Lessons not learned from the past. *International Journal for the Psychology of Religion, 3,* 29–31.

Gorsuch, R. L. (1994). Toward motivational theories of intrinsic religious commitment. *Journal for the Scientific Study of Religion, 28,* 315–325.

Gorsuch, R. L. (1995). Religious aspects of substance abuse and recovery. *Journal of Social Issues, 51,* 65–83.

Gorsuch, R. L. (2002). *Integrating psychology and spirituality.* Westport, CT: Praeger.

Gorsuch, R. L., & Aleshire, D. (1974). Christian faith and ethnic prejudice: A review and interpretation of research. *Journal for the Scientific Study of Religion, 13,* 281–307.

Gorsuch, R. L., & Butler, M. C. (1976). Initial drug abuse: A review of predisposing social psychological factors. *Psychological Bulletin, 83,* 120–137.

Gorsuch, R. L., & Hao, J. Y. (1993). Forgiveness: An exploratory factor analysis and its relationship to religious variables. *Review of Religious Research, 34,* 333–347.

Gorsuch, R. L., & McFarland, S. (1972). Single vs. multiple-item scales for measuring religious values. *Journal for the Scientific Study of Religion, 11,* 53–64.

Gorsuch, R. L., & McPherson, S. E. (1989). Intrinsic/Extrinsic measurement: I/E-revised and single-item scales. *Journal for the Scientific Study of Religion, 28,* 348–354.

Gorsuch, R. L., & Miller, W. R. (1999). Assessing spirituality. In W. R. Miller (Ed.), *Integrating spirituality into treatment* (pp. 47–64). Washington, DC: American Psychological Association.

Gorsuch, R. L., Mylvaganan, G., Gorsuch, K., & Johnson, R. (1997). Perceived religious motivation. *International Journal for the Psychology of Religion, 7,* 253–261.

Gorsuch, R. L., & Ortberg, J. (1983). Moral obligations and attitudes: Their relationship to behavioral intentions. *Journal of Personality and Social Psychology, 44,* 1025–1028.

Gorsuch, R. L., & Smith, C. S. (1983). Attributions of responsibility to God: An interaction of religious beliefs and outcomes. *Journal for the Scientific Study of Religion, 22,* 340–352.

Gorsuch, R. L., & Spilka, B. (1987). *The Varieties* in historical and contemporary contexts. *Contemporary Psychology, 32*(9), 773–778.

Gorsuch, R. L., & Wakeman, E. P. (1991). A test and expansion of the Fishbein model on religious attitudes and behavior in Thailand. *International Journal for the Psychology of Religion, 1,* 33–40.

Gottschalk, S. (1973). *The emergence of Christian Science in American religious life.* Berkeley: University of California Press.

Gould, S. J. (1978). Biological potential vs. biological determinism. In A. L. Caplan (Ed.), *The sociobiology debate* (pp. 343–351). New York: Harper & Row.

Gould, S. J. (1987, July 19). The verdict on creationism. *The New York Times Magazine,* pp. 32–34.

Gould, S. J. (1991). Exaptation: A crucial tool for an evolutionary psychology. *Journal of Social Issues, 47,* 43–65.

Gould, S. J. (1999). *Rocks of ages.* New York: Ballantine.

Graebner, O. E. (1964). Child concepts of God. *Religious Education, 59,* 234–241.

Grana Gomes, J. L., & Munoz-Rivas, M. (2000). Psychological risk and protection factors for drug use by adolescents/Factores psicologicos de riesgo y de proteccion para el consumo de drogas en adolescents. *Psicologia Conductual, 8,* 249–269.

Granqvist, P. (1998). Religiousness and perceived childhood attachment: On the question of compensation or correspondence. *Journal for the Scientific Study of Religion, 37,* 350–367.

Granqvist, P. (2002a). *Attachment and religion: An integrative framework* (Comprehensive Summaries of Uppsala Dissertations from the Faculty of Social Sciences, No. 116). Uppsala, Sweden: Uppsala University.

Granqvist, P. (2002b). Attachment and religiosity in adolescence: Cross-sectional and longitudinal evaluations. *Personality and Social Psychology Bulletin, 28,* 260–270.

Granqvist, P., & Hagekull, B. (1999). Religiousness and perceived childhood attachment: Profiling socialized correspondence and emotional compensation. *Journal for the Scientific Study of Religion, 38,* 254–273.

Granqvist, P., & Hagekull, B. (2001). Seeking security in the new age: On attachment and emotional compensation. *Journal for the Scientific Study of Religion, 40,* 527–545.

Grant, D., & Epp, L. (1998). The gay orientation: Does God mind? *Counseling and Values, 43,* 28–33.

Grasmick, H. G., Bursik, R. J., & Cochran, J. K. (1991). "Render unto Caesar what is Caesar's": Religiosity and taxpayers' inclinations to cheat. *Sociological Quarterly, 32,* 251–266.

Grasmick, H. G., Kinsey, K., & Cochran, J. K. (1991). Denomination, religiosity and compliance with the law: A study of adults. *Journal for the Scientific Study of Religion, 30,* 99–107.

Grasmick, H. G., Morgan, C. S., & Kennedy, M. B. (1992). Support for corporal punishment in the schools: A comparison of the effects of socioeconomic status and religion. *Social Science Quarterly, 73,* 177–187.

Graves, P. L., Wang, N.-Y., Mead, L. A., Johnson, J. V., & Klag, M. J. (1998). Youthful precursors of midlife social support. *Journal of Personality and Social Psychology, 74,* 1329–1336.

Greeley, A. M. (1963). *Religion and career: A study of college graduates.* New York: Sheed & Ward.

Greeley, A. M. (1967). *The changing Catholic college.* Chicago: Aldine.

Greeley, A. M. (1972a). *The denominational society.* Glenview, IL: Scott, Foresman.

Greeley, A. M. (1972b). *Unsecular man.* New York: Schocken Books.

Greeley, A. M. (1974). *Ecstasy: A way of knowing.* Englewood Cliffs, NJ: Prentice-Hall.

Greeley, A. M. (1975). *Sociology of the paranormal: A reconnaissance* (Sage Research Papers in the Social Sciences, Vol. 3, No. 90–023). Beverly Hills, CA: Sage.

Greeley, A. M. (1981). Religious musical chairs. In T. Robbins & D. Anthony (Eds.), *In gods we trust: New patterns of religious pluralism in America* (pp. 101–126). New Brunswick, NJ: Transaction Books.

Greeley, A. M. (1987, Spring). The "impossible": It's happening. *Noetic Sciences Review,* p. 7.

Greeley, A. M. (1993). How serious is the problem of sexual abuse by clergy? *America, 168,* 20–27.

Greeley, A. M. (2002). *Religion in Europe at the end of the second millenium.* New Brunswick, NJ: Transaction Books.

Greeley, A. M., & Gockel, G. L. (1971). The religious effects of parochial education. In M. P. Strommen (Ed.), *Research on religious development: A comprehensive handbook* (pp. 264–301). New York: Hawthorne Books.

Greeley, A. M., & Rossi, P. H. (1966). *The education of Catholic Americans.* Chicago: Aldine.

Green, J. C. (2000). Religion and politics in the 1990s: Confrontations and coalitions. In M. Silk (Ed.), *Religion and American politics: The 2000 election in context* (pp. 19–40). Hartford, CT: Trinity University Center for the Study of Religion in Public Life.

Green, J. C., Rozell, M. J., & Wilcox, C. (2001). The case of the Christian right. *Journal for the Scientific Study of Religion, 40,* 413–426.

Greenberg, D., & Witztum, E. (1992). Content and prevalence of psychopathology in world religions. In J. F. Schumaker (Ed.), *Religion and mental health* (pp. 300–314). New York: Oxford University Press.

Greenberg, S. (1960). Jewish educational institutions. In L. Finkelstein (Ed.), *The Jews: Their history, culture, and religion* (3rd ed., Vol. 2, pp. 1254–1287). New York: Jewish Publication Society of America.

Greenwald, A. G., & Banaji, M. (1995). Implicit social cognition: Attitudes, self-esteem, and stereotypes. *Psychological Review, 102,* 4–27.

Greenwood, S. F. (1995). Transpersonal theory and religious experience. In R. W. Hood, Jr. (Ed.), *Handbook of religious experience* (pp. 495–519). Birmingham, AL: Religious Education Press.

Greer, J. E. (1983). A critical study of "Thinking about the Bible." *British Journal of Religious Education, 5,* 113–125.

Greil, A. L. (1993). Explorations along the sacred frontier: Notes on para-religions, quasi-religions, and other boundary phenomena. In D. G. Bromley & J. K. Hadden (Eds.), *Handbook of cults and sects in America: Assessing two decades of research and theory development* (pp. 153–172). Greenwich, CT: JAI Press.

Greil, A. L., & Robbins, T. (1994). Introduction: Exploring the boundaries of the sacred. In A. L. Greil

& T. Robbins (Eds.), *Between sacred and secular: Research and theory on quasi-religion* (pp. 1–23). Greenwich, CT: JAI Press.

Greil, A. L., & Rudy, D. R. (1990). On the margins of the sacred. In T. Robbins & D. Anthony (Eds.), *In gods we trust: New patterns of religious pluralism in America* (pp. 219–232). New Brunswick, NJ: Transaction Books.

Greven, P. (1991). *Spare the child: The religious roots of punishment and the psychological impact of physical abuse.* New York: Knopf.

Grey, I. M., & Swain, R. B. (1996). Sexual and religious attitudes of Irish students. *Irish Journal of Psychology, 17,* 213–227.

Griffin, G. A. E., Gorsuch, R., & Davis, A.-L. (1987). A cross-cultural investigation of religious orientation, social norms, and prejudice. *Journal for the Scientific Study of Religion, 26,* 358–365.

Griffiths, A. J. F., Miller, J. H., Suzuki, D. T., Lewontin, R. C., & Gelbart, W. M. (2000). *An introduction to genetic analysis.* New York: Freeman.

Griffiths, B., Dixon, C., Stanley, G., & Weiland, R. (2001). Religious orientation and attitudes toward homosexuality: A functional analysis. *Australian Journal of Psychology, 53,* 12–17.

Grof, S. (1980). *LSD psychotherapy.* Pomona, CA: Hunter House.

Grootenhuis, M. A., & Last, B. F. (1997). Parents' emotional reactions related to different prospects for the survival of their children with cancer. *Journal of Psychosocial Oncology, 15*(1), 43–62.

Gross, L. (1982). *The last Jews in Berlin.* New York: Simon & Schuster.

Gross, M. L. (1978). *The psychological society.* New York: Random House.

Grossman, J. D. (1975). *The dark interval.* Nile, IL: Argus Communications.

Groth-Marnat, G. (1992). Buddhism and mental health: A comparative analysis. In J. F. Schumaker (Ed.), *Religion and mental health* (pp. 270–280). New York: Oxford University Press.

Group for the Advancement of Psychiatry (GAP). (1960). *Psychiatry and religion* (Report No. 48, formulated by the Committee on Psychiatry and Religion). New York: Author.

Group for the Advancement of Psychiatry (GAP). (1968, January). *The psychic function of religion in mental illness and health* (Report No. 67, formulated by the Committee on Psychiatry and Religion). New York: Author.

Group for the Advancement of Psychiatry (GAP). (1976, November). *Mysticism: Spiritual quest or psychic disorder* (Report No. 97, formulated by the Committee on Psychiatry and Religion). New York: Author.

Gruner, L. (1985). The correlation of private, religious devotional practices and marital adjustment. *Journal of Comparative Family Studies, 16,* 47–59.

Guertin, W. H., & Bailey, J. P. (1970). *Introduction to modern factor analysis.* Ann Arbor, MI: Edwards Brothers.

Guralnik, D. B. (Ed.). (1986). *Webster's new world dictionary of the American language* (2nd college ed.). New York: Prentice Hall Press.

Guthrie, S. E. (1993). *Faces in the clouds: A new theory of religion.* New York: Oxford University Press.

Guthrie, S. E. (1996a). Religion: What is it? *Journal for the Scientific Study of Religion, 35,* 412–419.

Guthrie, S. E. (1996b). [Book reviews of P. Boyer, *The naturalness of religious ideas,* and S. N. Balagangadhara, *"The heathen in his blindness"—Asia, the West, and the dynamic of religion*]. *American Anthropologist, 98,* 162–163.

Guttman, J. (1984). Cognitive morality and cheating behavior in religious and secular school children. *Journal of Educational Research, 77,* 249–254.

Hadaway, C. K. (1980). Denominational switching and religiosity. *Review of Religious Research, 21,* 451–461.

Hadaway, C. K. (1989). Identifying American apostates: A cluster analysis. *Journal for the Scientific Study of Religion, 28,* 201–215.

Hadaway, C. K., Elifson, K. W., & Petersen, D. M. (1984). Religious involvement and drug use among urban adolescents. *Journal for the Scientific Study of Religion, 23,* 109–128.

Hadaway, C. K., & Marler, P. L. (1993). All in the family: Religious mobility in America. *Review of Religious Research, 35,* 97–116.

Hadaway, C. K., Marler, P. L., & Chaves, M. (1993). What the polls don't show: A closer look at U.S. church attendance. *American Sociological Review, 58,* 741–752.

Hadaway, C. K., & Roof, W. C. (1988). Apostasy in American churches: Evidence from national survey data. In D. G. Bromley (Ed.), *Falling from the faith: Causes and consequences of religious apostasy* (pp. 29–46). Newbury Park, CA: Sage.

Haddock, G. M., Zanna, M. P., & Esses, V. M. (1993). Assessing the structure of prejudicial attitudes: The case of attitudes toward homosexuals. *Journal of Personality and Social Psychology, 65,* 1105–1118.

Haerich, P. (1992). Premarital sexual permissiveness and religious orientation: A preliminary investigation. *Journal for the Scientific Study of Religion, 31,* 361–365.

Haj-Yahia, M. M. (2002). Attitudes of Arab women toward different patterns of coping with wife abuse. *Journal of Interpersonal Violence, 17,* 721–745.

Haldane, J. B. S. (1931). In *Science and religion: A symposium* (pp. 37–53). New York: Scribner.

Haldeman, D. C. (1991). Sexual orientation conversion therapy for gay men and lesbians: A scientific examination. In J. Gonsiorek & J. D. Weinrich (Eds.), *Homosexuality: Research implications for public policy* (pp. 149–160). Thousand Oaks, CA: Sage.

Haldeman, D. C. (1994), The practice and ethics of sexual orientation conversion therapy. *Journal of Consulting and Clinical Psychology, 62,* 221–227.

Haldeman, D. C. (1996). Spirituality and religion in the lives of lesbians and gay men. In R. P. Cabaj & T. S. Stein (Eds.), *Textbook of homosexuality and mental health* (pp. 881–896). Washington, DC: American Psychiatric Press.

Hale, J. R. (1977). *Who are the unchurched?* Washington, DC: Glenmary Research Center.

Halford, L. J., Anderson, C. L., & Clark, E. (1981). Prophecy fails again and again: The Morrisites. *Free Inquiry in Creative Sociology, 9,* 5–10.

Hall, B. A. (1994). Ways of maintaining hope in HIV disease. *Research in Nursing and Health, 17,* 283–293.

Hall, G. S. (1900). The religious content of the child-mind. In N. M. Butler et al., *Principles of religious education* (pp. 161–189). New York: Longmans, Green.

Hall, G. S. (1904). *Adolescence: Its psychology and relations to physiology, anthropology, sociology, sex, crime, religion and education* (2 vols.). New York: Appleton.

Hall, G. S. (1917). *Jesus, the Christ, in light of psychology* (2 vols.). Garden City, NY: Doubleday.

Hall, J. K., Zilboorg, G., & Bunker, H. A. (1944). *One hundred years of American psychiatry.* New York: Columbia University Press.

Hall, J. R. (1989). *Gone from the promised land: Jonestown in American cultural history.* New Brunswick, NJ: Transaction Books.

Hall, T. A. (1995). Spiritual effects of childhood sexual abuse in adult Christian women. *Journal of Psychology and Theology, 23,* 129–134.

Hall, T. W., & Edwards, K. J. (1996). The initial development and factor analysis of the Spiritual Assessment Inventory. *Journal of Psychology and Theology, 24,* 233–246.

Halligan, F. R. (1995). Jungian theory and religious experience. In R. W. Hood, Jr. (Ed.), *Handbook of religious experience* (pp. 231–253). Birmingham, AL: Religious Education Press.

Hamberg, E. M. (1991). Stability and change in religious beliefs, practice, and attitudes: A Swedish panel study. *Journal for the Scientific Study of Religion, 30,* 63–80.

Hamlyn, D. W. (1967). Empiricism. In P. Edwards (Ed.), *The encylopaedia of philosophy* (Vol. 2, pp. 499–504). New York: Crowell, Collier & Macmillan.

Hammond, J. A., Cole, B. S., & Beck, S. H. (1993). Religious heritage and teenage marriage. *Review of Religious Research, 35,* 117–133.

Hands, D. (1992, Fall). Clergy sexual abuse. *Saint Barnabas Community Chronicle,* pp. 1–3.

Hanford, J. T. (1991). The relationship between faith development of James Fowler and moral development of Lawrence Kohlberg: A theoretical review. *Journal of Psychology and Christianity, 10,* 306–310.

Hansen, C. (1998). Long-term effects of religious upbringing. *Mental Health, Religion and Culture, 1,* 91–111.

Hansen, J. C., & Campbell, D. P. (1985). *Manual for the SVIB-SCII.* Stanford, CA: Stanford University Press.

Hansen, K. J. (1981). *Mormonism and the American experience.* Chicago: University of Chicago Press.

Hanson, R. A. (1991). The development of moral reasoning: Some observations about Christian fundamentalism. *Journal of Psychology and Theology, 19,* 249–256.

Hardt, H. D. (1963). *Mental health status and religious attitudes of hospitalized veterans.* Unpublished doctoral dissertation, University of Texas.

Hardy, A. (1965). *The living stream.* London: Collins

Hardy, A. (1966). *The divine flame.* London: Collins.

Hardy, A. (1975). *The biology of God.* New York: Taplinger.

Hardy, A. (1979). *The spiritual nature of man: A study of contemporary religious experience.* Oxford: Clarendon Press.

Hardy, K. R. (1974). Social origins of American scientists and scholars. *Science, 185,* 497–506.

Hardyck, J. A., & Braden, M. (1962). When prophecy fails again. A report of failure to replicate. *Journal of Abnormal and Social Psychology, 65,* 136–141.

Harley, B., & Firebaugh, G. (1993). Americans' belief in an afterlife: Trends over the past two decades. *Journal for the Scientific Study of Religion, 32,* 269–278.

Harms, E. (1944). The development of religious experience in children. *American Journal of Sociology, 50,* 112–122.

Harris, N. A., Spilka, B., & Emrick, C. (1990, August 12). *Religion and alcoholism: A multidimensional approach.* Paper presented at the annual convention of the American Psychological Association, Boston.

Harris, P. L. (2000). On not falling down to earth: Children's metaphysical questions. In K. S. Rosengren, C. N. Johnson, & P. L. Harris (Eds.), *Imagining the impossible: Magical, scientific, and religious thinking in children* (pp. 157–178). Cambridge, England: Cambridge University Press.

Hart, D., & Schneider, D. (1997). Spiritual care for children with cancer. *Seminar in Oncological Nursing, 13*(4), 263–270.

Hartocollis, P. (1976). Aggression and mysticism. *Contemporary Psychoanalysis, 12,* 214–226.

Hartshorne, H., & May, M. A. (1928). *Studies in the nature of character: Vol. 1: Studies in deceit.* New York: Macmillan.

Hartshorne, H., & May, M. A. (1929). *Studies in the nature of character: Vol. 2: Studies in service and self-control.* New York: Macmillan.

Hartshorne, H., May, M. A., & Shuttleworth, F. K. (1930). *Studies in the nature of character: Vol. 3: Studies in the organization of character.* New York: Macmillan.

Hartz, G. W., & Everett, H. C. (1989). Fundamentalist religion and its effect on mental health. *Journal of Religion and Health, 28,* 207–217.

Hassan, M. K., & Khalique, A. (1987). A study of prejudice in Hindu and Muslim college students. *Psychologia: An International Journal of Psychology in the Orient, 30,* 80–84.

Hastings, P. K., & Hoge, D. R. (1976). Changes in religion among college students, 1948 to 1974. *Journal for the Scientific Study of Religion, 15,* 237–249.

Hathaway, S. R., & McKinley, J. C. (1951). *The Minnesota Multiphastic Personality Inventory manual.* New York: Psychological Corporation.

Haun, D. L. (1977). Perceptons of the bereaved, clergy, and funeral directors concerning bereavement. *Dissertation Abstracts International, 37,* 6791A.

Havens, J. (1963). The changing climate of research on the college student and his religion. *Journal for the Scientific Study of Religion, 3,* 52–69.

Havighurst, R. J., & Keating, B. (1971). The religion of youth. In M. P. Strommen (Ed.), *Research on religious development: A comprehensive handbook* (pp. 686–723). New York: Hawthorne Books.

Hawley, J. S. (Ed.). (1994a). *Fundamentalism and gender.* New York: Oxford University Press.

Hawley, J. S. (1994b). Hinduism: *Sati* and its defenders. In J. S. Hawley (Ed.), *Fundamentalism and gender* (pp. 79–110). New York: Oxford University Press.

Hawley, J. S. (Ed.). (1994c). *Sati,the blessing and the curse.* New York: Oxford University Press.

Hay, D. (1979). Religious experience amongst a group of postgraduate students: A qualitative study. *Journal for the Scientific Study of Religion, 18,* 164–182.

Hay, D. (1987). *Exploring inner space: Scientists and religious experience* (2nd ed.). London: Mowbray.

Hay, D. (1994). "The biology of God": What is the current status of Hardy's hypothesis? *International Journal for the Psychology of Religion, 4,* 1–23.

Hay, D., & Heald, G. (1987). Religion is good for you. *New Society, 80,* 20–22.

Hay, D., & Morisy, A. (1978). Reports of ecstatic, paranormal, or religious experience in Great Britain and the United States: A comparison of trends. *Journal for the Scientific Study of Religion, 17,* 255–268.

Hay, D., & Morisy, A. (1985). Secular society, religious meanings: A contemporary paradox. *Review of Religious Research, 26,* 213–227.

Hayden, J. J. (1991, August 18). *Rheumatic disease and chronic pain: Religious and affective variables.* Paper presented at the annual convention of the American Psychological Association, San Francisco.

Hayes, B. C., & Hornsby-Smith, M. P. (1994). Religious identification and family attitudes: An international comparison. *Research in the Social Scientific Study of Religion, 6,* 167–186.

Hearn, W. R. (1968). Biological science. In R. H. Bube (Ed.), *The encounter between Christianity and science* (pp. 199–223). Grand Rapids, MI: W. B. Eerdmans.

Hearnshaw, C. S. (1987). *The shaping of modern psychology.* New York: Routledge.

Heelas, P. (1985). Social anthropology and the psychology of religion. In L. B. Brown (Ed.), *Advances in the psychology of religion* (pp. 34–51). New York: Pergamon Press.

Heider, F. (1958). *The psychology of interpersonal relations.* New York: Wiley.

Heiler, F. (1932). *Prayer: A study in the history and psychology of religion.* New York: Oxford University Press.

Heirich, M. (1977). Change of heart: A test of some widely held theories of religious conversion. *American Sociological Review, 83,* 653–680.

Helfaer, P. (1972). *The psychology of religious doubt.* Boston: Beacon Press.

Helman, C. G. (1994). *Culture, health, and illness* (3rd ed.). Oxford: Butterworth–Heinemann.

Helminiak, D. A. (1987). *Spiritual development: An interdisciplinary study.* Chicago: Loyola University Press.

Helminiak, D. A. (1994). *What the Bible really says about homosexuality.* San Francisco: Alamo Square Press.

Helminiak, D. A. (1995). Non-religious lesbians and gays facing AIDS: A fully psychological approach to spirituality. *Pastoral Psychology, 43,* 301–318.

Helminiak, D. A. (1996a). A scientific spirituality: The interface of psychology and theology. *International Journal for the Psychology of Religion, 6,* 1–19.

Helminiak, D. A. (1996b). *The human core of spirituality.* Albany: State University of New York Press.

Helminiak, D. A. (1998). *Religion and the human sciences.* Albany: State University of New York Press.

Herberg, W. (1960). *Protestant, Catholic, Jew.* Garden City, NY: Doubleday.

Herek, G. M. (1987). Religious orientation and prejudice: A comparison of racial and sexual attitudes. *Personality and Social Psychology Bulletin, 13,* 34–44.

Herek, G. M. (1988). Heterosexuals' attitudes toward lesbians and gay men: Correlates and gender differences. *Journal of Sex Research, 25,* 451–477.

Herold, E., Corbesi, B., & Collins, J. (1994). Psychosocial aspects of female topless behavior on Australian beaches. *Journal of Sex Research, 31,* 133–142.

Herrick, C. J. (1956). *The evolution of human nature.* Austin: University of Texas Press.

Hertel, B. R., & Donahue, M. J. (1995). Parental influences on God images among children: Testing Durkheim's metaphoric parallelism. *Journal for the Scientific Study of Religion, 34,* 186–199.

Herzbrun, M. B. (1993). Father–adolescent religious consensus in the Jewish community: A preliminary report. *Journal for the Scientific Study of Religion, 32,* 163–168.

Hewstone, M. (Ed.). (1983a). *Attribution theory: Social and functional extensions.* Oxford: Blackwell.

Hewstone, M. (1983b). Attribution theory and common-sense explanations: An introductory overview. In M. Hewstone (Ed.), *Attribution theory: Social and functional extensions* (pp. 1–27). Oxford: Blackwell.

Hewstone, M., Islam, M. R., & Judd, C. M. (1993). Models of crossed categorization and intergroup relations. *Journal of Personality and Social Psychology, 64,* 779–793.

Hick, J. (1989). *An interpretation of religion.* New Haven, CT: Yale University Press.

Hickman, F. S. (1926). *Introduction to the psychology of religion.* New York: Abingdon Press.

Higdon, J. F. (1986, September). *Association of fundamentalism with MPD.* Paper presented at the Third International Conference on Multiple Personality Disorder, Chicago.

Higgins, E. T. (1989). Continuities and discontinuities in self-regulatory and self-evaluative processes: A developmental theory relating self and affect. *Journal of Personality, 57,* 407–444.

Hightower, P. R. (1930). Biblical information in relation to character and conduct. *University of Iowa Studies in Character, 3*(2), 72.

Hilgard, E. R. (1973). A neodissociation interpretation of pain reduction in hypnosis. *Psychological Review, 80,* 396–411.

Hilgard, E. R. (1986). *Divided consciousness: Multiple controls in human thought and action.* New York: Wiley.

Hill, P. C. (1994). Toward an attitude process model of religious experience. *Journal for the Scientific Study of Religion, 33,* 303–314.

Hill, P. C. (1995). Affective theory and religious experience. In R. W. Hood, Jr. (Ed.), *Handbook of religious experience* (pp. 353–377). Birmingham, AL: Religious Education Press.

Hill, P. C., & Bassett, R. L. (1992). Getting to the heart of the matter: What the social-psychological study of attitudes has to offer psychology of religion. *Research in the Social Scientific Study of Religion, 4,* 159–182.

Hill, P. C., & Pargament, K. I. (2003). Advances in the conceptualization and measurement of religion and spirituality: Implications for physical and mental health research. *American Psychologist, 58,* 64–74.

Hill, P. C., Pargament, K. L., Hood, R. W., Jr., McCullough, M. E., Swyers, J. P., Larson, D. B., & Zinnbauer, B. J. (2000). Conceptualizing religion and spirituality: Points of commonality, points of departure. *Journal for the Theory of Social Behavior, 30,* 51–77.

Hill, P., & Hood, R. W., Jr. (1999a). *Measures of religiosity.* Birmingham, AL: Religious Education Press.

Hill, P., & Hood, R. W., Jr. (1999b). Religion, affect and the unconscious. *Journal of Personality, 67,* 1015–1046.

Hiltner, S. (1949). *Pastoral counseling.* New York: Abingdon–Cokesbury.

Hiltner, S. (1962). Conclusion: The dialogue on man's nature. In S. Doniger (Ed.), *The nature of man in theological and psychological perspective* (pp. 237–261). New York: Harper.

Himmelfarb, G. (1962). *Darwin and the Darwinian revolution.* Garden City, NY: Doubleday.

Himmelfarb, H. S. (1979). Agents of religious socialization among American Jews. *Sociological Quarterly, 20,* 477–494.

Hinde, R. A. (1999). *Why gods persist: A scientific approach to religion.* London: Routledge.

Hine, V. H. (1969). Pentecostal glossolalia: Toward a functional interpretation. *Journal for the Scientific Study of Religion, 8,* 211–226.

Hinkle, L. E., Jr., & Wolff, H. E. (1956). Communist interrogation and the indoctrination of "enemies of the states." *Archives of Neurology and Psychiatry, 76,* 117.

Hippocrates. (1952). The sacred disease. In R. M. Hutchins (Ed.), *Great books of the Western World* (Vol. 10, pp. 154–160). Chicago: Encyclopedia Britannica.

Hirschi, T., & Stark, R. (1969). Hellfire and delinquency. *Social Problems, 17,* 202–213.

Hirsley, M. (1993, May 18). Resurgent religion: 13–nation study finds belief in God. *The Denver Post,* pp. 2A, 4A.

Hochstein, L. M. (1986). Pastoral counselors: Their attitudes toward gay and lesbian clients. *Journal of Pastoral Care, 40,* 158–165.

Hodges, D. L. (1974). Breaking a scientific taboo: Putting assumptions about the supernatural into scientific theories of religion. *Journal for the Scientific Study of Religion, 13,* 393–408.

Hoebel, E. A. (1966). *Anthropology: The study of man.* New York: McGraw-Hill.

Hoelter, J. W., & Epley, R. J. (1979). Religious correlates of the fear of death. *Journal for the Scientific Study of Religion, 9,* 163–172.

Hoffman, S. J. (1992, November). *Prayers, piety and pigskins: Religion in modern sports.* Paper presented at the annual convention of the Society for the Scientific Study of Religion, Washington, DC.

Hoffman, V. J. (1995). Muslim fundamentalists: Psychosocial profiles. In M. E. Marty & R. S. Appleby (Eds.), *Fundamentalism comprehended* (pp. 199–230). Chicago: University of Chicago Press.

Hoge, D. R. (1981). *Converts, dropouts, returnees: A study of religious change among catholics.* New York: Pilgrim Press.

Hoge, D. R. (1988). Why Catholics drop out. In D. G. Bromley (Ed.), *Falling from the faith: Causes and consequences of religious apostasy* (pp. 81–99). Newbury Park, CA: Sage.

Hoge, D. R., & Carroll, J. W. (1973). Religiosity and prejudice in Northern and Southern churches. *Journal for the Scientific Study of Religion, 12,* 181–197.

Hoge, D. R., Heffernan, E., Hemrick, E. F., Nelsen, H. M., O'Connor, J. P., Philibert, P. J., & Thompson, A. D. (1982). Desired outcomes of religious education and youth ministry in six denominations. *Review of Religious Research, 23,* 230–254.

Hoge, D. R., Johnson, B., & Luidens, D. A. (1993). Determinants of church involvement of young adults who grew up in Presbyterian churches. *Journal for the Scientific Study of Religion, 32,* 242–255.

Hoge, D. R., Johnson, B., & Luidens, D. A. (1995). Types of denominational switching among Protestant young adults. *Journal for the Scientific Study of Religion, 34,* 253–258.

Hoge, D. R., & Keeter, L. G. (1976). Determinants of college teachers' religious beliefs and participation. *Journal for the Scientific Study of Religion, 15,* 221–235.

Hoge, D. R., with McGuire, K., & Stratman, B. F. (1981). *Converts, dropouts, returnees: A study of religious change among Catholics.* New York: Pilgrim Press.

Hoge, D. R., & Petrillo, G. H. (1978a). Determinants of church participation among high school youth. *Journal for the Scientific Study of Religion, 17,* 359–379.

Hoge, D. R., & Petrillo, G. H. (1978b). Development of religious thinking in adolescence: A test of Goldman's theories. *Journal for the Scientific Study of Religion, 17,* 139–154.

Hoge, D. R., Petrillo, G. H., & Smith, E. I. (1982). Transmission of religious and social values from parents to teenage children. *Journal of Marriage and the Family, 44,* 569–580.

Hoge, D. R., & Thompson, A. D. (1982). Different conceptualizations of goals of religious education and youth ministry in six denominations. *Review of Religious Research, 23,* 297–304.

Hoge, D. R., & Yang, F. (1994). Determinants of religious giving in religious denominations: Data from two nationwide surveys. *Review of Religious Research, 36,* 123–148.

Hoggatt, L., & Spilka, B. (1978). The nurse and the terminally ill patient. *Omega, 9,* 255–256.

Holahan, C. J., & Moos, R. H. (1987). Personal and contextual determinants of coping strategies. *Journal of Personality and Social Psychology, 52,* 946–955.

Holden, G. W., & Edwards, L. A. (1989). Parental attitudes toward child rearing: Instruments, issues, and implications. *Psychological Bulletin, 106,* 29–58.

Holder, D. W., Durant, R. H., Harris, T. L., Daniel, J. H., Obeidallah, D., & Goodman, E. (2000). The association between adolescent spirituality and voluntary sexual activity. *Journal of Adolescent Health, 26,* 295–302.

Holley, R. T. (1991). Assessing potential bias: The effects of adding religious content to the Defining Issues Test. *Journal of Psychology and Christianity, 10,* 323–336.

Hollingshead, A. B., & Redlich, F. C. (1958). *Social class and mental illness.* New York: Wiley.

Holm, N. G. (1982). Mysticism and intense experiences. *Journal for the Scientific Study of Religion, 21,* 268–276.

Holm, N. G. (1987a). *Scandinavian psychology of religion.* Åbo, Finland: Åbo Akademi.

Holm, N. G. (1987b). Sundén's role theory and glossolalia. *Journal for the Scientific Study of Religion, 26,* 383–389.

Holm, N. G. (1991). Pentecostalism: Conversion and charismata. *International Journal for the Psychology of Religion, 1,* 135–151.

Holm, N. G. (1995). Role theory and religious experience. In R. W. Hood, Jr. (Ed.), *Handbook of religious experience* (pp. 397–420). Birmingham, AL: Religious Education Press.

Holm, N. G., & Belzen, J. A. (Eds.). (1995). *Sundén's role theory: An impetus to contemporary psychology of religion.* Åbo, Finland: Åbo Akademi.

Holmes, U. T. (1980). *A history of Christian spirituality.* New York: Seabury Press.

Holt, J. (2002, April 14). 'Intelligent design creationism and its critics': Supernatural selection. *The New*

York Times [Online]. Available: http://www.nytimes.com/2002/04/14/books/review/14Holtlt. html?rd=hcmcp?p=042q [Retrieved April 14, 2002].

Holtz, T. H. (1998). Refugee trauma aversus torture trauma: A retrospective controlled cohort study of Tibetan refugees. *Journal of Nervous and Mental Disease, 186,* 24–34.

Homola, M., Knudsen, D., & Marshall, H. (1987). Religion and socioeconomic achievement. *Journal for the Scientific Study of Religion, 26,* 201–217.

Hong, G.-Y. (1995). Buddhism and religious experience. In R. W. Hood, Jr. (Ed.), *Handbook of religious experience* (pp. 87–121). Birmingham, AL: Religious Education Press.

Honigmann, J. J. (1959). *The world of man.* New York Harper & Row.

Hood, R. W., Jr. (1970). Religious orientation and the report of religious experience. *Journal for the Scientific Study of Religion, 9,* 285–291.

Hood, R. W., Jr. (1973a). Hypnotic susceptibility and reported religious experience. *Psychological Reports, 33,* 549–550.

Hood, R. W., Jr. (1973b). Religious orientation and the experience of transcendence. *Journal for the Scientific Study of Religion, 12,* 441–448.

Hood, R. W., Jr. (1974). Psychological strength and the report of intense religious experience. *Journal for the Scientific Study of Religion, 13,* 65–71.

Hood, R. W., Jr. (1975). The construction and preliminary validation of a measure of reported mystical experience. *Journal for the Scientific Study of Religion, 14,* 29–41.

Hood, R. W., Jr. (1976a). Conceptual criticisms of regressive explanations of mysticism. *Review of Religious Research, 7,* 179–188.

Hood, R. W., Jr. (1976b). Mystical experience as related to present and anticipated future church participation. *Psychological Reports, 39,* 1127–1136.

Hood, R. W., Jr. (1977). Eliciting mystical states of consciousness with semistructured nature experiences. *Journal for the Scientific Study of Religion, 16,* 155–163.

Hood, R. W., Jr. (1978a). Anticipatory set and setting: Stress incongruity as elicitors of mystical experience in solitary nature situations. *Journal for the Scientific Study of Religion, 17,* 278–287.

Hood, R. W., Jr. (1978b). The usefulness of the indiscriminatively pro and anti categories of religious orientation. *Journal for the Scientific Study of Religion, 17,* 419–431.

Hood, R. W., Jr. (1980). Social legitimacy, dogmatism, and the evaluation of intense experiences. *Review of Religious Research, 21,* 184–194.

Hood, R. W., Jr. (1983). Social psychology and religious fundamentalism. In A. W. Childs & G. B. Melton (Eds.), *Rural psychology* (pp. 169–198). New York: Plenum Press.

Hood, R. W., Jr. (1985). Mysticism. In P. Hammond (Ed.), *The sacred in a secular age* (pp. 285–297). Berkeley: University of California Press.

Hood, R. W., Jr. (1989). Mysticism, the unity thesis, and the paranormal. In G. K. Zollschan, J. F. Schumaker, & G. F. Walsh (Eds). *Exploring the paranormal: Perspectives on belief and experience* (pp. 117–130). New York: Avery.

Hood, R. W., Jr. (1991). Holm's use of role theory: Empirical and hermeneutical considerations of sacred text as a source of role adoption. *International Journal for the Psychology of Religion, 1,* 153–159.

Hood, R. W., Jr. (1992a). A Jamesean look at self and self loss in mysticism. *Journal of the Psychology of Religion, 1,* 1–14.

Hood, R. W., Jr. (1992b). Mysticism, reality, illusion and the Freudian critique of religion. *International Journal for the Psychology of Religion, 2,* 141–159.

Hood, R. W., Jr. (1992c). Sin and guilt in faith traditions: Issues for self-esteem. In J. F. Schumaker (Ed.), *Religion and mental health* (pp. 110–121). New York: Oxford Univerity Press.

Hood, R. W., Jr. (1994). Psychology and religion. In U. S. Ramachdran (Ed.), *Encyclopaedia of human behavior* (Vol. 3, pp. 619–629). New York: Academic Press.

Hood, R. W., Jr. (1995a). The facilitation of religious experience. In R. W. Hood, Jr. (Ed.), *Handbook of religious experience* (pp. 569–597). Birmingham, AL: Religious Education Press.

Hood, R. W., Jr. (Ed.). (1995b). *Handbook of religious experience.* Birmingham, AL: Religious Education Press.

Hood, R. W., Jr. (1995c). The soulful self of William James. In D. W. Capps & J. L. Jacobs (Eds.), *The struggle for life: A companion to William James's* The varieties of religious experience (Society for the Scientific Study of Religion Monograph Series, Whole No. 9, pp. 209–219). West Lafayette, IN: Society for the Scientific Study of Religion.

Hood, R. W., Jr. (1998). When the spirit maims and kills: Social psychological considerations of the history of serpent handling sects and the narrative of handlers. *International Journal for the Psychology of Religion, 8,* 71–86.

Hood, R. W., Jr. (2000a). American psychology of religion and the *Journal for the Scientific Study of Religion. Journal for the Scientific Study of Religion, 39,* 531–543.

Hood, R. W., Jr. (2000b, October). *The relationship between religion and spirituality.* Paper presented at the annual convention of the Society for the Scientific Study of Religion, Houston, TX.

Hood, R. W., Jr. (2002a). The mystical self: Lost and found. *International Journal for the Psychology of Religion, 12,* 1–14.

Hood, R. W., Jr. (2002b). *Dimensions of mystical experiences: Empirical studies and psychological links.* Amsterdam: Rhodopi.

Hood, R. W., Jr. (2003). The relationship between religion and spirituality. In D. Bromley (Series Ed.) & A. L. Greil & D. Bromley (Vol. Eds.), *Defining religion: Investigating the boundaries between the sacred and the secular: Vol. 10. Religion and the social order* (pp. 241–265). Amsterdam, The Netherlands: Elsevier Science.

Hood, R. W., Jr., Ghorbani, N., Watson, P. J., Ghramaleki, A. F., Bing, M. B., Davison, H. R., Morris, R. J., & Williamson, P. J. (2001). Dimensions of the Mysticism Scale: Confirming the three factor structure in the United States and Iran. *Journal for the Scientific Study of Religion, 40,* 691–705.

Hood, R. W., Jr., & Hall, J. R. (1977). Comparison of reported religious experience in Caucasian, American Indian, and two Mexican American samples. *Psychological Reports, 41,* 657–658.

Hood, R. W., Jr., & Hall, J. R. (1980). Gender differences in the description of erotic and mystical experience. *Review of Religious Research, 21,* 195–207.

Hood, R. W., Jr., & Kimbrough, D. (1995). Serpent-handling Holiness sects: Theoretical considerations. *Journal for the Scientific Study of Religion, 34,* 311–322.

Hood, R. W., Jr., & Morris, R. J. (1981). Knowledge and experience criteria in the report of mystical experience. *Review of Religious Research, 23,* 76–84.

Hood, R. W., Jr., & Morris, R. J. (1983). Toward a theory of death transcendence. *Journal for the Scientific Study of Religion, 22,* 353–365.

Hood, R. W., Jr., Morris, R. J., & Harvey, D. K. (1993, October). *Religiosity, prayer and their relationship to mystical experience.* Paper presented at the annual meeting of the Religious Research Association, Raleigh, NC.

Hood, R. W., Jr., Morris, R. J., Hickman, S. E., & Watson, P. J. (1995). Martin and Malcolm as cultural icons: An empirical study comparing lower class African American and white males. *Review of Religious Research, 36,* 382–388.

Hood, R. W., Jr., Morris, R. J., & Watson, P. J. (1985). Boundary maintenance, socio-political views, and presidential preference. *Review of Religious Research, 27,* 134–145.

Hood, R. W., Jr., Morris, R. J., & Watson, P. J. (1986). Maintenance of religious fundamentalism. *Psychological Reports, 9,* 547–559.

Hood, R. W., Jr., Morris, R. J., & Watson, P. J. (1987). Religious orientation and prayer experience. *Psychological Reports, 60,* 1201–1202.

Hood, R. W., Jr., Morris, R. J., & Watson, P. J. (1989). Prayer experience and religious orientation. *Review of Religious Research, 31,* 39–45.

Hood, R. W., Jr., Morris, R. J., & Watson, P. J. (1991). Male commitment to the cult of the Virgin Mary and the passion of Christ as a function of early maternal bonding. *International Journal for the Psychology of Religion, 1,* 221–231.

Hood, R. W., Jr., Morris, R. J., & Watson, P. J. (1993). Further factor analysis of Hood's Mysticism Scale. *Psychological Reports, 3,* 1176–1178.

Hood, R. W., Jr., Spilka, B., Hunsberger, B., & Gorsuch, R. L. (1996). *The psychology of religion: An empirical approach* (2nd ed.). New York: Guilford Press.

Hood, R. W., Jr., & Williamson, W. P. (2000). An empirical test of the unity thesis: The structure of mystical descriptors in various faith samples. *Journal of Christianity and Psychology, 19,* 222–244.

Hood, R. W., Jr., Williamson, W. P., & Morris, R. J. (1999). Evaluation of the legitimacy of conversion experience as a function of the five signs of Mark 16. *Review of Religious Research, 41,* 96–109.

Hood, R. W., Jr., Williamson, W. P., & Morris, R. J. (2000). Changing views of serpent handling: A quasi-experimental study. *Journal for the Scientific Study of Religion, 39,* 287–296.

Hooper, T. (1962). *Some meanings and correlates of future time and death among college students.* Unpublished doctoral dissertation, University of Denver.

Hooper, T., & Spilka, B. (1970). Some meanings and correlates of future time and death perspectives among college students. *Omega, 1,* 49–56.

Hope, L. C., & Cook, C. C. H. (2001). The role of Christian commitment in predicting drug use amongst church affiliated young people. *Mental Health, Religion and Culture, 4,* 109–117.

Horn, J. L. (1967). On subjectivity in factor analysis. *Educational and Psychological Measurement, 27,* 811–820.

Horner, J., & Dobb, E. (1997). *Dinosaur lives.* New York: HarperCollins.

Horowitz, I. L. (1983a). Symposium on scholarship and sponsorship: Universal standards, not universal beliefs. Further reflections on scientific method and religious sponsors. *Sociological Analysis, 44,* 179–182.

Horowitz, I. L. (1983b). A reply to critics and crusaders. *Sociological Analysis, 44,* 221–225.

Horstmann, M. J., & Tonigan, J. S. (2000). Faith development in Alcoholics Anonymous (AA): A study of two AA groups. *Alcoholism Treatment Quarterly, 18,* 75–84.

Horton, P. C. (1973). The mystical experience as a suicide preventative. *American Journal of Psychiatry, 130,* 294–296.

Hostetler, J. A. (1968). *Amish society* (rev. ed.). Baltimore: Johns Hopkins University Press.

Hostetler, J. A., & Huntington, G. E. (1967). *The Hutterites in North America.* New York: Holt, Rinehart & Winston.

Hoult, T. F. (1958). *The sociology of religion.* New York: Dryden.

Hout, M., & Greeley, A. M. (1990). The cohort doesn't hold: Comment on Chaves (1989). *Journal for the Scientific Study of Religion, 29,* 519–524.

Howkins, K. G. (1966). *Religious thinking and religious education.* London: Tyndale Press.

Hoyert, D. L., Kochanek, K. D., & Murphy, S. L. (1999). *Deaths: Final data for 1997* (National Vital Statistics Report 47(19), DHHS Publication No. 99-1120) [Online]. Available: http://www.cdc.gov/n;chs/data/nvs47_19.pdf [Retrieved February 16, 2002].

Huber, S., Reich, K. H., & Schenker, D. (2000, July). *Studying empirically religious development: Interview, repertory grid, and specific questionnaire techniques.* Paper presented at the Symposium for Psychologists of Religion, Sigtuna, Sweden.

Huck, D. M., & Armer, J. M. (1995). Affectivity and mental health among elderly religious. *Issues in Mental Health Nursing, 16,* 447–459.

Hudson, W. H. (1939). *Far away and long ago.* London: Dent.

Hufford, D. J. (1982). *The terror that comes in the night: An experience-centered study of supernatural assault traditions.* Philadelphia: University of Pennsylvania Press.

Hughes, P. (1954). *A popular history of the Catholic church.* Garden City, NY: Doubleday.

Hughes, P., Bellamy, J., Black, A., & Kaldor, P. (2000). Dropping out of church: The Australian experience. In L. J. Francis & Y. J. Katz (Eds.), *Joining and leaving religion: Research perspectives* (pp. 167–194). Leominster, England: Gracewing.

Hull, D. B., & Burke, J. (1991). The religious right, attitudes toward women, and tolerance for sexual abuse. *Journal of Offender Rehabilitation, 17,* 1–12.

Hundleby, J. D. (1987). Adolescent drug use in a behavioral matrix: A confirmation and comparison of the sexes. *Addictive Behaviors, 12,* 103–112.

Hunsberger, B. (1976). Background religious denomination, parental emphasis, and the religious orientation of university students. *Journal for the Scientific Study of Religion, 15,* 251–255.

Hunsberger, B. (1977). A reconsideration of parochial schools: The case of Mennonites and Roman Catholics. *Mennonite Quarterly Review, 51,* 140–151.

Hunsberger, B. (1978). The religiosity of college students: Stability and change over years at university. *Journal for the Scientific Study of Religion, 17,* 159–164.

Hunsberger, B. (1980). A reexamination of the antecedents of apostasy. *Review of Religious Research, 21,* 158–170.

Hunsberger, B. (1983a). Apostasy: A social learning perspective. *Review of Religious Research, 25,* 21–38.

Hunsberger, B. (1983b). *Current religious position and self-reports of religious socialization influences.* Paper presented at the annual convention of the Society for the Scientific Study of Religion, Knoxville, TN.

Hunsberger, B. (1983c). *Religion and attribution theory: A test of the actor–observer bias.* Paper presented at the annual convention for the Society for the Scientific Study of Religion, Knoxville, TN.

Hunsberger, B. (1985a). Parent–university student agreement on religious and nonreligious issues. *Journal for the Scientific Study of Religion, 24,* 314–320.

Hunsberger, B. (1985b). Religion, age, life satisfaction, and perceived sources of religiousness: A study of older persons. *Journal of Gerontology, 40,* 615–620

Hunsberger, B. (1995). Religion and prejudice: The role of religious fundamentalism, quest, and right-wing authoritarianism. *Journal of Social Issues, 51,* 113–129.

Hunsberger, B. (1996). Religious fundamentalism, right-wing authoritarianism, and hostility toward homosexuals in nonChristian religious groups. *International Journal for the Psychology of Religion, 6,* 39–49.

Hunsberger, B. (2000). Swimming against the current: Exceptional cases of apostates and converts. In L. J. Francis & Y. J. Katz (Eds.), *Joining and leaving religion: Research perspectives.* (pp. 233–248). Leominster, England: Gracewing.

Hunsberger, B., Alisat, S., Pancer, S. M., & Pratt, M. (1996). Religious fundamentalism and religious doubts: Content, connections, and complexity of thinking. *International Journal for the Psychology of Religion, 6,* 201–220.

Hunsberger, B., & Brown, L. B. (1984). Religious socialization, apostasy, and the impact of family background. *Journal for the Scientific Study of Religion, 23,* 239–251.

Hunsberger, B., & Ennis, J. (1982). Experimenter effects in studies of religious attitudes. *Journal for the Scientific Study of Religion, 21,* 131–137.

Hunsberger, B., & Jackson, L. (in press). Religion, meaning, and prejudice. *Journal of Social Issues.*

Hunsberger, B., Lea, J., Pancer, S. M., Pratt, M., & McKenzie, B. (1992). Making life complicated: Prompting the use of integratively complex thinking. *Journal of Personality, 60,* 95–114.

Hunsberger, B., McKenzie, B., Pratt, M., & Pancer, S. M. (1993). Religious doubt: A social psychological analysis. *Research in the Social Scientific Study of Religion, 5,* 27–51.

Hunsberger, B., Owusu, V., & Duck, R. (1999). Religion and prejudice in Ghana and Canada: Religious fundamentalism, right-wing authoritarianism and attitudes toward homosexuals and women. *International Journal for the Psychology of Religion, 9,* 181–194.

Hunsberger, B., Pancer, S. M., Pratt, M., & Alisat, S. (1996). The transition to university: Is religion related to adjustment? *Research in the Social Scientific Study of Religion, 7,* 181–199.

Hunsberger, B., & Platonow, E. (1986). Religion and helping charitable causes. *Journal of Psychology, 120,* 517–528.

Hunsberger, B., Pratt, M., & Pancer, S. M. (1994). Religious fundamentalism and integrative complexity of thought: A relationship for existential content only? *Journal for the Scientific Study of Religion, 33,* 335–346.

Hunsberger, B., Pratt, M., & Pancer, S. M. (2001a). Adolescent identity formation: Religious exploration and commitment. *Identity: An International Journal of Theory and Research, 1,* 365–387.

Hunsberger, B., Pratt, M., & Pancer, S. M. (2001b). Religious versus nonreligious socialization: Does religious background have implications for adjustment? *International Journal for the Psychology of Religion, 11,* 105–128.

Hunsberger, B., Pratt, M., & Pancer, S. M. (2002). A longitudinal study of religious doubts in high school and beyond: Relationships, stability, and searching for answers. *Journal for the Scientific Study of Religion, 41,* 255–266.

Hunsberger, B., & Watson, B. (1986, November). *The Devil made me do it: Attributions of responsibility to God and Satan.* Paper presented at the annual convention of the Society for the Scientific Study of Religion, Washington, DC.

Hunt, M. (1959). *The natural history of love.* New York: Knopf.

Hunt, R. A. (1972). Mythological–symbolic religious commitment: The LAM scales. *Journal for the Scientific Study of Religion, 11,* 42–52.

Hunt, R. A., & King, M. B. (1978). Religiosity and marriage. *Journal for the Scientific Study of Religion, 17,* 399–406.

Hunter, E. (1951). *Brainwashing in red China.* New York: Vanguard.

Hunter, J. A. (2001). Self-esteem and in-group bias among members of a religious social category. *Journal of Social Psychology, 141,* 401–411.

Hunter, W. F. (Ed.). (1989). The case for theological literacy in the psychology of religion [special issue]. *Journal of Psychology and Theology, 17.*

Hur, Y.-M., & Bouchard, T. J., Jr. (1997). The genetic correlation between impulsivity and sensation seeking traits. *Behavior Genetics, 27,* 455–463.

Hutch, R. A. (1980). The personal ritual of glossolalia. *Journal for the Scientific Study of Religion, 19,* 255–266.

Hutsebaut, D., & Verhoeven, D. (1995). Studying dimensions of God representation: Choosing closed or open-ended research questions. *International Journal for the Psychology of Religion, 5,* 49–60.

Huxley, J. (1966). A discussion on ritualization of behavior in animals and man: Introduction. *Philosophical Transactions of the Royal Society of London, Series B, Biological Sciences, 251,* 249–272.

Huxley, J. (1968). Ritual in human society. In D. R. Cutler (Ed.), *The religious situation: 1968* (pp. 696–711). Boston: Beacon Press.

Hyde, K. E. (1990). *Religion in childhood and adolescence: A comprehensive review of the research.* Brimingham, AL: Religious Education Press.

Hynam, C. A. (1970). The influence of superstition, religion and science upon anomie in a modern Western setting. *Revue Internationale de Sociologie, 6,* 190–215.

Iannaccone, L. (1994). Why strict churches are strong. *American Journal of Sociology, 99,* 1180–1211.

Iannaccone, L. (1996). Reassessing church growth: Statistical pitfalls and their consequences. *Journal for the Scientific Study of Religion, 36,* 141–157.

Ibrahim, S. E. (1980). Anatomy of Egypt's militant groups. *International Journal of Middle East Studies, 12,* 423–453.

Ibrahim, S. E. (1982). Islamic militancy as a social movement. In A. E. M. Dessouki (Ed.), *Islamic resurgence in the Arab world* (pp. 117–137). New York: Praeger.

Ice, M. L. (1987). *Clergy women and their worldviews.* New York: Praeger.

Idler, E. L., & Kasl, S. V. (1992). Religion, disability, depression and the timing of death. *American Journal of Sociology, 97,* 1052–1079.

Illich, I. (1976). *Medical nemesis: The expropriation of health.* New York: Pantheon Books.

Ineichen, B. (1998). The influence of religion on the suicide rate: Islam and Hinduism compared. *Mental Health, Religion, and Culture, 1,* 31–36.

Inge, D. (1899). *Christian mysticism.* London: Methuen.

Inglehart, R., & Baker, W. E. (2000). Modernization, cultural change, and the persistence of traditional values. *American Sociological Review, 65,* 19–51.

Insel, T. R. (1993). Oxytocin and the neuroendocrine basis of affiliation. In J. Schulkin (Ed.), *Hormonal induced change in mind and brain.* (pp. 225–251). San Diego, CA: Academic Press.

Institute for the Scientific Study of Meditation. (2001). *The effect of meditation on the brain activity in Tibetan meditators* [Online]. Available: http://www.members.aol.com/InstSSM/frontal.html [Retrieved June 20, 2001].

Irvine, W. (1955). *Apes, angels, and Victorians.* London: Weidenfeld, & Nicholson.

Isley, P. J. (1997). Child sexual abuse and the Catholic church: An historical and contemporary review. *Pastoral Psychology, 45,* 277–299.

Isralowitz, R. E., & Ong, T. (1990). Religious values and beliefs and place of residence as predictors of alcohol use among Chinese college students in Singapore. *International Journal of the Addictions, 25*, 515–529.

Jackman, M. R. (1994). *The velvet glove: Paternalism and conflict in gender, class, and race relations.* Berkeley, CA: University of California Press.

Jackson, C. W., Jr., & Kelly, E. L. (1962). Influence of suggestion and subject's prior knowledge in research on sensory deprivation. *Science, 132*, 211–212.

Jackson, G. (1908). *The fact of conversion: The Cole Lectures for 1908.* New York: Revell.

Jackson, L. M. (2001, May). Problems and promise in religious intergroup relations. In V. Saroglou (Chair), *Pluralism and Identity.* Symposium conducted at the University Catholique de Louvain, Belgium.

Jackson, L. M., & Esses, V. M. (1997). Of scripture and ascription: The relation between religious fundamentalism and intergroup helping. *Personality and Social Psychology Bulletin, 23*, 893–906.

Jackson, L. M., & Hunsberger, B. (1999). An intergroup perspective on religion and prejudice. *Journal for the Scientific Study of Religion, 38*, 509–523.

Jackson, N. J., & Spilka, B. (1980, April 10). *Correlates of religious mystical experience: A selective study.* Paper presented at the annual convention of the Rocky Mountain Psychological Association, Tucson, AZ.

Jacobs, D. M. (1992). *Secret life: First-hand accounts of UFO abductions.* New York: Simon & Schuster.

Jacobs, J. L. (1984). The economy of love in religious commitment: The deconversion of women from nontraditional religious movements. *Journal for the Scientific Study of Religion, 23*, 155–171.

Jacobs, J. L. (1987). Deconversion from religious movements: An analysis of charismatic bonding and spiritual commitment. *Journal for the Scientific Study of Religion, 26*, 294–308.

Jacobs, J. L. (1989). *Divine disenchantment.* Bloomington: Indiana University Press.

Jacobs, J. L. (1996). Women, ritual, and secrecy: The creation of crypto-Jewish culture. *Journal for the Scientific Study of Religion, 35*, 97–108.

Jacobson, C. (1999). Denominational and racial ethnic differences in fatalism. *Review of Religious Research, 41*, 3–20.

Jacobson, C. K. (1998). Religiosity and prejudice: An update and denominational analysis. *Review of Religious Research, 39*, 264–272.

Jacobson, E., & Bruno, J. (1994). Narrative variants and major psychiatric illnesses in close encounter and abduction narrators. In A. Pritchard, D. E. Prichard, J. E. Mack, P. Kasey, & C. Yapp (Eds.), *Alien discussions: Proceedings of the Abduction Study Conference, MIT* (pp. 304–309). Cambridge, MA: North Cambridge Press.

Jahreiss, W. O. (1942). Some influences of Catholic education and creed upon psychotic reactions. *Diseases of the Nervous System, 3*, 377–381.

James, W. (1950). *The principles of psychology* (2 vols.). New York: Dover. (Original work published 1890)

James, W. (1985). *The varieties of religious experience.* Cambridge, MA: Harvard University Press. (Original work published 1902)

Janssen, J., de Hart, J., & den Draak, C. (1990). A content analysis of the praying practices of Dutch youth. *Journal for the Scientific Study of Religion, 29*, 99–107.

Janssen, J., De Hart, J., & Gerardts, M. (1994). Images of God in adolescence. *International Journal for the Psychology of Religion, 4*, 105–121.

Jantzen, G. M. (1995). *Power, gender, and Christian mysticism.* Cambridge, England: Cambridge University Press.

Janus, S. S., & Janus, C. L. (1993). *The Janus report on sexual behavior.* New York: Wiley.

Jarusiewicz, B. (2000). Spirituality and addiction: Relationship to recovery and relapse. *Alcoholism Treatment Quarterly, 18*, 99–109.

Jaynes, J. (1976). *The origin of consciousness in the breakdown of the bicameral mind.* Boston: Houghton Mifflin.

Jeffers, F. C., Nichols, C. R., & Eisdorfer, C. (1961). Attitudes of older persons toward death: A preliminary study. *Journal of Gerontology, 16*, 53–56.

Jelen, T. G., & Wilcox, C. (1992). The effects of religious identification on support for the New Christian Right: An analysis of political activists. *Social Science Journal, 29,* 199–210.

Jenkins, R. A., & Pargament, K. I. (1988). The relationship between cognitive appraisals and psychological adjustment in cancer patients. *Social Science and Medicine, 26,* 625–633.

Jennings, T. W. (1990). Homosexuality. In R. J. Hunter, H. N. Malony, L. O. Mills, & J. Patton (Eds.), *Dictionary of pastoral care and counseling* (pp. 529–532). Nashville, TN: Abingdon Press.

Jensen, G. F., & Erickson, M. L. (1979). The religious factor and delinquency: Another look at the hellfire hypotheses. In R. Wuthnow (Ed.), *The religious dimension: New directions in quantitative research* (pp. 157–177). New York: Academic Press.

Jensen, I. K. K. (1989). Belief in God: Impetus for social action. In W. R. Garrett (Ed.), *Social consequences of religious belief* (pp. 90–99). New York: Paragon House.

Jernigan, H. L. (1976). Bringing together psychology and theology: Reflections on ministry to the bereaved. *Journal of Pastoral Care, 30,* 88–102.

Johnson, B. (1961). Do Holiness sects socialize in dominant values? *Social Forces, 39,* 309–317.

Johnson, B. (1963). On church and sect. *American Sociological Review, 28,* 539–549.

Johnson, B. (1971). Church and sect revisited. *Journal for the Scientific Study of Religion, 10,* 124–137.

Johnson, B. L., Eberly, S., Duke, J. T., & Sartain, D. H. (1988). Wives' employment status and marital happiness of religious couples. *Review of Religious Research, 29,* 259–270.

Johnson, B. R., Jang, S. J., Larson, D. B., & Li, S. D. (2001). Does adolescent religious commitment matter? A reexamination of the effects of religiosity on delinquency. *Journal of Research in Crime and Delinquency, 38,* 22–44.

Johnson, B. R., Jang, S. J., Li, S. D., & Larson, D. (2000). The 'invisible institution' and black youth crime: The church as an agency of local social control. *Journal of Youth and Adolescence, 29,* 479–498.

Johnson, D. M., Williams, J. S., & Bromley, D. G. (1986). Religion, health and healing: Findings from a southern city. *Sociological Analysis, 47,* 66–73.

Johnson, D. P. (1979). Dilemmas of charismatic leadership: The case of the People's Temple. *Sociological Analysis, 40,* 315–323.

Johnson, D. P., & Mullins, L. C. (1989). Subjective and social dimensions of religiosity and loneliness among the well elderly. *Review of Religious Research, 31,* 3–15.

Johnson, M. A. (1973). Family life and religious commitment. *Review of Religious Research, 14,* 144–150.

Johnson, M. A., Lohr, H., Wagner, J., & Barge, W. (1975). *The relationship between pastors' effectiveness and satisfaction and other psychological and sociological variables: The Growth in Ministry Research Project.* Philadelphia: Division for Professional Leadership, Lutheran Church in America.

Johnson, P. E. (1959). *Psychology of religion* (rev. ed.). New York: Abingdon Press.

Johnson, R. C., Danko, G. P., Darvill, R. J., Bochner, S., Bowers, J. K., & Huang, Y.-H. (1989). Cross-cultural assessment of altruism and its correlates. *Personality and Individual Differences, 10,* 855–868.

Johnson, S. D. (1987). Factors related to intolerance of AIDS victims. *Journal for the Scientific Study of Religion, 26,* 105–110.

Johnson, S., & Spilka, B. (1988, October 30). *Coping with breast cancer: The role of religion.* Paper presented at the annual convention of the Society for the Scientific Study of Religion, Chicago.

Johnson, S., & Spilka, B. (1991). Religion and the breast cancer patient: The roles of clergy and faith. *Journal of Religion and Health, 30,* 21–33.

Johnson, W. (1974). *The search for transcendence.* New York: Harper & Row.

Johnston, J. C., de Groot, H., & Spanos, N. P. (1995). The structure of paranormal belief: A factor-analytic investigation. *Imagination, Cognition and Personality, 14,* 165–174.

Johnston, L. D., O'Malley, P. M., & Bachman, J. G. (2001). *Monitoring the future: National results on adolescent drug use. Overview of key findings, 2000.* Ann Arbor: Institute for Social Research, University of Michigan.

Johnston, W. (1974). *Silent music.* New York: Harper.

Johnstone, R. L. (1966). *The effectiveness of Lutheran elementary and secondary schools as agencies of Christian education.* St. Louis, MO: Concordia Seminary Research Center.

Johnstone, R. L. (1988). *Religion in society: A sociology of religion* (3rd ed.). Englewood Cliffs, NJ: Prentice-Hall.

Jones, J. W. (1993). Living on the boundary between psychology and religion. *Psychology of Religion Newsletter, 18*(4), 1–7.

Jones, R. H. (1986). *Science and mysticism.* London: Associated Universities Press.

Jones, S. L. (1994). A constructive relationship for religion with the science and profession of psychology: Perhaps the boldest model yet. *American Psychologist, 49,* 184–199.

Jones, W. L. (1937). *A psychological study of conversion.* London: Epworth.

Jowett, B. (1907). *The dialogues of Plato* (Vol. 1). New York: Scribner.

Joyce, C. R. B., & Weldon, R. M. C. (1965). The objective efficacy of prayer: A double-blind clinical trial. *Journal of Chronic Diseases, 18,* 367–377.

Judah, J. S. (1974). *Hare Krishna and the counterculture.* New York: Wiley.

Juergensmeyer, M. (2000). *Terror in the mind of God: The global rise of religious violence.* Berkeley: University of California Press.

Jull-Johnson, D. S. (1995). The use of social bereavement rituals by gay men confronting HIV-related loss. *Dissertation Abstracts International, 56*(6), 3449B.

Jung, C. G. (1933). *Modern man in search of a soul* (W. S. Dell & C. F. Baynes, Trans.). New York: Harcourt, Brace.

Jung, C. G. (1938). *Psychology and religion.* New Haven, CT: Yale University Press.

Jung, C. G. (1964). Flying saucers: A modern myth of things seen in the skies. In H. Read, M. Fordham, & G. Adler (Eds.) & R. F. C. Hull (Trans.), *The collected works of C. G. Jung* (Vol. 10, pp. 309–433). Princeton, NJ: Princeton University Press. (Original work published 1958)

Jung, C. G. (1968). Archetypes of the collective unconscious. In H. Read, M. Fordham, & G. Adler (Eds.) and R. F. C. Hull (Trans.), *The collected works of C. G. Jung* (2nd ed., Vol. 9, Part I, pp. 3–41). Princeton, NJ: Princeton University Press. (Original work published 1954)

Jung, C. G. (1969). A psychological approach to the dogma of the Trinity. In H. Read, M. Fordham, & G. Adler (Eds.) & R. F. C. Hull (Trans.), *The collected works of C. G. Jung* (2nd ed., Vol. 11, pp. 107–200). Princeton, NJ: Princeton University Press. (Original work published 1948)

Junger, M., & Polder, W. (1993). Religiosity, religious climate, and delinquency among ethnic groups in the Netherlands. *British Journal of Criminology, 33,* 416–435.

Kagan, J. (1998). *Three seductive ideas.* Cambridge, MA: Harvard University Press.

Kaiser Family Foundation. (2001, November). *A report on the experiences of lesbians, gays, and bisexuals in America and the public's views on issues and policies related to sexual orientation.* (Report No. 3193). Menlo Park, CA: Author.

Kalish, R. A., & Dunn, L. (1976). Death and dying: A survey of credit offerings in theological schools and some possible implications. *Review of Religious Research, 17,* 134–140.

Kalish, R. A., & Reynolds, D. K. (1973). Phenomenological reality and post-death contact. *Journal for the Scientific Study of Religion, 12,* 209–221.

Kandel, D. B., & Sudit, M. (1982). Drinking practices among urban adults in Israel: A cross-cultural comparison. *Journal of Studies on Alcohol, 43,* 1–16.

Kane, D., Cheston, S. E., & Greer, J. (1993). Perceptions of God by survivors of childhood sexual abuse: An exploratory study in an underresearched area. *Journal of Psychology and Theology, 21,* 228–237.

Kanekar, S., & Merchant, S. M. (2001). Helping norms in relation to religious affiliation. *Journal of Social Psychology, 141,* 617–626.

Karasu, T. B. (1999). Spiritual psychotherapy. *American Journal of Psychotherapy, 53,* 143–162.

Karlsen, C. F. (1989). *The devil in the shape of a woman.* New York: Random House.

Karsh, E. (2002, December). Intifada II: The long trail of Arab anti-Semitism. *Commentary,* pp. 49–53.

Kasamatsu, M., & Hirai, T. (1969). An electroencephalographic study on the Zen meditation (*zazen*). In C. Tart (Ed.), *Altered states of consciousness* (pp. 489–501). New York: Wiley.

Kass, J. D., Friedman, R., Leserman, J., Zuttermeister, P. C., & Benson, H. (1991). Health outcomes and a new index of spiritual experience. *Journal for the Scientific Study of Religion, 30,* 203–211.

Kastenbaum, R. J. (1981). *Death, society, and human experience.* St. Louis, MO: C. V. Mosby.

Kastenbaum, R. J., & Aisenberg, R. (1972). *The psychology of death.* New York: Springer.

Katchadourian, H. A. (1989). *Fundamentals of human sexuality.* New York: Holt, Rinehart and Winston.

Katz, S. T. (1977). *Mysticism and philosophical analysis.* New York: Oxford University Press.

Katz, S. T. (1983). *Mysticism and religious traditions.* New York: Oxford University Press.

Katz, S. T. (1992). *Mysticism and language.* New York: Oxford University Press.

Kaufmann, W. (1958). *Critique of religion and philosophy.* New York: Harper.

Kay, W. K. (1996). Bringing child psychology to religious curricula: The cautionary tale of Goldman and Piaget. *Educational Review, 48,* 205–215.

Kazantzakis, N. (1961). *Report to Greco.* New York: Simon & Schuster.

Kearl, M. (1989). *Endings: A sociology of death and dying.* New York: Oxford University Press.

Kearl, M. (1997). You never have to die! On Mormons, NDEs, cryonics, the American immortalist ethos. In K. Charmaz, G. Howarth, & A. Kellehear (Eds.), *The unknown country: Experiences of death in Australia, Britain, and the USA* (pp. 212–228). London: Macmillan.

Kearl, M. (2002). *Euthanasia and the right to die* [Online]. Available: http://www.trinity.edu/~mkearl/dteuth.htlml [Retrieved February 21, 2002].

Kedem, P., & Cohen, D. W. (1987). The effects of religious education on moral judgment. *Journal of Psychology and Judaism, 11,* 4–14.

Kegeles, S. M., Coates, C. J., Christopher, T. A., & Lazarus, J. L., (1989). Perceptions of AIDS: The continuing saga of AIDS-related stigma. *AIDS, 3*(Suppl.), S253–S258.

Kelley, D. M. (1972). *Why conservative churches are growing.* New York: Harper & Row.

Kelley, H. H. (1967). Attribution theory in social psychology. In D. Levine (Ed.), *Nebraska Symposium on Motivation* (Vol. 15, pp. 192–238). Lincoln: University of Nebraska Press.

Kelley, M. L., Power, T. G., & Wimbush, D. D. (1992). Determinants of disciplinary practices in low-income black mothers. *Child Development, 63,* 573–582.

Kelley, Sister M. W. (1958). The incidence of hospitalized mental illness among religious sisters in the United States. *American Journal of Psychiatry, 115,* 72–75.

Kelley, Sister M. W. (1961). Depression in the psychoses of members of religious communities of women. *American Journal of Psychiatry, 118,* 423–425.

Kellstedt, L., & Smidt, C. (1991). Measuring fundamentalism: An analysis of different operational strategies. *Journal for the Scientific Study of Religion, 30,* 259–278.

Kelly, G. A. (1983). Faith, freedom, and disenchantment: Politics and the American religious establishment. In M. Douglas & S. Tipton (Eds.), *Religion and America* (pp. 207–228). Boston: Beacon Press.

Kelsey, M. T. (1964). *Tongue speaking: An experiment in spiritual experience.* Garden City, NY: Doubleday.

Kemper, T. D. (1978). *A social interaction theory of emotions.* New York: Wiley.

Kendler, K. S. Gardner, C. O., & Prescott, C. A. (1997). Religion, psychopathology, and substance abuse: A multimeasure, genetic–epidemiological study. *American Journal of Psychiatry, 154,* 322–329.

Keniston, K. (1968). *Young radicals.* New York: Harcourt, Brace & World.

Keniston, K. (1971). *Youth and dissent.* New York: Harcourt Brace Jovanovich.

Kennedy, G. (Ed.). (1957). *Evolution and religion.* Boston: D. C. Heath.

Kennedy, J. E., Rosati, K. G., Spann, L. H., Neelon, F. A., & Rosati, R. A. (n.d.). *Changing for the better: Spirituality supports healthy lifestyle choices.* Unpublished manuscript, Rice Diet Program and Department of Medicine, Duke University Medical Center, Durham, NC.

Kent, S. A. (2001). *From slogans to mantras: Social protest and religious conversion in the late Vietnam war era.* Syracuse, NY: Syracuse University Press.

Keysar, A., & Kosmin, B. A. (1995). The impact of religious identification on differences in educational attainment among American women in 1990. *Journal for the Scientific Study of Religion, 34,* 49–62.

Khavari, K. A., & Harmon, T. M. (1982). The relationship between the degree of professed religious belief and use of drugs. *International Journal of the Addictions, 17,* 847–857.

Kidorf, I. W. (1966). The shiva: A form of group psychotherapy. *Journal of Religion and Health, 5,* 43–46.

Kieren, D. K., & Munro, B. (1987). Following the leaders: Parents' influence on adolescent religious activity. *Journal for the Scientific Study of Religion, 26,* 249–255.

Kierniesky, N., & Groelinger, L. (1977). General anxiety and death imagery in Catholic seminarians and college students. *Journal of Psychology, 97,* 199–203.

Kiev, A. (1966). Prescientific psychiatry. In S. Arieti (Ed.), *American handbook of psychiatry* (Vol. 3, pp. 166–179). New York: Basic Books.

Kilbourne, B. K. (1983). The Conway and Siegelman claim against religious cults: An assessment of their data. *Journal for the Scientific Study of Religion, 22,* 380–385.

Kilbourne, B. K., & Richardson, J. T. (1984a). Psychotherapy and new religions in a pluralistic society. *American Psychologist, 39,* 237–251.

Kilbourne, B. K., & Richardson, J. T. (1984b). *The DSM-III and its relation to psychotherapy for cult-converts.* Unpublished manuscript.

Kilbourne, B. K., & Richardson, J. T. (1986). Cultphobia. *Thought, 61,* 258–266.

Kilbourne, B. K., & Richardson, J. T. (1989). Paradigm conflict, types of conversion, and conversion theories. *Sociological Analysis, 50,* 1–21.

Kildahl, J. P. (1965). The personalities of sudden religious converts. *Pastoral Psychology, 16,* 37–44.

Kildahl, J. P. (1972). *The psychology of speaking in tongues.* New York: Harper & Row.

Kim, B. (1979). Religious deprogramming and subjective reality. *Sociological Analysis, 40,* 197–207.

Kimbrough, D. L. (1995). *Taking up serpents: Snake handling in eastern Kentucky.* Chapel Hill: University of North Carolina Press.

King, D. G. (1990). Religion and health relationships: A review. *Journal of Religion and Health, 29,* 101–112.

King, P. E., Furrow, J. L., & Roth, N. (2002). The influence of families and peers on adolescent religiousness. *Journal of Psychology and Christianity, 21,* 109–120.

King, V., Elder, G. H., Jr., & Whitbeck, L. B. (1997). Religious involvement among rural youth: An ecological and life-course perspective. *Journal of Research on Adolescence, 7,* 431–456.

Kirk, S. A., & Kutchins, H. (1992). *The selling of DSM: The rhetoric of science in psychiatry.* New York: Aldine de Gruyter.

Kirkpatrick, L. A. (1986). *Empirical research on images of God: A methodological and conceptual critique.* Paper presented at the annual convention of the Society for the Scientific Study of Religion, Savannah, GA.

Kirkpatrick, L. A. (1988). The Conway–Siegelman data on religious cults: Kilbourne's analysis reassessed (again). *Journal for the Scientific Study of Religion, 27,* 117–121.

Kirkpatrick, L. A. (1989). A psychometric analysis of the Allport–Ross and Feagin measures of intrinsic–extrinsic religious orientation. In M. L. Lynn & D. O. Moberg (Eds.), *Research in the Social Scientific Study of Religion* (Vol. 1, pp. 1–31). Greenwich, CT: JAI Press.

Kirkpatrick, L. A. (1992). An attachment-theory approach to the psychology of religion. *International Journal for the Psychology of Religion, 2,* 3–28.

Kirkpatrick, L. A. (1993). Fundamentalism, Christian orthodoxy, and intrinsic religious orientation as predictors of discriminatory attitudes. *Journal for the Scientific Study of Religion, 32,* 256–268.

Kirkpatrick, L. A. (1994). The role of attachment in religious belief and behavior. *Advances in Personal Relationships, 5,* 239–265.

Kirkpatrick, L. A. (1995). Attachment theory and religious experience. In R. W. Hood, Jr. (Ed.), *Handbook of religious experience* (pp. 446–475). Birmingham, AL: Religious Education Press.

Kirkpatrick, L. A. (1997). A longitudinal study of changes in religious belief and behavior as a function of individual differences in attachment style. *Journal for the Scientific Study of Religion, 36,* 207–217.

Kirkpatrick, L. A. (1998). God as a substitute attachment figure: A longitudinal study of adult attachment style and religious change in college students. *Personality and Social Psychology Bulletin, 24,* 961–973.

Kirkpatrick, L. A. (1999). Attachment and religious representations and behavior. In J. Cassidy & P. R. Shaver (Eds.), *Handbook of attachment: Theory, research, and clinical applications* (pp. 803–822). New York: Guilford Press.

Kirkpatrick, L. A., & Hood, R. W., Jr. (1990). Intrinsic–extrinsic religious orientation: The boon or bane of contemporary psychology of religion? *Journal for the Scientific Study of Religion, 29,* 442–462.

Kirkpatrick, L. A., Hood, R. W., Jr., & Hartz, G. W. (1991). Fundamentalist religion conceptualized in terms of Rokeach's theory of the open and closed mind: New perspectives on some old ideas. in M. L. Lynn & D. O. Moberg (Eds.), *Research in the social scientific study of religion* (Vol. 3, pp. 157–179). Greenwich, CT: JAI Press.

Kirkpatrick, L. A., & Shaver, P. R. (1990). Attachment theory and religion: Childhood attachments, religious beliefs, and conversion. *Journal for the Scientific Study of Religion, 29,* 315–334.

Kirkpatrick, L. A., & Shaver, P. R. (1992). An attachment-theoretical approach to romantic love and religious belief. *Personality and Social Psychology Bulletin, 18,* 266–275.

Kittrie, N. (1971). *The right to be different.* Baltimore: John Hopkins University Press.

Klaczynski, P. A., & Gordon, D. H. (1996). Self-serving influences on adolescents' evaluations of belief-relevant evidence. *Journal of Experimental Child Psychology, 62,* 317–339.

Klass, D., & Heath, A. O. (1996–1997). Grief and abortion: *Mizuko kuyo,* the Japanese ritual solution. *Omega, 34,* 1–13.

Klassen, D. W., & McDonald, M. J. (2002). Quest and identity development: Re-examining pathways for existential research. *International Journal for the Psychology of Religion, 12,* 189–200.

Klausner, S. Z. (1964). *Psychiatry and religion.* New York: Free Press.

Kling, F. R. (1958). A study of testing related to the ministry. *Religious Education, 53,* 243–248.

Kling, F. R. (1959). *The motivation of ministerial candidates* (Research Bulletin No. 59–2). Princeton, NJ: Educational Testing Service.

Klingberg, G. (1959). A study of religious experience in children from nine to thirteen years of age. *Religious Education, 54,* 211–216.

Klinger, E. (1971). *Structure and functions of fantasy.* New York: Wiley.

Klopfer, F. J., & Price, W. F. (1979). Euthanasia acceptance as related to afterlife belief and other attitudes. *Omega, 9,* 245–253.

Kluegel, J. R. (1980). Denominational mobility: Current patterns and recent trends. *Journal for the Scientific Study of Religion, 19,* 26–39.

Kobasa, S. C. O., Maddi, S. R., & Kahn, S. (1982). Hardiness and health: A prospective study. *Journal of Personality and Social Psychology, 42,* 168–177.

Koch, P. (1994). *Solitude: A philosophical encounter.* Chicago: Open Court.

Koenig, H. G. (1988). Religious behaviors and death anxiety in later life. *Hospice Journal, 4,* 3–24.

Koenig, H. G. (1992). Religion and mental health in later life. In J. F. Schumaker (Ed.), *Religion and mental health* (pp. 177–188). New York: Oxford University Press.

Koenig, H. G. (1994a). *Aging and God: Spiritual pathways to mental health in midlife and later years.* New York: Haworth Press.

Koenig, H. G. (1994b). *Self-destructive behaviors related to death in physically ill elderly men: Pilot data.* Unpublished manuscript, Duke University Medical Center.

Koenig, H. G. (1995). Use of acute hospital services and mortality among religious and non-religious copers with medical illness. *Journal of Religious Gerontology, 9*(3), 1–22.

Koenig, H. G., George, L. K., & Siegler, I. C. (1988). The use of religion and other emotion-regulating coping strategies among older adults. *The Gerontologist, 28,* 303–310.

Koenig, H. G., Kvale, J. N., & Ferrel, C. (1988). Religion and well-being in later life. *The Gerontologist, 28,* 18–28.

Koenig, H. G., & Larson, D. B. (2001). Religion and mental health: Evidence for an association. *International Review of Psychiatry, 13,* 67–78.

Koenig, H. G., McCullough, M. E., & Larson, D. B. (2001). *Handbook of religion and health.* New York: Oxford University Press.

Koenig, H. G., Pargament, K. I., & Nielsen, J. (1998). Religious coping and health status in medically ill hospitalized older adults. *Journal of Nervous and Mental Disease, 186,* 513–521.

Kohlberg, L. (1964). Development of moral character and moral ideology. In M. L. Hoffman & L. W. Hoffman (Eds.), *Review of child development research* (pp. 383–431). New York: Russell Sage Foundation.

Kohlberg, L. (1969). Stage and sequence: The cognitive-developmental approach to socialization. In D. A. Goslin (Ed.), *Handbook of socialization theory and research* (pp. 347–480). Chicago: Rand McNally.

Kohlberg, L. (1980). Stages of moral development as a basis for moral education. In B. Munsey (Ed.), *Moral development, moral education, and Kohlberg* (pp. 15–98). Birmingham, AL: Religious Education Press.

Kohlberg, L. (1981). *Essays on moral development: Vol. 1. The philosophy of moral development: Moral stages and the idea of justice.* San Francisco: Harper & Row.

Kohlberg, L. (1984). *Essays on moral development: Vol. 2. The psychology of moral development: The nature and validity of moral stages.* San Francisco: Harper & Row.

Kojetin, B. A., McIntosh, D. N., Bridges, R. A., & Spilka, B. (1987). Quest: Constructive search or religious conflict? A research note. *Journal for the Scientific Study of Religion, 26,* 111–115.

Kolakowski, L. (1985). *Bergson.* New York: Oxford University Press.

Kolb, B., & Whishaw, I. Q. (1990). *Fundamentals of human neuropsychology* (3rd ed.). New York: Freeman.

Koltko, M. E. (1993, August 21). *Religion and vocational development: The neglected relationship.* Paper presented at the annual convention of the American Psychological Association, Toronto.

Konig, R., Eisinga, R., & Scheepers, P. (2000). Explaining the relationship between Christian religion and anti-Semitism in the Netherlands. *Review of Religious Research, 41,* 373–393.

Kooistra, W. P., & Pargament, K. I. (1999). Religious doubting in parochial school adolescents. *Journal of Psychology and Theology, 27,* 33–42.

Kopplin, D. (1976). *Religious orientations of college students and related personality characteristics.* Paper presented at the annual convention of the American Psychological Association, Washington, DC.

Köse, A. (1996a). *Conversion to Islam: A study of native British converts.* London: Kegan Paul.

Köse, A. (1996b). Religious conversion: Is it an adolescent phenomenon? The case of native British converts to Islam. *International Journal for the Psychology of Religion, 64,* 253–262.

Köse, A., & Loewenthal, K. M. (2000). Conversion motifs among British converts to Islam. *International Journal for the Psychology of Religion.*

Kosmin, B. A., & Lachman, S. P. (1993). *One nation under God.* New York: Harmony Books.

Kotre, J. N. (1971). *The view from the border.* Chicago: Aldine/Atherton.

Kraft-Ebing, R. von. (1904). *Textbook of insanity.* Philadelphia: F. A. Davis.

Kramrisch, S., Otto, J., Ruck, C., & Wasson, R. (1986). *Persephone's quest: Etheogens and the origin of religion.* New Haven, CT: Yale University Press.

Krause, N., & Ingersoll-Dayton, B. (2001). Religion and the process of forgiveness in late life. *Review of Religious Research, 42,* 252–276.

Krause, N., Ingersoll-Dayton, B., Ellison, C. G., & Wulff, K. M. (1999). Aging, religious doubt, and psychological well-being. *Gerontologist, 39,* 525–533.

Krause, N., & Van Tranh, T. (1989). Stress and religious involvement among older blacks. *Journal of Gerontology: Social Sciences, 44,* S4–S13.

Kraybill, D. B. (1977). *Ethnic education: The impact of Mennonite schooling.* San Francisco: R & E Research Associates.

Kraybill, D. B. (1994). Plotting social change across four afiliations. In D. B. Kraybill & M. A. Olshan (Eds.), *The Amish struggle with modernity* (pp. 53–74). Hanover, NH: University Press of New England.

Krejci, M. J. (1998). Gender comparison of God schemas: A multidimensional scaling analysis. *International Journal for the Psychology of Religion, 8,* 57–66.

Kripal, J. J. (2001). *Roads of excess, palaces of wisdom and the reflexivity in the study of mysticism.* Chicago: University of Chicago Press.

Krishnan, V. (1993). Gender of children and contraceptive use. *Journal of Biosocial Science, 25,* 213–221.

Kristensen, K. B., Pedersen, D. M., & Williams, R. N. (2001). Profiling religious maturity: The relationships of religious attitude components to religious orientations. *Journal for the Scientific Study of Religion, 40,* 75–86.

Kroeger, C. C., & Beck, J. R. (Eds.). (1996). *Women, abuse, and the Bible: How scripture can be used to hurt or to heal.* Grand Rapids, MI: Baker Books.

Kroll, J., & Bachrach, B. (1982). Visions and psychopathology in the Middle Ages. *Journal of Nervous and Mental Disease, 170,* 41–49.

Kroll, M. D. (1994). A commentary on optimism, fundamentalism, and egoism. *Psychological Science, 5,* 56.

Kroll-Smith, J. S. (1980). The testimony as performance: The relationship of an expressive event to the belief system of a Holiness sect. *Journal for the Scientific Study of Religion, 19,* 16–25.

Kruglanski, A. W., Hasmel, I. Z., Maides, S. A., & Schwartz, J. M. (1978). Attribution theory as a special case of lay epistemology. In J. H. Harvey, W. Ickes, & R. F. Kidd (Eds.), *New directions in attribution research* (Vol. 2, pp. 299–333). Hillsdale, NJ: Erlbaum.

Kuhn, M. H., & McPartland, T. S. (1954). An empirical investigation of self-attitudes. *American Sociological Review, 19,* 68–76.

Kuhn, T. (1962). *The structure of scientific revolutions.* Chicago: University of Chicago Press.

Kundera, M. (1983). *The unbearable lightness of being.* London: Faber & Faber.

Kunkel, L. E., & Temple, L. L. (1992). Attitudes towards AIDS and homosexuals: Gender, marital status, and religion. *Journal of Applied Social Psychology, 22,* 1030–1040.

Kunkel, M. A., Cook, S., Meshel, D. S., Daughtry, D., & Hauenstein, A. (1999). God images: A concept map. *Journal for the Scientific Study of Religion, 38,* 193–202.

Kupky, O. (1928). *The religious development of adolescents.* New York: Macmillan.

Kurth, C. J. (1961). Psychiatric and psychological selection of candidates for the sisterhood. *Guild of Catholic Psychiatrists Bulletin, 8,* 19–25.

Kushner, H. (1981). *When bad things happen to good people.* New York: Schocken Books.

Kutter, C. J., & McDermott, D. S. (1997). The role of the church in adolescent drug education. *Journal of Drug Education, 27,* 293–305.

LaBarre, W. (1969). *The peyote cult* (enlarged ed.) New York: Schocken Books.

LaBarre, W. (1972a). Hallucinations and the shamanantic origins of religion. In P. T. Furst (Ed.), *The flesh of the gods* (pp. 261–278). New York: Praeger.

LaBarre, W. (1972b). *The ghost dance: The origins of religion* (rev. ed.). New York: Delta.

Ladd, K. L., McIntosh, D. N., & Spilka, B. (1994, November). *The development of God schemata: The influence of denomination, age, and gender.* Paper presented at the annual convention of the Society for the Scientific Study of Religion, Albuquerque, NM.

Ladd, K. L., McIntosh, D. N., & Spilka, B. (1998). Children's God concepts: Influences of denomination, age, and gender. *International Journal for the Psychology of Religion, 8,* 49–56.

Ladd, K. L., Milmoe, S., & Spilka, B. (1994, April). *Religious schemata: Coping with breast cancer.* Paper presented at the annual convention of the Rocky Mountain Psychological Association, Las Vegas, NV.

Ladd, K. L., & Spilka, B. (2002). Inward, outward, and upward: Cognitive aspects of prayer. *Journal for the Scientific Study of Religion, 41,* 475–484.

Lafal, J., Monahan, J., & Richman, P. (1974). Communication of meaning in glossolalia. *Journal of Social Psychology, 92,* 277–291.

Lafferty, J. (1990). Religion and racism in South Africa: Conflict between faith and culture. *Social Thought, 16,* 36–49.

Lam, P.-Y. (2002). As the flocks gather: How religion affects voluntary association participation. *Journal for the Scientific Study of Religion, 41,* 405–422.

Lammers, C., Ireland, M., Resnick, M., & Blum, R. (2000). Influences on adolescents' decision to postpone onset of sexual intercourse: A survival analysis of virginity among youths aged 13 to 18 years. *Journal of Adolescent Health, 26,* 42–48.

Lamothe, R. (1998). Sacred objects as vital objects: Transitional objects reconsidered. *Journal of Psychology and Theology, 26,* 159–167.

Lane, R. E. (1969). *Political thinking and consciousness.* Chicago: Markham.

Langer, E. J. (1983). *The psychology of control.* Beverly Hills, CA: Sage.

Langford, B. J., & Langford, C. C. (1974). Review of the polls. *Journal for the Scientific Study of Religion, 13,* 221–222.

LaPierre, L. L. (1994). A model for describing spirituality. *Journal of Religion and Health, 33,* 153–161.

Larsen, K. S., & Long, E. (1988). Attitudes toward sex-roles: Traditional or egalitarian? *Sex Roles, 19,* 1–12.

Larsen, S. (1976). *The shaman's doorway.* New York: Harper & Row.

Larson, D. B., Koenig, H. G., Kaplan, B. H., Greenberg, R. S., Logue, E., & Tyroler, H. A. (1989). The impact of religion on men's blood pressure. *Journal of Religion and Health, 28,* 265–277.

Laski, M. (1961). *Ecstasy: A study of some secular and religious experiences.* Bloomington: University of Indiana Press.

Latkin, C. A. (1995). New directions in applying psychological theory to the study of new religions. *International Journal for the Psychology of Religion, 5,* 177–180.

Laurencelle, R. M., Abell, S. C., & Schwartz, D. J. (2002). The relation between intrinsic faith and psychological well-being. *International Journal for the Psychology of Religion, 12,* 109–123.

Lavery, J. V., Dickens, B. M., Boyle, J. M., & Singer, P. A. (1997). Bioethics for clinicians: II. Euthanasia and assisted suicide. *Canadian Medical Association Journal, 156,* 1405–1408.

Lawless, E. J. (1988). *Handmaidens of the Lord.* Philadelphia: University of Pennsylvania Press.

Lawrence, B. B. (1989). *Defenders of God.* New York: I. B. Tauris.

Lawson, R., Drebing, C., Berg, G., Vincellette, A., & Penk, W. (1998). The long term impact of child abuse on religious behavior and spirituality in men. *Child Abuse and Neglect, 22,* 369–380.

Lawton, L. E., & Bures, R. (2001). Parental divorce and the "switching" of religious identity. *Journal for the Scientific Study of Religion, 40,* 99–111.

Laythe, B., Finkel, D., & Kirkpatrick, L. A. (2001). Predicting prejudice from religious fundamentalism and right-wing authoritarianism: A multiple-regression approach. *Journal for the Scientific Study of Religion, 40,* 1–10.

Lazarus, R. S. (1990). Constructs of the mind in adaptation. In N. L. Stein, B. Leventhal, & T. Trabasso (Eds.), *Psychological and biological approaches to emotion* (pp. 3–20). Hillsdale, NJ: Erlbaum.

Lazarus, R. S., & Folkman, S. (1984). *Stress, appraisal, and coping.* New York: Springer.

Leach, E. R. (1966). Ritualization in man in relation to conceptual and social development. *Philosophical Transactions of the Royal Society of London, Series B, Biological Sciences, 251,* 403–408.

Leak, G. K., & Fish, S. (1989). Religious orientation, impression management, and self-deception: Toward a clarification of the link between religiosity and social desirability. *Journal for the Scientific Study of Religion, 28,* 355–359.

Leak, G. K., Loucks, A. A., & Bowlin, P. (1999). Development and initial validation of an objective measure of faith development. *International Journal for the Psychology of Religion, 9,* 105–124.

Leak, G. K., & Randall, B. A. (1995). Clarification of the link between right-wing authoritarianism and religiousness: The role of religious maturity. *Journal for the Scientific Study of Religion, 34,* 245–252.

Leane, W., & Shute, R. (1998). Youth suicide: The knowledge and attitudes of Australian teachers and clergy. *Suicide and Life-Threatening Behavior, 28,* 165–169.

Leary, T. (1964). Religious experience: Its production and interpretation. *Psychedelic Review, 1,* 324–346.

Lebacqz, K., & Barton, R. G. (1991). *Sex in the parish.* Louisville, KY: Westminster John Knox Press.

Lebra, T. S. (1970). Religious conversion as a breakthrough for transculturation: A Japanese sect in Hawaii. *Journal for the Scientific Study of Religion, 9,* 181–186.

Ledbetter, M. F., & Foster, J. D. (1989). Measuring spiritual giftedness: A factor analytic study of a Spiritual Gifts Inventory. *Journal of Psychology and Theology, 17,* 274–283.

Lee, J. W., Rice, G. T., & Gillespie, V. B. (1997). Family worship patterns and their correlation with adolescent behavior and beliefs. *Journal for the Scientific Study of Religion, 36,* 372–381.

Leech, K. (1985). *Experiencing God: Theology as spirituality.* New York: Harper & Row.

Lefcourt, H. M. (1973). The function of the illusions of control and freedom. *American Psychologist, 28,* 417–425.

Lehrer, E. L. (1996). Religion as a determinant of marital fertility. *Journal of Population Economics, 9,* 173–196.

Lehrer, E. L., & Chiswick, C. U. (1993). Religion as a determinant of marital stability. *Demography, 30,* 385–403.

Leming, M. R. (1979, October 27). *The effects of personal and institutionalized religion upon death attitudes.* Paper presented at the annual convention of the Society for the Scientific Study of Religion, San Antonio, TX.

Leming, M. R. (1980). Religion and death: A test of Homan's thesis. *Omega, 10,* 347–364.

Lemoult, J. (1978). Deprogramming members of religious sects. *Fordham Law Review, 46,* 599–640.

Lenski, G. E. (1961). *The religious factor: A sociological study of religious impact on politics, economics and family life.* Garden City, NY: Doubleday.

Lenz, F. (1995). *Surfing the Himalayas: A spiritual adventure.* New York: St. Martin's Press.

Lerner, M. (1957). *America as a civilization.* New York: Simon & Schuster.

Lerner, M. J. (1980). *The belief in a just world.* New York: Plenum Press.

Lerner, R. M., & Spanier, G. B. (1980). *Adolescent development: A life-span perspective.* New York: McGraw-Hill.

Lester, D. (1967). Experimental and correlational studies of the fear of death. *Psychological Bulletin, 67,* 27–36.

Lester, D. (1972). Religious behaviors and attitudes toward death. In A. Godin (Ed.), *Death and presence* (pp. 107–124). Brussels: Lumen Vitae Press.

Leuba, J. H. (1896). A study in the psychology of religious phenomena. *American Journal of Psychology, 7,* 309–385.

Leuba, J. H. (1925). *The psychology of religious mysticism.* New York: Hacourt, Brace.

Leuba, J. H. (1929). *The psychology of religious mysticism* (rev. ed.). London: Kegan, Paul, Trench, & Trubner.

Leuba, J. H. (1934). Religious beliefs of American scientists. *Harper's Magazine, 169,* 291–300.

Levenger, G. (1979). A social psychological perspective on marital dissolution. In G. Levenger & O. C. Moles (Eds.), *Divorce and separation: Contexts, causes, and consequences* (pp. 37–60). New York: Basic Books.

Levenson, H. (1973). Multidimensional locus of control in psychiatric patients. *Journal of Consulting and Clinical Psychology, 41,* 397–404.

Levin, J. S., & Chatters, L. M. (1998). Research on religion and mental health: An overview of empirical findings and theoretical issues. In H. G. Koenig (Ed.), *Handbook of religion and mental health* (pp. 33–51). San Diego, CA: Academic Press.

Levin, J. S., & Schiller, P. L. (1987). Is there a religious factor in health? *Journal of Religion and Health, 26,* 9–36.

Levin, J. S., & Vanderpool, H. Y. (1989). Is religion therapeutically significant for hypertension? *Social Sciences and Medicine, 29,* 69–78.

Levin, T. M., & Zegans, L. S. (1974). Adolescent identity and religious conversion: Implications for psychotherapy. *British Journal of Medical Psychology, 47,* 73–82.

Levinger, G. (1979). A social psychological perspective on marital dissolution. In G. Levinger & O. C. Moles (Eds.), *Divorce and separation: Contexts, causes, and consequences* (pp. 37–60). New York: Basic Books.

Levinson, D. J., Darrow, C. N., Klein, E. B., Levinson, M. H., & McKee, B. (1978). *The seasons of a man's life.* New York: Knopf.

Levitan, T. (1960). *The laureates: Jewish winners of the Nobel Prize.* New York: Twayne.

Levy, L. H., Martinkowski, K. S., & Derby, J. F. (1994). Differences in patterns of adaptation in conjugal bereavement: Their sources and potential significance. *Omega, 29,* 71–87.

Lewellen, T. C. (1979). Deviant religion and cultural evolution: The Aymara case. *Journal for the Scientific Study of Religion, 81,* 243–251.

Lewis, C. A., & Joseph, S. (1994). Religiosity: Psychoticism and obsessionality in Northern Irish university students. *Personality and Individual Differences, 17,* 685–687.

Lewis, C. A., & Maltby, J. (1995). Religiosity and personality among U.S. adults. *Personality and Individual Differences, 18,* 293–295.

Lewis, C. S. (1956). *Surprised by joy: The shape of my early life.* New York: Harcourt, Brace.

Lewis, I. M. (1971). *Ecstatic religion: An anthropological study of spirit possession and Shamanism.* Baltimore: Penguin.

Lewis, J. R. (1989). Apostates and the legitimation of repression: Some historical and empirical perspectives on the cult controversy. *Sociological Analysis, 49,* 386–396.

Lewis, J. R., & Bromley, D. G. (1987). The cult withdrawal syndrome: A case of misattribution of cause. *Journal for the Scientific Study of Religion, 26,* 508–522.

Leyn, R. M. (1976). Terminally ill children and their families: A study of the variety of responses to fatal illness. *Maternal–Child Nursing Journal, 5,* 179–188.

Lifton, R. J. (1961). *Thought reform and the psychology of totalism.* New York: Norton.

Lifton, R. J. (1973). The sense of immortality: On death and the continuity of life. *American Journal of Psychoanalysis, 33,* 3–15.

Lifton, R. J. (1985). Cult processes, religious liberty and religious totalism. In T. Robbins, W. Shepherd, & J. McBride (Eds.), *Cults, culture, and law* (pp. 59–70). Chico, CA: Scholars Press.

Lilly, J. C. (1956). Mental effects on reduction of ordinary levels of physical stimuli on intact healthy persons. *Psychiatric Research Reports, 5,* 1–19.

Lilly, J. C. (1977). *The deep self.* New York: Warner Books.

Lilly, J. C., & Lilly, A. (1976). *The dyadic cyclone.* New York: Simon & Schuster.

Linder Gunnoe, M., Hetherington, E. M., & Reiss, D. (1999). Parental religiosity, parenting style, and adolescent social responsibility. *Journal of Early Adolescence, 19,* 199–225.

Lindner, E. W. (Ed.). (2003). *Yearbook of American and Canadian churches and megachurches 2003.* New York: National Council of Churches of Christ.

Linville, P. W. (1985). Self-complexity and affective extremity: Don't put all of your eggs in one cognitive basket. *Social Cognition, 3,* 94–120.

Lippy, C. H. (1994). *Being religious, American style.* Westport, CT: Praeger.

Litchfield, A. W., Thomas, D. L., & Li, B. D. (1997). Dimensions of religiosity as mediators of the relations between parenting and adolescent deviant behavior. *Journal of Adolescent Research, 12,* 199–226.

Litke, J. (1983, August 5). Ideas about afterlife a heavenly mix, survey indicates. *The Denver Post,* p. 15D.

Loehr, F. (1959). *The power of prayer on plants.* Garden City, NY: Doubleday.

Loewenthal, K. M., & Cornwall, N. (1993). Religiosity and perceived control of life events. *International Journal for the Psychology of Religion, 3,* 39–45.

Lofland, J. (1977). *Doomsday cult* (rev. ed.) New York: Irvington Press.

Lofland, J., & Skonovd, N. (1981). Conversion motifs. *Journal for the Scientific Study of Religion, 20,* 373–385.

Lofland, J., & Stark, R. (1965). Becoming a world saver: A theory of conversion to a deviant perspective. *American Sociological Review, 30,* 862–874.

Loftus, E. F., & Guyer, M. J. (2002). Who abused Jane Doe?: The hazards of the single case history. Part 1. *Skeptical Inquirer, 26*(3), 24–32.

London, P. (1964). *The modes and morals of psychotherapy.* New York: Holt, Rinehart & Winston.

Long, D., Elkind, D., & Spilka, B. (1967). The child's conception of prayer. *Journal for the Scientific Study of Religion, 6,* 101–109.

Lorenz, K. S. (1966). Evolution of ritualization in the biological and cultural spheres. *Philosophical transactions of the Royal Society of London, Series B, Biological Sciences, 251,* 273–284.

Lottes, I., Weinberg, M., & Weller, I. (1993). Reactions to pornography on a college campus: For or against? *Sex Roles, 29,* 69–89.

Lovekin, A., & Malony, H. N. (1977). Religious glossolalia: A longitudinal study of personality changes. *Journal for the Scientific Study of Religion, 16,* 383–393.

Loveland, G. G. (1968). The effects of bereavement on certain religious attitudes. *Sociological Symposium, 1,* 17–27.

Lowe, C. M. (1955). Religious beliefs and religious delusions. *American Journal of Psychotherapy, 9,* 54–61.

Lowe, C. M., & Braaten, R. O. (1966). Differences in religious attitudes in mental illness. *Journal for the Scientific Study of Religion, 5,* 435–445.

Lown, E. A., & Vega, W. A. (2001). Prevalence and predictors of physical partner abuse among Mexican American women. *American Journal of Public Health, 91,* 441–445.

Lucknow, A., McIntosh, D. N., Spilka, B., & Ladd, K. (2000, February). *The multidimensionality of prayer.* Paper presented at the annual convention of the Society for Personality and Social Psychology, Nashville, TN.

Ludwig, D. J., Weber, T., & Iben, D. (1974). Letters to God: A study of children's religious concepts. *Journal of Psychology and Theology, 2,* 31–35.

Luft, G. A., & Sorell, G. T. (1987). Parenting style and parent–adolescent religious value consensus. *Journal of Adolescent Research, 2,* 53–68.

Lukoff, D., & Lu, F. G. (1988). Transpersonal psychology research review topic: Mystical experience. *Journal of Transpersonal Psychology, 20,* 161–184.

Lukoff, D., Lu, F., & Turner, R. (1992). Toward a more culturally sensitive DSM-IV: Psychoreligious and psychospiritual problems. *Journal of Nervous and Mental Disease. 180,* 673–682.

Lukoff, D., Zanger, R., & Lu, F. (1990). Transpersonal psychology research review: Psychoactive substances and transpersonal states. *Journal of Transpersonal Psychology, 22,* 107–148.

Lumsden, C. J., & Wilson, E. O. (1983). *Promethean fire: Reflections on the origin of mind.* Cambridge, MA: Harvard University Press.

Lupfer, M. B., Brock, K. F., & DePaola, S. J. (1992). The use of secular and religious attributions to explain everyday behavior. *Journal for the Scientific Study of Religion, 31,* 486–503.

Lupfer, M. B., DePaola, S., Brock, K. F., & Clement, L. (1994). Making secular and religious attributions: The availability hypothesis revisited. *Journal for the Scientific Study of Religion, 33,* 162–171.

Lupfer, M., & Wald, K. (1985). An exploration of adults' religious orientations and their philosophies of human nature. *Journal for the Scientific Study of Religion, 24,* 293–304.

Lynch, B. (1996). Religious and spirituality conflicts. In D. Davies & C. Neal (Eds.), *Pink therapy: A guide for counselors and therapists working with lesbian, gay and bisexual clients* (pp. 199–207). Bristol, PA: Open University.

Lynxwiler, J., & Gay, D. (2000). Moral boundaries and deviant music: Public attitudes toward heavy metal and rap. *Deviant Behavior, 21,* 63–85.

MacDonald, C. B., & Luckett, J. B. (1983). Religious affiliation and psychiatric diagnoses. *Journal for the Scientific Study of Religion, 22,* 15–37.

MacDonald, J. M. (1958). *Psychiatry and the criminal.* Springfield, IL: Charles Thomas.

MacDonald, W. L. (1992). Idionecrophanies: The social construction of perceived contact with the dead. *Journal for the Scientific Study of Religion, 31,* 215–223.

MacLean, P. D. (1989). *The triune brain in evolution: Role in paleocerebral functions.* New York: Plenum Press.

Madsen, G. E., & Vernon, G. M. (1983). Maintaining the faith during college: A study of campus religious group participation. *Review of Religious Research, 25,* 127–141.

Maeterlinck, M. (1912). *Death.* New York: Dodd, Mead.

Mafra, C. (2000). Shared accounts: Experiences of conversion to Pentecostalism among Brazilians and Portuguese. *Mana, 6,* 57–86.

Magnusson, D. (Ed.). (1981). *Toward a psychology of situations.* Hillsdale, NJ: Erlbaum.

Mahoney, A., Pargament, K. I., & Swank, A. B. (in press). Religion and the sanctification of the family. *Review of Religious Research.*

Mahoney, A., Pargament, K. I., Tarakeshwar, N., & Swank, A. B. (2001). Religion in the home in the 1980s and 1990s: A meta-analytic review and conceptual analysis of links between religion, marriage, and parenting. *Journal of Family Psychology, 15,* 559–596.

Makarec, K., & Persinger, M. A. (1985). Temporal lobe signs: Electroencephalographic validity and enhanced scores in special populations. *Perceptual and Motor Skills, 60,* 831–842.

Makela, K. (1975). Consumption level and cultural drinking patterns as determinants of alcohol problems. *Journal of Drug Issues, 5,* 433–357.

Makepeace, J. M. (1987). Social and victim–offender differences in courtship violence. *Family Relations Journal of Applied Family and Child Studies, 36,* 87–91.

Malinowski, B. (1965). The role of magic and religion. In W. A. Lessa & E. Z. Vogt (Eds.), *A reader in contemporary religion* (pp. 63–72). New York: Harper & Row.

Malony, H. N. (1978, June). Pastoring about death to dying persons. *Theology: News and Notes,* pp. 16–18.

Malony, H. N., & Lovekin, A. A. (1985). *Glossolalia: Behavioral science perspectives on speaking in tongues.* New York: Oxford University Press.

Maltby, J., & Day, L. (2000). Religious orientation and death obsession. *Journal of Genetic Psychology, 116,* 122–124.

Manfredi, C., & Pickett, M. (1987). Perceived stressful situations and coping strategies utilized by the elderly. *Journal of Community Mental Health Nursing, 4,* 99–110.

Manning, C. (1999). *God gave us the right: Conservative Catholic, evangelical Protestant, and Orthodox Jewish women grapple with feminism.* New Brunswick, NJ: Rutgers University Press.

Marceil, J. C. (1977). Implicit dimensions of idiography and nomothesis. *American Psychologist, 32,* 1046–1055.

Marcellino, E. M. (1996). Internalized homonegativity, self concept and images of God in gay and lesbian individuals. *Dissertation Abstracts International, 57*(1–A), 273.

Marcia, J. (1966). Development and validation of ego-identity status. *Journal of Personality and Social Psychology, 3,* 551–558.

Marcia, J., Waterman, A., Matteson, D., Archer, S., & Orlofsky, J. (Eds.). (1993). *Ego identity: A handbook for psychosocial research.* New York: Springer-Verlag.

Marcum, J. P. (1988). Religious affiliation, participation, and fertility: A cautionary note. *Journal for the Scientific Study of Religion, 27,* 621–629.

Marcum, J. P. (1999). Measuring church attendance: A further look. *Review of Religious Research, 41,* 121–129.

Marcum, J., & Woolever, C. (1999, September 27). 1998 survey of new members Presbyterian Church (U.S.A.). In *Research Services Presbyterian Church (U.S.A.)* [Online]. Available: http://www.pcusa.org/pcusa/cmd/rs/NEWMEMB.htm [Retrieved May 15, 2001].

Marcuse, H. (1955). *Eros and civilization: A philosophical inquiry into Freud.* Boston: Beacon.

Margaret Louise, Sister. (1961). Psychological problems of vocation candidates. *National Catholic Education Association Bulletin, 58,* 450–454.

Margolis, R. D., & Elifson, K. W. (1979). Typology of religious experience. *Journal for the Scientific Study of Religion, 18,* 61–67.

Marin, G. (1976). Social-psychological correlates of drug use among Colombian university students. *International Journal of the Addictions, 11,* 199–207.

Markstrom, C. A. (1999). Religious involvement and adolescent psychosocial development. *Journal of Adolescence, 22,* 205–221.

Markstrom-Adams, C., Hofstra, G., & Dougher, K. (1994). The ego-virtue of fidelity: A case for the study of religion and identity formation in adolescence. *Journal of Youth and Adolescence, 23,* 453–469.

Markstrom-Adams, C., & Smith, M. (1996). Identity formation and religious orientation among high school students from the United States and Canada. *Journal of Adolescence, 19,* 247–261.

Marlasch, C. (1979). The emotional consequences of arousal without reason. In C. E. Izard (Ed.), *Emotions in personality and psychophysiology* (pp. 565–590). New York: Plenum Press.

Marsden, M. J. (1983). Preachers of paradox: The Religious New Right in historical perspective. In M. Douglas & S. Tipton (Eds.), *Religion and America: Spiritual life in a secular age* (pp. 150–168). Boston, Beacon Press.

Marshall, J. L. (1996). Sexual identity and pastoral concerns: Caring with women who are developing lesbian identities. In J. S. Moessner (Ed.), *Through the eyes of women* (pp. 143–166). Minneapolis, MN: Fortress.

Marshall, S. K., & Markstrom-Adams, C. (1995). Attitudes on interfaith dating among Jewish adolescents: Contextual and developmental considerations. *Journal of Family Issues, 16,* 787–811.

Marsiglio, W. (1993). Attitudes toward homosexual activity and gays as friends: A national survey of heterosexual 15- to 19-year-old males. *Journal of Sex Research, 30,* 12–17.

Martin, D., & Wrightsman, L. S., Jr. (1964). Religion and fears about death: A critical review. *Religious Education, 59,* 174–176.

Martin, W. T. (1984). Religiosity and United States suicide rates, 1972–1978. *Journal of Clinical Psychology, 40,* 1166–1169.

Marty, M. E. (1975). *The pro & con book of religious America: A bicentennial argument.* Waco, TX: Word.

Marty, M. E. (1976). *A nation of behavers.* Chicago: University of Chicago Press.

Marty, M. E., & Appleby, R. S. (Eds.). (1991). *Fundamentalisms observed.* Chicago: University of Chicago Press.

Marty, M. E., & Appleby, R. S. (Eds.). (1994). *Accounting for fundamentalisms.* Chicago: University of Chicago Press.

Maslow, A. H. (1963). The need to know and the fear of knowing. *Journal of General Psychology, 68,* 111–125.

Maslow, A. H. (1964). *Religions, values, and peak experiences.* Columbus: Ohio State University Press.

Mason, W. A., & Windle, M. (2001). Family, religious, school and peer influences on adolescent alcohol use: A longitudinal study. *Journal of Studies on Alcohol, 62,* 44–53.

Mason, W. A., & Windle, M. (2002). A longitudinal study of the effects of religiosity on adolescent alcohol use and alcohol-related problems. *Journal of Adolescent Research, 17,* 346–363.

Masterman, M. (1970). The nature of paradigm. In I. Lakotos & A. Musgraves (Eds.), *Criticism and the growth of knowledge* (pp. 59–89). Cambridge, England: Cambridge University Press.

Masters, K. S., & Bergin, A. E. (1992). Religious orientation and mental health. In J. F. Schumaker (Ed.), *Religion and mental health* (pp. 221–232). New York: Oxford University Press.

Masters, R. E. L., & Houston, J. (1966). *The varieties of psychedelic experience.* New York: Delta.

Masters, R. E. L., & Houston, J. (1973). Subjective realities. In B. Schwartz (Ed.), *Human connection and the new media* (pp. 88–106). Englewood Cliffs, NJ: Prentice-Hall.

Masters, W. H., & Johnson, V. E. (1970). *Human sexual inadequacy.* Boston: Little, Brown.

Mathes, E. W. (1982). Mystical experience, romantic love, and hypnotic susceptibility. *Psychological Reports, 50,* 701–702.

Mathews, A. P. (1994). *The sexuality of submissive wives.* Paper presented at the annual convention of the Society for the Scientific Study of Religion, Albuquerque, NM.

Mathews, S., & Smith, G. B. (Eds.). (1923). *A dictionary of religion and ethics.* New York: Macmillan.

Maton, K. I. (1989). The stress-buffering role of spiritual support: Cross-sectional and prospective investigations. *Journal for the Scientific Study of Religion, 28,* 310–323

Maton, K. I., & Wells, E. A. (1995). Religion as a community resource for well-being: Prevention, healing and empowerment. *Journal of Social Issues, 51,* 177–193.

Mattlin, J. A., Wethington, E., & Kessler, R. C. (1990). Situational determinants of coping and coping effectiveness. *Journal of Health and Social Behavior, 31,* 103–122.

Maupin, E. W. (1965). Individual differences in response to a Zen meditation exercise. *Consulting Psychology, 29,* 139–143.

Maxwell, M., & Tschudin, V. (Eds.). (1990). *Seeing the invisible: Modern religious and other transcendent experiences.* London: Penguin.

May, C. L. (1956). A survey of glossolalia and related phenomena in non-Christian religions. *American Anthropologist, 58,* 75–96.

Mayer, A., & Sharp, H. (1962). Religious preference and worldly success. *American Sociological Review, 27,* 218–227.

Mayer, E. (1985). Children of intermarriage. In E. Mayer (Ed.), *Love tradition: Marriage between Jews and Christians* (pp. 245–277). New York: Plenum Press.

Maynard, E. A., Gorsuch, R. L., & Bjorck, J. P. (2001). Religious coping style, concept of God, and personal religious variables in threat, loss, and challenge situations. *Journal for the Scientific Study of Religion, 40,* 65–74.

McAdams, D. P., Booth, L., & Selvik, R. (1981). Religious identity among students at a private college: Social motives, ego stage, and development. *Merrill–Palmer Quarterly, 27,* 219–239.

McCallister, B. J. (1995). Cognitive theory and religious experience. In R. W. Hood, Jr. (Ed.), *Handbook of religious experience* (pp. 312–352). Birmingham, AL: Religious Education Press.

McCartin, R., & Freehill, M. (1986). Values of early adolescents compared by type of school. *Journal of Early Adolescence, 6,* 369–380.

McClelland, D. C. (1961). *The achieving society.* Princeton, NJ: Van Nostrand.

McClenon, J. (1984). *Deviant science.* Philadelphia: University of Pennsylvania Press.

McClenon, J. (1990). Chinese and American anomalous experiences. *Sociological Analysis, 51,* 53–67.

McClosky, H., & Brill, A. (1983). *Dimensions of tolerance: What Americans believe about civil liberties.* New York: Russell Sage Foundation.

McConahay, J. B. (1986). Modern racism, ambivalence, and the modern racism scale. In J. F. Dovidio & S. M. Gaeartner (Eds.), *Prejudice, discrimination, and racism* (pp. 91–124). Orlando, FL: Academic Press.

McConahay, J. B., & Hough, J. C., Jr. (1973). Love and guilt-oriented dimensions of Christian belief. *Journal for the Scientific Study of Religion, 12,* 53–64.

McCosh, J. (1890). *The religious aspect of evolution.* New York: Scribner.

McCrae, R. R. (Ed.). (1992). The five-factor model: Issues and applications [Special issue]. *Journal of Personality, 60.*

McCullough, M. E. (1995). Prayer and health: Conceptual issues, research review, and research agenda. *Journal of Psychology and Theology, 23,* 15–29.

McCullough, M. E. (2001). Religious involvement and mortality. In T. G. Plante & A. C. Sherman (Eds.), *Faith and health: Psychological perspectives* (pp. 53–74). New York: Guilford Press.

McCullough, M. E., Hoyt, W. T., Larson, D. B., Koenig, H. G., & Thoreson, C. (2000). Religious involvement and mortality: A meta-analytic view. *Health Psychology, 19,* 211–222.

McCullough, M. E., & Larson, D. B. (1999). Prayer. In W. R. Miller (Ed.), *Integrating spirituality into treatment* (pp. 85–110). Washington, DC: American Psychological Association.

McCullough, M. E., Pargament, K. I., & Thoresen, C. E. (Eds.). (2000). *Forgiveness: Theory, research, and practice.* New York: Guilford Press.

McCullough, M. E., & Worthington, E. L., Jr. (1999). Religion and the forgiving personality. *Journal of Personality, 67,* 1142–1164.

McCutcheon, A. L. (1988). Denominations and religious intermarriage: Trends among white Americans in the twentieth century. *Review of Religious Research, 29,* 213–227.

McDargh, J. (1983). *Psychoanalytic object relations theory and the study of religion.* Lanham, MD: University Press of America.

McDargh, J. (2001). Faith development theory and the postmodern problem of foundations. *International Journal for the Psychology of Religion, 11,* 185–199.

McDuff, E. M., & Mueller, C, W. (1999). Social support and compensating differentials in the ministry: Gender differences in two Protestant denominations. *Review of Religious Research, 40,* 307–330.

McFarland, S. G. (1989). Religious orientations and the targets of discrimination. *Journal for the Scientific Study of Religion, 28,* 324–336.

McFarland, S. G. (1990). *Religiously oriented prejudice in communism and Christianity: The role of Quest.* Paper presented at the annual convention of the Southeastern Psychological Association, Atlanta, GA.

McFarland, S. G., & Warren, J. C., Jr. (1992). Religious orientations and selective exposure among fundamentalist Christians. *Journal for the Scientific Study of Religion, 31,* 163–174.

McFatters, D. (2002, February 16). "Practical immortality": An intriguing concept. *Rocky Mountain News,* p. 1W.

McGinley, P. (1969). *Saint-watching.* New York: Viking.

McGinn, B. (1989). Preface. In M. Idel & B. McGinn (Eds.), *Mystical union and monotheistic faith: An ecumenical dialogue* (pp. vii–ix). New York: McMillan.

McGinn, B. (1991). Appendix: Theoretical foundations: The modern study of mysticism. In B. McGinn (Ed.), *The foundations of mysticism* (pp. 265–343). New York: Crossroads.

McGuire, M. B. (1990). Religion and the body: Rematerializing the human body in the social sciences of religion. *Journal for the Scientific Study of Religion, 29,* 283–296.

McGuire, M. B. (1992). *Religion: The social context* (3rd ed.). Belmont, CA: Wadsworth.

McIntosh, D. N. (1995). Religion-as-schema, with implications for the relation between religion and coping. *International Journal for the Psychology of Religion, 5,* 1–16.

McIntosh, D. N., Kojetin, B. A., & Spilka, B. (1985). *Form of personal faith and general and specific locus of control.* Paper presented at the annual convention of the Rocky Mountain Psychological Association, Tucson, AZ.

McIntosh, D. N., Silver, R. C., & Wortman, C. B. (1993). Religion's role in adjustment to a negative life event: Coping with the loss of a child. *Journal of Personality and Social Psychology, 65,* 812–821.

McIntosh, D. N., & Spilka, B. (1990). Religion and physical health: The role of personal faith and control beliefs. In M. L. Lynn & D. O. Moberg (Eds.), *Research in the social scientific study of religion* (Vol. 2, pp. 167–194). Greenwich, CT: JAI Press.

McKenna, R. H. (1976). Good Samaritanism in rural and urban settings: A nonreactive comparison of helping behavior of clergy and control subjects. *Representative Research in Social Psychology, 7,* 58–65.

McKeon, R. (Ed.). (1941). *The basic works of Aristotle.* New York: Random House.

McKinney, J. P., & McKinney, K. G. (1999). Prayer in the lives of late adolescents. *Journal of Adolescence, 22,* 279–290.

McKnight, L. R., & Loper, A. B. (2002). The effects of risk and resilience factors in the prediction of delinquency in adolescent girls. *School Psychology International, 23,* 186–198.

McLaughlin, E. C. (1974). Equality of souls, inequality of sexes: Women in medieval theology. In R. R. Ruether (Ed.), *Religion and sexism: Images of woman in the Jewish and Christian traditions* (pp. 213–266). New York: Simon and Schuster.

McLoughlin, W. F. (1978). *Revivals, awakenings, and reform.* Chicago: University of Chicago Press.

McNeill, J. T. (1951). *A history of the cure of souls.* New York: Harper.

McQuire, M. B. (1992). *Religion: The social context* (3rd ed.). Belmont, CA: Wadsworth.

McRae, R. R. (1984). Situational determinants of coping responses: Loss, threat, and challenge. *Journal of Personality and Social Psychology, 46,* 919–928.

McRae, R. R., & Costa, P. T. (1986). Personality, coping, and coping effectiveness in an adult sample. *Journal of Personality, 54,* 385–405.

Mead, F. S. (Ed.). (1965). *The encyclopedia of quotations.* Westwood, NJ: Revell.

Mead, G. H. (1934). *Mind, self, and society.* Chicago: University of Chicago Press.

Mead, M. (1972). Ritual expression of the cosmic sense. In M. Mead (Ed.), *Twentieth century faith* (pp. 153–170). New York: Harper & Row. (Original work published 1966)

Meadow, M. J., & Kahoe, R. D. (1984). *Psychology of religion: Religion in individual lives.* New York: Harper & Row.

Meadow, M. J., & Rayburn, C. A. (Eds.). (1985). *A time to weep, a time to sing.* Minneapolis, MN: Winston.

Meehl, P. E. (1954). *Clinical vs. statistical prediction.* Minneapolis, MN: University of Minnesota Press.

Meier, P. D. (1977). *Christian child-rearing and personality development.* Grand Rapids, MI: Baker House.

Meissner, W. W. (1961). *Annotated bibliography in religion and psychology.* New York: Academy of Religion and Health.

Melton, J. G. (1985). Spiritualization and reaffirmation: What really happens when prophecy fails. *American Studies, 26,* 17–29.

Menges, R. J., & Dittes, J. E. (1965). *Psychological studies of clergymen: Abstracts of research.* New York: Nelson.

Mercer, C., & Durham, T. W. (1999). Religious mysticism and gender orientation. *Journal for the Scientific Study of Religion, 38,* 175–182.

Merrill, R. M., Salazar, R. D., & Gardner, N. W. (2001). Relationship between family religiosity and drug use behavior among youth. *Social Behavior and Personality, 29,* 347–358.

Messer, B., & Harter, S. (1986). *Manual for the Adult Self-Perception Profile.* Denver, CO: University of Denver.

Meyer, M. S., Altmaier, E. M., & Burns, C. P. (1992). Religious orientation and coping with cancer. *Journal of Religion and Health, 31,* 273–279.

Miller, A. S., & Hoffman, J. P. (1995). Risk and religion: An explanation of gender differences in religiosity. *Journal for the Scientific Study of Religion, 34,* 63–75.

Miller, B. C., Norton, M. C., Curtis, T., Hill, E. J., Schvaneveldt, P., & Young, M. H. (1997). The timing of sexual intercourse among adolescents: Family, peer, and other antecedents. *Youth and Society, 29,* 54–83.

Miller, L., Weissman, M., Gur, M., & Adams, P. (2001). Religiousness and substance use in children of opiate addicts. *Journal of Substance Abuse, 13,* 232–236.

Miller, W. (1973). *Why do Christians break down?* Minneapolis, MN: Augsburg.

Miller, W. R. (Ed.). (1999). *Integrating spirituality into treatment.* Washington, DC: American Psychological Association.

Miller, W. R., & C' deBaca, J. (1994). Quantum change: Toward a psychology of transformation. In T. F. Heatherton & J. L. Weinberger (Eds.), *Can personality change?* (pp. 253–280). Washington, DC: American Psychological Association.

Mills, C. W. (1959). *The sociological imagination.* New York: Oxford University Press.

Minton, B., & Spilka, B. (1976). Perspectives on death in relation to powerlessness and form of personal religion. *Omega, 7,* 261–267.

Missoula Demonstration Project. (2001). *The quality of life's end: Annual report, 1999, Missoula, MT* [Online]. Available: http://www.missoulademonstration.org/annual report/ [Retrieved September 27, 2001].

Mitchell, C. E. (1988). Paralleling cognitive and moral development with spiritual development and denominational choice. *Psychology: A Quarterly Journal of Human Behavior, 25,* 1–9.

Mithen, S. (1996). *The prehistory of the mind: The cognitive origins of art, religion, and science.* London: Thames & Hudson.

Moberg, D. O. (1962). *The church as a social institution.* Englewood Cliffs, NJ: Prentice-Hall.

Moberg, D. O. (1965a). The integration of older members in the church congregation. In A. M. Rose & W. A. Peterson (Eds.), *Older people and their social worlds* (pp. 125–140). Philadelphia: Davis.

Moberg, D. O. (1965b). Religiosity in old age. *The Gerontologist, 5,* 78–88.

Moberg, D. O. (1971). Religious practices. In M. P. Strommen (Ed.), *Research on religious development: A comprehensive handbook* (pp. 551–598). New York: Hawthorn Books.

Moberg, D. O. (1979). *Spiritual well-being.* Washington, DC: University Press of America.

Moberg, D. O. (1984). Subjective measures of spiritual well-being. *Review of Religious Research, 25,* 351–364.

Moberg, D. O. (2002). Assessing and measuring spirituality: Confronting dilemmas of the universal and particular evaluative criteria. *Journal of Adult Development, 9,* 47–60.

Moberg, D. O., & Hoge, D. R. (1986). Catholic college students' religious and moral attitudes, 1961 to 1982: Effects of the sixties and seventies. *Review of Religious Research, 28,* 104–117.

Moberg, D. O., & Sears, H. T. (1971). *Spiritual well-being: Background and issues.* Washington, DC: White House Conference on Aging.

Moen, M. C. (1990). Ronald Reagan and the social issues: Rhetorical support for the Christian right. *Social Science Journal, 27,* 199–207.

Monaghan, R. R. (1967). Three faces of the true believer: Motivations for attending a fundamentalist church. *Journal for the Scientific Study of Religion, 6,* 236–245.

Montagu, A. (1950). *On being human.* New York: Henry Schuman.

Montgomery, R. L. (1991). The spread of religions and macrosocial relations. *Sociological Analysis, 52,* 14–22.

Moody, R. (1976). *Life after life.* New York: Bantam.

Moore, D. W. (2000, March). Two of three Americans feel religion can answer most of today's problems. *The Gallup Poll Monthly,* No. 414, 53–60.

Moore, K. A., & Glei, D. (1995). Taking the plunge: An examination of positive youth development. *Journal of Adolescent Research, 10,* 15–40.

Mora, G. (1969). The scrupulosity syndrome. In E. M. Pattison (Ed.), *Clinical psychiatry and religion* (pp. 163–174). Boston: Little, Brown.

Moracco, J. C., & Richardson, G. (1985). *Stress in the clergy: The relationship of demographic and personal variables on perceptions.* Paper presented at the annual convention of the American Psychological Association, Los Angeles.

Morin, R. (2000, April 2). Unconventional wisdom: New facts and hot stats from the social sciences. *The Washington Post,* p. B5.

Morin, S. M., & Welsh, L. A. (1996). Adolescents' perceptions and experiences of death and grieving. *Adolescence, 31,* 585–595.

Morinis, A. (1985). The religious experience: Pain and the transformation of consciousness in ordeals of initiation. *Ethos, 13,* 150–174.

Morreim, D. C. (1991). *Changed lives: The story of Alcoholics Anonymous.* Minneapolis, MN: Augsburg.

Morris, C. G., & Maisto, A. A. (1998). *Psychology: An introduction* (10th ed.). Upper Saddle River, NJ: Prentice-Hall.

Morris, R. J., Hood, R. W., & Watson, P. J. (1989). A second look at religious orientation, social desirability and prejudice. *Bulletin of the Psychonomic Society, 27,* 81–84.

Mowrer, O. H. (1958). Discussion: Symposium on relationships between religion and mental health. *American Psychologist, 13,* 576–579.

Mowrer, O. H. (1961). *The crisis in psychiatry and religion.* Princeton, NJ: Van Nostrand.

Mueller, D. J. (1967). Effects and effectiveness of parochial elementary schools: An empirical study. *Review of Religious Research, 9,* 48–51.

Mueller, G. H. (1978). The Protestant and the Catholic ethic. *Annual Review of the Social Sciences of Religion, 2,* 143–166.

Mullen, K., & Francis, L. J. (1995). Religiosity and attitudes towards drug use among Dutch school children. *Journal of Alcohol and Drug Education, 41,* 16–25.

Munnichs, J. M. A. (1980). *Old age and finitude.* New York: Arno Press.

Murphy, G., & Ballou, R. O. (1960). *William James on psychical research.* New York: Viking.

Murphy-Berman, V., Berman, J. J., Pachauri, A., & Kumar, P. (1985). Religious attitudes and perceptions of justice. *Psychologia: An International Journal of Psychology in the Orient, 18,* 29–34.

Musick, M., & Wilson, J. (1995). Religious switching for marital reasons. *Sociology of Religion, 56,* 257–270.

Myers, D. G. (1992). *The pursuit of happiness.* New York: Morrow.

Myers, D. G. (1998). *Psychology* (5th ed.). New York: Worth.

Myers, D., & Spencer, S. J. (2001). *Social psychology* (Canadian ed.). Toronto: McGraw-Hill.

Myers, F. W. H. (1961). *Human personality and its survival of bodily death.* New Hyde Park, NY: University Books. (Original work published 1903)

Myers, S. M. (1996). An interactive model of religiosity inheritance: The importance of family context. *American Sociological Review, 61,* 858–866.

Nagi, M. H., Pugh, M. D., & Lazerine, N. G. (1977–1978). Attitudes of Catholic and Protestant clergy toward euthanasia. *Omega, 8,* 153–164.

Nagy, M. (1948). The child's theories concerning death. *Journal of Genetic Psychology, 73,* 3–27.

Najman, J. M., Williams, G. M., Keeping, J. D., Morrison, J., & Anderson, M. L. (1988). Religious values, practices and pregnancy outcomes: A comparison of the impact of sect and mainstream Christian affiliation. *Social Science and Medicine, 26,* 401–407.

Naranjo, C., & Ornstein, R. E. (1971). *On the psychology of meditation.* New York: Viking.

Natera, G., Renconco, M., Alemendares, R., Rosowsky, H., & Alemendares, J. (1983). Patterns of alcohol consumption in two semirural areas between Honduras and Mexico. *Acta Psiquiatrica y Psicologica de America Latina, 29,* 116–127.

National Center for Education Statistics. (1993). *Youth indicators: Trends in the well-being of American youth.* Washington, DC: U.S. Government Printing Office.

National Center for Injury Prevention and Control. (2003). *Suicide in the United States.* Available: http://www.cdc.gov/ncipc/factsheets/suifacts.htm [Retrieved March 19, 2003].

National Clearinghouse for Mental Health Information. (1967). *Bibliography on religion and mental health 1960–1964.* Washington, DC: U. S. Department of Health, Education and Welfare.

Nauss, A. (1983). Seven profiles of effective ministers. *Review of Religious Research, 24,* 334–346.

Nauss, A. (1996). Assessing ministerial effectiveness: A review of measures and their use. In J. M. Greer, D. O. Moberg, & M. L. Lynn (Eds.), *Research in the social scientific study of religion* (Vol. 7, pp. 221–251). Greenwich, CT: JAI Press.

Nauta, R. (1988). Task performance and attributional biases in the ministry. *Journal for the Scientific Study of Religion, 27*, 609–620.

Needleman, J., & Baker, G. (Eds.). (1978). *Understanding the new religions.* New York: Seabury.

Nelsen, H. M. (1980). Religious transmission versus religious formation: Preadolescent-parent interaction. *Sociological Quarterly, 21*, 207–218.

Nelsen, H. M. (1981a). Gender differences in the effects of parental discord on preadolescent religiousness. *Journal for the Scientific Study of Religion, 20*, 351–360.

Nelsen, H. M. (1981b). Life without afterlife: Toward congruency of belief across generations. *Journal for the Scientific Study of Religion, 20*, 109–118.

Nelsen, H. M. (1981c). Religious conformity in an age of disbelief: Contextual effects of time, denomination, and family processes upon church decline and apostasy. *American Sociological Review, 46*, 632–640.

Nelsen, H. M. (1982). The influence of social and theological factors upon the goals of religious education. *Review of Religious Research, 23*, 255–263.

Nelsen, H. M. (1990). The religious identification of children of interfaith marriages. *Review of Religious Research, 32*, 122–134.

Nelsen, H. M., Cheek, N. H., & Au, P. (1985). Gender differences in images of God. *Journal for the Scientific Study of Religion, 24*, 396–402.

Nelsen, H. M., & Kroliczak, A. (1984). Parental use of the threat "God will punish": Replication and extension. *Journal for the Scientific Study of Religion, 23*, 267–277.

Nelsen, H. M., & Potvin, R. H. (1981). Gender and regional differences in the religiosity of Protestant adolescents. *Review of Religious Research, 22*, 268–285.

Nelsen, H. M., Potvin, R. H., & Shields, J. (1976). *The religion of children.* Unpublished manuscript, Catholic University of America.

Nelson, B. (2002, March 12). 6 days of creation: The search of evidence. *Newsday* [Online]. Available: http://www.newsday.com/news/health/ny-dsspdn262111mar12.story?coll=ny% [Retrieved March 12, 2002].

Nelson, L. D. (1988). Disaffiliation, desacralization, and political values. In D. G. Bromley (Ed.), *Falling from the faith: Causes and consequences of religious apostasy* (pp. 122–139). Newbury Park, CA: Sage.

Nelson, L. D., & Cantrell, C. H. (1980). Religiosity and death anxiety: A multidimensional analysis. *Review of Religious Research, 21*, 148–157.

Nelson, L. D., & Dynes, R. R. (1976). The impact of devotionalism and attendance on ordinary and emergency helping behavior. *Journal for the Scientific Study of Religion, 15*, 47–59.

Nelson, L. D., & Nelson, C. C. (1975). A factor-analytic investigation of the multidimensionality of death anxiety. *Omega, 6*, 171–178.

Nelson, M. O. (1971). The concept of God and feelings toward parents. *Journal of Individual Psychology, 27*, 46–49.

Nesbitt, P. D. (1997). Clergy feminization: Controlled labor or transformative change. *Journal for the Scientific Study of Religion, 36*, 585–598.

Neufeld, K. (1979). Child-rearing, religion and abusive parents. *Religious Education, 74*, 234–244.

New York Times [Online]. (2002, August 26). Confession had his signature; DNA did not. Available: http://www.nytimes.com [Accessed August 26, 2002].

Newberg, A. B., & d'Aquili, E. G. (2000). The neuropsychology of religious and spiritual experience. In J. Andresen & R. K. C. Forman (Eds.), *Cognitive models and spiritual maps: Interdisciplinary explorations of religious experience* (pp. 251–266). Bowling Green, OH: Imprint Academic.

Newman, B. M., & Newman, P. R. (1995). *Development through life: A psychosocial approach.* Pacific Grove, CA: Brooks/Cole.

Newman, J. S., & Pargament, K. I. (1990). The role of religion in the problem-solving process. *Review of Religious Research, 31*, 390–403.

Newport, F. (2001, June). American attitudes toward homosexuality continue to become more tolerant. *The Gallup Poll Monthly*, 5–9.

Newport, F., Moore, D. W., & Saad, L. (2000). Long term Gallup trends: A portrait of American public opinion through the century. *Gallup Poll Monthly: Year 2000 Review*, 20–32.

Niebuhr, H. R. (1929). *The social sources of denominationalism.* New York: Holt, Rinehart & Winston.

Nielsen, M. E. (1998). An assessment of religious conflicts and their resolution. *Journal for the Scientific Study of Religion, 37,* 181–190.

Nielsen, M. E. (2001, September 14). Religion's role in the terroristic attack of September 11, 2001 [Online]. Available: http://www.psywww.com/psyrelig/fundamental/html [Retrieved December 1, 2001].

Nielsen, M. E., & Fultz, J. (1997). An alternative view of religious complexity. *International Journal for the Psychology of Religion, 7,* 23–35.

Nipkow, K. E., & Schweitzer, F. (1991). Adolescents' justifications for faith or doubt in God: A study of fulfilled and unfulfilled expectations. In F. K. Oser & W. G. Scarlett (Eds.), *Religious development in childhood and adolescence* (New Directions for Child Development, No. 52, pp. 91–100). San Francisco: Jossey-Bass.

Nolan, W. M. (1990). Scrupulosity. In R. J. Hunter, H. N. Malony, L. O. Mills, & J. Patton (Eds.), *Dictionary of pastoral care and counseling* (p. 1120). Nashville, TN: Abingdon Press.

Nordquist, T. A. (1978). *Ananda cooperative village: A study in the beliefs, values and attitudes of a new age religious community.* Uppsala, Sweden: Borgstroms Tryckeri.

Nucci, L., & Turiel, E. (1993). God's word, religious rules, and their relation to Christian and Jewish children's concepts of morality. *Child Development, 64,* 1475–1491.

Nunn, C. Z. (1964). Child-control through a "coalition with God." *Child Development, 35,* 417–432.

Nunnally, J. C. (1961). *Popular conceptions of mental health.* New York: Holt, Rinehart & Winston.

Nye, W. C., & Carlson, J. S. (1984). The development of the concept of God in children. *Journal of Genetic Psychology, 145,* 137–142.

Oakes, K. E., Allen, J. P., & Ciarrocchi, J. W. (2000). Spirituality, religious problem-solving, and sobriety in Alcoholics Anonymous. *Alcoholism Treatment Quarterly, 18,* 37–50.

O'Brien, E. (Ed.). (1965). *The varieties of mystical experience.* Garden City, NY: Doubleday/Anchor.

O'Brien, C. R. (1979). Pastoral dimensionms in death education research. *Journal of Religion and Health, 18,* 74–77.

Ochsmann, R. (1984). Belief in an afterlife as a moderator of fear of death? *European Journal of Social Psychology, 14,* 53–67.

O'Connell, D. C. (1961). Is mental illness a result of sin? In A. Godin (Ed.), *Child and adult before God* (pp. 55–64). Brussels: Lumen Vitae Press.

O'Dea, T. F. (1957). *The Mormons.* Chicago: University of Chicago Press.

O'Donnell, J. P. (1993). Predicting tolerance for new religious movements: A multivariate analysis. *Journal for the Scientific Study of Religion, 32,* 356–365.

O'Faolain, J., & Martines, L. (Eds.). (1973). *Not in God's image.* New York: Harper & Row.

Ogata, A., & Miyakawa, T. (1998). Religious experiences in epileptic patients with a focus on ictus-related episodes. *Psychiatry and Clinical Neurosciences, 52,* 321–325.

O'Hara, J. P. (1980). A research note on the sources of adult church commitment among those who were regular attenders during childhood. *Review of Religious Research, 21,* 462–467.

Ojha, H., & Pramanick, M. (1992). Religio-cultural variation in childrearing practices. *Psychological Studies, 37,* 65–72.

Okagaki, L., & Bevis, C. (1999). Transmission of religious values: Relations between parents' and daughters' beliefs. *Journal of Genetic Psychology, 160,* 303–318.

Oksanen, A. (1994). *Religious conversion: A meta-analytical study.* Lund, Sweden: Lund University Press.

Oliner, S. P., & Oliner, P. M. (1988). *The altruistic personality: Rescuers of Jews in Nazi Europe.* New York: Free Press.

Olshan, M. A. (1994). Conclusion: What good are the Amish? In D. B. Kraybill & M. A. Olshan (Eds.), *The Amish struggle with modernity* (pp. 231–242). Hanover, NH: University Press of New England.

Olson, D. V. A. (1989). Church friendships: Boon or barrier to church growth? *Journal for the Scientific Study of Religion, 28,* 432–447.

Olson, D. V. A., & Perl, P. (2001). Variations in strictness and religious commitment among five denominations. *Journal for the Scientific Study of Religion, 40,* 757–764.

Olson, J. M., Vernon, P. A., Harris, J. A., & Jang, K. L. (2001). The heritability of attitudes: A study of twins. *Journal of Personality and Social Psychology, 80,* 845–860.

Onions, C. T. (Ed.). (1955). *The Oxford universal dictionary on historical principles* (3rd ed.). London: Oxford University Press.

Orbach, H. L. (1961). Aging and religion: A study of church attendance in the Detroit metropolitan area. *Geriatrics, 16,* 530–540.

Ornstein, R. O. (1986). *The psychology of human consciousness* (3rd ed.). New York: Viking Press.

Ortberg, J. C., Jr., Gorsuch, R. L., & Kim, G. J. (2001). Changing attitude and moral obligation: Their independent effects on behavior. *Journal for the Scientific Study of Religion, 40,* 489–496.

Osarchuk, M., & Tatz, S. J. (1973). Effect of induced fear of death on belief in an afterlife. *Journal of Personality and Social Psychology, 27,* 256–260.

Oser, F. K. (1991). The development of religious judgment. In F. K. Oser & W. G. Scarlett (Eds.), *Religious development in childhood and adolescence* (New Directions for Child Development, No. 52, pp. 5–25). San Francisco: Jossey-Bass.

Oser, F. K. (1994). The development of religious judgment. In B. Puka (Ed.), *Moral development: A compendium. Vol. 2. Fundamental research in moral development* (pp. 375–395). New York: Garland Press.

Oser, F. K., & Gmunder, P. (1991). *Religious judgment: A developmental approach* (H. F. Hahn, Trans.). Birmingham, AL: Religious Education Press.

Oser, F. K., & Reich, K. H. (1990). Moral judgment, religious judgment, worldview, and logical thought: A review of their relationship. *British Journal of Religious Education, 12,* 94–101.

Oser, F. K., & Reich, K. H. (1996). Psychological perspectives on religious development. *World Psychology, 2,* 365–396.

Oser, F. K., Reich, K. H., & Bucher, A. A. (1994). Development of belief and unbelief in childhood and adolescence. In J. Corveleyn & D. Hutsebaut (Eds.), *Belief and unbelief: Psychological perspectives* (Vol. 3, pp. 39–62). Atlanta, GA: Rodopi.

Oser, F. K., & Scarlett, W. G. (Eds.). (1991). *Religious development in childhood and adolescence* (New Directions for Child Development, No. 52). San Francisco: Jossey-Bass.

Oshodin, O. G. (1983). Alcohol abuse: A case study of secondary school students in a rural area of Benin District, Nigeria. *Journal of Alcohol and Drug Education, 29,* 40–47.

Osis, K., & Haraldson, E. (1977). *At the hour of death.* New York: Avon.

Ostow, M. (1990). The fundamentalist phenomenon: A psychological perspective. In N. J. Cohen (Ed.), *The fundamentalist phenomenon* (pp. 99–125). Grand Rapids, MI: Eerdmans.

Ostow, M., & Scharfstein, B.-A. (1954). *The need to believe.* New York: International Universities Press.

Ostrer, H. (2000). Genetic analysis of Jewish origins. *Avotaynu, 16*(1), 15–16.

Otto, R. (1932). *Mysticism East and West* (B. L. Bracey & R. C. Payne, Trans.). New York: Macmillan.

Otto, R. (1958). *The idea of the holy* (J. W. Harvey, Trans.). London: Oxford University Press. (Original work published 1917)

Overholser, W. (1963). Psychopathology in religious experience. In *Research in Religion and Mental Health: Proceedings of the Fifth Academy Symposium, 1961, of the Academy of Religion and Mental Health* (pp.100–116). New York: Fordham University Press.

Owens, C. M. (1972). The mystical experience: Facts and values. In J. White (Ed.), *The highest state of consciousness* (pp. 135–152). Garden City, NY: Doubleday/Anchor.

Oxford dictionary of quotations (2nd ed.). (1959). London: Oxford University Press.

Oxman, T. E., Rosenberg, S. D., Schnurr, P. P., Tucker, G. J., & Gala, G. G. (1988). The language of altered states. *Journal of Nervous and Mental Disease, 176,* 401–408.

Ozorak, E. (1989). Social and cognitive influences on the development of religious beliefs and commitment in adolescence. *Journal for the Scientific Study of Religion, 28,* 448–463.

Ozorak, E. W. (1996). The power, but not the glory: How women empower themselves through religion. *Journal for the Scientific Study of Religion, 35,* 17–29.

Pafford, M. (1973). *Inglorious Wordsworths: A study of some transcendental experiences in childhood and adolescence.* London: Hodder & Stoughton.

Pagelow, M. D., & Johnson, P. (1988). Abuse in the American family: The role of religion. In A. L.

Horton & J. A. Williamson (Eds.), *Abuse and religion: When praying isn't enough* (pp. 1–12). Lexington, MA: Lexington Books.

Pahnke, W. N. (1966). Drugs and mysticism. *International Journal of Parapsychology, 8,* 295–320.

Pahnke, W. N. (1969). Psychedelic drugs and mystical experience. In E. M. Pattison (Ed.), *Clinical psychiatry and religion* (pp. 149–162). Boston: Little, Brown.

Paine, T. (1897). *The political works of Thomas Paine.* Chicago: Donahue Brothers.

Palkovitz, R., & Palm, G. (1998). Fatherhood and faith in formation: The developmental effects of fathering on religiosity, morals, and values. *Journal of Men's Studies, 7,* 33–51.

Palmer, C. E., & Noble, D. N. (1986). Premature death: Dilemmas of infant mortality. *Social Casework, 67,* 332–339.

Paloutzian, R. F. (1981). Purpose-in-life and value changes following religious conversion. *Journal of Personality and Social Psychology, 41,* 1153–1168.

Paloutzian, R. F. (1996). *Invitation to the psychology of religion* (2nd ed.). Needham Heights, MA: Allyn & Bacon.

Paloutzian, R. F., Jackson, S. L., & Crandell, J. E. (1978). Conversion experience, belief system, and personal and ethical attitudes. *Journal of Psychology and Theology, 6,* 266–275.

Paloutzian, R. F., Richardson, J. T., & Rambo, L. R. (1999). Religious conversion and personality change. *Journal of Personality, 67,* 1047–1079.

Pancer, S. M., Jackson, L. M., Hunsberger, B., Pratt, M., & Lea, J. (1995). Religious orthodoxy and the complexity of thought about religious and non-religious issues. *Journal of Personality, 63,* 213–232.

Pancer, S. M., & Pratt, M. (1999). Social and family determinants of community service involvement in Canadians. In M. Yates & J. Youniss (Eds.), *Roots of civic identity: Intervention perspectives on community service and activism in youth* (pp. 32–55). New York: Cambridge University Press.

Pandey, R. E. (1974–1975). A factor-analytic study of attitudes toward death among college students. *International Journal of Social Psychiatry, 21,* 7–11.

Pardini, D. A., Plante, T. G., Sherman, A., & Stump, J. E. (2000). Religious faith and spirituality in substance abuse recovery: Determining the mental health benefits. *Journal of Substance Abuse Treatment, 19,* 347–354.

Pargament, K. I. (1992). Of means and ends: Religion and the search for significance. *International Journal for the Psychology of Religion, 2,* 201–229.

Pargament, K. I. (1997). *The psychology of religion and coping.* New York: Guilford Press.

Pargament, K. I. (1999). The psychology of religion and spirituality?: Yes and no. *International Journal for the Psychology of Religion, 9,* 3–16.

Pargament, K. I., & Brant, C. R. (1998). Religion and coping. In H. G. Koenig (Ed.), *Handbook of religion and mental health* (pp. 111–128). San Diego, CA: Academic Press.

Pargament, K. I., Ensing, D. S., Falgout, K., Olsen, H., Reilly, B., Van Haitsma, K., & Warren, R. (1990). God help me: I. Coping efforts as predictors of the outcomes to significant negative life events. *American Journal of Community Psychology, 18,* 793–824.

Pargament, K. I., Kennell, J., Hathaway, W., Grevengoed, N., Newman, J., & Jones, W. (1988). Religion and the problem-solving process: Three styles of coping. *Journal for the Scientific Study of Religion, 27,* 90–104.

Pargament, K. I., Koenig, H. G., & Perez, L. M. (2000). The many methods of religious coping: Development and initial validation of the RCOPE. *Journal of Clinical Psychology, 56,* 519–543.

Pargament, K. I., & Mahoney, A. (2002). Spirituality: Discovering and conserving the sacred. In C. R. Snyder & S. J. Lopez (Eds.), *Handbook of positive psychology* (pp. 646–659). New York: Oxford University Press.

Pargament, K. I., Poloma, M. M., & Tarakeshwar, N. (2001). Methods of coping from the religions of the world: The bar mitzvah, karma, and spiritual healing. In C. R. Snyder (Ed.), *Coping with stress: Effective people and processes* (pp. 259–284). New York: Oxford University Press.

Pargament, K. I., & Rye, M. S. (1998). Forgiveness as a method of religious coping. In E. L. Worthington, Jr. & M. E. McCullough (Eds.), *Psychological research and theoretical perspectives* (pp. 57–76). Philadelphia: Templeton Press.

Park, C., & Cohen, L. H. (1993). Religious and nonreligious coping with the death of a friend. *Cognitive Therapy and Research, 17,* 561–577.

Park, C., Cohen, L. H., & Herb, L. (1990). Intrinsic religiousness and religious coping as life stress moderators for Catholics versus Protestants. *Journal of Personality and Social Psychology, 59,* 562–574.

Park, H.-S., Bauer, S., & Oescher, J. (2001). Religiousness as a predictor of alcohol use in high school students. *Journal of Drug Education, 31,* 289–303.

Park, J. Z., & Smith, C. (2000). "To whom much has been given . . ." : Religious capital and community voluntarism among churchgoing Protestants. *Journal for the Scientific Study of Religion, 39,* 272–286.

Parker, C. A. (1971). Changes in religious beliefs of college students. In M. P. Strommen (Ed.), *Research on religious development: A comprehensive handbook* (pp. 724–776). New York: Hawthorn Books.

Parker, G. (1983). *Parental overprotection.* New York: Grune & Stratton.

Parker, G. B., & Brown, L. B. (1982). Coping behaviors that mediate between life events and depression. *Archives of General Psychiatry, 39,* 1386–1391.

Parker, G., Tupling, H., & Brown, L. B. (1979). A parental bonding instrument. *British Journal of Medical Psychology, 52,* 1–10.

Parker, I. (1989). *The crisis in social psychology and how to end it.* New York: Routledge.

Parker, I., & Shotter, J. (Eds.). (1987). *Deconstructing social psychology.* New York: Routledge.

Parker, M., & Gaier, E. L. (1980). Religion, religious beliefs, and religious practices among Conservative Jewish adolescents. *Adolescence, 15,* 361–374.

Parkes, C. M. (1972). *Bereavement: Studies of grief in later life.* New York: International Universities Press.

Parnell, J. O., & Sprinkle, R. L. (1990). Personality characteristics of persons who claim UFO experiences. *Journal of UFO Studies, 2,* 105–137.

Parrinder, G. (1980). *Sex in the world's religions.* New York: Oxford University Press.

Parsons, W. B. (1999). *The enigma of the oceanic feeling: Revisioning the psychoanalytic theory of mysticism.* New York: Oxford University Press.

Pastorino, E., Dunham, R. M., Kidwell, J., Bacho, R., & Lamborn, S. D. (1997). Domain-specific gender comparisons in identity development among college youth: Ideology and relationships. *Adolescence, 32,* 559–577.

Patrick, T., & Dulack, T. (1977). *Let our children go!* New York: Ballantine Books.

Pattison, M. (1968). Behavioral science research on the nature of glossolalia. *Journal of the American Scientific Affiliation, 20,* 73–86

Patton, J. (2000). Forgiveness in pastoral care and counseling. In M. E. McCullough, K. I. Pargament, & C. E. Thoresen (Eds.), *Forgiveness: Theory, research, and practice* (pp. 281–295) New York: Guilford Press.

Patton, M. S. (1988). Suffering and damage in Catholic sexuality. *Journal of Religion and Health, 27,* 129–142.

Paul, C., Fitzjohn, J., Eberhart-Phillips, J., Herbison, P., & Dickson, N. (2000). Sexual abstinence at age 21 in New Zealand: The importance of religion. *Social Science and Medicine, 51,* 1–10.

Payne, B. P. (1988). Religious patterns and participation of older adults: A sociological perspective. *Educational Gerontology, 14,* 255–267.

Payne, J. N. (1990). *A study of demographics, role stress, and hardiness in the prediction of burnout among ministers.* Unpublished doctoral dissertation, University of Mississippi.

Pearce, L. P., & Axinn, W. G. (1998). The impact of family religious life on the quality of mother–child relations. *American Sociological Review, 63,* 810–828.

Peatling, J. H. (1974). Cognitive development in pupils in grades four through twelve: The incidence of concrete and religious thinking. *Character Potential: A Record of Research, 7,* 52–61.

Peatling, J. H. (1977). Cognitive development: Religious thinking in children, youth and adults. *Character Potential: A Record of Research, 8,* 100–115.

Peatling, J. H., & Laabs, C. W. (1975). Cognitive development in pupils in grades four through twelve: The incidence of concrete and abstract religious thinking. *Character Potential: A Record of Research, 7,* 107–115.

Peatling, J. H., Laabs, C. W., & Newton, T. B. (1975). Cognitive development: A three-sample comparison of means on the Peatling Scale of Religious Thinking. *Character Potential: A Record of Research, 7,* 159–162.

Pederson, N. L., Gatz, M., Plomin, R., Nesselroade, J. R., & McClearn, G. E. (1989). Individual differences in locus of control during the second half of the life span for identical and fraternal twins reared apart and reared together. *Journal of Gerontology: Psychological Sciences, 44*(4), 100–105.

Peek, C. W., Curry, E. W., & Chalfant, H. P. (1985). Religiosity and delinquency over time: Deviance, deterrence and deviance amplification. *Social Science Quarterly, 66,* 120–131.

Peel, R. (1987). *Spiritual healing in a scientific age.* San Francisco: Harper & Row.

Pelletier, K. R., & Garfield, C. (1976). *Consciousness: East and West.* New York: Harper & Row.

Pelton, R. W., & Carden, K. W. (1974). *Snake handlers: God-fearers or fanatics?* Nashville, TN: Nelson.

Perez, R. L. (2000). Fiesta as tradition, fiesta as change: Ritual, alcohol and violence in a Mexican community. *Addiction, 95,* 365–373.

Perkins, H. W. (1991). Religious commitment, yuppie values, and well-being in post-collegiate life. *Review of Religious Research, 32,* 244–251.

Perkins, H. W. (1994). The contextual effect of secular norms on religiosity as moderator of student alcohol and other drug use. *Research in the Social Scientific Study of Religion, 6,* 187–208.

Perrin, R. D. (2000). Religiosity and honesty: Continuing the search for the consequential dimension. *Review of Religious Research, 41,* 534–544.

Perry, E. L., & Hoge, D. R. (1981). Faith priorities of pastor and laity as a factor in the growth and decline of Presbyterian congregations. *Review of Religious Research, 22,* 221–241.

Perry, E. L., Davis, J. H., Doyle, R. T., & Dyble, J. E. (1980). Toward a typology of unchurched Protestants. *Review of Religious Research, 21,* 388–404.

Perry, N., & Echeverría, L. (1988). *Under the heel of Mary.* London: Routledge & Kegan Paul.

Perry, R. B. (1935). *The thought and character of William James* (2 vols.). Boston: Little, Brown.

Persinger, M. A. (1987). *Neurophysiological basis of God beliefs.* New York: Praeger.

Persinger, M. A. (1993). Vectorial cerebral hemisphericity as differential sources for the sensed presence, mystical experiences, and religious conversions. *Perceptual and Motor Skills, 76,* 915–930.

Persinger, M. A., Bureau, Y. R. J., Peredery, O. P., & Richards, P. M. (1994). The sensed presence as right hemispheric intrusions into the left hemispheric awareness of self: An illustrative case study. *Perceptual and Motor Skills, 78,* 999–1009.

Persinger, M. A., & Makarec, K. (1987). Temporal lobe epileptic signs and correlative behaviors displayed by normal populations. *Journal of General Psychology, 114,* 179–195.

Peter, L. J. (Ed.).(1979). *Peter's quotations.* New York: Bantam.

Petersen, A. C. (1988). Adolescent development. *Annual Review of Psychology, 39,* 583–607.

Petersen, L. R., & Donnenwerth, G. V. (1997). Secularization and the influence of religion on beliefs about premarital sex. *Social Forces, 75,* 1071–1088.

Peterson, B. E., & Lane, M. D. (2001). Implications of authoritarianism for young adulthood: Longitudinal analysis of college experiences and future goals. *Personality and Social Psychology Bulletin, 27,* 678–690.

Peterson, C., Seligman, M. E. P., & Vaillant, G. E. (1988). Pessimistic explanatory style is a risk factor for physical illness: A thirty-five year longitudinal study. *Journal of Personality and Social Psychology, 55,* 23–27.

Petraitis, J., Flay, B. R., & Miller, T. Q. (1995). Reviewing theories of adolescent substance use: Organizing pieces in the puzzle. *Psychological Bulletin, 117,* 67–86.

Petsonk, J., & Remsen, J. (1988). *The intermarriage handbook: A guide for Jews and Christians.* New York: William Morrow/Quill.

Pettersson, T. (1991). Religion and criminality: Structural relationships between church involvement and crime rates in contemporary Sweden. *Journal for the Scientific Study of Religion, 30,* 279–291.

Pevey, C. (1994, November 4). *Submission and power among Southern Baptist ladies.* Paper presented at the annual convention of the Society for the Scientific Study of Religion, Albuquerque, NM.

Pfeiffer, J. E. (1992). The psychological framing of cults: Schematic representations and cult evaluations. *Journal of Applied Social Psychology, 22,* 531–544.

Phares, E. J. (1976). *Locus of control in personality.* Morristown, NJ: General Learning Press.

Philibert, P. J., & Hoge, D. R. (1982). Teachers, pedagogy and the process of religious education. *Review of Religious Research, 23,* 264–285.

Philipchalk, R., & Mueller, D. (2000). Glossolalia and temperature change in the right and left cerebral hemispheres. *International Journal for the Study of Religion, 10,* 181–185.

Piaget, J. (1948). *The moral judgment of the child* (M. Gabain, Trans.). Glencoe, IL: Free Press. (Original work published 1936)

Piaget, J. (1952). *The origins of intelligence in children* (M. Cook, Trans.). New York: International Universities Press. (Original work published 1936)

Piaget, J. (1954). *The construction of reality in the child* (M. Cook, Trans.). New York: Basic Books. (Original work published 1937)

Pierce, B. J., & Cox, W. F. (1995). Development of faith and religious understanding in children. *Psychological Reports, 76,* 957–958.

Pilarzyk, K. T. (1978). The origin, development and decline of a youth culture movement: An application of sectarianization theory. *Review of Religious Research, 20,* 23–43.

Pilkington, G. W., Poppleton, P. K., Gould, J. B., & McCourt, M. M. (1976). Changes in religious beliefs, practices and attitudes among university students over an eleven-year period in relation to sex differences, denominational differences and differences between faculties and years of study. *British Journal of Social and Clinical Psychology, 15,* 1–9.

Pinker, S. (1997). *How the mind works.* New York: Norton.

Plante, T. G. (1999). Introduction: What do we know about Roman Catholic priests who sexually abuse minors? In T. G. Plante (Ed.), *Bless me father for I have sinned: Perspectives on sexual abuse committed by Roman Catholic Priests* (pp. 1–6). Westport, CT: Praeger.

Plante, T. G., & Sharma, N. K. (2001). Religious faith and mental health outcomes. In T. G. Plante & A. C. Sherman (Eds.), *Faith and health: Psychological perspectives* (pp. 240–261). New York: Guilford Press.

Plante, T. G., & Sherman, A. C. (Eds.). (2001). *Faith and health: Psychological perspectives.* New York: Guilford Press.

Plaskow, J., & Romero, J. A. (Eds). (1974). *Women and religion* (ref. ed.). Missoula, MT: Scholars Press.

Ploch, D. R., & Hastings, D. W. (1994). Graphic presentations of church attendance using General Social Survey data. *Journal for the Scientific Study of Religion, 33,* 16–33.

Plutchik, R., & Ax, F. A. (1967). A critique of "Determinants of emotional state" by Schachter and Singer. *Psychophysiology, 4,* 79–82.

Pollner, M. (1987). *Mundane reason: Reality in everyday and sociological discourse.* Cambridge, England: Cambridge University Press.

Pollner, M. (1989). Divine relations, social relations, and well-being. *Journal of Health and Social Behavior, 30,* 92–104.

Poloma, M. M. (1991). A comparison of Christian Science and mainline Christian healing ideologies and practices. *Review of Religious Research, 32,* 337–350.

Poloma, M. M., & Gallup, G. H., Jr. (1991). *Varieties of prayer: A survey report.* Philadelphia: Trinity Press International.

Poloma, M. M., & Pendleton, B. F. (1989). Exploring types of prayer and quality of life research: A research note. *Review of Religious Research, 31,* 46–53.

Poloma, M. M., & Pendleton, B. F. (1991). *Exploring neglected dimensions of quality of life research.* Lewiston, NY: Mellen.

Ponton, M. O., & Gorsuch, R. L. (1988). Prejudice and religion revisited: A cross-cultural investigation with a Venezuelan sample. *Journal for the Scientific Study of Religion, 27,* 260–271.

Porges, S. W. (1998). Love: An emergent property of the mammalian autonomic nervous system. *Psychoneuroendocrinology, 23,* 837–861.

Porterfield, A. (2001). *The transformation of American religion.* New York: Oxford University Press.

Post, R. H. (1973). Jews, genetics, and disease. In A. Shiloh & I. C. Selavan (Eds.), *Ethnic groups of America: Their morbidity, mortality, and behavior disorders. Vol. 1. The Jews* (pp. 67–71). Springfield, IL: Charles Thomas.

Poston, L. (1992). *Islamic da 'wah in the West.* Oxford: Oxford University Press.

Potvin, R. H. (1977). Adolescent God images. *Review of Religious Research, 19,* 43–53.

Potvin, R. H., & Sloane, D. M. (1985). Parental control, age, and religious practice. *Review of Religious Research, 27,* 3–14.

Poulson, R. L., Eppler, M. A., Satterwhite, T. N., Wuensch, K. L., & Bass, L. A. (1998). Alcohol consumption, strength of religious beliefs and risky sexual behavior in college students. *Journal of American College Health, 46,* 227–232.

Pratt, J. B. (1920). *The religious consciousness: A psychological study.* New York: Macmillan.

Pratt, M. W., Hunsberger, B., Pancer, S. M., & Roth, D. (1992). Reflections on religion: Aging, belief orthodoxy, and interpersonal conflict in adult thinking about religious issues. *Journal for the Scientific Study of Religion, 31,* 514–522.

Prendergast, M. L. (1994). Substance use and abuse among college students: A review of recent literature. *Journal of American College Health, 43,* 99–113.

Pressman, P., Lyons, J. S., Larson, D. B., & Gartner, J. (1992). Religion, anxiety, and fear of death. In J. F. Schumaker (Ed.), *Religion and mental health* (pp. 98–109). New York: Oxford University Press.

Pressman, P., Lyons, J. S., Larson, D. B., & Strain, J. J. (1990). Religious belief, depression, and ambulation status in elderly women with broken hips. *American Journal of Psychiatry. 147,* 758–760.

Preston, D. L. (1981). Becoming a Zen practitioner. *Sociological Analysis, 42,* 47–55.

Preston, D. L. (1982). Meditative–ritual practice and spiritual conversion–commitment: Theoretical implications based upon the case of Zen. *Sociological Analysis, 43,* 257–270.

Preston, D. L. (1988). *The social organization of Zen practice.* Cambridge, England: Cambridge University Press.

Preus, J. S. (1987). *Explaining religion.* New Haven, CT: Yale University Press.

Preus, K. (1982). Tongues: an evaluation from a scientific perspective. *Concordia Theological Quarterly, 46,* 277–293.

Prince, R. H. (1992). Religious experience and psychopathology. In J. F. Schumaker (Ed.), *Religion and mental health* (pp. 281–290). New York: Oxford University Press.

Pritt, A. F. (1998). Spiritual correlates of reported sexual abuse among Mormon women. *Journal for the Scientific Study of Religion, 37,* 273–285.

Propst, L. B. (1988). *Psychotherapy in a religious framework.* New York: Human Sciences Press.

Proudfoot, W. (1985). *Religious experience.* Berkeley: University of California Press.

Proudfoot, W., & Shaver, P. (1975). Attribution theory and the psychology of religion. *Journal for the Scientific Study of Religion, 14,* 317–330.

Pruyser, P. W. (1968). *A dynamic psychology of religion.* New York: Harper & Row.

Pruyser, P. W. (1971). A psychological view of religion in the 1970s. *Bulletin of the Menninger Clinic, 35,* 77–97.

Pruyser, P. W. (1977). The seamy side of current religious beliefs. *Bulletin of the Menninger Clinic, 41,* 329–348.

Puhakka, K. (1995). Hinduism and religious experience. In R. W. Hood, Jr. (Ed.), *Handbook of religious experience* (pp. 122–143). Birmingham, AL: Religious Education Press.

Purves, W. K., Orians, G. H., & Heller, H. C. (1995). *Life: The science of biology.* Sunderland, MA: Sinauer.

Putnam, R. D. (2000). *Bowling alone: The collapse and revival of American community.* New York: Simon & Schuster.

Pylyshyn, Z. W. (1973). What a mind's eye tells the mind's brain. *Psychological Bulletin, 80,* 1–24.

Qin, J., Goodman, G. S., Bottoms, B. L., & Shaver, P. R. (1998). Repressed memories of ritualistic and religion-related abuse. In S. J. Lynn & K. M. McConkey (Eds.), *Truth in memory* (pp. 260–283). New York: Guilford Press.

Quinley, H. E., & Glock, C. Y. (1979). *Anti-Semitism in America.* New York: Free Press.

Qureshi, N. A., & Al-Habeeb, T. A. (2000). Sociodemographic parameters and clinical pattern of drug abuse in Al-Qassim region—Saudi Arabia. *Arab Journal of Psychiatry, 11,* 10–21.

Rabinowitz, S. (1969). Developmental problems in Catholic seminarians. *Psychiatry, 32,* 107–117.

Ragan, C., Malony, H. N., & Beit-Hallahmi, B. (1980). Psychologists and religion: Professional factors and personal belief. *Review of Religious Research, 21,* 208–217.

Ramachandran, V. S., & Blakeslee, S. (1999). *Phantoms in the brain.* New York: William Morrow.

Rambo, L. R. (1982). Current research on religious conversion. *Religious Studies Review, 8,* 146–159.

Rambo, L. R. (1992). The psychology of conversion. In H. N. Malony & S. Southard (Eds.), *Handbook of religious conversion* (pp. 159–177). Birmingham, AL: Religious Education Press.

Rambo, L. R. (1993). *Understanding religious conversion.* New Haven: CT: Yale University Press.

Ranck, J. G. (1961). Religious conservatism–liberalism and mental health. *Pastoral Psychology, 12,* 34–40.

Randall, T. M., & Desrosiers, M. (1980). Measurement of supernatural belief: Sex differences and locus of control. *Journal of Personality Assessment, 44,* 493–498.

Rappaport, R. A. (1999). *Ritual and religion in the making of humanity.* Cambridge, England: Cambridge University Press.

Rasmussen, C. H. & Johnson, M. E. (1994). Spirituality and religiosity: Relative relationships to death anxiety. *Omega, 29,* 313–318.

Rätsch, C. (Ed.). (1990). *Gateway to inner space: Sacred plants, mysticism and psychotherapy.* Dorset, England: Prism Press.

Rayburn, C. A., & Richmond, L. J. (1998). "Theobiology": Attempting to understand God and ourselves. *Journal of Religion and Health, 37,* 345–356.

Rayburn, C. A., & Richmond, L. J. (2000). Theobiology: Its relevance to deeper understanding. In S. M. Natale (Ed.), *On the threshold of the millennium* (pp. 281–288). New York: Oxford University Press.

Rayburn, C. A., Richmond, L. J., & Rogers, L. (1983). Stress among religious leaders. *Thought, 58,* 329–344.

Rayburn, C. A., Richmond, L. J., & Rogers, L. (1986). Men, women, and religion: Stress within leadership roles. *Journal of Clinical Psychology, 42,* 540–546.

Rea, M. P., Greenspoon, S., & Spilka, B. (1975). Physicians and the terminal patient: Some selected attitudes and behavior. *Omega, 6,* 291–302.

Redekop, C. A. (1974). A new look at sect development. *Journal for the Scientific Study of Religion, 13,* 345–352.

Reed, G. (1974). *The psychology of anomalous experience.* Boston: Houghton Mifflin.

Reeves, N. C., & Boersma, F. J. (1989–1990). The therapeutic use of ritual in maladaptive grieving. *Omega, 20,* 281–291.

Regnerus, M. D., Smith, C., & Sikkink, D. (1998). Who gives to the poor? The influence of religious tradition and political location on the personal generosity of Americans toward the poor. *Journal for the Scientific Study of Religion, 37,* 481–493.

Reich, K. H. (1989). Between religion and science: Complementarity in the religious thinking of young people. *British Journal of Religious Education, 11,* 62–69.

Reich, K. H. (1991). The role of complementarity reasoning in religious development. In F. K. Oser & W. G. Scarlett (Eds.), *Religious development in childhood and adolescence* (New Directions for Child Development, No. 52, pp. 77–89). San Francisco: Jossey-Bass.

Reich, K. H. (1992). Religious development across the lifespan: Conventional and cognitive developmental approaches. In D. L. Featherman, R. M. Lerner, & M. Perlmutter (Eds.), *Life-span development and behavior* (Vol. 11, pp. 145–188). Hillsdale, NJ: Erlbaum.

Reich, K. H. (1993a). Cognitive-developmental approaches to religiousness: Which version for which purpose? *International Journal for the Psychology of Religion, 3,* 145–171.

Reich, K. H. (1993b). Integrating differing theories: The case of religious development. *Journal of Empirical Theology, 6,* 39–49.

Reich, K. H. (1994). Can one rationally understand Christian doctrines? An empirical study. *British Journal of Religious Education, 16,* 114–126.

Reich, K. H. (1997). Do we need a theory for the religious development of women? *International Journal for the Psychology of Religion, 7,* 67–86.

Reich, K. H. (2000). Scientist vs. believer: On navigating between the Scilla of scientific norms and the Charybdis of personal experience. *Journal of Psychology and Theology, 28,* 190–200.

Reid, T. (1969). *The active powers of the human mind.* Cambridge, MA: MIT Press.

Reifsnyder, W. E., & Campbell, E. I. (1960). Religious attitudes of male neuropsychiatric patients: I. Most frequently expressed attitudes. *Journal of Pastoral Care, 14,* 92–97.

Reik, T. (1946). *Ritual: Psychoanalytic studies.* New York: Farrar, Straus.

Reineke, M. J. (1989). Out of order: A critical perspective on women in religion. In J. Freeman (Ed.), *Women: A feminist perspective* (4th ed., pp. 395–413). Mountain View, CA: Mayfield.

Reinert, D. F., & Smith, C. E. (1997). Childhood sexual abuse and female spiritual development. *Counseling and Values, 41,* 235–245.

Reinert, D. F., & Stifler, K. R. (1993). Hood's Mysticism Scale revisited: A factor-analytic replication. *Journal for the Scientific Study of Religion, 32,* 383–388.

Reisman, J. M. (1991). *A history of clinical psychology* (2nd ed.). New York: Hemisphere.

Reiss, I. L. (1976). *The family system in America* (2nd ed.). New York: Holt, Rinehart and Winston.

Religions for Peace (RFP). (2001). *Missions and activities.* [Online]. Available: http://www.wcrp.org/RforP/MISSION CONTENT.html [Retrieved August 12, 2002].

Rest, J. R. (1979). *Development in judging moral issues.* Minneapolis: University of Minnesota Press.

Rest, J. R. (1983). Morality. In J. H. Flavell & E. M. Markham (Vol. Eds.) & P. H. Mussen (Series Ed.), *Handbook of child psychology: Vol. 3. Cognitive development* (4th ed., pp. 556–629). New York: Wiley.

Rest, J. R., Cooper, D., Coder, R., Masanz, J., & Anderson, D. (1974). Judging the important issues in moral dilemmas: An objective measure of development. *Developmental Psychology, 10,* 491–501.

Rest, J. R., Narvaez, D., Thoma, S. J., & Bebeau, M. J. (1999). DIT2: Devising and testing a revised instrument of moral judgment. *Journal of Educational Psychology, 91,* 644–659.

Reynolds, D. I. (1994). Religious influence and premarital sexual experience: Critical observations on the validity of a relationship. *Journal for the Scientific Study of Religion, 33,* 382–387.

Reynolds, D. K., & Nelson, F. L. (1981). Personality, life situation, and life expectancy. *Suicide and Life-Threatening Behavior, 11,* 99–110.

Rhodewalt, F., & Smith, T. W. (1991). Current issues in Type A behavior, coronary proneness, and coronary heart disease. In C. R. Snyder & D. R. Forsyth (Eds.), *Handbook of social and clinical psychology* (pp. 197–220). New York: Pergamon Press.

Riccio, J. A. (1979). Religious affiliation and socioeconomic achievement. In R. Wuthnow (Ed.), *The religious dimension: New directions in quantitative research* (pp. 199–228). New York: Academic Press.

Richard, A. J., Bell, D. C., & Carlson, J. W. (2000). Individual religiosity, moral community and drug user treatment. *Journal for the Scientific Study of Religion, 39,* 240–246.

Richards, P. S. (1991). The relation between conservative religious ideology and principled moral reasoning: A review. *Review of Religious Research, 32,* 359–368.

Richards, P. S., & Bergin, A. E. (1997). *A spiritual strategy for counseling and psychotherapy.* Washington, DC: American Psychological Association.

Richards, P. S., & Bergin, A. E. (Eds.). (2000). *Handbook of psychotherapy and religious diversity.* Washington, DC: American Psychological Association.

Richards, P. S., & Bergin, A. E. (Eds.). (in press). *Spiritual strategy case studies.* Washington, DC: American Psychological Association.

Richards, P. S., & Davison, M. L. (1992). Religious bias in moral development research: A psychometric investigation. *Journal for the Scientific Study of Religion, 31,* 467–485.

Richards, T. A., Wrubel, J., & Folkman, S. (1999–2000). Death rites in the San Francisco gay community: Cultural developments of the AIDS epidemic. *Omega, 40,* 335–350.

Richardson, A. H. (1973). Social and medical correlates of survival among octogenarians: United Automobile Worker retirees and Spanish American War veterans. *Journal of Gerontology, 28,* 207–215.

Richardson, H. (Ed.). (1980). *New religions and mental health.* New York: Edwin Mellen Press.

Richardson, J. T. (1973). Psychological interpretation of glossolalia: A reexamination of research. *Journal for the Scientific Study of Religion, 12,* 199–207.

Richardson, J. T. (1978a). An oppositional and general conceptualization of cult. *Social Research, 41,* 299–327.

Richardson, J. T. (Ed.). (1978b). *Conversion careers: In and out of the new religions.* Beverly Hills, CA: Sage.

Richardson, J. T. (1979). From cult to sect: Creative eclecticism in new religious movements. *Pacific Sociological Review, 22,* 139–166.

Richardson, J. T. (1985a, October). *Legal and practical reasons for claiming to be a religion.* Paper presented at the annual meeting of the Society for the Scientific Study of Religion, Savannah, GA.

Richardson, J. T. (1985b). The active vs. passive convert: Paradigm conflict in conversion/recruitment research. *Journal for the Scientific Study of Religion, 24,* 163–179.

Richardson, J. T. (1992). Mental health of cult consumers. In J. F. Schumaker (Ed.), *Religion and mental health* (pp. 233–244). New York: Oxford University Press.

Richardson, J. T. (1993a). Definitions of cult: From sociological–technical to popular–negative. *Review of Religious Research, 34,* 348–356.

Richardson, J. T. (1993b). Religiosity as deviance: Negative religious bias in and misuse of the DSM-III. *Deviant Behaviors, 14,* 1–21.

Richardson, J. T. (1995). Clinical and personality assessment of participants in new religions. *International Journal for the Psychology of Religion, 5,* 145–170.

Richardson, J. T. (1999a). Social control of new religions: From "brainwashing" claims to sexual abuse accusations. In S. Palmer & C. Hardman (Eds.), *Children in new religions* (pp. 172–186). New Brunswick, NJ: Rutgers University Press.

Richardson, J. T. (1999b). Social justice and minority religions. *Social Justice Research, 12,* 241–252.

Richardson, J. T., Best, J., & Bromley, D. G. (Eds.). (1991). *The Satanism scare.* Hawthorne, NY: Aldine/de Gruyter.

Richardson, J. T., & Introvigne, M. (2001). "Brainwashing" theories in European parliamentary administrative reports. *Journal for the Scientific Study of Religion, 40,* 143–168.

Richardson, J. T., Stewart, T. M., & Simmonds, R. (1979). *Organized miracles: A study of a communal youth fundamentalist group.* New Brunswick, NJ: Transaction Books.

Richardson, J. T., & van Driel, B. (1984). Public support for anti-cult legislation. *Journal for the Scientific Study of Religion, 23,* 412–418.

Ring, K. (1984). Heading toward omega: In search of the meaning of the near death experience. New York: Morrow.

Ritzema, R. J. (1979). Religiosity and altruism: Faith without works? *Journal of Psychology and Theology, 7,* 105–113.

Rizzuto, A.-M. (1979). *The birth of the living God: A psychoanalytic study.* Chicago: University of Chicago Press.

Rizzuto, A.-M. (1991). Religious development: A psychoanalytic point of view. In F. K. Oser & W. G. Scarlett (Eds.), *Religious development in childhood and adolescence* (New Directions for Child Development, No. 52, pp. 47–60). San Francisco: Jossey-Bass.

Rizzuto, A.-M. (2001). Religious development beyond the modern paradigm discussion: The psychoanalytic point of view. *International Journal for the Psychology of Religion, 11,* 201–214.

Roach, J. L. (1990). *Coping with burnout: An ethnographic study of clergy in the Episcopal church.* Unpublished doctoral dissertation, University of Nebraska.

Robbins, A. (1985). New religious movements, brainwashing and deprogramming: The view from the law journals. *Religious Studies Review, 11,* 361–370.

Robbins, T. (1977, February 26). Even a Moonie has civil rights. *The Nation,* pp. 233–242.

Robbins, T. (1983). The beach is washing away: Controversial religion and the sociology of religion. *Sociological Analysis, 7,* 197–206.

Robbins, T. (2001). Combating "cults" and "brainwashing" in the United States and Western Europe: A comment on Richardson and Introvigne's report. *Journal for the Scientific Study of Religion, 40,* 169–175.

Robbins, T., & Anthony, D. (1979). Cults, brainwashing, and countersubversion. *Annals of the American Academy of Political and Social Science, 446,* 78–90.

Robbins, T., & Anthony, D. (1980). The limits of "coercive persuasion" as an explanation for conversion to authoritarian sects. *Political Psychology, 3,* 22–37.

Robbins, T., & Anthony, D. (1982). Deprogramming, brainwashing and the medicalization of deviant religious groups. *Social Problems, 29,* 284–296.

Roberts, A. E., Koch, J. R., & Johnson, D. P. (2001). Religious reference groups and the persistence of normative behavior: An empirical test. *Sociological Spectrum, 21,* 81–98.

Roberts, C. W. (1989). Imagining God: Who is created in whose image? *Review of Religious Research, 30,* 375–386.

Roberts, F. J. (1965). Some psychological factors in religious conversion. *British Journal of Social and Religious Psychology, 4,* 185–187.

Roberts, K. A. (1984). *Religion in sociological perspective.* Homewood, IL: Dorsey Press.

Roberts, M. K., & Davidson, J. D. (1984). The nature and sources of religious involvement. *Review of Religious Research, 25,* 334–350.

Roberts, T. B., & Hruby, P. J. (1995). *Religion and psychoactive sacraments: A bibliographic guide.* San Francisco: Council on Spiritual Practices.

Robertson, R. (1975). On the analysis of mysticism: Pre-Weberian, Weberian, and post-Weberian perspectives. *Sociological Analysis, 36,* 241–266.

Robinson, D. N. (1981). *An intellectual history of psychology.* New York: Macmillan.

Roche Report: Frontiers of Psychiatry. (1972, April 15). Search for mysticism held rejection of aggression. *2*(8), 1.

Rochford, E. B., Jr., Purvis, S., & NeMar, E. (1989). New religions, mental health, and social control. *Research in the Social Scientific Study of Religion, 1,* 57–82.

Roco, M., & Ticu, B. (1996). Preliminary research on the phases of religious judgment. *Revue Roumaine de Psychologie, 40,* 141–161.

Rodell, D. E., & Benda, B. B. (1999). Alcohol and crime among religious youth. *Alcoholism Treatment Quarterly, 17,* 53–66.

Roe, A. (1956). *The psychology of occupations.* New York: Wiley.

Roelofs, H. M. (1972). Dimensions of political alienation. In W. C. Bier (Ed.), *Alienation: Plight of modern man?* (pp. 85–93). New York: Fordham University Press.

Rogers, M. (Ed.). (1983). *Contradictory quotations.* Harlow, England: Longman.

Rohner, R. P. (1994). Patterns of parenting: The warmth dimension in worldwide perspective. In W. J. Lonner & R. Malpass (Eds.), *Psychology and culture* (pp. 113–120). Boston: Allyn & Bacon.

Rohrbaugh, J., & Jessor, R. (1975). Religiosity in youth: A personal control against deviant behavior. *Journal of Personality, 43,* 136–155.

Rokeach, M. (1964). *The three Christs of Ypsilanti: A psychological study.* New York: Knopf.

Rokeach, M. (1968). *Beliefs, attitudes, and values.* San Francisco: Jossey-Bass.

Rokeach, M. (1969). Value systems and religion. *Review of Religious Research, 11,* 24–38.

Rollins-Bohannon, J. (1991). Religiosity, related to grief levels of bereaved mothers and fathers. *Omega, 23,* 153–159.

Romme, M., & Escher, A. (1989). Hearing voices. *Schizophrenia Bulletin, 15,* 209–216.

Romme, M., & Escher, A. (1996). Empowering people who hear voices. In G. Haddock & P. D. Slade (Eds.), *Cognitive and behavioral interventions with psychotic disorders* (pp. 137–150). London: Routledge.

Roof, W. C. (1989). Multiple religious switching: A research note. *Journal for the Scientific Study of Religion, 28,* 530–535.

Roof, W. C. (1993). *A generation of seekers: The spiritual journeys of the boom generation.* San Francisco: HarperSanFrancisco.

Roof, W. C. (1999). *Spiritual marketplace.* Princeton, NJ: Princeton University Press.

Roof, W. C., & Hadaway, C. K. (1979). Denominational switching in the seventies: Going beyond Stark and Glock. *Journal for the Scientific Study of Religion, 18,* 363–379.

Roof, W. C., & McKinney, W. (1987). *American mainline religion: Its changing shape and future.* New Brunswick, NJ: Rutgers University Press.

Roozen, D. A. (1980). Church dropouts: Changing patterns of disengagement and re-entry. *Review of Religious Research, 21,* 427–450.

Rose, A. M. (1955). *Mental health and mental disorder.* New York: Norton.

Rosegrant, J. (1976). The impact of set and setting on religious experience in nature. *Journal for the Scientific Study of Religion, 15,* 301–310.

Rosen, B. C. (1950). Race, ethnicity, and the achievement syndrome. *American Sociological Review, 24,* 47–60.

Rosenau, P. M. (1992). *Postmodernism and the social sciences: Insights, inroads, and intrusions.* Princeton, NJ: University of Princeton Press.

Rosenberg, M. (1962). The dissonant religious context and emotional disturbance. *American Journal of Sociology, 68,* 1–10.

Rosengren, K. S., Johnson, C. N., & Harris, P. L. (Eds.). (2000). *Imagining the impossible: Magical, scientific, and religious thinking in children.* Cambridge, England: Cambridge University Press.

Rosenheim, E., & Muchnik, B. (1984–1985). Death concerns in differential levels of consciousness as functions of defense strategy and religious belief. *Omega, 15,* 15–23.

Roshdieh, S., Templer, D. I., Cannon, W. G., & Canfield, M. (1998–1999). The relationships of death anxiety and death depression to religion and civilian war-related experiences in Iranians. *Omega, 38,* 201–210

Ross, C. E. (1990). Religion and psychological distress. *Journal for the Scientific Study of Religion, 29,* 236–245

Ross, L., & Nisbett, R. E. (1991). *The person and the situation: Perspectives of social psychology.* New York: McGraw-Hill.

Ross, M. W. (1983). Clinical profiles of Hare Krishna devotees. *American Journal of Psychiatry, 140,* 416–420.

Rossetti, S. J. (1995). The impact of child sexual abuse on attitudes toward God and the Catholic Church. *Child Abuse and Neglect, 19,* 1469–1481.

Rossi, A. M., Sturrock, J. B., & Solomon, P. (1963). Suggestion effects on reported imagery in sensory deprivation. *Perceptual and Motor Skills, 16,* 39–45.

Roszak, T. (1968). *The making of a counterculture.* Garden City, NY: Doubleday.

Roszak, T. (1975). *The unfinished animal.* New York: Harper & Row.

Rotenberg, M. (1978). *Damnation and deviance: The Protestant ethic and the spirit of failure.* New York: Free Press.

Roth, P. A. (1987). *Meaning and method in the social sciences: The case for methodological pluralism.* Ithaca, NY: Cornell University Press.

Rothbaum, F., Weisz, J. R., & Snyder, S. S. (1982). Changing the world and changing the self: A two process model of perceived control. *Journal of Personality and Social Psychology. 42,* 5–37.

Rowe, D. C. (1987). Resolving the person–situation debate: Invitation to an interdisciplinary dialogue. *American Psychologist, 42,* 218–227.

Rubin, Z. (1970). Measurement of romantic love. *Journal of Personality and Social Psychology, 16,* 265–273.

Rudman, L. A., Greenwald, A. G., Mellott, D. S., & Schwartz, J. L. K. (1999). Measuring the automatic components of prejudice: Flexibility and generality of the Implicit Association Test. *Social Cognition, 17,* 437–465.

Ruether, R. R. (1972, September). *St. Augustine's penis: Sources of misogynism in Christian theology and prospects for liberation today.* Paper presented at the International Congress of Learned Societies in the Field of Religion, Los Angeles.

Ruether, R. R. (Ed.). (1974). *Religion and sexism: Images of women in the Jewish and Christian traditions.* New York: Simon & Schuster.

Ruether, R. R. (1975). *New woman, new earth: Sexist ideologies and human liberation.* Minneapolis, MN: Winston.

Ruether, R. R., & McLaughlin, E. (Eds.). (1979). *Women of spirit.* New York: Simon & Schuster.

Ruffing, J. K. (Ed.). (2001). *Mysticism and social transformation.* Syracuse, NY: Syracuse University Press.

Russell, B. (1935). *Religion and science.* London: Oxford University Press.

Ruthven, M. (1984). *Islam in the world.* New York: Oxford University Press.

Ryan, R. M., Rigby, S., & King, K. (1993). Two types of religious internalization and their relations to religious orientations and mental health. *Journal of Personality and Social Psychology, 65,* 586–596.

Sachs, S. (2002a, April 27). Anti-Semitism is deepening among Muslims. *The New York Times,* p. B9.

Sachs, S. (2002b, June 15). Baptist pastor attacks Islam, inciting cries of intolerance. *The New York Times,* p. A10.

Saigh, P. A. (1979). The effect of perceived examiner religion on the Digit Span performance of Lebanese elementary schoolchildren. *Journal of Social Psychology, 109,* 167–173.

Saigh, P. H., O'Keefe, T., & Antoun, F. (1984). Religious symbols and the WISC-R performance of Roman Catholic parochial school students. *Journal of Genetic Psychology, 145,* 159–166.

Salzman, L. (1953). The psychology of religious and ideological conversion. *Psychiatry, 16,* 177–187.

Samarin, W. J. (1959). Glossolalia as learned behavior. *Canadian Journal of Theology, 19,* 60–64.

Samarin, W. J. (1972). *Tongues of men and angels.* New York: Macmillan.

Sammon, S. D., Reznikoff, M., & Geisinger, K. F. (1985). Psychosocial development and stressful life events among religious professionals. *Journal of Personality and Social Psychology, 48,* 676–687.

Sanders, C. M. (1979–1980). A comparison of adult bereavement in the death of a spouse, child, and parent. *Omega, 10,* 303–322.

Sanderson, C., & Linehan, M. M. (1999). Acceptance and forgiveness. In W. R. Miller (Ed.), *Integrating spirituality into treatment* (pp. 199–216). Washington, DC: American Psychological Association.

Sandomirsky, S., & Wilson, J. (1990). Process of disaffiliation: Religious mobility among men and women. *Social Forces, 68,* 1211–1299.

Sanford, J. A. (1982). *Ministry burnout.* New York: Paulist Press.

Sapp, G. L. (1986). Moral judgment and religious orientation. In G. L. Sapp (Ed.), *Handbook of moral development* (pp. 271–286). Birmingham, AL: Religious Education Press.

Sarafino, E. P. (1990). *Health psychology.* New York: Wiley.

Sargent, W. (1957). *Battle for the mind.* London: Heinemann.

Saroyan, W. (1937). *My name is Aram.* New York: Harcourt, Brace.

Sasaki, M. A. (1979). Status inconsistency and religious commitment. In R. Wuthnow (Ed.), *The religious dimension: New directions in quantitative research* (pp. 135–156). New York: Academic Press.

Saunders, J. (2001, July 6). Furor erupts as police seize spanked children. *Globe and Mail* [Toronto], p. A1.

Scarboro, A., Campbell, N., & Stave, S. (1994). *Living witchcraft: An American coven.* Westport, CT: Praeger.

Scarlett, W. G. (1994). Cognitive-developmental and psychoanalytic comments on Tamminen's essay. *International Journal for the Psychology of Religion, 4,* 87–90.

Scarlett, W. G., & Perriello, L. (1991). The development of prayer in adolescence. In F. K. Oser & W. G. Scarlett (Eds.), *Religious development in childhood and adolescence* (New Directions for Child Development, No. 52, pp. 63–76). San Francisco: Jossey-Bass.

Schachter, S. (1951). Deviation, rejection, and communication. *Journal of Abnormal and Social Psychology, 46,* 190–207.

Schachter, S. (1964). The interaction of cognitive and physiological determinants of emotional states. In L. Berkowitz (Ed.), *Advances in experimental social psychology* (Vol. 1, pp. 49–80). New York: Academic Press.

Schachter, S. (1971). *Emotion, obesity, and crime.* New York: Academic Press.

Schachter, S., & Singer, J. E. (1962). Cognitive, social, and physiological determinants of emotional states. *Psychological Review, 69,* 379–399.

Schaefer, C. A., & Gorsuch, R. L. (1991). Psychological adjustment and religiousness: The multivariate belief–motivation theory of religiousness. *Journal for the Scientific Study of Religion, 30,* 448–461.

Schaefer, C. A., & Gorsuch, R. L. (1992). Dimensionality of religion: Belief and motivation as predictors of behavior. *Journal of Psychology and Christianity, 11,* 244–254.

Schaffer, M. D. (1990, August 15). Sex a special challenge for many clergy members. *The Denver Post,* p. 6B.

Scharfstein, B.-A. (1973). *Mystical experience.* Indianapolis, IN: Bobbs-Merrill.

Scharfstein, B.-A. (1993). *Ineffability.* Albany: State University of New York Press.

Scheepers, P. Gijsberts, M., & Hello, E. (2002). Religiosity and prejudice against ethnic minorities in Europe: Cross-national tests on a controversial relationship. *Review of Religious Research, 43,* 242–265.

Scheffel, D. (1991). *In the shadow of the antichrist: The Old Believers of Alberta.* Lewiston, NY: Broadview Press.

Scheflen, A. E. (1972). *Body language and social order.* Englewood Cliffs, NJ: Prentice-Hall.

Scheflin, A., & Opton, E. (1978). *The mind manipulators.* New York: Paddington.

Schein, E., Schneier, I., & Barker, C. H. (1971). *Coercive persuasion.* New York: Norton.

Schellenberg, J. A. (1990). William James and symbolic interactionism. *Personality and Social Psychology Bulletin, 16,* 769–773.

Schlagel, R. H. (1986). *Contextual realism: A metaphysical framework for modern science.* New York: Paragon House.

Schmeidler, G. R. (1992). William James: Pioneering ancestor of modern parapsychology. In M. E. Donnelly (Ed.), *Reinterpreting the legacy of William James* (pp. 339–352). Washington, DC: American Psychological Association.

Schmidt, L. A. (1995). "A battle not man's but God's": Origins of the American temperance crusade in the struggle for religious authority. *Journal of Studies on Alcohol, 56,* 110–121.

Schoenfeld, E. (1978). Image of man: The effect of religion on trust. *Review of Religious Research, 20,* 61–67.

Schoenrade, P., Ludwig, C., Atkinson, T., & Shane, R. (1990, November). *Whose loss?: Intrinsic religion and the consideration of one's own or another's death.* Paper presented at the annual convention of the Society for the Scientific Study of Religion, Virginia Beach, VA.

Scholem, G. G. (1969). *On the Kabbalah and its symbolism* (R. Manheim, Trans.). New York: Schocken Books.

Schuller, D. S. (1980). Sixty-four core clusters and their profiles. In D. S. Schuller, M. P. Strommen, & M. L. Brekke (Eds.), *Ministry in America* (pp. 90–223). San Francisco: Harper & Row.

Schumaker, J. F. (1995). *The corruption of reality.* Amherst, NY: Prometheus Books.

Schuon, F. (1975). *The transcendent unity of religion* (rev. ed., P. Townsend, Trans.). New York: Harper & Row.

Schur, E. (1976). *The awareness trap: Self absorption instead of social change.* Chicago: Quadrangle.

Schwartz, L. L., & Kaslow, F. W. (1979). Religious cults, the individual and the family. *Journal of Marital and Family Therapy, 5,* 15–26.

Schweitzer, F. (1997). Why we might still need a theory for the religious development of women. *International Journal for the Psychology of Religion, 7,* 87–91.

Schweitzer, F. (2000). Religious affiliation and disaffiliation in late adolescence and early adulthood: The impact of a neglected period of life. In L. J. Francis & Y. J. Katz (Eds.), *Joining and leaving religion: Research perspectives* (pp. 87–101). Leominster, England: Gracewing.

Scioli, A., Stavely, T., Stevenson, R., Chace, A., Topolski, C., & St. Amand, M. (1997). *Contrasting spirituality and intrinsic religiousness.* Paper presented at the annual convention of the American Psychological Association, Chicago.

Scobie, G. E. W. (1973). Types of religious conversion. *Journal of Behavioral Science, 1,* 265–271.

Scobie, G. E. W. (1975). *Psychology of religion.* New York: Wiley.

Scobie, G. E. W. (1999). Belief positive and negative: When believing is not believing. *Journal of Psychology and Christianity, 18,* 27–42.

Scott, J. (1989). Conflicting beliefs about abortion: Legal approval and moral doubts. *Social Psychology Quarterly, 52,* 319–326.

Seals, B. F., Ekwo, E. E., Williamson, R. A., & Hanson, J. W. (1985). Moral and religious influences on the amniocentesis decision. *Social Biology, 32,* 13–30.

Sears, C. E. (1924). *Days of delusion: A strange bit of history.* Boston: Houghton Mifflin.

Sears, D. O. (1988). Symbolic racism. In P. A. Katz & D. A. Taylor (Eds.), *Eliminating racism* (pp. 53–84). New York: Plenum Press.

Seeman, M. (1959). The meaning of alienation. *American Sociological Review, 24,* 783–790.

Segal, R. A. (1985). Have the social sciences been converted? *Journal for the Scientific Study of Religion, 24,* 321–324.

Segalowitz, S. J. (1983). *Two sides of the brain: Brain lateralization explained.* Englewood Cliffs, NJ: Prentice-Hall.

Seggar, J., & Kunz, P. (1972). Conversion: Analysis of a step-like process for problem solving. *Review of Religious Research, 13,* 178–184.

Seidlitz, L., Abernethy, A. D., Duberstein, P. R., Evinger, J. S., Chang, T. H., & Lewis, B. (2002). Development of the Spiritual Transcendence Index. *Journal for the Scientific Study of Religion, 41,* 439–453.

Selig, S., & Teller, G. (1975). The moral development of children in three different school settings. *Religious Education, 70,* 406–415.

Seligman, M. E. P. (1975). *Helplessness: On depression, development, and death.* San Francisco: Freeman.

Sensky, T. (1983). Religiosity, mystical experience and epilepsy. In F. C. Rose (Ed.), *Research in epilepsy* (pp. 214–220). New York: Pitman.

Sethi, S., & Seligman, M. E. P. (1993). Optimism and fundamentalism. *Psychological Science, 4,* 256–259.

Sethi, S., & Seligman, M. E. P. (1994). The hope of fundamentalists. *Psychological Science, 5,* 58.

Seybold, K. S., & Hill, P. C. (2001). The role of religion and spirituality in mental and physical health. *Current Directions in Psychological Science, 10,* 21–24.

Shafranske, E. (1995). Freudian theory and religious experience. In R. W. Hood, Jr. (Ed.), *Handbook of religious experience* (pp. 200–232). Birmingham, AL: Religious Education Press.

Shafranske, E. (1996). Religious beliefs, practices and affiliations of clinical psychologists. In E. Shanfranske (Ed.), *Religion and the clinical practice of psychology* (pp. 149–164). Washington DC: American Psychological Association.

Shafranske, E. P. (1992). Religion and mental health in early life. In J. F. Schumaker (Ed.), *Religion and mental health* (pp. 163–176). New York: Oxford University Press.

Shafranske, E. P. (Ed.). (1996). *Religion and the clinical practice of psychology.* New York: Human Sciences Press.

Shafranske, E. P., & Malony, H. N. (1985, February). *Religion, spirituality, and psychotherapy: A study of California psychologists.* Paper presented at the meeting of the California State Psychological Association, San Francisco.

Shakespeare, W. (1964). *Measure for measure.* New York: New American Library. (Original work produced 1604)

Shand, J. D. (1990). A forty-year followup of the religious beliefs and attitudes of a sample of Amherst College grads. In M. L. Lynn & D. O. Moberg (Eds.), *Research in the social scientific study of religion* (Vol. 2, pp. 117–136) Greenwich, CT: JAI Press.

Shapiro, E. (1977). Destructive cultism. *American Family Physician,15,* 80–83.

Sharf, R. H. (2000). The rhetoric of religion in the study of religious experience. In J. Andresen & R. K. Forman (Eds.). *Cognitive models and spiritual maps: Interdisciplinary explorations of religious experience* (pp. 267–287). Bowling Green, OH: Imprint Academic.

Shaver, K. G. (1975). *An introduction to attribution processes.* Cambridge, MA: Winthrop.

Shaw, G. B. (1931). Briefer views. In A. M. Drummond & R. H. Wagner, (Eds.), *Problems and opinions* (p. 378). New York: Century.

Shea, J. (1992). Religion and sexual adjustment. In J. F. Schumaker (Ed.), *Religion and mental health* (pp. 70–84). New York: Oxford University Press.

Sheeran, P., Spears, R., Abraham, S. C. S., & Abrams, D. (1996). Religiosity, gender, and the double standard. *Journal of Psychology, 130,* 23–33.

Sheldon, J. P., & Parent, S. L. (2002). Clergy's attitudes and attributions of blame toward female rape victims. *Violence against Women, 8,* 233–256.

Shephard, R. N. (1978). The mental image. *American Psychologist, 33,* 125–137.

Sherif, M. (1953). *Groups in harmony and tension.* New York: Harper & Row.

Sherif, M. (1966). *In common predicament: Social psychology of intergoup conflict and cooperation.* Boston: Houghton Mifflin.

Sherkat, D. E. (2000). "That they be keepers of the home"; The effect of conservative religion on early and late transitions into housewifery. *Review of Religious Research, 41,* 344–358.

Sherkat, D. E. (2001). Investigating the sect–church–sect cycle: Cohort-specific attendance differences across African-American denominations. *Journal for the Scientific Study of Religion, 40,* 221–233.

Sherkat, D. E., & Darnell, A. (1999). The effect of parents' fundamentalism on children's educational attainment: Examining differences by gender and children's fundamentalism. *Journal for the Scientific Study of Religion, 38,* 23–35.

Shermer, M. (2000). *How we believe: The search for God in an age of science.* New York: Freeman.

Sheskin, A., & Wallace, S. E. (1980). Differing bereavements: Suicide, natural, and accidental death. In R. A. Kalish (Ed.), *Death, dying, transcending* (pp. 74–87). Farmingdale, NY: Baywood.

Shiloh, A., & Selavan, I. C. (Eds.). (1973). *Ethnic groups of America: Their morbidity, mortality, and behavior disorders. Vol. 1. The Jews.* Springfield, IL: Charles Thomas.

Shor, R. E., & Orne, E. C. (1962). *Harvard Group Scale of Hypnotic Susceptibility.* Palo Alto, CA: Consulting Psychologists Press.

Shortz, J. L., & Worthington, E. L. (1994). Young adults' recall of religiosity, attributions, and coping in a parental divorce. *Journal for the Scientific Study of Religion, 33,* 173–179.

Shrauger, J. S., & Silverman, R. E. (1971). The relationship of religious background and participation to locus of control. *Journal for the Scientific Study of Religion, 10,* 11–16.

Shreeve, J. (1996, August 4). Design for living. *The New York Times Book Review,* p. 8.

Shuman, C. R., Fournet, G. P., Zelhart, P. F., Roland, B. C., & Estes, R. E. (1992). Attitudes of registered nurses toward euthanasia. *Death Studies, 16,* 1–15.

Shupe, A. D., Jr., & Bromley, D. (1985). Social response to cults. In P. Hammond (Ed.), *The sacred in a secular age* (pp. 58–69). Berkeley: University of California Press.

Shupe, A. D., Jr., Bromley, D. G., & Oliver, D. L. (1984). *The anti-cult movement in America.* New York: Garland Press.

Shupe, A. D., Jr., Spielman, R., & Stigall, S. (1977). Deprogramming. *American Behavioral Scientist, 20,* 941–956.

Sidgewick, H. A. (1894). Report of the census on hallucinations. *Proceedings of the Society for Psychical Research, 26,* 259–394.

Sieben, I. (2001). Schooling or social origin? The impact of educational attainment on religious, political, and social orientations after controlling for family background. *Mens en Maatschappij, 76,* 22–43.

Siegel, R. K. (1977). Religious behavior in animals and man: Drug-induced effects. *Journal of Drug Issues, 7,* 219–236.

Siglag, M. A. (1987, August 30). *Schizophrenic and mystical experiences.* Paper presented at the annual convention of the American Psychological Association, New York.

Sigmund, K., & Nowak, M. A. (2000). A tale of two selves. *Science, 290,* 949–950.

Silberman, C. E. (1985). *A certain people: American Jews and their lives today.* New York: Summit Books.

Silverman, M. K., & Pargament, K. I. (1990). *God help me: III. Longitudinal and prospective studies on effects of religious coping efforts on the outcomes of significant negative life events.* Paper presented at the annual convention of the American Psychological Association, San Francisco.

Silverstein, S. A. (1988). A study of religious conversion in North America. *Genetic, Social, and General Psychological Monographs, 114,* 261–305.

Silvestri, P. J. (1979). Locus of control and God dependence. *Psychological Reports, 45,* 89–90.

Simmonds, R. B. (1977a). Conversion or addiction? *American Behavioral Scientist, 20,* 909–924.

Simmonds, R. B. (1977b). *The people of the Jesus movement: A personality assessment of members of a fundamentalist religious community.* Unpublished doctoral dissertation, University of Nevada at Reno.

Simpkinson, A. A. (1996, November–December). Soul betrayal. *Common Boundary,* pp. 24–37.

Simpson, J. B. (Ed.). (1964). *Contemporary quotations.* New York: Galahad Books.

Singer, J. L. (1966). *Daydreaming: An introduction to the experimental study of inner experience.* New York: Random House.

Singer, M. T. (1978a, January). Coming out of the cults. *Psychology Today,* pp. 72–82.

Singer, M. T. (1978b). Therapy with ex-cult members. *Journal of the National Association of Private Psychiatric Hospitals, 9,* 14–18.

Singer, M. T., & Ofshe, R. (1990). Thought reform programs and the production of psychiatric casualties. *Psychiatric Annals, 20,* 188–193.

Singer, M. T., & West, L. J. (1980). Cults, quacks, and non-professional therapies. In H. I. Kaplan & J. B. Sadock (Eds.) *Comprehensive textbook of psychiatry* (Vol. 3, pp. 3245–3258). Baltimore: Williams & Wilkins.

Sipe, A. W. R. (1990). *A secret world: Sexuality and the search for celibacy.* New York: Brunner/Mazel.

Sipe, A. W. R. (1995). *Sex, priests, and power: Anatomy of a crisis.* New York: Brunner/Mazel.

Skal, D. J. (1998). *Screams of reason.* New York: Norton.

Skidmore, D. (1993, October). 8000 from world religions look for unity. *Episcopal Life,* p. 15.

Skinner, B. F. (1948). "Superstition" in the pigeon. *Journal of Experimental Psychology, 38,* 168–172.

Skinner, B. F. (1969). *Contingencies of reinforcement.* New York: Appleton-Century-Crofts.

Skinner, E. (1996). A guide to constructs of control. *Journal of Personality and Social Psychology, 71,* 549–570.

Skonovd, N. (1983). Leaving the cultic religious milieu. In D. Bromley & J. Richardson (Eds.), *The brainwashing/deprogramming controversy: Sociological, psychological, legal and historical perspectives* (pp. 91–105). Lewiston, NY: Edward Mellon.

Skorikov, V., & Vondracek, F. W. (1998). Vocational identity development: Its relationship to other identity domains and to overall identity development. *Journal of Career Assessment, 6,* 13–35.

Slaughter-Defoe, D. T. (1995). Revisiting the concept of socialization: Caregiving and teaching in the 90s—a personal perspective. *American Psychologist, 50,* 276–286.

Slawson, P. F. (1973). Treatment of a clergyman: Anxiety neurosis in a celibate. *American Journal of Psychotherapy, 27,* 52–60.

Sleek, S. (1994, June). Spiritual problems included in DSM-IV. *APA Monitor,* p. 8.

Sloan, R. P., & Bagiella, E. (2002). Claims about religious involvement and health outcomes. *Annals of Behavioral Medicine, 24,* 14–21.

Smart, N. (Ed.). (1964). *Philosophers and religious truth.* New York: Macmillan.

Smart, N. (1978). Understanding religious experience. In S. Katz (Ed.), *Mysticism and philosophical analysis* (pp. 10–21). New York: Oxford University Press.

Smith, C., Lundquist Denton, M. L., Faris, R., & Regnerus, M. (2002). Mapping American adolescent religious participation. *Journal for the Scientific Study of Religion, 41,* 597–612.

Smith, D. L. (1996). Private prayer, public worship, and personality among 11–15-year-old adolescents. *Personality and Individual Differences, 21,* 1063–1065.

Smith, E. R., & Mackie, D. M. (1995). *Social psychology.* New York: Worth.

Smith, H. (2000). *Cleansing the doors of perception: The religious significance of entheogenic plants and chemicals.* New York: Tarcher/Putnam.

Smith, J. H., & Handelman, S. A. (1990). *Psychoanalysis and religion.* Baltimore: Johns Hopkins University Press.

Smith, J. Z. (1996). The bare facts of ritual. In R. L. Grimes (Ed.), *Readings in ritual studies* (pp. 473–483). Upper Saddle River, NJ: Prentice-Hall. (Original work published 1982)

Smith, M. (1977). *An introduction to mysticism.* New York: Oxford University Press.

Smith, P. C., Range, L. M., & Ulmer, A. (1991–1992). Belief in afterlife as a buffer in suicidal and other bereavement. *Omega, 24,* 217–225.

Smith, R. E., Wheeler, G., & Diener, E. (1975). Faith without works: Jesus people, resistance to temptation, and altruism. *Journal of Applied Social Psychology, 5,* 320–330.

Snarey, J. R. (1985). Cross-cultural universality of social–moral development: A critical review of Kohlbergian research. *Psychological Bulletin, 97,* 202–233.

Snelling, C. H., & Whitley, O. R. (1974). Problem-solving behavior in religious and para-religious groups: An initial report. In A. W. Eister (Ed.), *Changing perspectives in the scientific study of religion* (pp. 315–334). New York: Wiley.

Snook, J. B. (1974). An alternative to church–sect. *Journal for the Scientific Study of Religion, 13,* 191–204.

Snook, S. C., & Gorsuch, R. L. (1985). *Religion and racial prejudice in South Africa.* Paper presented at the annual convention of the American Psychological Association, Los Angeles.

Snow, D. A., & Machalek, R. (1983). The convert as a social type. In R. Collins (Ed.), *Sociological theory* (pp. 259–289). San Francisco: Jossey-Bass.

Snow, D. A., & Machalek, R. (1984). The sociology of conversion. *Annual Review of Sociology, 10,* 167–190.

Snow, D. A., Zurcher, L. A., Jr., & Ekland-Olson, S. (1980). Social networks and social movements: A microstructural approach to differential recruitment. *American Sociological Review, 45,* 797–801.

Snow, D. A., Zurcher, L. A., Jr., & Ekland-Olson, S. (1983). Further thoughts on social networks and movement recruitment. *Sociology, 17,* 112–120.

Socha, P. (1999). The existential human situation: Spirituality as a way of coping. In K. H. Reich, F. Oser, & W. G. Scarlett (Eds.), *Psychological studies on spiritual and religious development: Vol. 2. Being human: The case of religion* (pp. 50–56). Berlin: Pabst Science.

Somit, A. (1968). Brainwashing. In D. Solls (Ed.), *International encyclopaedia of the social sciences* (Vol. 2, pp. 138–143). New York: Macmillan.

Southard, S. (1956). Religious concern in the psychoses. *Journal of Pastoral Care, 10,* 226–233.

Spanos, N. P., & Moretti, P. (1988). Correlates of mystical and diabolical experiences in a sample of female university students. *Journal for the Scientific Study of Religion, 27,* 105–116.

Sparks, G. G. (2001, September–October). The relationship between paranormal beliefs and religious beliefs. *Skeptical Inquirer,* pp. 50–56.

Sparrow, G. S. (1995). *I am with you always: True stories of encounters with Jesus.* New York: Bantam.

Spellman, C. M., Baskett, G. D., & Byrne, D. (1971). Manifest anxiety as a contributing factor in religious conversion. *Journal of Consulting and Clinical Psychology, 36,* 245–247.

Spencer, C., & Agahi, C. (1982). Social background, personal relationships, and self-descriptions as predictors of drug-user status: A study of adolescents in post-revolutionary Iran. *Drug and Alcohol Dependence, 10,* 77–84.

Spencer, J. (1975). The mental health of Jehovah's Witnesses. *British Journal of Psychiatry, 126,* 556–559.

Spielberger, C. D. (1966). The effects of anxiety on complex learning and academic achievement. In C. D. Spielberger (Ed.), *Anxiety and behavior* (pp. 361–398). New York: Academic Press.

Spilka, B. (1970). Images of man and dimensions of personal religion: Values for an empirical psychology of religion. *Review of Religious Research, 11,* 171–182.

Spilka, B. (1976). The compleat person: Some theoretical views and research findings for a theological-psychology of religion. *Journal of Psychology and Theology, 4,* 15–24.

Spilka, B. (1977). Utilitarianism and personal faith. *Journal of Psychology and Theology, 5,* 226–233.

Spilka, B. (1993, August). *Spirituality: Problems and directions in operationalizing a fuzzy concept.* Paper presented at the annual meeting of the American Psychological Association, Toronto.

Spilka, B. (1999, August). *Towards a theory of religious origins: Evolutionary and genetic considerations.* Paper presented at the annual convention of the American Psychological Association, Boston.

Spilka, B., Addison, J., & Rosensohn, M. (1975). Parents, self, and God: A test of competing theories of individual–religion relationships. *Review of Religious Research, 16,* 154–165.

Spilka, B., Armatas, P., & Nussbaum, J. (1964). The concept of God: A factor analytic approach. *Review of Religious Research, 6,* 28–36.

Spilka, B., Brown, G. A. & Cassidy, S. E. (1993). The structure of mystical experience in relation to pre- and post-experience lifestyle correlates. *International Journal for the Psychology of Religion, 2,* 241–257.

Spilka, B., & Hartman, S. (2000). Religion, cancer, and the family. In L. Baider, C. L. Cooper, & A. K. De-Nour (Eds.), *Cancer and the family* (2nd ed., pp. 443–455). New York: Wiley.

Spilka, B., Hood, R. W., Jr., & Gorsuch, R. L. (1985). *The psychology of religion: An empirical approach.* Englewood Cliffs, NJ: Prentice-Hall.

Spilka, B., Kojetin, B., & McIntosh, D. (1985). Forms and measures of personal faith: Questions, correlates and distinctions. *Journal for the Scientific Study of Religion, 24,* 437–442.

Spilka, B., Ladd, K. L., McIntosh, D. N., & Milmoe, S. (1996). The content of religious experience: The roles of expectancy and desirability. *International Journal for the Psychology of Religion, 6,* 95–105.

Spilka, B., & Loffredo, L. (1982). *Classroom cheating among religious students: Some factors affecting perspectives, actions and justifications.* Paper presented at the annual convention of the Rocky Mountain Psychological Association, Albuquerque, NM.

Spilka, B., & McIntosh, D. (1995). Attribution theory and religious experience. In R. W. Hood, Jr. (Ed.), *Handbook of religious experience* (pp. 421–445). Birmingham, AL: Religious Education Press.

Spilka, B., & McIntosh, D. N. (1996, August). *Religion and spirituality: The known and the unknown.* Paper presented at the Convention of the American Psychological Association, Toronto.

Spilka, B., & McIntosh, D. N. (Eds.). (1997). *The psychology of religion: Theoretical approaches.* Boulder, CO: Westview/Harper.

Spilka, B., & Schmidt, G. (1983a). General attribution theory for the psychology of religion: The influence of event-character on attributions to God. *Journal for the Scientific Study of Religion, 22,* 326–339.

Spilka, B., & Schmidt, G. (1983b). *Stylistic factors in attributions: The role of religion and locus of control.* Paper presented at the annual convention of the Rocky Mountain Psychological Association, Snowbird, UT.

Spilka, B., Shaver, P., & Kirkpatrick, L. A. (1985). A general attribution theory for the psychology of religion. *Journal for the Scientific Study of Religion, 24,* 1–20.

Spilka, B., & Spangler, J. (1979, October 31). *Spiritual support in life-threatening illness.* Paper presented at the annual convention of the Society for the Scientific Study of Religion, San Antonio, TX.

Spilka, B., Spangler, J. D., & Nelson, C. B. (1983). Spiritual support in life-threatening illness. *Journal of Religion and Health, 22,* 98–104.

Spilka, B., Spangler, J. D., & Rea, M. P. (1981). The role of theology in pastoral care for the dying. *Theology Today, 38,* 16–29.

Spilka, B., Spangler, J. D., Rea, M. P., & Nelson, C. B. (1981). Religion and death: The clerical perspective. *Journal of Religion and Health, 20,* 299–306.

Spilka, B., Stout, L., Minton, B., & Sizemore, D. (1977). Death and personal faith: A psychometric investigation. *Journal for the Scientific Study of Religion, 16,* 169–178.

Spilka, B., & Werme, P. (1971). Religion and mental disorder: A critical review and theoretical perspective. In M. Strommen (Ed.), *Research on religious development: A comprehensive handbook* (pp. 461–484). New York: Hawthorn Books.

Spilka, B., Zwartjes, W. J., & Zwartjes, G. M. (1991). The role of religion in coping with childhood cancer. *Pastoral Psychology, 39,* 285–304.

Spinetta, J. J. (1977). Adjustment in children with cancer. *Journal of Pediatric Psychology, 2*(2), 49–51.

Spiro, M. (1966). Religion: Problems of definition and explanation. In M. Banton (Ed.), *Anthropological approaches to the study of religion* (pp. 85–126). London: Tavistock.

Springer, S. P., & Deutsch, G. (1981). *Left brain, right brain.* San Francisco: W. H. Freeman.

Sprinthall, N. A., & Collins, W. A. (1995). *Adolescent psychology: A developmental view* (3rd ed.). New York: McGraw-Hill.

Srole, L., Langner, T. S., Michael, S. T., Opler, M. K., & Rennie, T. A. C. (1962). *Mental health in the metropolis.* New York: McGraw-Hill.

Stace, W. T. (1960). *Mysticism and philosophy.* Philadelphia: Lippincott.

Stack, S. (1983). The effect of religious commitment on suicide: A cross-national analysis. *Journal of Health and Social Behavior, 24,* 362–374.

Stack, S., & Wasserman, I. (1992). The effect of religion on suicide ideology: An analysis of the networks perspective. *Journal for the Scientific Study of Religion, 31,* 457–466.

Stambrook, M., & Parker, K. C. H. (1987). The development of the concept of death in childhood: A review of the literature. *Merrill–Palmer Quarterly, 33,* 133–157.

Stander, F. (1987). Some rigors of our time: The First Amendment and real life and death. *Cultic Studies Journal, 4,* 1–17.

Stanford, C. T. (2001). *Significant others.* New York: Basic Books.

Starbuck, E. D. (1897). A study of conversion. *American Journal of Psychology, 8,* 268–308.

Starbuck, E. D. (1899). *The psychology of religion.* New York: Scribner.

Starbuck, E. D. (1904). The varieties of religious experience. *The Biblical World, 24*(N.S.), 100–111.

Stark, R. (1963). On the incompatibility of religion and science: A survey of American graduate students. *Journal for the Scientific Study of Religion, 3,* 3–20.

Stark, R. (1968). Age and faith: A changing outlook or an old process? *Sociological Analysis, 29,* 1–10.

Stark, R. (1972). The economics of piety: Religious commitment and social class. In G. W. Thielbar & S. D. Feldman (Eds.), *Issues in social inequality* (pp. 483–503). Boston: Little, Brown.

Stark, R. (1984). Religion and conformity: Reaffirming a *sociology* of religion. *Sociological Analysis, 45,* 273–282.

Stark, R. (1985a). Church and sect. In P. E. Hammond (Ed.), *The sacred in a secular age* (pp. 139–149). Berkeley: University of California Press.

Stark, R. (Ed.). (1985b). *Religious movements.* New York: Paragon House.

Stark, R. (1996). Religion as context: Hellfire and delinquency one more time. *Sociology of Religion, 57,* 163–173.

Stark, R. (1998). *Sociology* (7th ed.). Belmont, CA: Wadsworth.

Stark, R. (1999). A theory of revelations. *Journal for the Scientific Study of Religion, 38,* 287–308.

Stark, R., & Bainbridge, W. S. (1979). Of churches, sects and cults: Preliminary concepts for a theory of religious movements. *Journal for the Scientific Study of Religion, 18,* 117–133.

Stark, R., & Bainbridge, W. S. (1980a). Networks of faith: Interpersonal bonds and recruitment to cults and sects. *American Journal of Sociology, 85,* 1376–1395.

Stark, R., & Bainbridge, W. S. (1980b). Towards a theory of religion. *Journal for the Scientific Study of Religion, 19,* 114–128.

Stark, R., & Bainbridge, W. S. (1985). *The future of religion.* Berkeley: University of California Press.

Stark, R., & Bainbridge, W. S. (1987). *A theory of religion.* New York: Peter Lang.

Stark, R., Foster, B. D., Glock, C. Y., & Quinley, H. (1970, April). Sounds of silence. *Psychology Today,* pp. 38–41, 60–61.

Stark, R., & Glock, C. Y. (1968). *American piety: The nature of religious commitment.* Berkeley: University of California Press.

Stark, R. A. (1965). A taxonomy of religious experience. *Journal for the Scientific Study of Religion, 5,* 97–116.

Stark, R. A. (1971). Psychopathology and religious commitment. *Review of Religious Research, 12,* 165–176.

Steele, B. F., & Pollock, C. B. (1968). A psychiatric study of parents who abuse infants and small children. In R. E. Helfer & C. H. Kempe (Eds.), *The battered child* (pp. 103–147). Chicago: University of Chicago Press.

Steeman, T. M. (1975). Church, sect, mysticism, denomination: Periodological aspects of Troeltsch's types. *Sociological Analysis, 26,* 181–204.

Steinberg, L. (1983). *The sexuality of Christ in Renaissance art and in modern oblivion.* New York: Pantheon.

Steinberg, L., Lamborn, S. D., Dornbusch, S. M., & Darling, N. (1992). Impact of parenting practices on adolescent achievement: Authoritative parenting, school involvement, and encouragement to succeed. *Child Development, 63,* 1266–1281.

Stengel, E. (1964). *Suicide and attempted suicide.* Baltimore: Penguin.

Stephan, C. W., & Stephan, W. G. (1985). *Two social psychologies.* Homewood, IL: Dorsey Press.

Stern, E. M., & Marino, B. G. (1970). *Psychotheology.* New York: Newman.

Stevens, J. (1987). *Storming heaven: LSD and the American dream.* New York: Harper & Row.

Stewart, C. (2001). The influence of spirituality on substance use of college students. *Journal of Drug Education, 31,* 343–351.

Stewart, C. W. (1974). *Person and profession: Career development in the ministry.* Nashville, TN: Abingdon Press.

Stifler, K., Greer, J., Sneck, W., & Dovenmuehle, R. (1993). An empirical investigation of the discriminability of reported mystical experiences among religious contemplatives, psychotic inpatients, and normal adults. *Journal for the Scientific Study of Religion, 32,* 366–372.

Stifoss-Hanssen, H. (1994). Rigid religiosity and mental health: An empirical study. In L. B. Brown (Ed.), *Religion, personality, and mental health* (pp. 138–143). New York: Springer-Verlag.

Stobart, St. C. (1971). *Torchbearers of spiritualism.* New York: Kennikat.

Stolzenberg, R. M., Blair-Loy, M., & Waite, L. J. (1995). Religious participation in early adulthood: Age and family life cycle effects on church membership. *American Sociological Review, 60,* 84–103.

Stone, J. R. (2000). *Expecting Armageddon: Essential readings in failed prophecy.* New York: Routledge.

Stone, P. J., Dunphy, D. C., Smith, M. S., & Ogilvie, D. M. (1966). *The general inquirer: A computer approach to content analysis.* Cambridge, MA: MIT Press.

Stone, W. F. (1974). *The psychology of politics.* New York: Free Press.

Stoppler, M. C. (n.d). *Cortisol: The "stress" hormone* [Online]. Available: http://www.stress.about.com/library/weeklyaa012901a.htm [Retrieved April 29, 2002].

Storch, E. A., & Storch, J. B. (2001). Organizational, nonorganizational, and intrinsic religiosity and academic dishonesty. *Psychological Reports, 88,* 548–552.

Storr, A. (1988). *Solitude: A return to the self.* New York: Ballantine Books.

Stouffer, S. (1955). *Communism, conformity, and civil liberty.* Garden City, NY: Doubleday.

Stout, L., Minton, B., & Spilka, B., (1976, May 14). *The construction and validation of multidimensional measures of death anxiety and death perspectives.* Paper presented at the annual convention of the Rocky Mountain Psychological Association, Phoenix, AZ.

Stout-Miller, R., Miller, L. S., & Langenbrunner, M. R. (1997). Religiosity and child sexual abuse. A risk factor assessment. *Journal of Child Sexual Abuse, 6,* 15–34.

Strassman, R. (2001). *DMT: The spirit molecule.* Rochester, VT: Park Street Press.

Straus, R. A. (1976). Changing oneself: Seekers and the creative transformation of experience. In J. Lofland (Ed.), *Doing social life* (pp. 252–272). New York: Wiley.

Straus, R. A. (1979). Religious conversion as a personal and collective accomplishment. *Sociological Analysis, 40,* 158–165.

Strauss, H. (1959). Epileptic disroders. In S. Arieti (Ed.), *American handbook of psychiatry: Vol. 2* (pp. 1109–1143). New York: Basic Books.

Strawbridge, W. J., Shema, S. J., Cohen, R. D., & Kaplan, G. A. (2001). Religious attendance increases survival by improving and maintaining good health behaviors, mental health, and social relationships. *Annals of Behavioral Medicine, 23,* 68–74.

Streib, H. (2001a). Faith development theory revisited: The religious styles perspective. *International Journal for the Psychology of Religion, 11,* 143–158.

Streib, H. (2001b). Fundamentalism as a challenge to religious education. *Religious Education, 96,* 227–244.

Strength, J. M. (1999). Grieving the loss of a child. *Journal of Psychology and Christianity, 18,* 338–353.

Strickland, M. P. (1924). *Psychology of religious experience.* New York: Abingdon Press.

Strommen, M. P. (Ed.). (1971). *Research on religious development: A comprehensive handbook.* New York: Hawthorn Books.

Strommen, M. P., Brekke, M. L., Underwager, R. C., & Johnson, A. L. (1972). *A study of generations.* Minneapolis, MN: Augsburg.

Strote, J., Lee, J. E., & Wechsler, H. (2002). Increasing MDMA use among college students: Results of a national survey. *Journal of Adolescent Health, 30,* 64–72.

Struch, N., & Schwartz, S. H. (1989). Intergroup aggression: Its predictors and distinctness from ingroup bias. *Journal of Personality and Social Psychology, 56,* 364–373.

Strunk, O., Jr. (1959). Interests and personality patterns of pre-ministerial students. *Psychological Reports, 5,* 740.

Suedfeld, P. (1975). The benefits of boredom: Sensory deprivation reconsidered. *American Scientist, 63,* 60–69.

Suedfeld, P., & Vernon, J. (1964). Visual hallucination in sensory deprivation: A problem of criteria. *Science, 145,* 412–413.

Sullivan, J. L., Pierson, J. E., & Marcus, G. E. (1982). *Political tolerance in American democracy.* Chicago: University of Chicago Press.

Summerlin, F. A. (1980). *Religion and mental health: A bibliography.* Rockville, MD: National Institute of Mental Health.

Surwillo, W. W., & Hobson, D. P. (1978). Brain electrical activity during prayer. *Psychological Reports, 43,* 135–143.

Sutherland, I., & Shepherd, J. P. (2001). Social dimensions of adolescent substance use. *Addiction, 96,* 445–458.

Sutherland, P. (1988). A longitudinal study of religious and moral values in late adolescence. *British Educational Research Journal, 14,* 73–78.

Suttie, I. D. (1952). *The origins of loved and hate.* New York: Julian Press.

Swanson, J. L., & Byrd, K. R. (1998). Death anxiety in young adults as a function of religious orientation, guilt, and separation–individuation conflict. *Death Studies, 22,* 257–268.

Swatos, W. H. (1976). Weber or Troeltsch?: Methodology, syndrome, and the development of church–sect theory. *Journal for the Scientific Study of Religion, 15,* 129–144.

Swatos, W. H. (1981). Church, sect and cult: Bringing mysticism back in. *Sociological Analysis, 42,* 17–26.

Swatos, W. H., Jr. (1992). Adolescent Satanism: A research note on exploratory survey data. *Review of Religious Research, 34,* 161–169.

Swenson, W. M. (1965). Attitudes toward death among the aged. In R. Fulton (Ed.), *Death and identity* (pp. 108–111). New York: Wiley.

Swinburne, R. (1981). The evidential value of religious experience. In A. R. Peacoke (Ed.), *The sciences and theology in the twentieth century* (pp. 182–196). Notre Dame, IN: University of Notre Dame Press.

Symonds, P. M. (1946). *Dynamics of human adjustment.* New York: Appleton-Century.

Szasz, T. (1960). The myth of mental illness. *American Psychologist, 15,* 113–118.

Szasz, T. (1970). *Ideology and insanity: Essays on the psychiatric dehumanization of man.* Garden City, NY: Doubleday.

Szasz, T. (1983). *The manufacture of madness.* New York: Harper & Row.

Szasz, T. (1984). *The therapeutic states: Psychiatry in the mirror of current events.* Buffalo, NY: Prometheus Books.

Taft, R. (1970). The measurement of the dimensions of ego permissiveness. *Personality: An International Journal, 1,* 163–184.

Tageson, C. W. (1982). *Humanistic psychology: A synthesis.* Homewood, IL: Dorsey Press.

Tajfel, H., & Turner, J. C. (1986). The social identity theory of intergroup behavior. In S. Worchel & W. G. Austin (Eds.), *Psychology of intergroup relations* (pp. 7–24). Chicago: Nelson-Hall.

Tamminen, K. (1976). Research concerning the development of religious thinking in Finnish students: A report of results. *Character Potential: A Record of Research, 7,* 206–219.

Tamminen, K. (1991). *Religious development in childhood and youth: An empirical study.* Helsinki: Suomalainen Tiedeakatemia.

Tamminen, K. (1994). Religious experiences in childhood and adolescence: A viewpoint of religious development between the ages of 7 and 20. *International Journal for the Psychology of Religion, 4,* 61–85.

Tamminen, K., & Nurmi, K. E. (1995). Developmental theories and religious experience. In R. W. Hood, Jr. (Ed.), *Handbook of religious experience* (pp. 169–311). Birmingham, AL: Religious Education Press.

Tamminen, K., Vianello, R., Jaspard, J.-M., & Ratcliff, D. (1988). The religious concepts of preschoolers. In D. Ratcliff (Ed.), *Handbook of preschool religious education* (pp. 97–108). Birmingham, AL: Religious Education Press.

Targ, E., Schlitz, M., & Irwin, H. J. (2000). Psi-related experiences. In E. Cardeña, S. J. Lynn, & S. Krippner (Eds.), *Varieties of anomalous experience* (pp. 219–252). Washington, DC: American Psychological Association.

Tart, C. (1975). Science, state of consciousness, and spiritual experiences: The need for state-specific sciences. In C. Tart (Ed.), *Transpersonal psychologies* (pp. 9–58). New York: Harper & Row.

Taslimi, C. R., Hood, R. W., Jr., & Watson, P. J. (1991). Assessment of former members of Shiloh: The adjective check list 17 years later. *Journal for the Scientific Study of Religion, 30,* 306–311.

Tate, E. D., & Miller, G. R. (1971). Differences in value systems of persons with varying religious orientations. *Journal for the Scientific Study of Religion, 10,* 357–365.

Taves, A. (1999). *Fits, trances, and visions: Experiencing religion and explaining experience from Wesley to James.* Princeton, NJ: Princeton University Press.

Tavris, C., & Sadd, S. (1977). *The Redbook report on female sexuality.* New York: Dell.

Tawney, R. H. (1926). *Religion and the rise of capitalism.* New York: Harcourt, Brace.

Taylor, H. (1998, August 12). *Large majority of people believe they will go to heaven; only one in fifty thinks they will go to hell* (The Harris Poll No. 41) [Online]. Available: http://www.harrisinteractive.com/harris poll/index.asp?PID=167 [Retrieved December 21, 2001].

Taylor, J., Rogers, J. A., Jackson-Lowman, H., Zhang, X., & Zhao, Y. (1995). *Refining a measure of spiritual orientation.* Unpublished manuscript.

Taylor, M., & Carlson, S. M. (2000). The influence of religious beliefs and parental attitudes about children's fantasy behavior. In K. S. Rosengren, C. N. Johnson, & P. L. Harris (Eds.), *Imagining the impossible: Magical, scientific, and religious thinking in children* (pp. 247–268). Cambridge, England: Cambridge University Press.

Taylor, S. E. (1991). *Health psychology* (2nd ed.). New York: McGraw-Hill.

Taylor, T. S. (2000). Is God good for you, good for your neighbor?: The influence of religious orientation on demoralization and attitudes towards lesbians and gays. *Dissertation Abstracts International, 60*(12), 4472A.

Tellegen, A., & Atkinson, G. (1974). Openness to absorbing and self-altering experiences ("absorption"), a trait related to hypnotic susceptibility. *Journal of Abnormal Psychology, 83,* 268–277.

Templin, D. P., & Martin, M. J. (1999). The relationship between religious orientation, gender, and drinking patterns among Catholic college students. *College Student Journal, 33,* 488–495.

TenElshof, J. K., & Furrow, J. L. (2000). The role of secure attachment in predicting spiritual maturity of students at a conservative seminary. *Journal of Psychology and Theology, 28,* 99–108.

Tennant, F. (1968). *The sources of the doctrine of the fall and original sin.* New York: Schocken Books. (Original work published 1903)

Tennyson, A. L. (1899). To J. S. In *The poetic and dramatic works of Alfred Lord Tennyson.* Boston: Houghton Mifflin.

ter Voert, M., Felling, A., & Peters, J. (1994). The effect of religion on self-interest morality. *Review of Religious Research, 35,* 302–323.

Teshome, M. J. (1992, August). *Separation–individuation among glossolalics and nonglossolalics.* Paper presented at the annual convention of the American Psychological Association, Washington, DC.

Thalbourne, M. A., & Delin, P. S. (1999). Transliminality: Its relation to dream life, religiosity, and mystical experience. *International Journal for the Psychology of Religion, 9,* 35–43.

Thalburne, M. A., Bartemucci, L., Delin, P. S., Fox, B., & Nofi, O. (1997). Transliminality: Its nature and correlates. *Journal of the American Society for Psychical Research, 91,* 305–331.

Thearle, M. J., Vance, J. C., Najman, J. M., Embelton, G., & Foster, W. J. (1995). Church attendance, religious affiliation and parental responses to sudden infant death, neonatal death and stillbirth. *Omega, 31,* 51–58.

Thomas, L. E. (1974). Generational discontinuity in beliefs: An exploration of the generation gap. *Journal of Social Issues, 30,* 1–22.

Thomas, L. E., & Cooper, P. E. (1978). Measurement and incidence of mystical experiences: An exploratory study. *Journal for the Scientific Study of Religion, 17,* 433–437.

Thomas, L. E., & Cooper, P. E. (1980). Incidence and psychological correlates of intense spiritual experiences. *Journal of Transpersonal Psychology,12,* 75–85.

Thompson, W. I. (1981). *The time falling bodies take to light.* New York: St. Martin's Press.

Thoresen, C. E., Harris, A. H. S., & Luskin, F. (2000). Forgiveness and health: An unanswered question. In M. E. McCullough, K. I. Pargament, & C. E. Thoresen (Eds.), *Forgiveness: Theory, research, and practice* (pp. 54–78). New York: Guilford Press.

Thorner, I. (1966). Prophetic and mystic experiences: Comparisons and consequences. *Journal for the Scientific Study of Religion, 5,* 2–96.

Thornton, A., & Camburn, D. (1989). Religious participation and adolescent sexual behavior. *Journal of Marriage and the Family, 51,* 641–654.

Thornton, E. E. (1970). *Professional education for the ministry: A history of clinical pastoral education.* Nashville, TN: Abingdon Press.

Thorson, J. A. (1991). Afterlife constructs, death anxiety, and life reviewing: The importance of religion as a moderating variable. *Journal of Psychology and Theology, 19,* 278–284.

Tien, A. Y. (1991). Distribution of hallucinations in the population. *Social Psychiatry and Psychiatric Epidemiology, 26,* 287–292.

Tillich, P. (1952). *The courage to be.* New Haven, CT: Yale University Press.

Tillich, P. (1957). *Dynamics of faith.* New York: Harper & Row.

Tippett, A. R. (1977). Conversion as a dynamic process in Christian mission. *Missiology, 2,* 203–221.

Tipton, R. M., Harrison, B. M., & Mahoney, J. (1980). Faith and locus of control. *Psychological Reports, 46,* 1151–1154.

Tipton, S. M. (1982). *Getting saved from the sixties: Moral meaning in conversion and cultural change.* Berkeley: University of California Press.

Tobin, S. S., Fullmer, E. M., & Smith, G. C. (1994). Religiosity and fear of death in non-normative aging. In L. E. Thomas & S. A. Eisenhandler (Eds.), *Aging and the religious dimension* (pp. 183–202). Westport, CT: Auburn House.

Travisano, R. (1970). Alternation and conversion as qualitatively different transformations. In G. P. Stone & H. A. Faberman (Eds.), *Social psychology through symbolic interaction* (pp. 594–606). Waltham, MA: Ginn-Blaisdell.

Trew, A. (1971). The religious factor in mental illness. *Pastoral Psychology, 22,* 21–28.

Trier, K. K., & Shupe, A. (1991). Prayer, religiosity and healing in the heartland, USA: A research note. *Review of Religious Research, 32,* 351–358.

Troeltsch, E. (1931). *The social teachings of the Christian churches* (2 vols., O. Wyon, Trans.). New York: Macmillan.

Tumminia, D. (1998). How prophecy never fails: Interpretive reason in a flying suacer group. *Sociology of Religion, 59,* 157–170.

Turiel, E., & Neff, K. (2000). Religion, culture, and beliefs about reality in moral reasoning. In K. S. Rosengren, C. N. Johnson, & P. L. Harris (Eds.), *Imagining the impossible: Magical, scientific, and religious thinking in children* (pp. 269–304). Cambridge, England: Cambridge University Press.

Turner, P. R. (1979). Religious conversion and community development. *Journal for the Scientific Study of Religion, 18,* 252–269.

Tyrrell, B. J. (1985). Christotherapy: An approach to facilitating psychospiritual healing and growth. In R. J. Wicks, R. D. Parsons, & D. Capps (Eds.), *Clinical handbook of pastoral counseling* (pp. 58–75). New York: Paulist Press.

Tzuriel, D. (1984). Sex role typing and ego identity in Israeli, Oriental, and Western adolescents. *Journal of Personality and Social Psychology, 46,* 440–457.

U.S. Bureau of the Census. (2000). *Statistical abstract of the United States: 2000.* Washington, DC: U.S. Government Printing Office.

U.S. Bureau of the Census. (2001). *Statistical abstract of the United States: 2001*. Washington, DC: U.S. Government Printing Office.

U.S. Office of the Surgeon General. (1999). *The Surgeon General's call to action to prevent suicide, 1999* [Online]. Available: http://www.surgeongeneral.gov/library/calltoaction/fact2.htm [Retrieved March 15, 2002].

U.S. Public Health Service. (1999). *The Surgeon's General call to action to prevent suicide*. Available: http://www.mentalhealth.org/suicideprevention/calltoaction.asp [Retrieved March 19, 2003].

Udry, J. R. (1971). *The social context of marriage* (2nd ed.). Philadelphia: Lippincott.

Ullman, C. (1982). Cognitive and emotional antecedents of religious conversion. *Journal of Personality and Social Psychology, 43*, 183–192.

Unamuno, M. de. (1954). *The tragic sense of life* (J. E. Crawford Fitch, Trans.). New York: Dover. (Original work published 1921)

Underhill, E. (1933). *The golden sequence: A fourfold study of the spiritual life* (3rd ed.). London: Methuen.

Underhill, R. M. (1936). *The autobiography of a Papago woman* (Memoirs of the American Anthropological Association, No. 46). Menasha, WI: American Anthropological Association.

Ungerleider, J. T., & Welish, D. K. (1979). Coercive persuasion (brainwashing), religious cults, and deprogramming. *American Journal of Psychiatry, 136*, 279–282.

Uslaner, E. M. (2002). Religion and civic engagement in Canada and the United States. *Journal for the Scientific Study of Religion, 41*, 239–254.

van der Lans, J. (1985). Frame of reference as a prerequisite for the induction of religious experience through meditation: An experimental study. In L. B. Brown (Ed.), *Advances in the psychology of religion* (pp. 127–134). Oxford: Pergamon Press.

van der Lans, J. (1987). The value of Sunden's role-theory demonstrated and tested with respect to religious experiences in meditation. *Journal for the Scientific Study of Religion, 26*, 401–412.

van der Lans, J. M. (1991). Interpretation of religious language and cognitive style: A pilot study with the LAM scale. *International Journal for the Psychology of Religion, 1*, 107–123.

van Driel, B., & Richardson, J. T. (1988). Categorization of new religions in American print media. *Sociological Analysis, 49*, 171–183.

Van Fossen, A. B. (1988). How do movements survive failures of prophecy? *Research in Social Movements, Conflicts and Change, 10*, 193–202.

Vande Kemp, H. (1976). Teaching psychology/religion in the seventies: Monopoly or cooperation? *Teaching of Psychology, 3*, 15–18.

Vandecreek, L., & Nye, C. (1993). Testing the Death Transcendence Scale. *Journal for the Scientific Study of Religion, 32*, 279–283.

VanderStoep, S. W., & Green, C. W. (1988). Religiosity and homonegativism: A path-analytic study. *Basic and Applied Social Psychology, 9*, 135–147.

Verdieck, M. J., Shields, J. J., & Hoge, D. R. (1988). Role commitment processes revisited: American Catholic priests 1970 and 1985. *Journal for the Scientific Study of Religion, 27*, 524–535.

Verdier, P. (1977). *Brainwashing and the cults*. Redondo Beach, CA: Institute of Behavioral Conditioning.

Vergote, A. (1993). What the psychology of religion is and what it is not. *International Journal for the Psychology of Religion, 3*, 73–86.

Vergote, A., & Tamayo, A. (Eds.). (1981). *The parental figures and the representation of God: A psychological and cross-cultural study*. The Hague: Mouton.

Vernon, G. M. (1968). The religious "nones": A neglected category. *Journal for the Scientific Study of Religion, 7*, 219–229.

Vernon, G. M., & Waddell, C. E. (1974). Dying as social behavior. *Omega, 5*, 199–206.

Vitz, P. C. (1977). *Psychology as religion*. Grand Rapids, MI: Eerdmans.

Volcano Press. (1995). *Family violence and religion*. Volcano, CA: Author.

Volinn, E. (1985). Eastern meditative groups: Why join? *Sociological Analysis, 46*, 147–156.

Volken, L. (1961). *Vision, revelations, and the church*. New York: J. P. Kennedy.

Vyse, S. A. (1997). *Believing in magic: The psychology of superstition*. New York: Oxford University Press.

Wade, N. (2002, July 4). Schizophrenia may be tied to two genes, research finds. *The New York Times*

[Online]. Available: http://www.nytimes.com/2002/07/04GENE.html?todaysheadlines [Retrieved July 4, 2002].

Wagenaar, T. C., & Bartos, P. E. (1977). Orthodoxy and attitudes of clergymen towards homosexuality and abortion. *Review of Religious Research, 18,* 114–125.

Wagner, G. J., Serafini, J., Rabkin, J., Remien, R., & Williams, J. (1994). Integration of one's religion and homosexuality: A weapon against internalized homophobia? *Journal of Homosexuality, 26,* 91–110.

Walinsky, A. (1995, July). The crisis of public order. *The Atlantic Monthly,* pp. 39–54.

Walker, S. R., Tonigan, J. S., Miller, W. R., Comer, S., & Kahlich, L. (1997). Intercessory prayer in the treatment of alcohol abuse and dependence: A pilot investigation. *Alternative Therapies, 3,* 79–86.

Wallace, A. F. C. (1956). Revitalization movements. *American Anthropologist, 58,* 264–281.

Wallace, C. W. (1966). *Religion: An anthropological view.* New York: Random House.

Wallace, J. M., Jr., & Forman, T. A. (1998). Religion's role in promoting health and reducing risk among American youth. *Health Education and Behavior, 25,* 721–741.

Wallace, J. M., Jr., & Williams, D. R. (1997). Religion and adolescent health-compromising behavior. In J. Schulenberg, J. Maggs, & K. Hurrelmann (Eds.), *Health risks and developmental transitions during adolescence* (pp. 444–468). Cambridge, England: Cambridge University Press.

Waller, N. G., Kojetin, B. A., Bouchard, T. J., Jr., Lykken, D. T., & Tellegen, A. (1990). Genetic and environmental influences on religious interests, attitudes, and values: A study of twins reared apart and together. *Psychological Science, 1,* 138–142.

Waller, N. G., Lykken, D. T., & Tellegen, A. (1995). Occupational interests, leisure time interests, and personality: Three domains or one? Findings from the Minnesota Twin Registry. In D. Lubinski & R. W. Dawis (Eds.), *Assessing individual differences in human behavior: New concepts, methods, and findings* (pp. 233–259). Palo Alto, CA: Davies-Black.

Wallis, R. (1974). Ideology, authority, and the development of cultic movements. *Social Research, 41,* 299–327.

Wallis, R. (1976). *The road to total freedom: A sociological analysis of Scientology.* New York: Columbia University Press.

Wallis, R. (1986). Figuring out cult receptivity. *Journal for the Scientific Study of Religion, 25,* 494–503.

Wallston, K. A., Wallston, B. S., & DeVellis, R. (1978). Development of the Multidimensional Health Locus of Control (MHLC) Scale. *Health Education Monographs, 6,* 161–170.

Walsh, A. (2002). Returning to normalcy. *Religion in the News, 5,* 26–28.

Walsh, R. (1982). Psychedelics and psychological well-being. *Journal of Humanistic Psychology, 22,* 22–32.

Walsh, W. J. (1906). *The apparitions of the shrines of heaven's bright queen* (4 vols.). New York: Cary-Stafford.

Wangerin, R. (1993). *The children of God.* Westport, CT: Bergin & Garvey.

Ware, A. P. (Ed.). (1985). *Midwives of the future.* Kansas City, MO: Leaven Press.

Warner, M. (1976). *Alone of all her sex: The myth and the cult of the Virgin Mary.* New York: Knopf.

Wass, H. (1984). Concepts of death: A developmental perspective. In H. Wass & C. A. Corr (Eds.), *Childhood and death* (pp. 3–24). Washington, DC: Hemisphere.

Wasserman, I., & Stack, S. (1993). The effect of religion on suicide: An analysis of cultural context. *Omega, 27,* 295–305.

Wasson, R. G. (1969). *Soma: Divine mushroom of immortality.* New York: Harcourt Brace Jovanovich.

Wasson, R. G., Hofmann, A., & Ruck, C. (1978). *The road to Eleusis: Unveiling the secret of mysteries.* New York: Harcourt Brace Jovanovich.

Waterman, A. (1985). *Identity in adolescence: Processes and contents.* San Francisco: Jossey-Bass.

Waters, E., & Cummings, E. M. (2000). A secure base from which to explore close relationships. *Child Development, 71,* 1–13.

Watkins, M. M. (1976). *Waking dreams.* New York: Harper & Row.

Watson, P. J. (1993). Apologetics and ethnocentricism: Psychology and religion within an ideological surround. *International Journal for the Psychology of Religion, 3,* 1–20.

Watson, P. J., Hood, R. W., Jr., & Morris, R. J. (1985). Dimensions of religiosity and empathy. *Journal of Psychology and Christianity, 4*, 73–85.

Watson, P. J., Hood, R. W., Jr., Morris, R. J., & Hall, J. R. (1984). Empathy, religious orientation, and social desirability. *Journal of Psychology, 117*, 211–216.

Watson, P. J., Howard, R., Hood, R. W., Jr., & Morris, R. J. (1988). Age and religious orientation. *Review of Religious Research, 29*, 271–280.

Watson, P. J., Morris, R. J., Foster, J. E., & Hood, R. W., Jr. (1986). Religiosity and social desirability. *Journal for the Scientific Study of Religion, 25*, 215–232.

Watson, P. J., Morris, R. J., & Hood, R. W., Jr. (1987). Antireligious humanistic values, guilt, and self esteem. *Journal for the Scientific Study of Religion, 26*, 535–546.

Watson, P. J., Morris, R. J., & Hood, R. W., Jr. (1990a). Attributional complexity, religious orientation, and indiscriminate proreligiousness. *Review of Religious Research, 32*, 110–121.

Watson, P. J., Morris, R. J., & Hood, R. W., Jr. (1990b). Intrinsicness, self-actualization and the ideological surround. *Journal of Psychology and Theology, 18*, 40–53.

Watson, P. J., Morris, R. J., & Hood, R. W., Jr. (1993). Mental health, religion and the ideology of irrationality. In M. L. Lynn & D. O. Moberg (Eds.), *Research in the social scientific study of religion* (Vol. 5, pp. 53–88). Greenwich, CT: JAI Press.

Watson, P. J., Sawyers, P., Morris, R. J., Carpenter, M. J., Jimenez, R. S., Jonas, K. A., & Robinson, D. L. (in press). Reanalysis within a Christian ideological surround: Relationship of intrinsic religious orientation with fundamentalism and right-wing authoritarianism. *Journal of Psychology and Theology.*

Wauck, L. (1957). *An investigation into the use of psychological tests as an aid in the selection of candidates for the diocesan priesthood.* Unpublished doctoral dissertation, Loyola University, Chicago.

Wax, M. L. (1984). Religion as universal: Tribulations of an anthropological enterprise. *Zygon, 19*, 5–20

Waxman, C. I. (1994). Religious and ethnic patterns of Jewish baby boomers. *Journal for the Scientific Study of Religion, 33*, 74–80.

Weaver, A. J., Berry, J. W., & Pittel, S. M. (1994). Ego development in fundamentalist and non-fundamentalist Protestants. *Journal of Psychology and Theology, 22*, 215–225.

Webb, M., & Otto Whitmer, K. J. (2001). Abuse history, world assumptions, and religious problem solving. *Journal for the Scientific Study of Religion, 40*, 445–453.

Weber, C. (n.d.). *The purpose of cortisol and corticosterone* [Online]. Available: http://www.member.tripod.com/~Charles_W/cortisol.html [Retrieved July 12, 2002].

Weber, M. (1930). *The Protestant ethic and the spirit of capitalism* (T. Parsons, Trans.). New York: Scribner. (Original work published 1904)

Weber, M. (1963). *The sociology of religion* (E. Frischoff, Trans.). Boston: Beacon Press. (Original work published 1922)

Webster, A. C. (1967). Patterns and relations of dogmatism, mental health, and psychological health in selected religious groups. *Dissertation Abstracts, 27*, 4142A.

Webster, H., Freedman, M., & Heist, P. (1962). Personality changes in college students. In N. Sanford (Ed.), *The American college: A psychological and social interpretation of the higher learning* (pp. 811–846). New York: Wiley.

Weigert, A. J., & Thomas, D. L. (1969). Religiosity in 5-D: A critical note. *Social Forces, 48*, 260–263.

Weigert, A. J., D'Antonio, W. V., & Rubel, A. J. (1971). Protestantism and assimilation among Mexican Americans: An exploratory study of minister's reports. *Journal for the Scientific Study of Religion, 10*, 219–232.

Weil, A. (1986). *The natural mind* (rev. ed.). Boston: Houghton Mifflin.

Weiner, B., Frieze, I, Kukla, A., Reed, L., Rest, S., & Rosenbaum, R. M. (1971). *Perceiving the causes of success and failure.* Morristown, NJ: General Learning Press.

Weisner, N. (1974). The effect of prophetic disconfirmation of the committee. *Review of Religious Research, 16*, 19–30.

Weisner, T. S., Beizer, L., & Stolze, L. (1991). Religion and families of children with developmental delays. *American Journal on Mental Retardation, 95*(6), 647–662.

Weisner, W. M., & Riffel, P. A. (1960). Scrupulosity: Religion and obsessive compulsive behavior in children. *American Journal of Psychiatry, 117,* 314–318.

Weiss, A. P. (1929). *A theoretical basis of human behavior* (2nd ed.). Columbus, OH: R. G. Adams.

Weiss, R. S. (1982). Attachment in adult life. In C. M. Parkes & J. Stevenson-Hinde (Eds.), *The place of attachment in human behavior* (pp. 171–184). New York: Basic Books.

Welch, M. R. (1977). Empirical examination of Wilson's sect typology. *Journal for the Scientific Study of Religion, 16,* 125–139.

Welch, M. R. (1978). Religious non-affiliation and worldly success. *Journal for the Scientific Study of Religion, 17,* 59–61.

Welch, M. R., Tittle, C. R., & Petee, T. (1991). Religion and deviance among adult Catholics: A test of the "moral communities" hypothesis. *Journal for the Scientific Study of Religion, 30,* 159–172.

Welch, R. R., & Leege, D. C. (1988). Religious predictors of Catholic parishioners' sociopolitical attitudes, devotional style, closeness to God, imagery, and agentic/communal religious identity. *Journal for the Scientific Study of Religion, 27,* 536–552.

Wells, M. G. (1999). Religion. In W. K. Silverman & T. H. Ollendick (Eds.), *Developmental issues in the clinical treatment of children* (pp. 199–212). Boston: Allyn & Bacon.

Wells, T., & Triplett, W. (1992). *Drug wars: An oral history from the trenches.* New York: William Morrow.

Wernik, U. (1975). Frustrated beliefs and early Christianity: A psychological enquiry into the gospels of the New Testament. *Numen, 22,* 96–130.

Westermeyer, J., & Walzer, V. (1975). Drug usage: An alternative to religion? *Diseases of the Nervous System, 36,* 492–495.

Whalen, J., & Flacks, R. (1989). *Beyond the barricades: The sixties generation grows up.* Philadelphia: Temple University Press.

Wheeler, H. (1971, March–April). The phenomenon of God. *The Center Magazine,* pp. 7–12.

White, C. (1991). *Clergy attitudes about death and response to those who are dying or bereaved.* Unpublished doctoral dissertation, University of Cincinnati.

White, R. W., & Watt, N. F. (1981). *The abnormal personality* (5th ed.). New York: Wiley.

Whitehead, A. N. (1926). *Religion in the making.* New York: Macmillan.

Whiteley, J., & Loxley, J. (1980). A curriculum for the development of character and community in college students. In L. Erickson & J. Whiteley (Eds.), *Developmental counseling and teaching* (pp. 262–297). Monterey, CA: Brooks/Cole.

Whitman, W. (1942). Starting from Paumanok. In *Leaves of grass.* Garden City, NY: Doubleday, Doran. (Original work published 1855)

Whitney, G. (1976). Genetic substrates for the initial evolution of human sociality. I. Sex chromosome mechanisms. *American Naturalist, 110,* 867–875.

Wicks, R. J., Parsons, R. D., & Capps, D. (Eds.). (1985). *Clinical handbook of pastoral counseling.* New York: Paulist Press.

Wiebe, P. H. (1997). *Visions of Jesus: Direct encounters from the New Testament to today.* New York: Oxford University Press.

Wiebe, P. H. (2000). Critical reflections on Christic visions. In J. Andresen & R. K. Forman (Eds.). *Cognitive models and spiritual maps: Interdisciplinary explorations of religious experience* (pp. 119–141). Bowling Green, OH: Imprint Academic.

Wiehe, V. R. (1990). Religious influence on parental attitudes toward the use of corporal punishment. *Journal of Family Violence, 5,* 173–186.

Wiesenthal, S. (1976). *The sunflower.* New York: Schocken Books.

Wiggins, J. S. (1966). Substantive dimensions of self-report on the MMPI item pool. *Psychological Monographs, 80*(Whole No. 630).

Wikstrom, O. (1987). Attribution, roles and religion: A theoretical analysis of Sunden's role theory of religion and the attributional approach to religious experience. *Journal for the Scientific Study of Religion, 26,* 390–400.

Wilcox, C. (1989). Popular support for the new Christian right. *Social Science Journal, 26,* 55–63.

Wilcox, C. (1996). *Onward Christian soldiers: The religious right in American politics,* Boulder, CO: Westview Press.

Wilcox, C., Ferrara, J., O'Donnell, J., Bendyna, M., Gehan, S., & Taylor, R. (1992). Public attitudes toward church–state issues: Elite–masses differences. *Journal of Church and State, 34,* 259–277.

Wilcox, C., & Jelen, T. G. (1991). The effects of employment and religion on women's feminist attitudes. *International Journal for the Psychology of Religion, 1,* 161–171.

Wilcox, W. B. (1998). Conservative Protestant childrearing: Authoritarian or authoritative? *American Sociological Review, 63,* 796–809.

Williams, R. (1971). A theory of God-concept readiness: From Piagetetian theories of child artificialism and the origin of religious feeling in children. *Religious Education, 66,* 62–66.

Williams, R. N., & Faulconer, J. E. (1994). Religion and mental health: A hermeneutic reconsideration. *Review of Religious Research, 35,* 335–349.

Williamson, P. (1995). *An attributional basis of the Church of God's rejection of serpent handling.* Paper presented at the annual convention of the Southeastern Psychological Association, Savannah, GA.

Williamson, W. P., & Pollio, H. R. (1999). The phenomenology of religious serpent handling: A rationale and thematic study of extemporaneous sermons. *Journal for the Scientific Study of Religion, 38,* 203–218.

Willits, F. K., & Crider, D. M. (1989). Church attendance and traditional religious beliefs in adolescence and young adulthood: A panel study. *Review of Religious Research, 31,* 68–81.

Wills, G. (1990). *Under God: Religion and American politics.* New York: Simon & Schuster.

Wilson, B. R. (1970). *Religious sects.* New York: McGraw-Hill.

Wilson, B. R. (1983). Sympathetic detachment and disinterested involvement: A note on academic integrity. *Sociological Analysis, 44,* 183–188.

Wilson, E. O. (1978). *On human nature.* Cambridge, MA: Harvard University Press.

Wilson, J. (2000). Locating religion in American politics. In M. Silk (Ed.), *Religion and American politics: The 2000 election in context* (pp. 7–18). Hartford, CT: Trinity University Center for the Study of Religion in Public Life.

Wilson, J., & Sherkat, D. E. (1994). Returning to the fold. *Journal for the Scientific Study of Religion, 33,* 148–161.

Wilson, J. Q. (1993). *The moral sense.* New York: Free Press.

Wilson, S. R. (1982). In pursuit of spiritual energy: Spiritual growth in a yoga ashram. *Journal of Humanistic Psychology, 22,* 43–55.

Wilson, W. P. (1998). Religion and psychoses. In H. G. Koenig (Ed.), *Handbook of religion and mental health* (pp. 161–173). San Diego, CA: Academic Press.

Wimberley, R. C. (1978). Dimensions of commitment generalizing from religion to politics. *Journal for the Scientific Study of Religion, 17,* 225–240.

Wimberley, R. C., & Christenson, J. A. (1981). Civil religion and other religious identities. *Sociological Analysis, 42,* 91–100.

Winfield, L. (2002, January 23). Reparative therapy doesn't work. *The Denver Post,* p. 11B.

Winokuer, H. R. (2000). The impact of expected versus unexpected death on the surviving spouse. *Dissertation Abstracts International, 61,* 553B.

Winter, T., Karvonen, S., & Rose, R. J. (2002). Does religiousness explain regional differences in alcohol use in Finland? *Alcohol and Alcoholism, 37,* 330–339.

Winzelberg, A., & Humphreys, K. (1999). Should patients' religiosity influence clinicians' referral to 12–step self-help groups?: Evidence from a study of 3,018 male substance abuse patients. *Journal of Consulting and Clinical Psychology, 67,* 790–794.

Wirth, L. (1928). *The ghetto.* Chicago: University of Chicago Press.

Wittberg, P. (1996). *Pathways to re-creating religious communities.* Mahwah, NJ: Paulist Press.

Witter, R. A., Stock, W. A., Okun, M. A., & Haring, M. J. (1985). Religion and subjective well-being in adulthood: A quantitative analysis. *Review of Religious Research, 26,* 332–342.

Wittgenstein, L. (1953). *Philosophical investigations* (G. E. M. Anscombe, Trans.). New York: Routledge & Kegan Paul. (Original work published 1945–1949)

Witvliet, C. V., & Ludwig, T. E. (1999, August). *Forgiveness and unforgiveness: Responses to interper-*

sonal offenses influence health. Poster presented at the annual convention of the American Psychological Association, Boston.

Wolcott, H. F. (1994). *Transforming qualitative data: Description, analysis, and interpretation.* Thousand Oaks, CA: Sage.

Wong, P. T. P. (1979). Frustration, exploration, and learning. *Canadian Psychological Review, 20,* 133–144.

Wong, P. T. P., & Weiner, B. (1981). When people ask 'why' questions, and the heuristics of attributional search. *Journal of Personality and Social Psychology, 40,* 650–663.

Wong-McDonald, A., & Gorsuch, R. (1997). *Surrender to God: An additional coping style?* Paper presented at the annual convention of the Society for the Scientific Study of Religion, San Diego, CA.

Wood, J. (1976). The structure of concern: Ministry in death-related situations. In L. H. Lofland (Ed.), *Toward a sociology of death and dying* (pp. 135–150). Beverly Hills, CA: Sage.

Wood, W. W. (1965). *Culture and personality aspects of the pentecostal holiness religion.* The Hague: Mouton.

Woodberry, J. D. (1992). Conversion in Islam. In H. N. Malony & S. Southard (Eds.), *Handbook of religious conversion* (pp. 22–40). Birmingham, AL: Religious Education Press.

Woodroof, J. T. (1985). Premarital sexual behavior and religious adolescents. *Journal for the Scientific Study of Religion, 24,* 343–366.

Woodruff, M. L. (1993). Report: Electroencephalograph taken from Pastor Liston Pack, 4:00 p.m., 7 Nov. 1985. In T. Burton, *Serpent-handling believers* (pp. 142–144). Knoxville: University of Tennessee Press.

Woodward, K. L. (1970, April 6). How America lives with death. *Time,* pp. 81–88.

Woody, J. D., Russel, R., D'Souza, H. J., & Woody, J. K. (2000). Adolescent non-coital sexual activity: Comparisons of virgins and non-virgins. *Journal of Sex Education and Therapy, 25,* 261–268.

Woolcott, P., Jr. (1969). Pathological processes in religion. In E. M. Pattison (Ed.), *Clinical psychiatry and religion* (pp. 61–76). Boston: Little, Brown.

Woolley, J. D. (2000). The development of beliefs about direct mental–physical causality in imagination, magic, and religion. In K. S. Rosengren, C. N. Johnson, & P. L. Harris (Eds.), *Imagining the impossible: Magical, scientific, and religious thinking in children* (pp. 99–129). Cambridge, England: Cambridge University Press.

Woolley, J. D., & Phelps, K. E. (2001). The development of children's beliefs about prayer. *Journal of Cognition and Culture, 1,* 139–167.

World Health Organization. (2001, October). *Suicide rates* [Online]. Available: http://www.who.int/mental health/Topic Suicide/suicide rates.html [Retrieved January 20, 2002].

Worten, S. A., & Dollinger, S. J. (1986). Mothers' intrinsic religious motivation, disciplinary preferences, and children's conceptions of prayer. *Psychological Reports, 58,* 218.

Worthington, E. L., Jr., Berry, J. W., & Parrott, L., III. (2001). Unforgiveness, forgiveness, religion, and health. In T. G. Plante & A. C. Sherman (Eds.), *Faith and health: Psychological perspectives* (pp. 107–138). New York: Guilford Press.

Wortman, C. B. (1976). Causal attributions and personal control. In J. H. Harvey, W. J. Ickes, & R. F. Kidd (Eds.), *New directions in attribution research* (Vol. 1, pp. 23–52). Hillsdale, NJ: Erlbaum.

Wright, J. E.. Jr. (1982). *Erikson: Identity and religion.* New York: Seabury Press.

Wright, L. S., Frost, C. J., & Wisecarver, S. J. (1993). Church attendance, meaningfulness of religion, and depressive symptomatology among adolescents. *Journal of Youth and Adolescence, 22,* 559–568.

Wright, S. A. (1986). Dyadic intimacy and social control in three cult movements. *Sociological Analysis, 47,* 137–150.

Wright, S. A. (1987). *Leaving cults: The dynamics of defection* (Monograph No. 7). Washington, DC: Society for the Scientific Study of Religion.

Wright, S. A. (1997). Media coverage of unconventional religion: Any "good news" for minority faiths? *Review of Religious Research, 39,* 101–115.

Wright, S. D., Pratt, C. C., & Schmall, V. L. (1985). Spiritual support for caregivers of dementia patients. *Journal of Religion and Health, 24,* 31–38.

Wright, W. (1999). *Born that way: Genes, behavior, personality.* New York: Routledge.

Wu, Z., Detels, R., Zhang, J., & Duan, S. (1996). Risk factors for intravenous drug use and sharing equipment among young male drug users in Lonchuan County, south-west China. *AIDS, 10,* 1017–1024.

Wulf, J., Prentice, D., Hansum, D., Ferrar, A., & Spilka, B. (1984). Religiosity, and sexual attitudes and behavior among evangelical Christian singles. *Review of Religious Research, 26,* 119–131.

Wulff, D. M. (1993). On the origins and goals of religious development. *International Journal for the Psychology of Religion, 3,* 181–186.

Wulff, D. M. (1995). Phenomenological psychology. In R. W. Hood, Jr. (Ed.), *Handbook of religious experience* (pp. 183–199). Birmingham, AL: Religious Education Press.

Wulff, D. M. (1997). *Psychology of religion: Classic and contemporary views* (2nd ed.). New York: Wiley.

Wulff, D. M. (2000). Mystical experience. In E. Cardeña, S. J. Lynn, & S. S. Krippner (Eds.), *Varieties of anomalous experience* (pp. 397–440). Washington DC: American Psychological Association.

Wundt, W. (1901). *Lectures on human and animal psychology* (J. E. Creighton & E. B. Titchener, Trans.). New York: Macmillan.

Wundt, W. (1916). *Elements of folk psychology.* London: Allen & Unwin.

Wuthnow, R. (1978). *Experimentation in American religion.* Berkeley: University of California Press.

Wuthnow, R. (1993). *Christianity in the twenty-first century.* New York: Oxford University Press.

Wuthnow, R. (1994). *God and mammon in America.* New York: Free Press.

Wuthnow, R. (2000). How religious groups promote forgiving: A national study. *Journal for the Scientific Study of Religion, 39,* 125–139.

Wuthnow, R., & Glock, C. Y. (1973). Religious loyalty, defection, and experimentation among college youth. *Journal for the Scientific Study of Religion, 12,* 157–180.

Wuthnow, R., & Mellinger, G. (1978). Religious loyalty, defection, and experimentation: A longitudinal analysis of university men. *Review of Religious Research, 19,* 231–245.

Wylie, L., & Forest, J. (1992). Religious fundamentalism, right-wing authoritarianism and prejudice. *Psychological Reports, 71,* 1291–1298.

Wylie, R. C. (1979). *The self concept* (2 vols., 2nd ed.). Lincoln: University of Nebraska Press.

Yamane, D. (2000). Narrative and religious experience. *Sociology of Religion, 61,* 171–189.

Yamane, D., & Polzer, M. (1994). Ways of seeing ecstasy in modern society: Experimental–expressive and cultural–linguistic views. *Sociology of Religion, 55,* 1–25.

Yates, J. W., Chalmer, B. J., St. James, P., Follansbee, M., & McKegney, F. P. (1981). Religion in patients with advanced cancer. *Medical and Pediatric Oncology, 9,* 121–128.

Yensen, R. (1990). LSD and psychotherapy. *Journal of Psychoactive Drugs, 17,* 267–277.

Yinger, J. M. (1967). Pluralism, religion, and secularism. *Journal for the Scientific Study of Religion, 6,* 17–28,

Yinger, J. M. (1970). *The scientific study of religion.* New York: Macmillan.

Yinon, Y., & Sharon, I. (1985). Similarity in religiousness of the solicitor, the potential helper, and the recipient as determinants of donating behavior. *Journal of Applied Social Psychology, 15,* 726–734.

Youniss, J., McLellan, J. A., & Yates, M. (1999). Religion, community service, and identity in American youth. *Journal of Adolescence, 22,* 243–253.

Youniss, J., McLellan, J. A., Su, Y., & Yates, M. (1999). The role of community service in identity development: Normative, unconventional, and deviant orientations. *Journal of Adolescent Research, 14,* 248–261.

Yudell, C. (1978, November). Are clergy afraid to die too? *U.S. Catholic,* pp. 33–39.

Zachry, W. H. (1990). Correlation of abstract religious thought and formal operations in high school and college students. *Review of Religious Research, 31,* 405–412.

Zaehner, R. C. (1957). *Mysticism, sacred and profane: An inquiry into some varieties of praenatural experience.* London: Oxford University Press.

Zaehner, R. C. (1972). *Zen, drugs and mysticism.* New York: Pantheon.

Zaehner, R. C. (1974). *Our savage God.* New York: Sheed & Ward.

Zaleski, C. (1987). *Otherworld journeys: Accounts of near-death experience in medieval and modern times.* New York: Oxford University Press.

Zaleski, E. H., & Schiaffino, K. M. (2000). Religiosity and sexual risk-taking behavior during the transition to college. *Journal of Adolescence, 23*, 223–227.

Zborowski, M., & Herzog, E. (1952). *Life is with people.* New York: International Universities Press.

Zern, D. (1997). The attitudes of present and future teachers to the teaching of values (in general) and of certain values (in particular). *Journal of Genetic Psychology, 158*, 505–507.

Zern, D. S. (1984). Religiousness related to cultural complexity and pressures to obey cultural norms. *Genetic Psychology Monographs, 110*, 207–227.

Zern, D. S. (1987). Positive links among obedience pressure, religiosity, and measures of cognitive accomplishment: Evidence for the secular value of being religious. *Journal of Psychology and Theology, 15*, 31–39.

Zilboorg, G., & Henry, G. W. (1941). *A history of medical psychology.* New York: Norton.

Zimbardo, P. G., & Hartley, C.F. (1985). Cults go to high school: A theoretical and empirical analysis of the initial stage in the recruitment process. *Cultic Studies Journal, 2*, 91–147.

Zinberg, N. (Ed.). (1977). *Alternate states of consciousness.* New York: Free Press.

Zinnbauer, B., & Pargament, K. I. (1998). Spiritual conversion: A study of religious change among college students. *Journal for the Scientific Study of Religion, 37*, 161–180.

Zinnbauer, B. J., Pargament, K. I., Cole, B., Rye, M. S., Butter, E. M., Belavich, T. G., et al. (1997). Religion and spirituality: Unfuzzying the fuzzy. *Journal for the Scientific Study of Religion, 36*, 549–564.

Zinnbauer, B. J., Pargament, K. I., Cowell, B., & Scott, A. B. (1996, August). *Religion and spirituality: Unfuzzying the fuzzy.* Paper presented at the annual convention of the American Psychological Association, Toronto.

Zinnbauer, B. J., Pargament, K. I., & Scott, A. B. (1999). The emerging meanings of religiousness and spirituality: Problems and prospects. *Journal of Personality, 67*, 889–919.

Zollschan, G. K., Schumaker, J. F., & Walsh, G. F. (Eds.). (1995). *Exploring the paranormal.* Great Britain: Prism Press.

Zondag, H. J., & Belzen, J. A. (1999). Between reduction of uncertainty and reflection: The range and dynamics of religious judgment. *International Journal for the Psychology of Religion, 9*, 63–81.

Zubeck, J. P. (Ed.). (1969). *Sensory deprivation: Fifty years of research.* New York: Appleton-Century-Crofts.

Zuckerman, D. M., Kasl, S. V., & Ostfeld, A. M. (1984). Psychosocial predictors of mortality among the elderly poor. *American Journal of Epidemiology, 119*, 410–423.

Zusne, L., & Jones, W. H. (1989). *Anomalistic thinking: A study of magical thinking* (2nd ed.). Hillsdale, NJ: Erlbaum.

Zwartjes, W. J., Spilka, B., Zwartjes, G. M., Heideman, D. R., & Cilli, K. A. (1979). *School problems of children with malignant neoplasms* (Final Report, Project No. 212–46–1061). Washington, DC: National Cancer Institute.

Zygmunt, J. F. (1972). When prophecy fails. A theoretical perspective on the comparative evidence. *American Behavioral Scientist, 16*, 245–268.

AUTHOR INDEX

SUBJECT INDEX